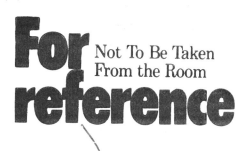

For Not To Be Taken
From the Room
reference

A BIBLIOGRAPHY OF
NURSING LITERATURE
1971–1975

A
BIBLIOGRAPHY OF NURSING LITERATURE

THE HOLDINGS OF THE ROYAL COLLEGE OF NURSING
1971–1975

Edited and compiled by Frances Walsh

The Library Association
London

© The Royal College of Nursing 1985. Published by Library Association Publishing
Limited, 7 Ridgmount Street, London WC1 E7AE and printed and bound in Great
Britain by The University Press, Cambridge. Designed by Geoff Green. Phototypeset by
Input Typesetting Limited, London.

First published 1985

British Cataloguing in Publication Data
Walsh, Frances
  A bibliography of nursing literature: the holdings of the Royal College of Nursing
1971–1975.
  1. Nursing—Bibliography
  I. Title II. Royal College of Nursing
  016.61073   Z6675.N7

ISBN 0 85365 623 1

CONTENTS

FOREWORD

This is the third volume of A Bibliography of Nursing Literature and covers the period from 1971 to 1975. The success of the first two volumes (Volume 1: 1859–1960, and Volume 2: 1961–1970) has clearly demonstrated the need for this comprehensive source of reference to nursing literature.

The enormous expansion in the publication of nursing literature continues from year to year and refects the growth and development of the profession of nursing. All progress is dependent upon the ability to establish foundations from the past, to develop in the present and plan for the future. Nursing is both an art and a science and is engaged in the essential process of formulating and refining its knowledge base and advancing levels of practice. The need to communicate increases commensurately and it has become vital that nurses, and others who have reason to understand nursing, have access to a comprehensive, yet compact, bibliography of nursing.

The Royal College of Nursing has committed its resources to the production of this bibliography and believes that it should be an essential resource in every library that provides a service to nurses and related professions.

Margaret D. Green
Director of Education
Royal College of Nursing

INTRODUCTION

Cumulation

This volume is a sequel to 'A Bibliography of Nursing Literature, 1961–70', and serves as a cumulation to 'Nursing Bibliography', which has been published monthly by The Royal College of Nursing since 1972.

Scope

In addition to the core material relating to nursing, this bibliography covers a high percentage of fringe material, where nursing touches upon the complexities of social life: the care of old people, child health, home/community care of the sick and disabled, and preventive medicine, etc.

Arrangement

This bibliography is arranged into 14 main subject areas producing 99 numbered leading headings which are further subdivided by lower case letters to accommodate specific topics. Study of the subject listings and the index to these listings, which both precede the bibliography proper, will guide readers to the relevant material.

SUBJECT LISTINGS

DISEASES AND TREATMENT

INDEX TO SUBJECT LISTINGS

The arrangement of terms within this index is alphabetical, the terms being filed using the word-by-word method with punctuation filing before a space. Any cross references, for example, *Nursing see also Intensive Care*, file after the single topic of *Nursing* but before any of the punctuated subdivisions.

Two forms of punctuation are used: the colon and the comma. The colon is used to convey concepts expressing the notion of 'by means of . . .'; 'for . . .'; 'in . . .'; and 'topic of . . .' etc; thus *Nursing : Alcoholism* means 'nursing in the treatment of alcoholism'. The comma is used to mean 'types . . .'; thus *Nursing, District* means 'District nursing'.

An example taken from some of the entries which appear under 'Nursing' illustrates the structure of the order:

NURSING AS A PROFESSION

1 BIBLIOGRAPHY AND REFERENCE BOOKS

a BIBLIOGRAPHIES

1 Cumulative index to nursing and allied health literature Glendale: Seventh Day Adventist Hospital Association, 1956.

2 Hospital abstracts HMSO, 1960–1961. Monthly with annual index.

3 International nursing index. New York: American Journal of Nursing Company in co-operation with the National Library of Medicine, 1966— .

4 Nursing bibliography A monthly list of current publications on nursing and allied subjects. Royal College of Nursing Library, 1972– .

5 Nursing studies index Prepared by Yale University School of Nursing under the direction of Virginia Henderson. Philadelphia: Lippincott.
Vol 1 1900–1929   1972
Vol 2 1930–1949   1970
Vol 3 1950–1956   1966
Vol 4 1957–1959   1963

6 Royal College of Nursing Library of Nursing Books and journals for nurse training school libraries. Rcn, 1971.

7 Thompson, A. M. C. A bibliography of nursing literature 1961–1970. Library Association for Rcn, 1974. Previous volume 1859–1960 published 1968.

b DICTIONARIES AND DIRECTORIES

1 Baillière's nurses' dictionary Edited by Barbara F. Cape and Pamela Dobson. 18th ed. Baillière Tindall, 1974.

2 Davies, P. M. Medical terminology in hospital practice: a guide for all those engaged in professions allied to medicine. 2nd ed. Heinemann Medical, 1974.

3 Miller, B. F. and Keane, C. B. Encyclopedia and dictionary of medicine and nursing. Philadelphia: Saunders, 1972.

4 Pearce, E. C. Medical and nursing dictionary and encyclopedia. 14th ed. Faber, 1975.

5 Roper, N. compiler Livingstone's dictionary for nurses, 14th ed. Edinburgh: Churchill Livingstone, 1973.

6 Royal College of Nursing Directory of nursing funds and trusts. Rcn, 1975.

7 Royal College of Nursing Directory of nursing scholarships, bursaries and grants. Rcn, 1974.

c INFORMATION NEEDS AND RESOURCES

1 Closurdo, J. S. Teaching library skills. [Program designed to teach library users independent search methods organized by the library staff of St. Joseph Mercy Hospital, Pontiac, Michigan.] Hospital Progress, 55 (9), Sep 1974, 36, 40, 42.

2 Colledge, M. Information retrieval. [One week's course in information retrieval and research appreciation at Newcastle Polytechnic.] Nursing Times, 70, 4 Apr 1974, 521–522.

3 Gauvain, S., editor Occupational health: a guide to sources of information. Heinemann, 1974.

4 Glass, L. Nursing research abstracts – a users' study. Nursing Research, 20 (2), Mar/Apr 1971, 152–158.

5 Hill, P. A. Filing and retrieving information. Nursing Times, 68, 30 Nov 1972, Occ. papers, 189–191.

6 Interagency Council on Library Resources for Nursing Reference sources for nursing. Nursing Outlook, 20 (5), May 1972, 338–343.

7 Interagency Council on Library Resources for Nursing Reference sources for nursing. Eighth revision. Nursing Outlook, 22 (5), May 1974, 331–337.

8 Medline: newest service in the medical information network. Nursing Research, 21 (2), Mar/Apr 1972, 101.

9 Medline. Lancet, 1, 24 Mar 1973, 650.

10 Nevill, A. D. and Parkin, M. L. Medlars and you. Canadian Nurse, 67 (1), Jan 1971, 46–47.

11 Parkin, M. L. Information resources for nursing research. Canadian Nurse, 68 (3), Mar 1972, 40–43.

12 Sherer, R. and Kratz, E. Medline: research tool aids health care delivery. [Medline terminal in a medical library.] Hospital Progress, 56 (7), Jul 1975, 38.

13 Stephenson, J. The use of nursing information. [Courses for nurses at Newcastle Polytechnic.] Nursing Mirror, 137, 17 Aug 1973, 46–47.

14 Steudtner, C. and Swertz, P. Documentation of the literature of hospital care in Europe. World Hospitals, 9 (1), Jan 1973, 28–30.

15 Taylor, S. D. ANF abstracting service, 1962–1971. Nursing Research Report, 6 (2), Jun 1971, 1–2, 4–8.

16 Taylor, S. D. How to search the literature. American Journal of Nursing. 74 (8), Aug 1974, 1457–1459.

17 University of Aston. Safety and Hygiene Group Where to find out. [Information needs.] Occupational Health, 25 (12), Dec 1973, 470–471.

d NURSING LITERATURE

1 American Journal of Nursing AJN 1900-1975. [Mainly illustrations.] American Journal of Nursing, 75 (10), Oct 1975, 1610, 1612, 1614, 1619.

2 Christie, H. A. Hospital journal club. [Multi-disciplinary club formed at Dingleton Hospital, Melrose, to keep up to date with current developments.] Nursing Times, 71, 17 Apr 1975, 631.

3 Collart, M. and others Books of the year, selected by nursing experts as significant reading for nurses. American Journal of Nursing. 74 (1), Jan 1974, 83–95.

4 Cooper, S. S. The book review: a significant educational resource. Journal of Nursing Education, 13, Aug 1974, 41–44.

5 Fisher, R. F. and Strank, R. A. Investigation into the reading habits of qualified nurses. Nursing Times, 67, 25 Feb 1971, 245–247.

6 Moudgil, A. C. and Sampson, P. The Nursing Journal of India: a study in content analysis (1961 to 1970). Nursing Journal of India, 64 (6), Jun 1973, 193–194.

7 O'Farrell, E. K. Write for the reader, he may need to know what you have to say. [Guidance for nurses on writing articles for journals.] Canadian Nurse, 71 (3), Mar 1975, 24–27.

8 Rouslin, S. On 'Getting into print'. [Hints for nurse authors.] Perspectives in Psychiatric Care, 8 (2), Apr/Jun 1975, 56–57.

9 Smith, R. Publish and be damned! [Experiences of a nurse author.] Nursing Mirror, 140, 3 Apr 1975, 71.

10 Woodford, J. and Fricker, R. That nursing journal. Can you afford to throw it away? How to set up a personal reference library at minimum cost. Nursing Times, 68, 21 Sep 1972, 1197–1198.

e LIBRARIES

1 Abdellah, F. G. The Nursing Archives at the National Library of Medicine. [Letters.] Nursing Research, 24 (5), Sep/Oct 1975, 389.

2 Bloomquist, H. and others, editors Library practice in hospitals:, a basic guide. Cleveland: Case Western Reserve University, 1972.

3 Cooper, B. Library services at Rampton Hospital. Health and Welfare Libraries Quarterly, 1 (3), Sep 1974, 46–59.

4 Faktor, F. M. QIDN Library. Health and Social Service Journal, 83, 17 Nov 1973, 2686.

5 Gillespie, S. Scottish health science libraries. Health and Welfare Libraries Quarterly, 1 (4), Dec 1974, 92–95.

6 Going, M. E., editor Hospital libraries and work with the disabled. 2nd ed. Library Association, 1973.

7 **Going, M. E.** Small beginnings – a history of the Kent and Sussex Hospital Library, Tunbridge Wells. Health and Welfare Libraries Quarterly, 2, Mar 1975, 4–6.

8 **Health Visitor** Health department libraries. Health Visitor, 44 (6), Jun 1971, 187.

9 **The Janet Geister Memorial Library** Occupational Health Nursing, 19 (1), Jan 1971, 17.

10 **Lewington, K. R. and others** Hospital librarians. [Correspondence.] Lancet, 1, 23 Mar 1974, 510–511.

11 **Library Association** The chartered librarian in the hospital. The Association, [1973].

12 **Library Association** Hospital libraries: recommended standards for libraries in hospitals. The Association, 1972.

13 **Likeman, C.** Libraries for nurses. [Two hospitals in the Wessex Region.] Nursing Mirror, 135, 25 Aug 1972, 40–41.

14 **Lorenz, C. J.** Is the hospital library a luxury or a necessity? Mercy Medical Center, Dubuque, Ia. has consolidated its doctors' and school of nursing libraries into a health science library. Hospital Progress, 55 (7), Jul 1974, 24–26.

15 **Matthews, D.** The re-organization of local government and of the National Health Service in England and Wales: a report from the Hospital Libraries and Handicapped Readers Group Conference – with comments. Book Trolley, 3 (9), Mar 1973, 3–9.

16 **Mowbray, D.** Library facilities for the health care system. Book Trolley, 3 (9), Mar 1973, 10–17.

17 **Murray, S.** Reference room on wheels shows how even small hospitals can improve their medical libraries. Modern Hospital, 120 (4), Apr 1973, 119–120.

18 **Nursing Times** Shared libraries. [Editorial.] Nursing Times, 69, 4 Oct 1973, 1269.

19 **Nursing Times** Ward library. [Ward information service for trained staff in the mental subnormality division of the former East Birmingham Hospital Group.] Nursing Times, 70, 25 Jul 1974, 1157.

20 **Oxford Joint Medical Libraries Committee** Oxford united: library co-operation in the Oxford hospital region. [Reprinted from a report.] Book Trolley, 3 (12), Dec 1973, 12–16.

21 **Parkhouse, R. E.** Automatic library. [Running a small library for pupil midwives without a librarian.] Nursing Times, 69, 26 Apr 1973, 550–551.

22 **Partington, W.** Queen Elizabeth II Hospital Library. Hertfordshire Library Service. Health and Welfare Libraries Quarterly, 2 (1), Mar 1975, 6–9.

23 **Paulin, L. V.** Reorganization – a prescription for better hospital libraries? Nursing Mirror, 136, 2 Mar 1973, 26–28; 23 Feb 1973, 14–17.

24 **Porth, C. and May, K. E.** The mobile library cart – practical aid to learning. [Small mobile reference libraries in areas of clinical instruction used in the University of Wisconsin-Milwaukee School of Nursing.] Nursing Outlook, 19 (9), Sep 1971, 602–603.

25 **Queen's Nursing Institute** The QNI library and information department. [Mainly illustrations.] Queen's Nursing Journal, 18 (3), Jun 1975, 78–79.

26 **Raybould, E.** Organizing a nursing school library. Nursing Mirror, 132, 7 May 1971, 29–35.

27 **Smith, D.** Basingstoke District Hospital Library Health and Welfare Libraries Quarterly. 1 (1), Mar 1974, 6–9.

28 **Sophia F. Palmer Library** Catalog of the Sophia F. Palmer Memorial Library, American Journal of Nursing Company, New York City. Boston: G. K. Hall, 1973, 2 vols.

29 **Stewart, C. C.** Your hospital library – an awakening giant. Hospital Topics, 53 (3), May/Jun 1975, 6, 46–47.

30 **Tabor, R. B.** Libraries and information for nurses. 1. The function of the library. 2. Libraries in miniature. 3. Techniques of information handling. Nursing Times, 67, 11 Mar 1971, 283–286; 18 Mar 1971, 321–323; 25 Mar 1971, 352–354.

31 **Wade, J. R.** The library services at Lister Hospital, Stevenage. Health and Welfare Libraries Quarterly, 1 (1), Mar 1974, 4–6.

2 BIOGRAPHY

1 ALKIN, E. **Gordon, J. E.** Distinguished British nurses of the past 1. Elizabeth Alkin – nurse and secret agent, 1616–1655. Midwife, Health Visitor and Community Nurse, 11 (3), Mar 1975, 77–81.

2 **Applebee, R.** No greater calling: the story of a nursing sister. Cornwall: United Writers, 1974.

3 AUSTEN, J. **Cope, Z.** The ailments and the last illness of Jane Austen. Nursing Mirror, 141, 25 Dec 1975, 50–52.

4 BEDFORD FENWICK, E. G. **Hector, W.** The work of Mrs. Bedford Fenwick and the rise of professional nursing. Rcn, 1973. (Research series.)

5 BOURGEOIS, L. **Hatcher, J.** Mme Louise Bourgeois – Royal Midwife and remarkable character. Midwives Chronicle, 84, Jan 1971, 26–27.

6 BRIDGES, D. Leading article on Daisy Bridges. Canadian Nurse, 69 (2), Feb 1973, 3. (Obituary 47).

7 BRIDGES, D. – a tribute. International Nursing Review, 20 (2), Mar/Apr 1973, 35–36.

8 BRIDGES, D. Vale – Miss Daisy Bridges [Obituary and tributes. Portrait, 12.] UNA Nursing Journal, 71, Jan/Feb 1973, 12–14.

9 BRIGGS, A. **Evagorou, D.** Asa Briggs: a profile, [and an account of the Briggs Committee]. Nursing Times, 66, 28 May 1970, 698–699.

10 CARRE, J. Profile – Miss Johanna Carre. [Chief Medical Nursing Officer, Essex County Council.] Midwife and Health Visitor, 8 (2), Feb 1972, 66.

11 CAVELL, E. **Harrison, E.** Memories of a childhood friendship. Nursing Mirror, 141, 9 Oct 1975, 51–52.

12 CAVELL, E. **Hellyer, R.** My matron. Nursing Mirror, 141, 9 Oct 1975, 50–51.

13 CAVELL, E. How much did she care? Nursing Times, 70, 10 Oct 1974, 1585–1587.

14 CAVELL, E. **Major, A.** 'The Poor Man's Nightingale'. [Edith Cavell at the Queen's District Home, Manchester.] Queen's Nursing Journal, 18, Oct 1975, 198.

15 CAVELL, E. **Mussallem, H. K.** Mount Edith Cavell: Canada's tribute to a gallant nurse. [Mount Edith Cavell in Alberta.] Canadian Nurse, 68, Feb 1972, 23–26.

16 CAVELL, E. **Ryder, R.** Edith Cavell. H. Hamilton, 1975.

17 CAVELL, E. **Ryder, R.** Edith Cavell – an appreciation. Nursing Mirror, 141, 9 Oct 1975, 47–49.

18 CELLIER, E. **Gordon, J. E.** Distinguished British nurses of the past. 3. Mrs. Elizabeth Cellier – 'the Popish Midwife' of the Restoration. Midwife Health Visitor and Community Nurse, 11 (5), May 1975, 139–142.

19 CHARLEY, I. Death of Irene Charley. International Nursing Review, 20 (4), Jul/Aug 1973, 128.

20 CHILD, J. C. **Stratford, D. O.** The South African Nursing Association and Miss J. C. Child. SA Nursing Journal, 38 (11), Nov 1971, 36–37.

21 **Cotterill, E.** A Black Country nurse at large. Tipton: Black Country Society, 1973.

22 COWELL, B. Profile of Miss B. Cowell. Midwife and Health Visitor, 7 (1), Jan 1971, 22.

23 DEANE, N. B. Miss Nora Bryan Deane, CBE, MA, SRN, SCM. [Obituary.] Midwives Chronicle, 86, Jun 1973, 180.

24 DEMPSEY, C. R. Eulogy. Catherine R. Dempsey, RN. First President of the American Association of Industrial Nurses, Inc. Occupational Health Nursing, 22, Jul 1974, 9–10.

25 EMORY, F. H. M. **Kotlarsky, C.** A pioneer in nursing education.[Florence Emory.] Canadian Nurse, 67 (11), Nov 1971, 33–35.

26 FARRER, M. I. Margaret I. Farrer. Chief Nursing Officer, Thames Group HMC. Midwife and Health Visitor, 9 (6), Jun 1973, 194.

27 FRIEND, P. M. Profile – Miss Phyllis M. Friend, CBE, SRN, RNT. Chief Nursing Officer, Department of Health and Social Security. Midwife and Health Visitor, 9 (1), Jan 1973, 24.

28 GANDHI C. M. Gandhiji's interest in nursing, medicine and health. Nursing Journal of India, 66 (10), Oct 1975, 225–238.

29 **Hale, C. B.** A good long time: the autobiography of an octogenarian. Regency Press, 1973.

30 HALKETT, Lady A. **Gordon, J. E.** Distinguished British nurses of the past. 2. Lady Anne Halkett 1622–1699. Midwife, Health Visitor and Community Nurse, 11 (4), Apr 1975, 114–117.

31 HEBDITCH, N. VSO's oldest volunteer returns home. [Miss Nora Hebditch who has been working in India.] Nursing Times, 67, 2 Dec 1971, 1506.

32 HECTOR, W. **Cullinan, J.** Careers extraordinary: 'in my end is my beginning'. [The working life of Miss Winifred Hector.] Nursing Times, 68, 7 Sep 1972, 1113–1114.

33 HECTOR, W. Personal view. [The author's work as consultant to the BBC for a series of television programmes on nursing.] British Medical Journal, 4, (5836), 11 Nov 1972, 358.

34 HEVEY, M. **Anstice, E.** 'Lifeline – can I help you?' [Maureen Hevey's previous career and present work with an advice and counselling service for those with unplanned pregnancies.] Nursing Times, 68, 28 Sep 1972, 1222–1223.

35 HOLDER, S. Profile – Stanley Holder. Midwife and Health Visitor, 8 (4), April 1972, 142.

36 HULL J. and ISAACS, B. **Cullinan, J.** Progress of a partnership. [Joan Hull and Betty Isaacs, writers of programmed textbooks for nurses.] Nursing Times, 68, 20 Apr 1972, 460–462.

37 JOSEPH, Sir K. **Bosanquet, N.** The Joseph legend. [Sir Keith Joseph's record as Secretary of State and his recent speech on population.] Nursing Times, 70, 7 Nov 1974, 1722–1723.

38 **King, E.** Rushed off my feet. Heinemann, 1971.

39 KINGSLEY, C. **Mooney, M.** Charles Kingsley – public health reformer. Midwife, Health Visitor and Community Nurse, 11 (1), Jan 1975, 7–8.

40 LAMBIE, M. **Alexander, A.** Miss Mary Lambie

strove for better conditions. New Zealand Nursing Journal, 64 (3), Mar 1971, 8–10.

41 LAWSON, M. G. Elder statesman – doctor before she was a nurse, [Mabel Gordon Lawson.] Nursing Times, 68, 17 Aug 1972, 1016.

42 LOVELAND, M. K. Profile. Midwife and Health Visitor, 7 (6), Jun 1971, 225.

43 McFARLANE, J. 'A dramatic day for nursing': England's first nursing professor appointed. Nursing Times, 70, 20 Jun 1974, 933.

44 Markham, J. The lamp was dimmed: the story of a nurse's training. Hale, 1975.

45 Markham, J. My little black bag: the story of a district nurse. Hale, 1973.

46 MARTIN, M. **Bailey, A.** The passing to the Great Beyond of a gallant nurse and a lover of Africans. Tribute to Mother Mary Martin. Nigerian Nurse, 7, Apr–Jun 1975, 28.

47 NIGHTINGALE, F. Letters of Florence Nightingale in the History of Nursing Archive, Special Collections, Boston University Libraries. Edited by Lois A. Monteiro. Boston, Mass.: Boston University Libraries, 1974.

48 NIGHTINGALE, F. Letters to a friend. Nursing Times, 69, 8 Nov 1973, 1474–1476.

49 NIGHTINGALE, F. **Barritt, E. R. compiler** Florence Nightingale: her work and wisdom. New York: Peter Pauper Press, 1975.

50 NIGHTINGALE, F. **Baylen, J. O.** The Florence Nightingale/Mary Stanley controversy: some unpublished letters. Medical History, 18 (2), Mar 1974, 186–193.

51 NIGHTINGALE, F. **Clayton, R. E.** How men may live and not die in India. [Florence Nightingale.] Australasian Nurses' Journal, 2, Apr 1974, 10–11. Extracts in Nursing Journal of India, 65 (10), Oct 1974, 261–262, 282–284.

52 NIGHTINGALE, F. **Coxhead, E.** Miss Nightingale's Country Hospital. [Royal Buckinghamshire Hospital, Aylesbury.] (Reprinted from Country Life, 23 Nov 1972). Nursing Times, 69, 10 May 1973, 615–617.

53 NIGHTINGALE, F. **Gordon, J. E.** Nurses and nursing in Britain. 23. The work of Florence Nightingale – 3: Her influence throughout the world. Midwife and Health Visitor, 9, Jan 1973, 17–22.

54 NIGHTINGALE, F. **Huxley, E.** Florence Nightingale. Weidenfeld & Nicholson, 1975.

55 NIGHTINGALE, F. **James, P. D.** A breath of fresh air. [Review of the 1975 reprint of 'Notes on nursing'.] Times Literary Supplement, 9 May 1975, 517.

56 NIGHTINGALE, F. **Monteiro, L.** Research into things past: tracking down one of Miss Nightingale's correspondents. Nursing Research, 21 (6), Nov/Dec 1972, 526–529.

57 NIGHTINGALE, F. **Rao Rameswara, G. A. J.** Florence Nightingale. Nursing Journal of India, 62 (6), Jun 1971, 179.

58 NIGHTINGALE, F. **Stewart, P.** Florence Nightingale. Wayland Publishers, 1973. (Eye witness history book.)

59 NIGHTINGALE, F. **Tinckler, L. F.** The barracks at Scutari: start of a nursing legend. Nursing Times, 69, 2 Aug 1973, 1006–1007.

60 PALMER, S. F. **Christy, T. E.** Portrait of a leader: Sophia F. Palmer. Nursing Outlook, 23 (12), Dec 1975, 746–751.

61 PATTISON, D. **Manton, J.** Sister Dora: the life of Dorothy Pattison. Methuen, 1971.

62 PEARCE, E. Evelyn Pearce: an appreciation. Nursing Times, 133, 22 Oct 1971, 5.

63 PREECE, E. **Gordon, J. E.** Distinguished British nurses of the past. 4. Mrs. Elizabeth Preece 1778–1790, Matron, Bristol Infirmary. Midwife, Health Visitor and Community Nurse, 11 (7), Jul 1975, 218, 220–223.

64 RODMELL, J. **Boorer, D.** A nurse and her hospital. A profile of Joyce Rodmell. [Matron of Sydney Hospital.] Nursing Times, 69, 10 May 1973, 606–607.

65 SEACOLE, M. **Gordon, J. E.** Mary Seacole – a forgotten nurse heroine of the Crimea. Midwife, Health Visitor and Community Nurse, 11 (2), Feb 1975, 47–50.

66 SIMPSON, M. Marjorie Simpson: focus on a pioneer. [Tributes from colleagues.] Nursing Times, 70, 4 Apr 1974, 518–519.

67 Smith, M. On my toes. Muller, 1972.

68 STOBIE, B. **Kavalier, F.** A rebellious community nurse. [Betty Stobie, Dingleton Hospital's community nurse in the Berwickshire area]. Nursing Times, 68, 5 Oct 1972, 1252–1254.

69 STRONG, R. **Gordon, J. E.** Distinguished British nurses of the past. 6. Mrs. Rebecca Strong – pioneer and centenarian, 1843–1944. Midwife, Health Visitor and Community Nurse, 11 (12), Dec 1975, 395–398, 409.

70 WALD, L. D. Lillian D. Wald. 'Our first public health nurse'. Nursing Outlook, 19 (10), Oct 1971, 659–660.

71 Walker, L. M. Heart to heart: being the true life story of a retired nurse and midwife. Nottingham: Duprint Service, 1971.

72 WARDROPER, S. **Gordon, J. E.** Distinguished British nurses of the past. 5. Mrs. Sarah Wardroper – Florence Nightingale's collaborator. Midwife, Health Visitor and Community Nurse, 11 (9), Sep 1975, 293–298, 300–301.

73 Wilson, E. Gone with the Raj. Wymondham: Reeve, 1974.

74 WYNDHAM-KAYE, J. Profile of Mrs. J. Wyndham-Kaye, General Secretary, Health Visitors' Association. Midwife and Health Visitor, 8 (9), Sep 1972, 319.

3 BRIGGS REPORT

a GENERAL

1 Briggs, A. Briggs on nursing. Nursing Times, 66, 3 Dec 1970, 1556–1567.

2 Briggs, A. The 'Committee on Nursing' and its significance for the future of the profession. District Nursing, 14 (9), Dec 1971, 192–194.

3 Briggs, A. Health and education. [Includes a section on nursing education and his experience as Chairman of the Committee on Nursing.] Royal Society of Health Journal, 94 (4), Aug 1974, 155–160.

4 Committee on Nursing Report. HMSO, 1972, Chairman: Professor Asa Briggs.

5 Committee on Nursing List of Committee members with details. Nursing Mirror, 12 Jun 1970, 9; Nursing Times, 21 May 1970, 643, 667.

6 Hallas, C. H. Briggs report. [Report of a talk]. Hospital and Health Services Review, 69 (2), Feb 1973, 73.

7 Hansard Announcement of the setting up of the committee by Richard Crossman. Hansard, 2 Mar 1970, col. 36–43.

b EVIDENCE

1 British Association of Social Workers The 'Briggs' Committee on nursing. Social Work Today, 2, 12 Aug 1971, 16–17; 2, 9 Sep 1971, 13–16.

2 British Medical Association A discussion of evidence for the Briggs Committee and the effect of the Salmon report. British Medical Journal, 1, 20 Feb 1971, Supplement 47–48. Evidence. British Medical Journal, 2, 1 May 1971, Supplement 36–39. Summarized in Nursing Times, 67, 13 May 1971, 562.

3 Council for the Training of Health Visitors Evidence to Briggs Committee. Nursing Times, 67, 11 Feb 1971, 162.

4 Health Visitors' Association Memorandum to the committee on nursing. Health Visitor, 44 (3), Mar 1971, 88–92.

5 Queen's Institute of District Nursing Evidence summarised in District Nursing, 13 (12), Mar 1971, 245; Nursing Times, 67, 4 Feb 1971, 131.

6 Royal College of Midwives Summary of evidence. Midwives Chronicle, Apr 1971, 116.

7 Royal College of Nursing Rcn evidence to the Committee on nursing. Rcn, 1971. (Summarized in Nursing Times, 67, 15 Jul 1971, 872–873.)

8 Royal College of Nursing The future pattern of nursing? [Rcn evidence to the Briggs Committee.] Hospital, 67 (8), Aug 1971, 261–262. Correspondence from Miss Prentice and Mr. Hart, 67 (10) Oct 1971, 366.

9 Watkin, B. Sense and nonsense from the Rcn. [Evidence to Briggs.] British Hospital Journal and Social Service Review, 81, 25 Sep 1971, 1979.

c COMMENTS AND REACTIONS

1 Bendall, E. Bendall on Briggs: a blueprint for the future which is both possible and worthwhile. Nursing Times, 68, 9 Nov 1972, 1403.

2 Boyd, E. A. A look at the Briggs Report. New Zealand Nursing Journal, 66 (6), Jun 1973, 27–32.

3 British Hospital Journal and Social Service Review Briggs in the community. [Editorial comment on proposals for health visitor status and training.] British Hospital Journal and Social Service Review, 82, 11 Nov 1972, 2503–2504.

4 British Hospital Journal and Social Service Review Comment on the Briggs Report is slowly forthcoming from the community nursing services. British Hospital Journal and Social Service Review, 82, 16 Dec 1972, 2800.

5 British Medical Journal New thoughts on nursing. [Comments on the Briggs Report.] British Medical Journal, 4, 28 Oct 1972, 191–192.

6 Collins, S. Briggs. Educating the nurse and midwife of the future. [Text of an address given at the Rcn conference on the Briggs Report.] Nursing Times, 68, 14 Dec 1972, 1592–1595.

7 Crossley, J. A. Nursing and midwifery resources. [Address to Rcn National Conference on the Briggs Report, Dec 1972.] Nursing Times, 69, 11 Jan 1973, Occ. Papers, 5–7.

8 Cullinan, J. Briggs' new nurse-making process. [Summary of Briggs proposals on nurse education.] Nursing Times, 68, 7 Dec 1972, 1562–1563.

9 Dack, P. Aide-memoire to Briggs. [Summary of Briggs Committee's main recommendations.] Nursing Mirror, 138, 17 May 1974, 38–40.

10 District Nursing Nursing: its future. [The Rcn conference on the Briggs Report.] District Nursing, 15 (11), Feb 1973, 248, 250.

11 Few, E. Role and rigmarole. [Comments on the Briggs Report.] Nursing Times, 68, 16 Nov 1972, 1465–1466.

12 Frost, W. Briggs and the health visitor. Nursing Times, 69, 8 Feb 1973, 170–171.

13 Hall, C. Briggs could herald a new era. Nursing Times, 68, 26 Oct 1972, 1338.

14 Health and Social Service Journal A greater medical profession? [Editorial comment.] Health and Social Service Journal, 83, 27 Jan 1973, 181–182.

15 Health and Social Service Journal Health visiting. [Reactions to the Briggs Report.] Health and Social Service Journal, 83, 3 Mar 1973, 471–472.

16 Health and Social Service Journal Nurses react to Briggs Report. [Reactions of Society of Chief Nursing Officers (Public Health) Health Visitors' Association, and National Nursing Staff Committee.] Health and Social Service Journal, 83, 17 Feb 1973, 358.

17 Health Visitor Family health sisters. [Briggs Report.] Health Visitor, 45 (11), Nov 1972, 351–352.

18 Health Visitor Other people's views on Briggs. Health Visitor, 46, Apr 1973, 113.

19 Health Visitor A reply to Miss Frost on 'Briggs'. [Editorial.] Health Visitor, 46 (3), Mar 1973, 75. Correspondence, 89–93.

20 Health Visitors' Association The Briggs report. Comments. Health Visitor, 46 (2), Feb 1973, 45–47.

21 Hospital and Health Services Review Changes for nursing. [Leading article on the Briggs Report.] Hospital and Health Services Review, 68 (12), Dec 1972, 431–433.

22 Hulme, J. Comment on Briggs. Health Services, 26, Jul/Aug 1973, 136–137.

23 Leach, D. Why educate nurses? How Briggs missed the point. Nursing Times, 69, 19 Jul 1973, 939–940.

24 Markham, J. What the nurses say . . . Some senior nurses comment on the Briggs Report. Nursing Mirror, 135, 17 Nov 1972, 21–22.

25 Midwife and Health Visitor The Briggs Report – a weighty document. [Comment on proposals for midwives and health visitors.] Midwife and Health Visitor, 8 (12), Dec 1972, 412–413.

26 Midwives Chronicle Collective thoughts on the Briggs report. By a Principal Nursing Officer of the Maternity wing following a study day. Midwives Chronicle, 86, Mar 1973, 76–77.

27 Nursing Mirror Welcome to Briggs. [Summary of and extracts from the report with comments.] Nursing Mirror, 135, 17 Nov 1972, 18–20; 24 Nov 1972, 20–22; 1 Dec 1972, 16–18.

28 Nursing Times Briggs reports. Standards, training, careers, staffing: the main recommendations. Nursing Times, 68, 19 Oct 1972, 1306–1307.

29 Nursing Times Briggs – the image and the reality. Nursing Times, 68, 9 Nov 1972, Supplement, 1–4.

30 Nursing Times Briggs: summary of recommendations. Nursing Times, 68, 26 Oct 1972, Supplement, 1–4.

31 Nursing Times Correspondence on the Briggs Report. Nursing Times, 68, 28 Dec 1972, 1654–1655; 69, 18 Jan 1973, 92–93; 25 Jan 1973, 124–125.

32 Nursing Times The school of experience. [Editorial on the educational implications of the Briggs Report.] Nursing Times, 68, 14 Dec 1972, 1567.

33 Nursing Times What they say about Briggs. [Comments from Bernard Finn, Albert Spanswick, Constance Biddulph, Miss G. M. Francis, and Miss M. I. Farrer and others.] Nursing Times, 68, 26 Oct 1972, 1342–1343; 2 Nov 1972, 1373–1375.

34 Page, J. and others Training, titles and 'tinted spectacles'. [Comments on the Briggs Report.] Nursing Times, 68, 9 Nov 1972, 1406–1407.

35 Pennell, A. D. A CNO in a mental subnormality group looks at Briggs. Nursing Times, 69, 22 Mar 1973, 390–391.

36 Royal College of Midwives RCM report on the Committee of Nursing. Midwives Chronicle, 86, Mar 1973, 68–69.

37 Royal College of Nursing Briggs. Briggs' explains. [Report of Conference.] Nursing Times, 69, 4 Jan 1973, 26–28.

38 Royal College of Nursing Rcn comment on the report of the Committee on Nursing. Rcn 1973.

39 Times Briggs Report. [Leading article.] Times, 18 Oct 1972, 17.

40 Watson, V. Asa Briggs Report as it affects midwives. Nursing Mirror, 136, 20 Apr 1973, 22–26.

41 Winiecki, G. Briggs Report: a qualified welcome. British Hospital Journal and Social Service Review, 82, 11 Nov 1972, 2508.

d IMPLEMENTATION

1 Bosanquet, N. Briggs in three years? Talking point. Nicholas Bosanquet talks to David Owen. Nursing Times, 70, 21 Nov 1974, 1799.

2 Bosanquet, N. and Clifton, R. Briggs: the context. 1. Resources for training. Nursing Times, 69, 10 May 1973, Occ. papers, 74–76.

3 Bosanquet, N. and Clifton, R. Briggs: the context. 2. Fresh start in pay. Nursing Times, 69, 17 May 1973, Occ. papers, 77–80.

4 Bosanquet, N. and Clifton, R. Briggs: the context. 3. Nursing work: some impressions. Nursing Times, 69, 24 May 1973, Occ. papers, 81–84.

5 Bosanquet, N. and Clifton, R. Briggs: the context. 4. Nursing work: some impressions. Nursing Times, 69, 31 May 1973, Occ. papers, 85–87.

6 Chisholm, M. K. Design, drift and directive. [Changes in the NHS and the recommendations of the Briggs Report as they will affect nurses.] Nursing Mirror, 137, 3 Aug 1973, 33–34.

7 Harrold, A. Planning for Briggs. 1. Nursing Times, 70, 23 May 1974, Occ. papers, 9–12.

8 Harrold, A. E. and Pace, A. J. Planning for Briggs. 2. Nurse allocation. [Three possible allocation plans for introducing training for the Certificate in Nursing Practice.] Nursing Times, 70, 30 May 1974, Occ. papers, 13–16.

9 Her Majesty's Government Briggs Committee on Nursing: the government's proposals. The Government, 1974. (Consultative document.)

10 Lancet Nothing much for the nurses. [The implementation of Briggs, and the case for better pay.] Lancet, 1, 18 May 1974, 971.

11 Nursing Times First moves on Briggs. Nursing Times, 70, 3 Oct 1974, 1529.

12 Nursing Times Health service priorities. Mrs Castle 'regrets' delay on Briggs. Nursing Times, 72, 5 Feb 1975, 160.

13 Owen, D. Owen on Briggs: the future of nurse training in the light of the present financial constraints. Nursing Mirror, 141, 16 Oct 1975, 40–41.

14 Stevenson, J. The year of the tiger. [Nursing developments in 1974 covering Halsbury and the progress of Briggs.] Nursing Mirror, 139, 19 Dec 1974, 37–39.

4 HISTORY

a GENERAL

1 Baly, M. E. Nursing and social change. Heinemann, 1973.

2 Broadley, M. E. It's different now 1–6. [Nurse training at the London Hospital in 1923.] Nursing Times, 71: 20 Nov 1975, 1844–1847; 27 Nov 1975, 1900–1901; 4 Dec 1975, 1940–1941; 11 Dec 1975; 1982–1983; 18 Dec 1975, 2024–2025; 25 Dec 1975, 2064–2065.

3 Calder, J. McKinley The story of nursing. 5th ed. Methuen, 1971.

4 Clarke, D. G. Nurse in the '30s. Nursing Mirror, 132, 7 May 1971, 44–45.

5 Coleman, V. Early nursing. [Comparative status of the medical and nursing professions in the nineteenth century.] Nursing Mirror, 140, 24 Apr 1975, 72.

6 Dolan, J. A. Nursing in society: a historical perspective. 13th ed. Philadelphia: Saunders, 1973.

7 Dopson, L. The wreck of the Rohilla. [Four nurses involved in the wreck of a hospital ship, October 1914.] Nursing Times, 70, 31 Oct 1974, 1706–1707.

8 Ellis, A. Superstitions. Nursing Times, 57, 23 Dec 1971, 1590–1591.

9 Farmborough, F. Nurse at the Russian Front: a diary 1914–1918. Constable, 1974.

10 Gordon, J. E. Nurses and nursing in Britain. 1. Roman times. Midwife and Health Visitor, 6 (6), Jun 1970, 215–218.

11 Gordon, J. E. Nurses and nursing in Britain. 2. The Saxon centuries. Midwife and Health Visitor, 6 (7), Jul 1970, 252–257.

12 Gordon, J. E. Nurses and nursing in Britain. 3. The mediaeval monastic tradition. Midwife and Health Visitor, 6 (8), Aug 1970, 294–295, 298–301.

13 Gordon, J. E. Nurses and nursing in Britain. 4. Domestic nursing from the Saxons to the Stuarts. Midwife and Health Visitor, 6 (9), Sep 1970, 333–339.

14 Gordon, J. E. Nurses and nursing in Britain. 5. The professional nurse to the 18th century. Midwife and Health Visitor, 6 (10), Oct 1970, 380–386.

15 Gordon, J. E. Nurses and nursing in Britain. 6. The nurse in war from the 12th to the 18th century. Midwife and Health Visitor, 6 (11), Nov 1970, 419–424.

16 Gordon, J. E. Nurses and nursing in Britain. 7. The hospital tradition from the Reformation to the 18th century. Midwife and Health Visitor, 6 (12) Dec 1970, 457–462.

17 Gordon, J. E. Nurses and nursing in Britain. 9 and 10. Through pestilence and plague to public health. Midwife and Health Visitor, 7 (9), Sep 1971, 354–359; (10), Oct 1971, 392–397.

18 Gordon, J. E. Nurses and nursing in Britain. 11 and 12. The hospital nurse in the 18th century. Midwife and Health Visitor, 7 (11) Nov 1971, 434–437; (12), Dec 1971, 467–471.

19 Gordon, J. E. Nurses and nursing in Britain. 16. The 19th century – voluntary hospitals and workhouse infirmaries. Midwife and Health Visitor, 8 (5), May 1972, 174–179.

20 Gordon, J. E. Nurses and nursing in Britain. 17 and 18. The nurse in war in the 18th and 19th centuries 1. In the navy. 2. In the army. Midwife and Health Visitor, 8 (6), Jun 1972, 214–217; (7), Jul 1972, 248–247.

21 Gordon, J. E. Nurses and nursing in Britain. 19 and 20. Nursing in the home in the 19th century. Midwife and Health Visitor, 8 (8) Aug 1972, 284–287; (9), Sep 1972, 320–323.

22 Gordon, J. E. Nurses and nursing in Britain. 21. The work of Florence Nightingale. 1. For the health of the army. Midwife and Health Visitor, 8 (10), Oct 1972, 351, 354–359.

23 Green, A. Hospital hauntings. Nursing Times, 71, 29 May 1975, 849–851. (See also correspondence on Ghosts in hospital, 71, 10 Jul 1975, 1104–1105.)

24 Griffin, G. J. and Griffin, J. K. History and trends of professional nursing. 7th ed. St. Louis: Mosby, 1973.

25 Holcombe, D. Victorian ladies at work. David and Charles, 1973, 68–102.

26 McCarrick, H. It's the same old story . . . [Nursing news of 1910.] Nursing Times, 67, 1 Apr 1971, 394–395.

27 Nelson, S. The influence of Christianity on the care of the sick up to the end of the Middle Ages. SA Nursing Journal, 40 (8), Aug 1973, 18–19, 34.

28 Nettleton, R. A nurse's life in the 1900s. Nursing Times, 68, 21 Dec 1972, 1615.

29 Nursing Times Fifty years ago. A selection of news and pictures from Nursing Times in 1925, when the magazine was just 20 years old. Nursing Times, 71, 2 Jan 1975, 11–13.

30 Royal Infirmary of Edinburgh Mistresses of the Royal Infirmary. [History of nursing in the Royal Infirmary of Edinburgh.] Nursing Times, 68, 5 Oct 1972, 1240–1241.

31 Ruddock, E. A room of one's own. [Conditions in a nurses' home during the Second World War.] Nursing Mirror, 137, 27 Jul 1973, 9.

32 Schofield, M. T. On a summer day in 1879. [When the author started training at Westminster Hospital.] Nursing Mirror, 132, 4 Jun 1971, 30–31.

b OVERSEAS COUNTRIES

1 Austin, A. L. Nurses in American history. Wartime volunteers – 1861–1865. American Journal of Nursing, 75 (5), May 1975, 816–818.

2 Benson, E. Nursing in Serbia – early days. [History of nursing in Yugoslavia.] American Journal of Nursing, 74 (3), Mar 1974, 472–474.

3 Bull, M. R. Kimberley – a century of nursing. Nursing Mirror, 133, 17 Dec 1972, 27–30.

4 Christy, T. E. Nurses in American history. The fateful decade 1890–1900. American Journal of Nursing, 75 (7), Jul 1975, 1163–1165.

5 Donnelley, P. G. Royal Hobart Hospital Centenary of Nursing 1875–1975. [Brief history of the provision of nursing care.] Australian Nurses' Journal, 5 (4), Oct 1975, 7–9.

6 Fitzpatrick, M. L. Nurses in American history. Nursing and the Great Depression. American Journal of Nursing, 75 (12), Dec 1975, 2188–2190.

7 The Frontier Nursing Service 1925–1975. Fifty years of care. [Kentucky.] Midwives Chronicle, 88, May 1975, 166–167.

8 Galiano, S. Brief history of nursing in Nicaragua. International Journal of Nursing Studies, 12 (4), 1975, 223–229.

9 Kalisch, B. J. and Kalisch, P. A. Slaves, servants or saints? An analysis of the system of nurse training in the United States 1873–1948. Nursing Forum, 14 (3), 1975, 222–263.

10 Kalisch, P. A. Heroines of '98: female Army nurses in the Spanish–American War. Nursing Research, 24 (6), Nov/Dec 1975, 411–429.

11 Kalisch, P. A. and Kalisch, B. J. The women's draft: an analysis of the controversy over the Nurses Selective Service Bill of 1945, pertaining to the need to draft nurses during World War II. Nursing Research, 22 (5), Sep/Oct 1973, 402–413.

12 Marais, J. Nursing in Mau Mau time [on the slopes of Mount Kenya]. SA Nursing Journal, 40 (11), Nov 1973, 25–26.

13 Milena, P. The development of nursing in the northern part of Jugoslavija. (SR – Slovenija.) International Journal of Nursing Studies, 9 (3), Aug 1972, 151–156.

14 Mills, T. M. Nursing sourdoughs in the Klondike. [Four Victorian Order nurses.] Canadian Nurse, 68 (4), Apr 1972, 51–54.

15 Morris, K. N. Those unsinkable Nightingale nurses. [Nursing history in Sydney.] Australian Nurses' Journal, 1 (2), Aug 1971, 22–23, 32–33.

16 Ndirangu, S. Early days of medical and nursing service in Kenya in relation to the CSM – Church of Scotland Mission. Kenya Nursing Journal, 1 (1), Jun 1972, 44–47.

17 Rawnsley, M. M. The Goldmark Report: mid-point in nursing history. [Report of the Committee for the Study of Nursing Education, 1923 shows the similarities in nursing issues then and now.] Nursing Outlook, 21 (6), Jun 1973, 380–383.

18 Reidy, M. The history of nursing in Ireland. International Nursing Review, 18 (4), 1971, 326–331.

19 RN Magazine Civil War nurses, North and South. RN Magazine, 34 (4), Apr 1971, 46–47.

20 Saint, N. Reflections – a 92 year old nurse reminisces. SA Nurses Journal, 5 (15), Mar/Apr, 1971, 8–9.

21 Selavan, I. C. Nurses in American history. The Revolution. American Journal of Nursing, 75 (4), Apr 1975, 592–594.

22 Shannon, M. C. Nurses in American history. Our first four licensure laws. [North Carolina, New Jersey, New York and Virginia.] American Journal of Nursing, 75 (8), Aug 1975, 1327–1329.

23 Tirpak, H. The Frontier Nursing Service: fifty years in the mountains. [Kentucky.] Nursing Outlook, 23, (5), May 1975, 308–310.

24 Wakeford, J. Address given by Dr. J. Wakeford to commemorate the 70th anniversary of the first Rhodesian trained nurse. Rhodesian Nurse, 5 (2), Jun 1972, 7–10.

25 White, G. A nurse in Asia. Nursing Times, 70, 14 Nov 1974, 1766–1768.

c SPECIAL AREAS

1 Aronovitch, B. Give it time: an experience of hospital, 1928-32. Deutsch, 1974.

2 Clemons, B. The operating room, nursing's first specialty. [History of operating room nursing and training for it.] RN Magazine, 36 (2), Feb 1973, OR 1–2, 4, 6, 9.

3 Corbally, M. The health visitor's role twenty-five years ago. Midwife and Health Visitor, 9 (2), Feb 1973, 45–46.

4 Dicker, K. Six days to Sunday. [The author's experiences as a child patient in 1932.] Nursing Times, 69, 8 Mar 1973, 309.

5 Dowling, W. C. Health visiting. 1. The beginning. 2. Expansion. 3. Latter days. Health Visitor, 46 (10) Oct 1973, 337–338; 46 (11), Nov 1973, 371–373; 46 (12), Dec 1973, 410–413.

6 Fletcher, H. In our day we had to . . . [Operating room procedures of the past.] NATNews, 10 (4), Aug 1973, 26.

7 Gordon, J. E. Nurses and nursing in Britain. 8. Care of the psychiatric patient. Midwife and Health Visitor, 7 (8), Aug 1971, 307–312.

8 Gordon, J. E. Nurses and nursing in Britain. 13 and 14. The children's nurse. Midwife and Health Visitor, 8 (1), Jan 1972, 25–29; (2), Feb 1972, 57–61.

9 Greene, B. The rise and fall of the Asylum Workers' Association. Nursing Mirror, 141, 25 Dec 1975, 53–55.

10 Hawkyard, E. A. On district half-a-century ago. District Nursing, 13 (12), Mar 1971, 241.

11 Martin, M. W. A postal gallery of nursing art. [Stamps of nursing interest.] Nursing Times, 68, 2 Nov 1972, 1386–1387; Journal of Practical Nursing, 23 (7), Jul 1973, 28–29.

12 Scharlibe, M. The Health Visitor 1919. [Extract from 'The Welfare of the Expectant Mother', published in 1919.] Health Visitor, 46 (5), May 1973, 163, 165.

13 White, R. The development of the poor law nursing service and the social, medical and political factors that influenced it, 1848 to 1948. MSc thesis, Manchester University, 1975.

5 NURSING AS A PROFESSION

a GENERAL

1 Abdellah, F. G. Evolution of nursing as a profession: perspective on manpower development. International Nursing Review, 19 (3), 1972, 219–235.

2 Ashley, A. Power, freedom and professional practice in nursing. Supervisor Nurse, 6 (1), Jan 1975, 12–14, 17, 19–20, 22–24, 29.

3 Ashley, J. A. This I believe. About power in nursing. Nursing Outlook, 21 (10), Oct 1973, 637–641.

4 Bajaj, S. Is nursing an independent profession? Nursing Journal of India, 65 (6), Jun 1974, 167, 172.

5 Besel, L. The private self and the professional self. Canadian Nurse, 70 (11), Nov 1974, 21–23.

6 Bowman, M. P. The hallmark of the nurse. How to develop a professional approach: Some notes for first year nurses. Nursing Times, 69, 8 Mar 1973, 318.

7 Bowman, R. A. and Culpepper, R. C. Power: Rx for change. [The power of the nursing profession.] American Journal of Nursing, 74 (6), Jun 1974, 1053–1056.

8 Catellier, E. Nursing: putting the pieces together. [Active role of the nurse in professional affairs.] Hospital Progress, 56 (7), Jul 1975, 76–77.

9 Cross, Y. Rogue nurses. Professional loyalty: what is it, and to whom is it owed? Nursing Mirror, 134, 31 Mar 1972, 14–16.

10 De Leon, S. A. P. Goals and value for the profession. [Paper given at the ICN Congress, Mexico.] Hong Kong Nursing Journal, 16, May 1974, 47–52.

11 Dugan, A. B. Nursing autonomy: key to quality nurturance. Journal of Nursing Administration, 1 (4), Jul/Aug 1971, 50–54.

12 Eaton, S. The cult of professionalism. Nursing Times, 70, 18 Jul 1974, 1122.

13 Elliott, F. N. What does society expect of its nurses? Hospitals, 46, 1 Jun 1972, 82, 85, 88, 149.

14 Everley, G. S. and Schabdach, G. M. Specialization: the road to professionalism. Supervisor Nurse, 6 (10), Oct 1975, 39, 41.

15 Goodwin, J. L. Titles – and professional status. Nursing Mirror, 133, 2 Jul 1971, 9–10.

16 Gordon, R. and Grime, J. Where lies the future? [Professionalization in nursing.] Nursing Times, 67, 25 Nov 1971, 1459–1461.

17 Gortner, S. R. Scientific accountability in nursing. [The consequences of nursing activities evaluated in a systematic way.] Nursing Outlook, 22 (12), Dec 1974, 764–768.

18 Hohman, J. Accountability: what it's all about. [Conference on the relationship of accountability to nursing service and education.] Hospitals, 49, 16 Mar 1975, 145–146, 150.

19 Holmes, B. Nursing as a profession: a comparative approach. Nursing Times, 68, 25 May 1972, 655–656.

20 Hunter, T. D. Nurses' professional future. Nursing Times, 67, 3 Jun 1971, 682–683.

21 Jacox, A. K. The pursuit of excellence as a professional goal. AORN Journal, 21 (7), Jun 1975, 1290–1291, 1293, 1295–1296, 1298, 1300, 1302, 1306, 1308.

22 Journal of the Royal College of General Practitioners Nursing comes of age. [Position of the nursing profession.] Journal of the Royal College of General Practitioners, 24, Apr 1974, 220.

23 Klein, R. Nursing. [Comment on the Rcn document 'The state of nursing' and the nurses case.] New Society, 28, 16 May 1974, 384.

24 Kovacs, A. R. Towards professionalization of nurses. International Nursing Review, 18 (3), 1971, 272–279.

25 Kujore, O. O. The nursing profession and you. [Professionalism in nursing.] Nigerian Nurse, 6 (1), Jan/Mar 1974, 11–12, 16.

26 Maas, M. L. Nurse autonomy and accountability in organized nursing services [as means for improved patient care]. Nursing Forum, 12 (3), 1973, 237–259.

27 McAuley, M. J. The constitution of the competent member: a study of nurses in their natural setting. MA (Econ) thesis, Manchester University, 1974.

28 McPherson, D. Problems of professionalism with particular reference to nursing. Jamaican Nurse, 13 (2), Aug/Sep 1973, 26–27.

29 Meehan, E. Integrity and openness: concept of professionalism. World of Irish Nursing, 4 (11), Nov 1975, 4–5.

30 Mulcahy, R. The nursing profession: responsibilities and privileges. Irish Nurses' Journal, 4 (2/3), Feb/Mar 1971, 5, 7–10.

31 Mullane, M. K. The challenge to professional nursing. Occupational Health Nursing, 19 (9), Sep 1971, 7–10.

32 Nursing Times Quandary. Who controls nursing? Nursing Times, 69, 4 Oct 1973, 1298.

33 O'Dwyer, E. M. Concept of professionalism. World of Irish Nursing, 4 (12), Dec 1975, 9.

34 Passos, J. Y. Accountability: myth or mandate? Journal of Nursing Administration, 3 (3), May/Jun 1973, 17–21.

35 Raven, K. A. Nursing, change, and the nursing division, DHSS.1. Nursing Times, 67, 7 Jan 1971, Occ. papers, 1–4; 14 Jan 1971, Occ. papers, 5–8.

36 Rinneard, B. Nurses' professional image and collective bargaining. Hospital Administration in Canada, 17 (6), Jun 1975, 64.

37 Royal College of Nursing The state of nursing. Rcn, 1974. [Document submitted to Mrs Castle. See report by J. Cullinan, Nursing Times, 70, 23 May 1974, 778–782.]

38 Rule, J. B. A crisis of identity: the Nursing Lecture 1974. Rcn, 1974.

39 Schlotfeldt, R. M. On the professional status of nursing. Nursing Forum, 13 (1), 1974, 16–31.

40 Schlotfeldt, R. M. Planning for progress. [Discrepancy between the philosophy and practice of nursing.] Nursing Outlook, 21 (12), Dec 1973, 766–769.

41 Scott Wright, M. Nursing – present perspectives and future prospects. From a lecture given at the 59th London Nursing Exhibition and Conference on Thursday, 24 October, 1974. Nursing Mirror, 139, 31 Oct 1974, 53–56.

42 Sutherland, A. H. The nurse as a citizen. Nursing Mirror, 131, 20 Nov/11 Dec 1970, 44–45.

43 Taaffe, T. C. A concept of professionalism: accountability and responsibility. World of Irish Nursing, 4 (11), Nov 1975, 1–2.

b ATTITUDES

1 Barham, V. Z. Changing the attitudes of hospital nurses. Nursing Outlook, 19 (8), Aug 1971, 538–540.

2 Bendall, E. Nursing attitudes in the health care team. Nursing Times, 69, 15 Feb 1973, Occ. papers, 25–27.

3 Bond, J. The construction of a scale to measure nurses' attitudes. International Journal of Nursing Studies, 2 (11), Jul 1974, 75–84.

4 Boorer, D. The study of attitudes – a vital problem for all nurses. Nursing Times, 67, 26 Aug 1971, 1045–1047.

5 Dulewicz, S. V. A study of nurses' job attitudes. MPhil thesis, Department of Occupational Psychology, Birbeck College, London University, 1972.

6 Frost, D. A question of attitudes. [A review of the King's Fund report.] Nursing Times, 67, 26 Aug 1971, 1047–1048.

7 Ghioto, B. R. Action and reaction. Occupational Health Nursing, 19 (3), Mar 1971, 11–13.

8 Group, T. M. and Roberts, J. I. Exorcising the ghosts of the Crimea. [The prevailing milieu continues to be authoritarian, male-dominated, and militaristic.] Nursing Outlook, 22 (6), Jun 1974, 368–372.

9 Kings Fund Centre Attitudes and assessment. [Projects at six hospitals.] The Centre, 1973. (KFC reprint, no 756.)

10 McKay, H. Nursing blues. [Survey of 223 nurses in Bedfordshire and Hertfordshire, showing their views on professional status, pay and their work.] New Society, 28, 20 Jun 1974, 705.

11 Moody, P. M. Attitudes of cynicism and humanitarianism in nursing students and staff nurses. Journal of Nursing Education, 12 (3), Aug 1973, 9–13.

12 Norris, C. M. Delusions that trap nurses . . . into dead end alleys away from growth, relevance, and impact on health care. Nursing Outlook, 21 (1), Jan 1973, 18–21; Canadian Nurse, 69 (6), Jun 1973, 37–40.

13 Rowe, K. H. Attitudes of nursing staff in three maternity hospitals. [Research project into the effect of change resulting from the implementation of the Salmon recommendations.] Nursing Times, 69, 22 Feb 1973, Occ. papers, 29–32.

14 Singh, A. and MacGuire, J. Occupational values and stereotypes in a group of trained nurses. Nursing Times, 67, 21 Oct 1971, Occ. papers, 165–168.

15 Stone, R. Help me. Self evaluation in nursing. Journal of Practical Nursing, 24 (5), May 1974, 29, 31.

c ETHICS

1 Adote, A. M. and Bwire, T. L. Ethics and nursing. Kenya Nursing Journal, 4 (2), Dec 1975, 14–15.

2 Agate, J. Ethical questions in geriatric care. 1. Nursing Mirror, 133, 5 Nov 1971, 17–18.

3 Agate, J. Ethical questions in geriatric care. 2. Rights and obligations of elderly patients. Nursing Mirror, 133, 12 Nov 1971, 42–43.

4 Agate, J. Ethical questions in geriatric care. 3. Family conflicts in the management of old people. Nursing Mirror, 133, 19 Nov 1971, 40–41.

5 Andrews, J. Aspects of nursing: the nurse and the ethical committee. The Wick Journal of Northwick Park HMC and Clinical Research Centre, Dec 1973.

6 Ashworth, P. Ethics in the Intensive Care Therapy Unit. Nursing Mirror, 139, 14 Nov 1974, 57–60, 63.

7 Aydelotte, M. K. Medical ethics and the nurse: mutual endorsement and support. Australian Nurses' Journal, 3 (1), Jul 1973, 9–11, 22.

8 Baker, E. On teaching ethics to nurses. Nursing Times, 69, 24 May 1973, 683–684.

9 Bergman, R. Ethics – concepts and practice. International Nursing Review, 20 (5), Sep/Oct 1973, 140–141.

10 Black, D. Ethical problems in hospital practice. Community Health, 6 (1), Jul/Aug 1974, 22–28.

11 Campbell, A. V. Moral dilemmas in medicine: a coursebook in ethics for doctors and nurses. Churchill Livingstone, 1972. 2nd ed. 1975.

12 Cannon, P. J. Ethics and nursing. World of Irish Nursing, 4 (9), Sep 1975, 1–2.

13 Carpenter, W. T. and Langsner, C. A. The nurse's role in informed consent. Nursing Times, 71, 3 Jul 1975, 1049–1051.

14 Crooks, L. C. Are nurses abdicating their obligations? [Nursing responsibilities in terms of the patient, the law and moral obligation.] AORN Journal, 22 (4), Oct 1975, 523–529.

15 Crowe, Rev. M. B. Christian values in nursing. Irish Nursing News, Jun 1972, 33–35.

16 Denison, J. M. Which brothers do we keep? The ethics and politics of caring. Canadian Nurse, 68, May 1971, 19–20.

17 Donaghue, S. Humanist traditions in nursing development. Australian Nurses' Journal, 4 (11), Jun 1975, 26–30.

18 Griffiths, N. The responsibilities and influence of the Catholic nurse in the profession. UNA Nursing Journal, 71, Mar/Apr 1973, 9–13.

19 Hanid, T. K. Ethical dilemmas in obstetric and newborn care. Midwife, Health Visitor and Community Nurse, 11 (1), Jan 1975, 9–11.

20 International Council of Nurses Code for nurses: ethical concepts applied to nursing. Revised edition. Geneva: ICN, 1973.

21 Jegede S. A. Nurses code of ethics and legal implications in nursing practice. [Including the work of the Nursing Council of Nigeria.] Nigerian Nurse, 6 (3), Jul/Sep 1974, 34–41.

22 Journal of Medical Ethics Ethics and the professions. [Including a section on nursing by P. Nuttall.] Journal of Medical Ethics, 1 (1), Apr 1975, 2–4.

23 Khan, P. Origin of nursing and Christian ideals. Nursing Journal of India, 63 (2), Feb 1972, 48, 58.

24 Mackenzie, N. The professional ethic and the hospital service. English Universities Press, 1971.

25 Mackenzie, N. and Cross, Y. Life and living it. [Yvonne Cross discusses ethics with Norah Mackenzie]. Nursing Mirror, 133, 15 Oct 1971, 49–51.

26 Patey, E. H. Matters of life and death. The manipulative society. [Important issues facing society today particularly those which affect nurses in their role as a caring profession.] Nursing Mirror, 139, 5 Dec 1974, 40–41.

27 Schorr, T. M. Magna Carta for nurses everywhere. [Editorial on the ICN code of ethics.] American Journal of Nursing, 73 (8), Aug 1973, 1329.

28 Silva, M. C. Science, ethics, and nursing. American Journal of Nursing, 74 (11), Nov 1974, 2004–2007.

29 Swaby, Gertrude What's in the nurses' new code. Jamaican Nurse, 14 (3), Dec 1974, 21–22.

d IMAGE

1 Atkinson, P. Kind hearts and curettes. [Medicine and nursing in romantic fiction.] New Society, 21, 27 Jul 1972, 178–180.

2 Beletz, E. E. Is nursing's public image up to date? Nursing Outlook, 22 (7), Jul 1974, 432–435.

3 Bergman, R. and others Opinion on nursing. 1. Research study with nurses and medical students. 2. Self image of the nurse. International Nursing Review, 18 (3), 1971, 195–227; 19 (2), 1972, 116–124.

4 Brookes, P. Two conceptions of nursing assessed. [An account of a paper by Miss C. Mordaque delivered at the WHO symposium.] Nursing Times, 69, 12 Apr 1973, 482.

5 Brown, J. S. and others Baccalaureate students' image of nursing: a replication. Nursing Research, 23 (1), Jan/Feb 1974, 53–59.

6 Carew, H. M. Forward – where? How? [Image of the registered nurse.] Occupational Health Nursing, 23 (9), Sep 1975, 17–19.

7 Friedman, W. Changes in diploma nursing students' perceptions of a good nurse. Nursing Forum, 10 (1), 1971, 72–79.

8 Hinds, G. H. Nursing image. New Zealand Nursing Journal, 66 (7), Jul 1973, 14–15.

9 Macinnes, C. Nurse wonderful. [Image of the nurse.] New Society, 28, 23 May 1974, 454.

10 Nursing Times The image. [Editorial on the entry under 'Nursing' in the 'NUT Careers Advice for Careers Teachers'.] Nursing Times, 68, 7 Dec 1972, 1535.

11 Richter, L. and Richter, E. Nurses in fiction. American Journal of Nursing, 74 (7), Jul 1974, 1280–1281.

12 Turcotte, C. How children see the nurse. [Interviews with school children to discover their image of nursing.] Canadian Nurse, 71 (4), Apr 1978, 41–42.

e LAW: GENERAL

1 Adelowo, E. O. Nursing practice and the law. Nigerian Nurse, 4 (2), Apr/Jun 1972, 28, 30–32; (3), Jul/Sep 1972, 27–31; (4), Oct/Dec 1972, 28–30.

2 Bernzwig, H. P. The nurse's liability for malpractice: a programmed course. 2nd ed. New York: McGraw-Hill, 1975.

3 Bullough, B. editor The law and the expanding nursing role. New York: Appleton-Century-Crofts, 1975.

4 Creighton, H. Changes in the legal aspects of nursing. Hospital Progress, 52 (9), Sep 1971, 87–94.

5 Creighton, H. Changing legal attitudes: the effect of the law on nursing. New York: National League for Nursing, 1974.

6 Creighton, H. Law every nurse should know. 3rd ed. Philadelphia: Saunders, 1975.

7 Das, D. M. H. Jurisprudence for nurses. Delhi: Atma Ram, 1974.

8 Das, D. M. H. Medico-legal aspects in nursing. Delhi: Atma Ram, 1973.

9 Driscoll, V. Liberating nursing practice. [From its legal subservience to the medical profession.] Nursing Outlook, 20 (1), Jan 1972, 24–28.

10 Germaine, A. Survival in a lawsuit prone society. [Legal responsibilities of the nurse.] Hospital Administration in Canada, 17 (7), Jul 1975, 18–19.

11 Good, S. R. and Kerr, J. C. Contemporary issues in Canadian law for nurses. Toronto: Holt, Rinehart and Winston, 1973.

12 Health Law Centre and Streiff, C. J. editors Nursing and the law. 2nd ed. Rockville, Maryland: Aspen Systems Corporation, 1975.

13 Hershey, N. The law and the nurse: the patient doesn't always win. American Journal of Nursing, 71 (5), May 1971, 967–969.

14 Hershey, N. Nursing practice acts and professional delusion. [Nursing law in the USA.] Journal of Nursing Administration, 4 (4), Jul/Aug 1974, 36–39.

15 International Council of Nurses Florence Nightingale International Foundation. Report of an international seminar on nursing legislation, Warsaw, 6–16 Jul. Basle: Karger, 1971.

16 Jegede, S. A. Nurses code of ethics and legal implications in nursing practice. [Including the work of the Nursing Council of Nigeria.] Nigerian Nurse, 6 (3), Jul/Sep 1974, 34–41.

17 Kellogg, N. Will Congress declare independence for nurses? [Legislation to establish registered nurses as independent professionals.] RN Magazine, 38 (7), Jul 1975, 30–35.

18 Kelly, L. Y. Nursing practice acts. American Journal of Nursing, 74 (7), Jul 1974, 1310–1319.

19 Lipman, M. Challenging physicians' orders. RN Magazine, 35 (5), May 1972, 54–55, 84, 86.

20 Lipman, M. Defamation: a rash comment could get you sued. [The problems of slander for the nursing profession.] RN Magazine, 38 (2), Feb 1975, 48–51.

21 Nursing Clinics of North America Symposium on current legal and professional problems [with particular reference to the extended role of the nurse]. Nursing Clinics of North America, 9 (3), Sep 1974, 395–585.

22 Parsons, R. The New South Wales College of Nursing nurse educators' seminar – October 1971. Notes on professional negligence. Lamp, 29 (3), Mar 1972, 19–21.

23 Revington, P. W. Nurses at law – cautionary tales. Nursing Times, 67, 20 May 1971, 620–621.

24 Rowe, G. A. When is a nurse legally liable? Hospital Administration in Canada, 13 (1), Jan 1971, 38, 40.

25 Rozovsky, L. E. The doctor, the nurse and the law. Canadian Hospital, 48 (1), Jan 1971, 32–33.

26 Speller, S. R. Law notes for nurses: with supplement for Scotland by R. A. Bennett. 7th ed. Rcn, 1972.

27 Speller, S. R. Law relating to hospitals and kindred institutions. 5th ed. H. K. Lewis, 1971.

28 Wakeford, R. E. The law and the nurse. English Universities Press, 1973.

f LAW: SPECIAL AREAS

1 Adriani, J. Nurse anesthetists and the law. Journal of the American Association of Nurse Anesthetists, 41 (4), Aug 1973, 307–329.

2 Boname, J. R. Changing attitudes create health care dilemma. [Legal vulnerability in the operating room.] AORN Journal, 22 (4), Oct 1975, 543–548.

3 Bromberg, M. J. Legal problems and safeguards in the ED. RN Magazine, 36 (5), May 1973, 49, 66, 68, 70, 72, 74, 76.

4 Creighton, H. Legal aspects of expanding LP/VN roles. Journal of Practical Nursing, 23 (8), Aug 1973, 16–19.

5 Dickens, B. M. The 'conscience clause' and the law on abortion. Nursing Times, 70, 20 Jun 1974, 968–969.

6 Dryden, K. G. The district nurse and the law. Queen's Nursing Journal, 18 (4), Jul 1975, 119, 124.

7 Dryden, K. G. The law, the nurse and the violent patient. Nursing Mirror, 133, 1 Oct 1971, 39–41.

8 Dryden, K. G. Professional negligence. [District nurse and the law.] Queen's Nursing Journal, 18 (5), Aug 1975, 139–140.

9 Ede, L. Legal aspects of occupational mental health nursing. Occupational Health Nursing, 21 (1), Jan 1973, 12–17.

10 Ede, L. and Nelson, R. A. Emergency care and the nurse. [Legal aspects.] Nursing Care, 6 (9), Sep 1973, 23–27.

11 Feld, L. G. The nurse's liability for faulty injections. Nursing Care, 7 (4), Apr 1974, 25.

12 Gouge, R. L. OR nurses face potential liabilities. [Medico-legal problems of nursing in the operating theatre.] AORN Journal, 20 (4), Oct 1974, 660–661, 664–665.

13 Hershey, N. Standards of performance in expanded practice. [Legal implications of nurse's role of physician's assistant]. American Journal of Nursing, 72 (1), Jan 1972, 86–87.

14 Langley, L. Law and the district nurse. Queen's Nursing Journal, 16 (3), Jun 1973, 66, 68.

15 McKechnie, F. B. Legal aspects of anesthesia. Journal of the American Association of Nurse Anesthetists, 41 (5), Oct 1973, 407–410.

16 Mostyn, F. E. The health visitor and the law. Health Visitor, 45 (4), Apr 1972, 102–103.

17 Murchison, I. A. Law – an element of quality control in occupational health nursing practice. [Effect of the increasing independence of the nursing profession from medical supervision.] Occupational Health Nursing, 22 (11), Nov 1974, 9–14.

18 Murchison, I. A. Role of law in the decision making process in occupational health nursing. Occupational Health Nursing, 21 (7), Jul 1973, 15–19.

19 Occupational Health To tell or not to tell? Occupational Health, 24 (1), Jan 1972, 1–2.

20 Orriss, H. D. Secondment of nurses and the legal hazards. Nursing Times, 67, 22 Apr 1971, 488–489.

21 Whincup, M. Confidentiality and the law. [Ethical problems in occupational health nursing.] Occupational Health, 24 (10), Oct 1972, 352–353.

22 Whincup, M. Legal aspects of occupational health nursing. 3. The nurse's duties. Nursing Times, 69, 9 Aug 1973, Occ. papers, 125–128.

23 Whincup, M. Legal aspects of occupational health nursing. 4. The nurse's duties. Nursing Times, 69, 16 Aug 1973, Occ. papers, 129–132.

24 Whincup, M. Letter of the law. 2. Negligence in medical practice. Nursing Mirror, 135, 6 Oct 1972, 42–43.

g ORGANIZATIONS

1 Bowman, R. A. The nursing organization as a political pressure group. Nursing Forum, 12 (1), 1973, 72–81.

2 Christie, L. S. A chance for the nursing profession? [Professional organization.] Nursing Times, 67, 4 Nov 1971, 1375–1376.

3 Collins, J. M. The making of an organization. Occupational Health Nursing, 20 (11), Nov 1972, 14–17.

4 Evans, A. The need for a strong nurses' organization. Australian Nurses' Journal, 4 (2), Aug 1974, 27.

5 Gilchrist, J. M. Freedom: an outmoded tradition. [Social freedom in education and professional organizations.] Canadian Nurse, 69 (4), Apr 1973, 25–27.

6 Grant, N. Trade union or professional association? Health Services, 26, Oct 1973, 162.

7 Hall, C. M. Who controls the nursing profession? The role of the professional association. Nursing Times, 69, 7 Jun 1973, Occ. papers, 89–92; Australian Nurses' Journal, 3 (2), Aug 1973, 29–52.

8 Jarrett, L. The modern student nurse and her professional organization. [Australia.] International Nursing Review, 18 (1), 1971, 31–37.

9 McKay, H. Membership patterns and attitudes of hospital nurses. [Membership of the Rcn and trade unions, and attitudes of nurses towards militancy.] Nursing Times, 70, 3 Oct 1974, 1547–1549.

10 Neall, R. The nursing conference: a sociological view. SA Nursing Journal, 40 (3), Mar 1973, 24, 33.

11 Newcomb, R. F. Nursing finds a new national voice. [Meeting of representatives from 20 nursing organizations.] RN Magazine, 36 (3), Mar 1973, 60, 64, 67–68.

12 Yergan, L. H. The preparation of the nurses for active participation in the professional organization. Jamaican Nurse, 11 (1), Apr 1971, 20.

h ORGANIZATIONS, INDIVIDUAL

1 Cowdray Club Dunn, A. The Cowdray goes 'In and Out.' Nursing Times, 71, 24 Jul 1975, 1160–1162.

2 Florence Nightingale Memorial Committee Ross, T. A visit to Florence Nightingale House. [Visit of Princess Alexandra.] Nursing Mirror, 140, 10 Apr 1975, 39–41.

GENERAL NURSING COUNCIL FOR ENGLAND AND WALES

3 Barry, N. Norman Barry – the new chairman of the General Nursing Council for England and Wales

talks to Nursing Times. Nursing Times, 71, 20 Feb 1975, 284–285.

4 Bendall, E. There but for the grace of God. . . . [The Disciplinary Committee of the GNC.] Nursing Mirror, 138, 10 May 1974, 44–47.

5 General Nursing Council for England and Wales A brief explanation of its development, responsibilities and structure. GNC, 1974.

6 General Nursing Council for England and Wales Functions, procedure and disciplinary jurisdiction. GNC, 1972.

7 General Nursing Council for England and Wales Report submitted to the Secretary of State for Social Services, 1970/1971–1974/1975. GNC, 1971–1975.

8 General Nursing Council for England and Wales What it is, what it does, how it works, how it affects you. GNC, 1974.

9 Nursing Times GNC election fiasco. [Editorial on the GNC elections.] Nursing Times, 71, 31 Jul 1975, 1191.

ROYAL COLLEGE OF NURSING

10 Dack, P. Rcn: reorganisation of membership structure. Nursing Mirror, 138, 12 Apr 1974, 38–39.

11 Nursing Times Care and unity, the central themes. Nursing Times, 68, 6 Apr. 1972, 412–414.

12 Nursing Times Plain speaking from the grass roots. Nursing Times, 69, 19 Apr 1973, 519–521.

13 Occupational Health Royal College or trade union: what can they offer the nurse? Occupational Health, 24 (3), Mar 1972, 90–91.

14 Sampson, G. R. Who speaks for the nurse? [Rcn policy on nurse training and the Salmon report.] British Hospital Journal and Social Service Review, 82, 19 Feb 1972, 411. Correspondence in reply from C. M. Hall and others, 82, 11 Mar 1972, 547.

15 Wakeley, J. Professionalism under threat. Rcn v. the unions. Supervisor Nurse, 6 (12), Dec 1975, 39.

i WOMEN AND NURSING

1 Bailon, S. V. G. Women's rights and the nurses. Philippine Journal of Nursing, 44 (1), Jan/Mar 1975, 23–31.

2 Bayer, M. and Brandner, P. Feminism and nursing. Australian Nurses' Journal, 4 (8), Mar 1975, 32–33.

3 Brand, K. L. and Glass, L. K. Perils and parallels of women and nursing. [Influence of the status and freedom of women on nursing development.] Nursing Forum, 14 (2), 1975, 160–174.

4 Bullough, B. and Bullough, V. L. Sex discrimination in health care: masculine bias. Nursing Outlook, 23 (1), Jan 1975, 40–45.

5 Canadian Nurse Is there sex discrimination in health care? [Results of questionnaire among Canadian nurses.] Canadian Nurse, 71 (12), Dec 1975, 15–22.

6 Cleland, V. Sex discrimination: nursing's most pervasive problem. American Journal of Nursing, 71 (8), Aug 1971, 1542–1547.

7 Fagin, C. M. Nurses' rights. [How they differ from human rights and women's rights.] American Journal of Nursing, 75 (1), Jan 1975, 82–85.

8 Heide, W. S. Nursing and women's liberation – a parallel. American Journal of Nursing, 73 (5), May 1973, 824–827.

9 Jamaican Nurse Issue focusing on International Women's Year. Jamaican Nurse, 15 (1), May 1975, 14–21.

10 Lamb, K. T. Freedom for our sister, freedom for ourselves: nursing confronts social change. Nursing Forum, 12 (4), 1973, 328–352.

11 Roberts, J. T. and Group, T. M. The women's movement and nursing. Nursing Forum, 12 (3), 1973, 303–322.

12 Royal College of Midwives Royal College of Midwives comments on equal opportunities for men and women and equality for women. Midwives Chronicle, 87, Jan 1974, 6–7; Nursing Mirror, 139, 21 Nov 1974, 40–41.

13 Starr, D. S. Poor baby: the nurse and feminism. [The inability of nurses to fight for women's rights.] Canadian Nurse, 70 (3), Mar 1974, 20–23.

14 World Health Issue on the position of women in the health professions. World Health, Jun 1975, 2–14.

6 NURSE'S ROLE

a GENERAL

1 Anderson, E. R. The role of the nurse: views of the patient, nurse and doctor in some general hospitals in England. Royal College of Nursing and National Council of Nurses of the United Kingdom, 1973. (Study of nursing care research project series 2, no. 1) [Based on PhD thesis Surrey University 1972.]

2 Awtrey, J. S. Teaching the expanded role. Nursing Outlook, 22 (2), Feb 1974, 98–102.

3 Badouaille, M. L. Why nursing is different. New Zealand Nursing Journal, 66 (7), Jul 1973, 29–30.

4 Bailey, D. H. Nursing in transition. International Nursing Review, 18 (1), 1971, 59–64.

5 Brookes, P. An expanding role for nurses. [Health and the practice of medicine in the future.] Nursing Times, 68, 30 Nov 1972, 1531.

6 Brophy, E. B. Relationships among self-role congruences and nursing experience. Nursing Research, 20 (5), Sep/Oct 1971, 447–450.

7 Browning, M. H. and Lewis, E. P., compilers The expanded role of the nurse. New York: American Journal of Nursing Co., 1973. (Contemporary nursing series.)

8 Canadian Nurses Association and Canadian Medical Association The expanded role of the nurse: a joint statement. Canadian Nurse, 69 (5), May 1973, 23–25.

9 Christensen, V. A. Nursing in a changing world. [An international view of current trends prepared for the World Health Organization.] Journal of Psychiatric Nursing and Mental Health Services, 12 (6), Nov/Dec 1974, 39–43.

10 Dodd, A. P. Towards an understanding of nursing. PhD thesis, Goldsmiths College, London University, 1973.

11 Durrant, K. J. and Christie, E. How relevant is the nurse. [The nurse's role in the hospital.] Nursing Times, 70, 28 Mar 1974, 479–480.

12 Evans, M. Locals and cosmopolitans: a latent role analysis of nurses during professional socialization. MA thesis, Liverpool University, 1974.

13 Ferguson, M. Nurse or feldscher. [Role of the nurse with examples drawn from the developing countries.] Nursing Times, 69, 11 Jan 1973, 40–41.

14 Ford, L. C. Nursing – evolution or revolution? Canadian Nurse, 67 (1), Jan 1971, 32–37.

15 Freeman, R. The expanding role of nursing: some implications. International Nursing Review, 19 (4), 1972, 351–357.

16 Hancock, C. Comment on forthcoming Royal College of Nursing Conference, 'Nursing and the future'. New Society, 18, 23 Sep 1971, 568–569.

17 Harris, G. A. Open forum. Nursing – present and future trends. Nursing Mirror, 140, 6 Feb 1975, 68.

18 Irish Nurses Organisation and Irish Medical Association Statement on the duties and position of the nurse. Dublin: The Organisation, 1974. Reprinted in World of Irish Nursing, 4 (1), Jan 1975, 1–2.

19 Leedham, C. L. The nurse's role in meeting the challenges of medical care. Occupational Health Nursing, 19 (11), Nov 1971, 7–8, 44.

20 Lester, J. Nursing of the future – a time of opportunity. A report from the Royal Society of Health Congress at Brighton. Nursing Mirror, 138, 3 May 1974, 41–44.

21 Leydon, I. Future trends in nursing. World of Irish Nursing, 1 (5), May 1972, 101, 103.

22 Longest, V. B. Expanded roles for VA nurses. [Veterans Administration.] American Journal of Nursing, 73 (12), Dec 1973, 2087–2089.

23 McFarlane, J. and Scott Wright, M. Royal Colleges discuss the future of clinical nursing. [Report of a conference of the Royal Colleges of Nursing, Midwives, Physicians, Surgeons, Obstetricians and Gynaecologists.] Nursing Times, 70, 5 Dec 1974, 1875. See also Is Salmon a scapegoat. British Medical Journal, 4, 7 Dec 1974, 550–551.

24 Morgan, D. M. The future expanded role of the nurse. Canadian Hospital, 49 (5). May 1972, 75–80.

25 Mussallem, H. K. 'What is nursing'? [Goals in nursing education conference address.] Australian Nurses' Journal, 5 (2), Aug 1975, 8–12.

26 Nuckolls, K. B. Who decides what the nurse can do? [Development of new nursing jobs and the relationship between medicine and nursing.] Rhodesian Nurse, 8 (1), Mar 1975, 7–13.

27 Nurses Association of Jamaica [Report of a conference discussing the expanded role of the nurse.] Jamaican Nurse, 14 (3), Dec 1974, 6–7.

28 Nursing Outlook A nurse is a nurse – or is she? [Editorial]. Nursing Outlook, 20 (1), Jan 1972, 21.

29 Nursing Papers Issue on the expanding role of the nurse: her preparation and practice. [Includes some articles on nurse practitioners.] Nursing Papers, 6 (2), Summer 1974.

30 Nuttall, P. Nursing in the year AD 2000. Summary of the first Battersea Memorial Lecture. Nursing Mirror, 141, 20 Nov 1975, 41–42.

31 Rayner, C. Tomorrow's nursing. Nursing Mirror, 139, 26 Dec 1974, 42–43.

32 Reifsteck, S. W. Expanding RN roles: at the grass-roots level. RN Magazine, 38 (5), May 1975, 91–93, 97–98.

33 Royal College of Nursing The extending role of the nurse Rcn conference report. Nursing Mirror, 138, 5 Apr 1974, 37–40.

34 Rule, J. B. A crisis of identity: the Nursing Lecture, 1974. Royal College of Nursing, 1974. Reprinted in Nursing Mirror, 139, 28 Nov 1974, 40–41.

35 Schlotfeldt, R. M. This I believe . . . nursing is health care. Nursing Outlook, 20 (4), Apr 1972, 245–246.

36 Scott Wright, M. On entering the fourth quarter. [Nursing in 1975.] Nursing Mirror, 139, 26 Dec 1974, 25–27.

37 Sheahan, D. The game of the name: nurse professional or nurse technician. Nursing Outlook, 20 (7), Jul 1972, 440–444.

38 Starr, S. The modern nurse, applied scientist or ministering angel. Nursing Mirror, 140, 26 Jun 1975, 56–58.

39 Stevens, B. J. New York State definition of the practice of nursing: implications for nursing education. Journal of Nursing Administration, 4 (3), May/Jun 1974, 37–41.

40 Sutherland, A. H. The common core of nursing. Nursing Times, 67, 27 May 1971, 650–651.

41 Talbot, D. M. Revolution in nursing. Occupational Health Nursing, 20 (6), Jun 1972, 7–13.

42 Tolliday, H. Defining the nurse's role: the use of defined organizational concepts in considering the content of nursing roles. Nursing Times, 68, 6 Apr 1972, Occ. papers, 53–56.

43 United States. Department of Health, Education and Welfare Extending the scope of nursing practice: a report of the Secretary's Committee to study extended roles for nurses. Washington: US Government Printing Office, 1972. See also Nursing Outlook, 20 (1), Jan 1972, 46–52.

42 Williamson, J. The conflict-producing role of the professionally socialized nurse-faculty member. [Discussion by Dorothy Smith, 367–373.] Nursing Forum, 11 (4), 1972, 357–366.

43 Yelverton, N. M. The role of nursing in a changing society. International Nursing Review, 19 (4), 1972, 328–332.

b CHANGE

1 Bendall, E. R. D. Education for change. [The need to reformulate nursing objectives.] Nursing Mirror, 137, 14 Sep 1973, 39–41.

2 Biddulph, C. The changing face of nursing. Nursing Times, 67, 28 Oct 1971, 1354–1355.

3 Burd, M. Changing responsibilities [of the nurse]. World of Irish Nursing, 3 (2), Dec 1974, 218–200.

4 Chisholm, M. K. Change – an occupational hazard. Nursing Mirror, 132, 15 Jan 1971, 46–48.

5 Copp, L. A. Professional change: which trends do nurses endorse? International Journal of Nursing Studies, 10 (1), Jan 1973, 55–62.

6 DeMarsh, K. G. The impact of change on the nursing profession. Hospital Administration in Canada, 13 (7), Jul 1971, 35–36.

7 Edelstein, R. R. G. Reaction to permanence and change in five hierarchical nursing groups. Nursing Research, 21 (2), Mar/Apr 1972, 154–158.

8 Fashina, E. M. The changing role of the nurse. Nigerian Nurse, 7 (4), Oct/Dec 1975, 16–17.

9 Levin, L. S. Time to hear a different drum. Far reaching changes in nursing and the health care system could stem from a partnership between nurses and consumers. American Journal of Nursing, 72 (11), Nov 1972, 2007–2010.

10 Montag, M. L. Changing patterns of nursing education and practice. Lamp, 30 (12), Dec 1973, 23–28.

11 Neall, R. Changes in nursing: some futuristic ideas. S.A. Nursing Journal, 41 (8), Aug 1974, 24–25.

12 Noth, M. T. Complex relationships and traditional barriers challenge nursing. [Change within the nursing profession.] Hospital Progress, 54 (11), Nov 1973, 52–55, 69, 72.

13 Philip, Sister M. Health services and nursing: changing patterns. [Changing role of nurse.] Australian Nurses Journal, 2 (3), Sep 1972, 33–34.

14 Rodgers, J. A. Theoretical considerations involved in the process of change. Nursing Forum, 12 (2), 1973, 160–174.

15 Ruano, B. J. This I believe . . . about nurses innovating change. Nursing Outlook, 19 (6), Jun 1971, 416–418.

16 Shetland, M. L. Changing needs and changing roles. Occupational Health Nursing, 20 (10), Oct 1972, 17–19.

17 Smoyak, S. A. The changing role of nursing today. Occupational Health Nursing, 22 (10), Oct 1974, 9–13.

c CONCEPTS AND PHILOSOPHY

1 Adam, E. T. A conceptual model for nursing. Canadian Nurse, 71 (9), Sep 1975, 40–41.

2 Ajadi, T. A. My philosophy of nursing. Nigerian Nurse, 7 (2), Apr/Jun 1975, 36–37, 40.

3 Armiger, B. Scholarship in nursing. Nursing Outlook, 22 (3), Mar 1974, 160–164.

4 Bachand, M. Wanted: a definition of nursing practice. Canadian Nurse, 70 (5), May 1974, 26–29.

5 Bergman, R. Translating a nursing belief into nursing practice. Hong Kong Nursing Journal, 17, Nov 1974, 11–16.

6 Bloch, D. Some crucial terms in nursing. What do they really mean? Nursing Outlook, 22 (11), Nov 1974, 689–694.

7 Boylan, A. An approach to nursing. 1. Developing clinical expertise. [Framework of knowledge on which the nurse can base a clinical judgement.] Nursing Times, 70, 14 Nov 1974, 1780–1781.

8 Cantor, M. M. JONA refresher: Philosophy, purpose and objectives: why do we have them? Journal of Nursing Administration, 3 (4), Jul/Aug 1973, 21–25.

9 Chapman, C. M. Clarify the concepts. [Theoretical framework for nursing.] Nursing Times, 68, 22 Jun 1972, 775–776.

10 Chapman, C. M. Still clarifying. [Nursing theory and education in relation to bedside skills.] Nursing Times, 68, 28 Sep 1972, 1230–1231.

11 Colaizzi, J. The proper object of nursing science. International Journal of Nursing Studies, 12 (4), 1975, 197–200.

12 Foley, J. Wanted: a theory of nursing. International Nursing Review, 18 (2), 1971, 138–147. Canadian Nurse, 67 (11), Nov 1971, 28–32.

13 Graham, S. Just clarify . . . A reply to Christine Chapman's article, Clarify the concepts. [Theoretical framework of nursing.] Nursing Times, 68, 6 Jul 1972, 849–850.

14 Hardy, M. E. Theories: components, development, evaluation. Nursing Research, 23 (2), Mar/Apr 1974, 100–106.

15 Hardy, M. E., editor Theoretical foundations for nursing. New York: MSS Information Corporation, 1973.

16 Meleis, A. I. Role insufficiency and role supplementation: a conceptual framework. Nursing Research, 24 (4), Jul/Aug 1975, 264–271.

17 Jacox, A. Theory construction in nursing: an overview. Nursing Research, 23 (1), Jan/Feb 1974, 4–13.

18 Johnson, D. E. Development of theory: a requisite for nursing as a primary health profession. Nursing Research, 23 (5), Sep/Oct 1974, 372–377.

19 Journal of Nursing Administration Fundamental issues in nursing. Wakefield, Massachusetts: Contemporary Publishing, 1975.

20 Ketefian, S., editor Translation of theory into nursing practice and education, with a bibliography on change: proceedings of the 7th annual clinical sessions. New York University, 1975.

21 King, I. M. Towards a theory of nursing: general concepts of human behaviour. New York: Wiley, 1971.

22 McFarlane, J. K. The science and art of nursing. 23rd annual oration, New South Wales College of Nursing, 17 September. The College, 1975. Lamp, 32 (10), Oct 1975, 11, 20.

23 MacQueen, J. A phenomenology of nursing. Nursing Papers, 6 (3), Fall 1974, 9.

24 Murphy, J. F., editor Theoretical issues in professional nursing. New York: Appleton-Century-Crofts, 1971.

25 Newman, M. A. Nursing's theoretical evolution. Nursing Outlook, 20 (7), Jul 1972, 449–453.

26 Nursing Development Conference Group Concept formalization in nursing: process and product. Boston: Little, Brown, 1973.

27 Orem, D. E. Nursing: concepts of practice. New York: McGraw-Hill, 1971.

28 Paterson, J. G. From a philosophy of clinical nursing to a method of nursology. Nursing Research, 20 (2), Mar/Apr 1971, 143–146.

29 Riehl, J. P. and Roy, C. Conceptual models for nursing practice. New York: Appleton-Century-Crofts, 1974.

30 Roy, C. Adaptation: a basis for nursing practice. Nursing Outlook, 19 (4), Apr 1971, 254–257.

31 Roy, C. A diagnostic classification for nursing. [Implications for practice, education and research.] Nursing Outlook, 23 (2), Feb 1975, 90–94.

32 Salmon, B. Pragmatic axles turn on emptiness. [Development of the art and science of nursing.] New Zealand Nursing Journal, 68 (3), Mar 1975, 24–28; UNA Nursing Journal, 4, Jul/Aug 1974, 29–35.

33 Scott Wright, M. Needs and goals in nursing. District Nursing, 15 (10), Jan 1973, 214–217. Reprinted in Community Health, 5 (1), Jul/Aug 1973, 24–30.

34 Tubi, A. M. Philosophy and objectives: their place in the nursing profession. Nigerian Nurse, 7 (1), Jan/Mar 1975, 26–28.

35 Vincent, P. Some crucial terms in nursing – a second opinion. [Reply to an article by Doris Bloch, Nursing Outlook, Nov 1974, with her response.] Nursing Outlook, 23 (1), Jan 1975, 46–48.

36 Walker, L. O. Toward a clearer understanding of the concept of nursing theory. Nursing Research, 20 (5), Sep/Oct 1971, 428–435; 21 (1), Jan/Feb 1972, 59–62. [Commentary, 20 (6) Nov/Dec 1971, 493–502.]

37 Williams, K. Ideologies of nursing: their meanings and implications. Nursing Times, 70, 8 Aug 1974, Occ. papers, 49–51.

7 HEALTH AND WELFARE

a SICKNESS AND ABSENCE

1 Bosanquet, N. Awayaday. [Sickness absence.] Nursing Times, 70, 24 Oct 1974, 1647.

2 Brookes, R. G. and Gardner, J. C. Sickness and absence levels of nursing staff for the mentally handicapped in the Birmingham region. Nursing Times, 68, 20 Jan 1972, Occ. papers, 9–12.

3 Cohen, A. The hazards of nursing. Health Services, 25 (6), Jun 1972, 14.

4 Cormack, D. Sickness and absence amongst nursing staffs in a psychiatric/mental deficiency hospital group. Dundee: Royal Dundee Liff hospital, 1973.

5 Elyath, E. A common disease among nurses. [Varicose veins.] Nursing Journal of India, 62 (12), Dec 1971, 398, 407.

6 Franks, G. L. Off sick – who? where and why? [Control of sickness absenteeism among nursing staff.] Nursing Times, 68, 14 Dec 1972, 1596–1597.

7 Kirtane, M. Analyzing absenteeism: a first step toward control. [Study to compare habits of RNs, LPNs and aides using two statistical techniques.] Hospital Progress, 56 (3), Mar 1975, 71–73.

8 Lampwick, D. How much does charity begin at home? [Neglect of nurses' health problems.] Nursing Mirror, 134, 16 Jun 1972, 30–31.

9 Lancet Hazards for pregnant nurses. Lancet, 1, 28 Feb 1970, 458–459.

10 Longest, B. B. and others A study of absenteeism. Hospital Progress, 54 (6), Jun 1973, 48, 50–52.

11 Lunn, J. A. Absenteeism: an occupational hazard. [High absence rate among student and pupil nurses.] Nursing Mirror, 140, 22/29 May 1975, 65–66.

12 Mammen, S. The concept of self-care. [The health of nurses in India.] Nursing Journal of India, 64 (11), Mar 1974, 375, 386.

13 Mann, K. J. and others Sickness absenteeism in a hospital in Israel. Hospital, 67 (9), Sep 1971, 307–311.

14 Meates, D. Nursing staff sickness and absenteeism in the medical and paediatrics unit. Nursing Times, 67, 16 Dec 1971, Occ. papers, 197–200.

15 Poole, F. T. Consequences of delaying claims for injuries in hospital. Nursing Mirror, 141 (3), 17 Jul 1975, 67–68.

16 Pounds, F. J. The sick nurse. 3. A review of the years 1969–1973 in the King's College Hospital Group. The Hospital, 1974.

17 Ramsay, L. E. and MacLeod, M. A. Incidence of idiopathic venous thromboembolism in nurses. British Medical Journal, 4, 24 Nov 1973, 446–448. Correspondence: 4, 22 Dec 1973, 737; 1, 9 Feb 1974, 248.

18 Rushworth, V. 'Not in today': absence survey. [Study of 300 nurses in a district general hospital.] Nursing Times, 71, 11 Dec 1975, Occ. papers, 121–124.

19 Vahey, P. G. Sickness and absence: study of absence rates of full-time nurses at a psychiatric hospital. [In relation to hours of duty.] Nursing Mirror, 133, 20 Aug 1971, 14–15.

20 Vegh, R. Why should nurses know better? [Nurses who have abortions.] World Medicine, 9 (8), 16 Jan 1974, 48, 51, 55.

21 Watkin, B. Management topics. Sickness and absence. Nursing Mirror, 138, 17 May 1974, 70.

b ADDICTION

1 Carr, A. Smoking habits of nurses. Nursing Times, 68, 1 Jun 1972, 672–673.

2 Elaine, B. and others Helping the nurse who misuses drugs. American Journal of Nursing, 74 (9), Sep 1974, 1665–1671.

3 Jefferys, M. A study of the relationship between situational stress and the smoking habits of nurses in three selected hospitals. Bedford College, 1974.

4 Levine, D. G. and others A special program for nurse addicts. American Journal of Nursing, 74 (9), Sep 1974, 1672–1673.

5 Lipp, M. R. and others Marijuana use by nurses and nursing students. American Journal of Nursing, 71 (12), Dec 1971, 2339–2341.

6 Nursing Mirror This downhill path is easy. [A nurse who became a drug addict.] Nursing Mirror, 139, 12 Jul 1974, 47–48.

7 Price, J. L. and Collins, J. R. Smoking among baccalaureate nursing students. Nursing Research, 22 (4), Jul/Aug 1973, 347–350.

8 Razzell, M. 'No thanks, I've quit smoking.' [A nurse's experience of giving up smoking.] Canadian Nurse, 71 (9), Sep 1975, 23–25.

9 Wood, V. The drug incident – a case study. [A student nurse experiments with drugs.] Canadian Nurse, 68 (7), Jul 1972, 21–26. Reprinted in Nursing Times, 68, 23 Nov 1972, 1495–1498.

c BACK DISORDERS

1 Abelson, I. Forward on backs. [Developments in 1975 relating to compensation for back injury.] Nursing Times, 71, 6 Nov 1975, 1762.

2 Canadian Nurse Lumber pain linked to hypokinesia. [A survey of 100 nurses.] Canadian Nurse, 70 (11), Nov 1974, 27–31.

3 Cust, G. and others The prevalence of low back pain in nurses. International Nursing Review, 19 (2), 1972, 169–178.

4 Dixon, M. Career in jeopardy. [Back injuries among nurses.] Nursing Mirror, 139, 7 Nov 1974, 72.

5 Glover, J. R. Occupational health research and the problem of back pain. [Includes nurses.] Transactions of the Society of Occupational Medicine, 21 (1), Jan 1971, 2–12.

6 Hoover, S. A. Job-related back injuries in a hospital. [Physical therapist teaches lifting techniques to all nursing employees.] American Journal of Nursing, 73 (12), Dec 1973, 2078–2079.

7 Nursing Times Back injuries claims. Successful case, 71, 28 Aug 1975, 1355; Lost claim, 71, 4 Dec 1975, 1921.

8 Nursing Times Issue on back injury among nurses. [Includes experiences of three nurses, comment on lack of information and problems of getting compensation.] Nursing Times, 70, Nov 1974, 1724–1745.

d COUNSELLING, WELFARE AND STRESS

1 Bendall, E. A caring profession. [GNC Welfare Service.] Nursing Mirror, 139, 14 Nov 1974, 39–40.

2 Blyth, J. The case for the home sister. SA Nursing Journal, 39 (2), Feb 1972, 31–32.

3 Breitung, J. Distress signal. [A nurse's suicide attempt.] Nursing Care, 8 (10), Oct 1975, 28–29.

4 Charing Cross amenities centre. Health and Social Service Journal, 83, 3 Mar 1973, 479.

5 Davitz, L. J. Identification of stressful situations in a Nigerian school of nursing. Nursing Research, 21 (4), Jul/Aug 1972, 352–357.

6 Downs, F. S. The ombudsman is a nurse. Nursing Outlook, 19 (7), Jul 1971, 473–475.

7 Duff, J. S. Hospital nurses at risk. [Stress in nurses.] Occupational Health, 26 (5), May 1974, 164–172.

8 Endersby, H. Nurses at work. Nurse Counsellor. Australian Nurses' Journal, 1 (7), Jan 1972, 5–6.

9 Frost, M. Caring for those who care. [The Royal College of Nursing's Welfare and Advisory Service.] Nursing Times, 70, 31 Jan 1974, 162–163.

10 Goodwin, P. The long road back, achieved. [Return to nursing after a mental breakdown.] Nursing Mirror, 135, 8 Dec 1972, 41–42.

11 Hambling, E. How do you feel? [Report of the first course in counselling for nurses at William Rathbone Staff College.] Nursing Times, 71, 19 Jun 1975, 986–987.

12 Hawkins, G. M. Counselling: the nurse's role. [Tavistock Centre Counselling Course.] Occupational Health, 25 (6), Jun 1973, 223–226.

13 Holgate, P. Stress affects nurses too. [Psychological stress in occupational health nurses.] Occupational Health, 24 (6), Jun 1972, 198–199.

14 Hopkins, M. Counselling service. [For nurses and other hospital staff.] New Zealand Nursing Journal, 66 (11), Nov 1973, 16–17.

15 Hugill, J. Nurse counselling. [Service set up at the Thomas Guy School of Nursing.] Nursing Mirror, 140, 10 Apr 1975, 58–61.

16 Humphreys, D. Window on student welfare. [Student welfare department in the United Manchester Hospitals.] Nursing Times, 68, 30 Mar 1972, 380–382.

17 Ivers, E. Self-understanding in counselling. Occupational Health Nursing, 19 (3), Mar 1971, 7–10.

18 Kearns, J. L. and others. What is counselling? Occupational Health, 25 (5), May 1973, 176–181.

19 King's Fund Centre The need for counselling for nurses working in the health service: reports of meetings Dec 1972–Jul 1973. The Fund, 1972–1973. (Reprints THC 742, 760, KFC 783, 784, 803, 815).

20 Linn, L. S. Primex trainees under stress. [Research project to examine the incidence of stress among students on a family nurse practitioner program at Los Angeles University.] Journal of Nursing Education, 14 (2), Apr 1975, 10–19.

21 Longbottom, F. Care for the caring professions. [Need for counselling.] Health and Social Service Journal, 85, 9 Aug 1975, 1730.

22 McCarrick, H. The sweet and sour of living in. Nursing Times, 69, 13 Sep 1973, 1175–1177.

23 Marriott, M. H. Nurses and their homes. [Summary of findings of a survey to evaluate residential accommodation at Charing Cross Hospital, conducted by M. H. Marriott.] British Hospital Journal and Social Service Review, 82, 22 Jul 1972, 1627.

24 Nash, P. Nursing stress. Nursing Times, 71, 20 Mar 1975, 476.

25 Oberst, M. T. The crisis-prone staff nurse. [Crisis in the nurse, factors leading up to it and ways to intervene.] American Journal of Nursing, 73, (11) Nov 1973, 1917–1921.

26 Robinson, W. The lively role of the Royal Free Hospital's Social Secretary. Nursing Times, 69, 31 May 1973, 713–714.

27 Rudd, T. N. Anxiety in nursing. Health and Social Service Journal, 83, 22 Dec 1973, 2999–3000.

28 Sayle, D. Nurses' use of leisure. Nursing Times, 68, 22 Jun 1972, Occ. papers, 97–99.

29 Sayle, D. Nurses' use of leisure. 2. Analysis of questionnaires. Nursing Times, 68, 29 Jun 1972, Occ. papers, 101–104.

30 Schreier, A. The need for counselling with nurses. SA Nursing Journal, 38 (5), May 1971, 11, 14.

31 Skellern, E. Nurses and stress. World Hospitals, 10 (3), Summer 1974, 137–140.

32 Tustin, J. Guidance and counselling versus nurse wastage. SA Nursing Journal, 41 (8), Aug 1974, 17.

33 Wood, V. Case method in nurse teacher education. [Use of case study in examining student nurse problems.] Nursing Times, 71, 24 Apr 1975, Occ. papers, 37–40.

34 Wood, V. Student nurse problems: the case of Mary Ellen Waters. [Psychological problems of a student nurse.] International Nursing Review, 22 (5), Sep/Oct 1975, 150–155.

e RETIRED NURSES

1 Brammall, R. Retirement benefits for nurses. 1. Midwives Chronicle, 85, Dec 1971, 410.

2 Evagorou, D. One day this could be your home. [Elderly Nurses National Home, Holdenhurst, Bournemouth.] Nursing Times, 66, 16 Apr 1970, 491–493.

3 Joan Nightingale House [A block of flatlets for elderly nurses.] District Nursing, 15 (11), Feb 1973, 252.

4 Nursing Mirror Remember your gifts to Howard House? Things are still happening there at Gerrards Cross where the Perseverance Trust has opened another house for retired nurses. [Margaret Smyth House; mainly illustrations.] Nursing Mirror, 135, 1 Dec 1972, 36–39.

5 Nursing Times South East. Fonthill. [A description of a home for retired nurses in Reigate.] Nursing Times, 71, 20 Mar 1975, 456–457.

6 Wolff, I. S. Retirement: a different season. [Views of retired nurse] Nursing Outlook, 21 (12), Dec 1973, 763–765.

8 SALARIES AND CONDITIONS OF SERVICE

a GENERAL

1 Crossman, R. Letter sent to Chairmen of Boards of Governors and Hospital Management Committees to ask that the best use is made of nurses' skills and that their working conditions are good. Nursing Times, 66, 21 May 1970, 671. Nursing Mirror, 130, 19 Jun 1970, 8–9.

2 International Labour Organization International Labour Conference, 61st 1976. Employment and conditions of work and life of nursing personnel. Geneva: ILO, 1975. Report VII (1).

3 International Labour Organization and World Health Organization Joint meeting on conditions of work and life of nursing personnel. (Geneva 19–30 November 1973): report. Geneva: ILO/WHO, 1973.

4 Lloyd, P. What about the nurse's health? Special factors affecting the working environment of nurses considered by the WHO/ILO expert committee. Occupational Health 26 (7) Jul 1974 249–253.

5 Nursing Times New international code on nurses' working conditions? [ILO report.] Nursing Times, 71, 21 Aug 1975, 1315.

6 Whincup, M. Legal aspects of occupational health nursing. Security of employment. Nursing Times, 69, 26 Jul 1973, Occ. papers, 117–120.

b LABOUR RELATIONS

1 American Association of Industrial Nurses Industry's nurses and collective bargaining. A statement by the American Association of Industrial Nurses, Inc. Occupational Health Nursing, 22 (12), Dec 1974, 16–17.

2 American Nurses Association Taft-Hartley amended: implications for nursing. [Implications of the Act protecting collective bargaining for employees discussed at an ANA emergency Board Meeting.] American Journal of Nursing, 75 (2), Feb 1975, 285–296.

3 American Nurses' Association The ANA: can a professional association be a trade union, too? [Commitment to collective bargaining.] Hospitals, 48 (17), 1 Sep 1974, 103, 106, 110, 114–115.

4 Amundson, N. E. Labor relations and the nursing leader. Alternatives to the strike in collective bargaining. Journal of Nursing Administration, 5 (1), Jan 1975, 11–12.

5 Amundson, N. E. Labor relations and the nursing leader. Bitterness and anger: residues of a strike in the hospital setting. Journal of Nursing Administration, 3 (2), Mar/Apr 1973, 8, 60–61.

6 Amundson, N. E. Labor relations and the nursing leader. [Dealing with a union.] Journal of Nursing Administration, 11 (3), May/Jun 1972, 10–11, 62.

7 Amundson, N. E. Labor relations and the nursing leader. 'Past practice is killing us!' Journal of Nursing Administration, 3 (6), Nov/Dec 1973, 12–13.

8 Bloom, I. Strike with honor. (Nurses' strike in Redwood, California, 18 June 1974.] Journal of Nursing Administration, 5 (4), May 1975, 19–20.

9 Carpenter, M. Changing work attachments and trade union activity among nurses in three hospitals. MA thesis, Warwick University, 1974.

10 Cleary, D. M. A nonstrike for patient care. [Nurses at St. Agnes Hospital, Philadelphia, strike for more professional recognition.] Modern Healthcare, 3 (6), Jun 1975, 43–44.

11 Cleland, V. S. The supervisor in collective bargaining. [USA practice.] Journal of Nursing Administration, 4 (5), Sep/Oct 1974, 33–35.

12 Conta, A. L. Bargaining by professionals. American Journal of Nursing, 72 (2), Feb 1972, 309–312.

13 Dickenson, M. Industrial relations in the Queensland Nursing Service: the anatomy of an attitude. Australian Nurses' Journal, 5 (1), Jul 1975, 23–27.

14 Dickenson, M. Nurses and their unions. [Development of trade union activities in Australia.] Lamp, 32 (4), Apr 1975, 11, 13.

15 Erickson, E. H. Collective bargaining: an inappropriate technique for professionals. Nursing Forum, 10 (3), 1971. Reprinted in Journal of Nursing Administration, 3 (2), Mar/Apr 1973, 55–58.

16 Jacox, A. Collective bargaining in Academe. Background and perspective. [Collective bargaining in American Universities, and its potential impact on the nurse faculty.] Nursing Outlook, 21 (11), Nov 1973, 700–704.

17 Journal of Nursing Administration Labor relations. Wakefield, Mass.: Contemporary Publishing, 1975.

18 Lewis, E. P. The Cedars of Lebanon story. [An account of a nurses' strike.] American Journal of Nursing, 69 (11), Nov 1969, 2385–2390.

19 Lihach, N. San Francisco: winners and losers. [Nursing strikes at San Francisco Hospitals.] Modern Healthcare, 2 (4), Oct 1974, 32–34.

20 McColl, B. H. RNs belong at the bargaining table. [Is collective bargaining inconsistent with professionalism?] Canadian Nurse, 70 (7), Jul 1974, 15–16.

21 Miller, M. H. Nurses' right to strike. [Historical development in USA] Journal of Nursing Administration, 5 (2), Feb 1975, 35–39.

22 Nursing Forum Issue on collective bargaining in nursing. [On practice in USA.] Nursing Forum, 10 (3), 1971, 229–332.

23 Nursing Mirror Rogue nurses: Striking. [Interview with a theatre sister.] Nursing Mirror, 134, 3 Mar 1972, 12–13.

24 Otterbridge, M. Thoughts on collective bargaining. [And nurses' involvement.] Jamaican Nurse, 13 (1), Apr/May 1973, 11–13.

25 Phillips, D. F. New demands of nurses. [The problems arising from the nurses strike in San Francisco.] Hospitals, 48 (16), 16 Aug 1974, 31–34; 48 (18), 16 Sep 1974, 41–43.

26 Rosasco, L. C. Collective bargaining: what's a director of nursing to do? Hospitals, 48 (18), 16 Sep 1974, 79–80, 83–84.

27 Rosmann, J. One year under Taft-Hartley. [A high level of union activity has occurred as a result of hospital coverage by Taft-Hartley law.] Hospitals, 49 (24), 16 Dec 1975, 64–68.

28 Saxton, D. F. Collective bargaining in Academe: a personal appraisal. [Collective bargaining in American Universities from the point of view of a nurse.] Nursing Outlook, 21 (11), Nov 1973, 704–707.

29 Wenham, D. To strike or not to strike? – The R.P.N. and collective bargaining. Canadian Journal of Psychiatric Nursing, 15 (2), Mar/Apr 1974, 8–9.

30 Woods, N. S. Organisation of industrial relations. New Zealand Nursing Journal, 66 (5), May 1973, 6–8.

c HALSBURY REPORT

1 Bosanquet, N. Talking point. The test of time. [The Halsbury report.] Nursing Times, 70, 26 Sep 1974, 1489.

2 Castle, B. Barbara Castle talks to Nursing Mirror, by P. Young. Nursing Mirror, 138, 28 Jun 1974, 33–34.

3 Clarke, R. V. Status of ward sisters. [Letter on the position of the ward sister since the Halsbury Report.] British Medical Journal, 4, 12 Oct 1974, 105.

4 Department of Health and Social Security. Committee of Inquiry into the Pay and Related Conditions of Service of Nurses and Midwives Report HMSO, 1974. Chairman: Earl of Halsbury. Supplement. HMSO, 1975. Extracts and summary of the report in Nursing Mirror, 139, 26 Sep 1974, i–viii; Nursing Times, 70, 26 Sep 1974, 1490–1495.

5 Halsbury, Earl of A job worth doing: Alison Dunn talks to the Earl of Halsbury. Nursing Times, 70, 26 Sep 1974, 1488.

6 Hammond, G. Letter from the chairman of the OH Section of the Rcn to Lord Halsbury. Occupational Health, 26 (11), Nov 1974, 425–426.

7 Hospital and Health Services Review The Halsbury report. [Leading article.] Hospital and Health Services Review, 70 (11), Nov 1974, 381–383.

8 Lancet Talking politics. The nurses – and others. Lancet, 1, 1 June 1974, 1103.

9 Lester, J. A kind of unity. [Nurses' rally in Hyde Park on 6 June]. Nursing Mirror, 138, 14 Jun 1974, 36–38.

10 Midwives Chronicle The Halsbury Report. [Editorial.] Midwives Chronicle, 87, Nov 1974, 376–377.

11 National Union of Public Employees NUPE submits evidence to the Halsbury Committee. Nursing Mirror, 139, 5 Jul 1974, 41–42.

12 Nurses and Midwives Whitley Council Staff Side. Evidence to the Halsbury Committee. Nursing Mirror, 139, 12 Jul 1974, i–viii.

13 Nursing Mirror Nurses' reactions to the Halsbury Report. Nursing Mirror, 139, 26 Sep 1974, 36–39.

14 Nursing Mirror Unions and colleges give evidence to Lord Halsbury. [Summary of evidence.] Nursing Mirror, 139, 12 Jul 1974, 43.

15 Nursing Times Not so fine a tune. [Editorial on the Halsbury recommendations for tutors.] Nursing Times, 71, 27 Feb 1975, 319.

16 Nursing Times Taking leave. [Editorial on the guidance given on the implementation of the extra leave awarded by Halsbury.] Nursing Times, 71, 23 Jan 1975, 123.

17 Nuttall, P. Nurse unrest troubles UK Health Service. American Journal of Nursing, 74, Oct 1974, 1777, 1779–1780.

18 Paulley, J. and Clay, T. What are the issues? [Factors behind the current unrest in the nursing profession.] Nursing Times, 70, 27 Jun 1974, 982–983.

19 Price, I. Status of ward sisters. [Letter commenting on the Halsbury Report.] British Medical Journal, 4, 9 Nov 1974, 345.

20 Royal College of Nursing Rcn Council calls for talks now on 'crisis' in nurse education. [In the light of the Halsbury Report.] Nursing Times, 70, 28 Nov 1974, 1832.

21 Royal College of Nursing Submission to the Halsbury Committee of Enquiry. Rcn, 1974.

22 Shattock, F. M. The nurses' reward. [Letter commenting on the Halsbury Report.] Lancet, 2, 9 Nov 1974, 1137–1138.

23 Stevenson, J. Lord Halsbury – the gentle Wizard of Oz. Nursing Mirror, 139, 26 Sep 1974, 34–35.

24 Stevenson, J. The year of the Tiger. [Nursing developments in 1974, covering Halsbury and the progress of Briggs.] Nursing Mirror, 139, 19 Dec 1974, 37–39.

d HOURS OF WORK

1 Bajnok, I. The 12 hour shift. 'It's good for nurses, but is it good for the patients'? [Experiment at University Hospital, London, Ontario.] Hospital Administration in Canada, 17 (10), Oct 1975, 25–26.

2 Bauer, J. Clinical staffing with a 10-hour day, 4-day work week. Journal of Nursing Administration, 1 (6), Nov/Dec 1971, 12–14.

3 Beaumont, D. W. Never late. [Flexitime at Nottingham's new teaching hospital.] Health and Social Service Journal, 84, 15 Jun 1974, 1338.

4 Children's Medical Centre, Dallas The good and the bad of 12 hour shifts. RN Magazine, 38 (9), Sep 1975, 47–48, 51–52.

5 Cavill, E. Open forum. Internal rotation: a way of eliminating split shifts and encouraging staff to work unpopular hours. Nursing Mirror, 137, 5 Oct 1973, 16.

6 Cleveland, R. T. and Hutchins, C. L. Seven days vacation every other week. A 10 hour a day, seven day a week, staffing pattern means improved continuity of care and greater satisfaction for nurses. Hospitals, 48 (15), 1 Aug 1974, 81–82, 84–85.

7 Colt, A. M. and Corley, T. F. What nurses think of the 10-hour shift. Hospitals, 48 (3), 1 Feb 1974, 134, 136, 138, 140–142.

8 Crump, C. K. and Newson, E. F. P. Implementing the 12 hour shift: a case history. Results of a study conducted at the University Hospital in London, Ontario. Hospital Administration in Canada, 17 (10), Oct 1975, 20–24.

9 Deans, J. H. and McSwain, G. Nurses have more time on, more time off, with seven-day week scheduling. Modern Hospital, 118 (6), Jun 1972, 107–108.

10 DeMarsh, K. G. and McLellan, E. I. The seven-day fortnight. [Experiment in Winnipeg General Hospital.] Canadian Nurse, 68 (1), Jan 1972, 37–38. See also Nursing Mirror, 135, 15 Sep 1972, 43.

11 DeMarsh, K. G. and McLellan, E. I. The seven day fortnight – 18 months after. Hospital Administration in Canada, 14 (10), Oct 1972, 33–34, 36.

12 Dicker, K. Reduce nurses' hours to thirty-six a week. Nursing Mirror, 139, 2 Aug 1974, 41.

13 Dufour, N. M. The system needs to be changed. [The relationship between shift work patterns and job satisfaction.] Canadian Nurse, 70 (11), Nov 1974, 13.

14 Evans, R. Recording nurses' overtime – for the 40 hour week. Nursing Times, 68, 6 Jan 1972, Occ. papers, 1–4.

15 Fisher, D. W. and Thomas, E. A 'Premium Day' approach to weekend staff nursing. [A pilot scheme at Rochester Methodist Hospital enabling nurses to have an additional 8 hours leave every 4 weeks.] Journal of Nursing Administration, 4 (5), Sep/Oct 1974, 59–60.

16 Fraser, L. P. The reconstructed work week: one answer to the scheduling dilemma. Journal of Nursing Administration, 11 (5), Sep/Oct 1972, 12–16.

17 Gahan, K. and Talley, R. A block scheduling system: [for staff nurses and para-professionals at Nebraska Psychiatric Institute]. Journal of Nursing Administration, 5 (9), Nov–Dec 1975, 39–41.

18 Hibberd, J. M. 12-hour shifts for nursing staff: a field experiment. Hospital Administration in Canada, 15 (1), Jan 1973, 26, 28–30.

19 Kent, L. A. The 4-40 workweek on trial. American Journal of Nursing, 72 (4), Apr 1972, 683–686.

20 Kogi, K. Social aspects of shift work in Japan. [Reference to nurses – p. 427–30.] International Labour Review, 104 (5), Nov 1971, 415–433.

21 Larsen, C. A four-day week for nurses. Nursing Outlook, 21 (10), Oct 1973, 650–651.

22 Maynes, J. The hours question. Lamp, 28 (2), Feb 1971, 24–27.

23 Minor, M. A. and Heldstab, B. 10 and 6 hour nursing shifts solve staffing problem. Hospital Progress, 52 (7), Jul 1971, 62–63, 66.

24 Morrish, A. R. and O'Connor, A. R. Cyclic scheduling. Journal of Nursing Administration, 1 (5), Sep/Oct 1971, 49–54.

25 Price, E. M. A study of innovative staffing. [Cyclical scheduling staffing.] Hospital Progress, 53 (1), Jan 1972, 67–72.

26 Ryan, S. M. The modified work week for nursing staff on two pediatric units. [Analysis of the process by which a trail scheme was evaluated and then adopted permanently.] Journal of Nursing Administration, 5 (6), Jul/Aug 1975, 31–34.

27 Scottish Hospital Centre Scottish nurses discuss forty-hour week. [Report of a conference.] British Hospital Journal and Social Service Review, 82, 15 Apr 1972, 832.

28 Sellars. T. V. The 4/40; does it raise personnel costs? At Norfolk General Hospital the four-day workweek has proved to be no more expensive – and perhaps less expensive – than usual staffing patterns. Hospitals, 47 (17), 1 Sep 1973, 94, 96, 100–101.

29 Staples, S. and Curtis, B. L. Extended work day – two years later. At St. Paul's Hospital, Vancouver,

NURSING AS A PROFESSION

it has resulted in increased patient care and employee leisure time. Hospital Administration in Canada, 17 (1), Jan 1975, 32, 34.

30 Stinson, S. M. and Hazlett, C. B. Nurse and physician opinion of a modified work week trial. [Seven day fortnight.] Journal of Nursing Administration, 5 (7), Sep 1975, 21–26.

31 Underwood, A. B. What a 12-hour shift offers. American Journal of Nursing, 75 (7), Jul 1975, 1176–1178.

32 Warstler, M. E. Cycle work schedules and a non-nurse co-ordinator of staffing. Journal of Nursing Administration, 3 (6), Nov/Dec 1973, 45–51.

e NIGHT DUTY

1 Felton, G. Body rhythm effects on rotating work shifts. [A research study of 39 nurses with implications for the nursing service.] Journal of Nursing Administration, 5 (3), Mar/Apr 1975, 16–19.

2 Felton, G. and Patterson, M. G. Shift rotation is against nature. American Journal of Nursing, 71 (4), Apr 1971, 760–763.

3 Goucher, J. Salmon and patient care at night. [Organization of night nursing service in a group of hospitals in Birmingham.] Nursing Times, 69, 29 Mar 1973, 418–420.

4 Jolles, K. E. Biorhythmics. Nursing Times, 69, 15 Feb 1973, 206–208.

5 Lyons, B. Keep in step with your circadian rhythms. [With a brief reference to the effect of night duty on nurses in New South Wales.] Australian Nurses' Journal, 5 (5), Nov 1975, 22–23.

6 McCarrick, H. Flexitime in East Birmingham. [Night duty hours.] Nursing Times, 68, 14 Dec 1972, 1576–1577.

7 O'Dell, M. L. Human biorhythmology implications for nursing practice [in relation to patient schedules]. Nursing Forum, 14 (1), 1975, 43–47.

8 Ostberg, O. Interindividual differences in circadian fatigue patterns of shift workers. British Journal of Industrial Medicine, 30 (4), Oct 1973, 341–351.

9 Oswald, I. The biological clock and shift work. [With reference to nurses and night duty.] Nursing Times, 67, 30 Sep 1971, 1207–1208.

10 RN Magazine RN survey of night nurses. RN Magazine, 37 (11), Nov 1974, 37–47; 37 (12), Dec 1974, 46–51; 38 (1), Jan 1975, 30–35.

11 Storlie, F. A day nurse looks at night nurses. RN Magazine, 37 (11), Nov 1974, 46–47.

12 Tooraen, L. A. Physiological effects of shift rotation on ICU nurses. Nursing Research, 21 (5), Sep/Oct 1972, 398–405.

f SALARIES AND SUPERANNUATION

1 Bosanquet, N. and Clifton, R. Briggs: The Context. 2. Fresh start in pay. Nursing Times, 69, 17 May 1973, Occ. papers, 77–80.

2 Bosanquet, N. Community cares. [Problems of conditions of work and allowances for community staff.] Nursing Times, 70, 19/26 Dec 1974, 1961.

3 Bosanquet, N. The last of the exceptions. [Nurses and inflation.] Nursing Times, 70, 11 Jul 1974, 1057.

4 Bosanquet, N. Talking point. Keep on pushing. [The case for better pay for nurses.] Nursing Times, 70, 16 May 1974, 734.

5 Bosanquet, N. Words can win more pay. Nursing Times, 70, 21 Feb 1974, 256–257.

6 Frye, J. Phase 2 and you. [Nursing salaries and economic policy.] American Journal of Nursing, 72 (3), Mar 1972, 474–476.

7 Hanrahan, K. A. Salaries for nurse tutors and clinical teachers. World of Irish Nursing, 3 (9), Sep 1974, 164–165.

8 Hospital and Health Services Review Rising expectations. [Grievances of nurses concerning salaries and conditions.] Hospital and Health Services Review, 70 (6), 1974, 185–187.

9 Humphreys, D. Doctor – what is a ward sister worth? Nursing Times, 68, 11 May 1972, 559.

10 Kavalier, F. Move to see PM over 'top jobs' salary deadlock. Nursing Times, 69, 31 May 1973, 688–689.

11 Lancet Nothing much for the nurses. [The implementation of Briggs, and the case for better pay.] Lancet, 1, 18 May 1974, 971.

12 Lancet Nurses and consultants. [Increases in pay for nurses and consultants.] Lancet, 1, 18 May 1974, 983.

13 Lemin, B. Sister how much are you worth? [Survey conducted among sisters attending a series of study days in a hospital group.] Nursing Times, 70, 16 May 1974, 766–767.

14 Lloyd, P. OH nurse advisers and managers on the cheap. [Analysis of an Rcn salary survey.] Occupational Health, 27 (8), Aug 1975, 324–329.

15 New Zealand Nursing Journal Night duty payment. [Representations from the New Zealand Nurses' Association.] New Zealand Nursing Journal, 65 (8), Aug 1972, 26–27.

16 Nurses and Midwives Whitley Council Salaries for NHS nurses and midwives [April 1, 1974]. Nursing Mirror, 139, 19 Jul 1974, 71–79.

17 Nursing Times Student nurses – what is a ward sister worth? Nursing Times, 68, 25 May 1972, 630–631.

18 Rose, H. W. Superannuation. 1. Swindle or bargain? Nursing Times, 71, 2 Oct 1975, 1564–1566.

19 Rose, H. W. Superannuation. 2. Claiming contributions back. Nursing Times, 71, 9 Oct 1975, 1632–1633.

g WHITLEY COUNCIL

1 Bosanquet, N. Revitalising Whitley. Nursing Times, 70, 22 Aug 1974, 1295.

2 Bosanquet, N. Talking point. Reforming Whitley. Nursing Times, 71, 20 Mar 1975, 448–449.

3 Confederation of Health Service Employees COHSE demands trade unions only on reformed Whitley. [Evidence to McCarthy review.] Nursing Times, 71, 25 Sep 1975, 1520.

4 Dimmock, S. and Farnham, D. Working with Whitley in today's NHS. Personnel Management, 7 (1), Jan 1975, 35–37.

5 Institute of Health Service Administrators NHS Whitley machinery. [Paper submitted to Dr. McCarthy for the review of Whitley.] Hospital and Health Services Review, 71 (10), Oct 1975, 356–360.

6 Naylor, M. IHSA president stresses weaknesses of Whitley. [Institute of Health Service Administrators conference.] Nursing Times, 71, 8 May 1975, 712.

7 Nurses and Midwives Whitley Council Nurses and Midwives. Evidence to the Pay Board. Health Services, 26, Oct 1973, 164–167. Nursing Times, 69, 9 Aug 1973, 1012.

8 Nursing Mirror Whitley under the microscope. [Views on the workings of Whitley by the Rcn, RCM and COHSE.] Nursing Mirror, 141, 20 Nov 1975, 36.

9 Royal College of Midwives Review of the NHS Whitley machinery. [Comments sent to DHSS.] Midwives Chronicle, 88, Nov 1975, 379.

10 Young, P. The Whitley Council machinery – has it failed? Nursing Mirror, 139, 9 Aug 1974, 47–48.

h UNIFORMS

1 American Journal of Nursing Function over fashion. [Nurses' attitudes to uniforms.] American Journal of Nursing, 71 (11), Nov 1971, 2167.

2 Ewing, E. Women in uniform through the centuries. Batsford, 1975.

3 Goodwin, P. Oars are not provided. [Shoes for nurses.] Nursing Times, 70, 29 Aug 1974, 1360–1361.

4 Ingram, P. Do we or don't we? A successful campaign by nursing staff to introduce disposable aprons. Nursing Times, 69, 31 May 1973, 715.

5 Kilby-Kelberg, S. Caps – wearable or unbearable? American Journal of Nursing, 74 (5), May 1974, 897–899.

6 McCarrick, H. Changing gear: should a nurse's uniform denote her status or act as protection? Nursing Times, 69, 11 Oct 1973, 1320–1321.

7 Nursing Times Uniformly stylish. [Illustrations of nursing uniform currently worn in Manchester.] Nursing Times, 68, 4 May 1972, 534–545.

8 Occupational Health What shall I wear today? [Some views on uniforms for occupational health nurses.] Occupational Health, 26 (9), Sep 1974, 339–345.

9 O'Connell, C. All the gear: a presentation, denunciation and appreciation of the nurse's uniform and adornments. Nursing Mirror, 132, 9 Apr 1971, 20–23.

10 Pinel, C. Controversy corner. Are uniforms necessary? Nursing Mirror, 139, 14 Nov 1974, 41.

11 Roeschlaub, E. L. Pantsuits may solve 'exposure problems'. Hospital Topics, 49, Jan 1971, 43–47.

12 Walsh, P. A. and Ashcroft, J. B. Nurses' uniforms – do they affect patient staff interaction. [Pilot study at the Benedict Clinic, Rainhill Hospital, Lancashire.] Nursing Times, 70, 7 Mar 1974, 363.

13 White, D. A uniform attraction. [Observations on uniforms in general.] New Society, 28, 4 Apr 1974, 5–6.

14 Wiggins, L. R. A nurse's cap – symbol of a proud profession. Journal of Practical Nursing, 23 (1), Jan 1973, 22–23.

i UNIFORMS: PSYCHIATRIC

1 Brands, J. Uniform and the psychiatric nurse. Nursing Mirror, 133, 24 Sep 1971, 29–31.

2 Lebensohn, Z. M. The case of the defrocked nurse. [Practice of not wearing uniform in psychiatric nursing.] Journal of Psychiatric Nursing, 10 (1), Jan/Feb 1972, 16–18.

3 Psyche Starch or slapdash? Uniform or mufti? [In a psychiatric hospital.] Nursing Times, 67, 13 May 1971, 583.

4 Sharpe, D. Uniform or mufti? A hospital survey. [Warlingham Park Hospital, Surrey.] Nursing Times, 69, 11 Oct 1973, 1317–1319.

5 Webster, C. The uniform image. [Uniforms in mental handicap hospitals.] Nursing Mirror, 141, 4 Dec 1975, 67.

MANPOWER AND MANAGEMENT

9 MANPOWER

a GENERAL

1 Abdellah, F. G. Evolution of nursing as a profession: perspective on manpower development. International Nursing Review, 19 (3), 1972, 219–235.

2 Beard, T. C. Observations on the shortage of trained nurses. Medical Journal of Australia, 2, 26 Jul 1975, 137–140.

3 Bergman, R. Nursing manpower: issues and trends. [Long term planning for manpower.] Journal of Nursing Administration, 5 (4), May 1975, 21–25.

4 Borgmeyer, U. A. E. Charting manpower. [Techniques of manpower planning for nursing administrators.] Health and Social Service Journal, 85, 20/27 Dec 1975, 2788.

5 Bosanquet, N. Behind the headlines. [Difficulties of newly qualified nurses finding post.] Nursing Times, 71, 4 Dec 1975, 1924–1925.

6 Cuming, M. W. Population trends and nursing womanpower. Nursing Times, 68, 4 May 1972, 551–552.

7 Gish, O. Nursing migration. Contained in: Doctor migration and world health. Bell, 1971, Appendix 2, 133–143.

8 Knopf, L. Debunking a myth. [A Nurse Career Pattern Study – a long-range longitudinal study of nurses – being considered by the National League for Nursing to estimate nursing manpower.] American Journal of Nursing, 74 (8), Aug 1974, 1418–1421.

9 Nursing Times Shortage of nurses over? Workers seek safe jobs in economic crisis. Nursing Times, 71, 7 Aug 1975, 1232.

10 RN Magazine Nursing at the crossroads: numbers aren't the answer. RN Magazine, 37 (7), Jul 1974, 40–43.

11 RN Magazine The nurse supply: shortage or surplus? [Results of a questionnaire sent to directors of nursing of general and special hospitals throughout the United States.] RN Magazine, 37 (6), Jun 1974, 34–35.

12 Scottish Home and Health Department The movements of hospital nursing staff in Scotland. Edinburgh: The Department, 1975. (Nursing manpower planning report no. 5.)

13 Scottish Home and Health Department National nursing manpower policies in Scotland. Edinburgh: The Department, 1974. (Nursing manpower planning report no. 1.)

14 Scottish Home and Health Department Nurse staffing (community) survey: book of tables. Edinburgh: The Department, 1975. (Nursing manpower planning report no. 4.)

15 Scottish Home and Health Department Nurse staffing (hospital) survey: book of tables. Edinburgh: The Department, 1975. (Nursing manpower planning report no. 3.)

16 Scottish Home and Health Department Practical manpower planning for nurses. Edinburgh: The Department, 1974. (Nursing manpower planning report no. 2.)

17 United States Department of Health Education and Welfare. Division of Medicine International migration of physicians and nurses: an annotated bibliography. United States Department of Health Education and Welfare, 1975.

18 Watkin, B. Management topics. Manpower planning. Nursing Mirror, 139, 2 Aug 1974, 61.

19 World Health Organization Nursing Unit. Nursing manpower development: a review of methods prepared . . . for the Scientific Group on the Development of Studies in Health, Manpower held in Geneva, 2–10 November 1970. Geneva: WHO, 1971.

b NURSING AS A CAREER

1 Abdellah, F. G. Research on career development in the health professions: nursing. Occupational Health Nursing, 21 (5), May 1973, 12–16.

2 Allen, B. Nursing as a career. Nursing Mirror, 133, 27 Aug 1971, 7.

3 American Hospital Association Career goals of hospital school of nursing seniors: report of a survey. Chicago: The Association, 1975.

4 Barrett, W. Assessing the need for career guidance for nurses. Nursing Times, 70, 8 Aug 1974, 1248–1249.

5 Bullough, B. and Bullough, V. A career ladder in nursing. American Journal of Nursing. Reprinted in Australian Nurses' Journal, 2 (2), Aug 1972, 29–32.

6 Employment Service Agency. Careers and Occupational Information Centre Nursing for men and women. HMSO, 1975 (Choice of careers series no. 82).

7 Imrie, V. J. Basic nursing careers. British Hospital Journal and Social Science Review, 81, 31 Jul 1971, 1545.

8 King, C. Nursing. Glasgow: Blackie, 1974. (People at work.)

9 Mordacq, C. Constraints and opportunities in a nursing career. International Nursing Review, 20 (4), Jul/Aug 1973, 112–122.

10 Powell, M. Patients are people: nursing. Reading: Educational Explorers, 1975. (My life and my work series.)

11 Sheahan, J. Your career in nursing. MacMillan Journals, 1975.

12 Wood, L. Proposal: a career plan for nursing. American Journal of Nursing, 73 (5), May 1973, 832–835.

c RECRUITMENT

1 Accetta, J. W. Hospital employment can be 'sold'. Hospital proves that the same marketing techniques used successfully by industry can be used to attract new employees. Hospitals, 46, 1 Jun 1972, 73–76.

2 Bates, M. and Lea, D. A. Organizing a hospital open day and careers exhibition. Hospital and Health Services Review, 69 (12), Dec 1973, 456–458.

3 Bright, K. Research into schoolgirls' interest in nursing. Lamp, 28 (11), Nov 1971, 7, 9, 11, 13.

4 Callard, R. Penny plain tuppence coloured – consumer reaction. Nursing Cadet Ruth Callard, 16½ reviews three recruitment booklets prepared by the DHSS, the Welsh Board and the Central Office of Information. Nursing Times, 68, 3 Aug 1972, 980–981.

5 Cleland, V. and others Inducements for nursing employment. [Survey to find relative importance of salaries, hours and holidays in nurse recruitment.] Nursing Research, 22 (5), Sep/Oct 1973, 414–422.

6 Clifton, R. F. and others Hospital nurse recruitment. Health and Social Service Journal, 83, 16 Jun 1973, 1369–1370.

7 Cuskelly, C. E. A changing world – a changing role. [The author's work as Nurse Careers Advisor for the Hospital Commission of New South Wales.] Lamp, 29 (11), Nov 1972, 39–41.

8 Cuskelly, C. Nursing advertisement and literature for 1974. Lamp, 30 (12), Dec 1973, 35–36.

9 Cuskelly, C. Recruitment of nursing staff. [In New South Wales.] Lamp, 31 (1), Jan 1974, 13, 15.

10 Drew, M. E. Expo or expire. [A humorous account of an exhibition designed to recruit sixthformers to the nursing profession.] Nursing Times, 69, 29 Mar 1973, 421.

11 Finn, A. and Penney, M. J. Recruit. retrain . . . retain . . . A suggested solution to the nursing shortage. Hospital Administration in Canada, 17 (7), Jul 1975, 29–30.

12 Funke, J. and others Slide-tape helps recruitment. [At University of Alberta School of Nursing.] Canadian Nurse, 71 (7), Jul 1975, 27.

13 Hampton, P. J. Why they choose nursing. Journal of Nursing Education, 11 (1), Jan 1972, 2–7.

14 Hess, J. and Coon, B. How to recruit and retain applicants in nursing. Nursing Outlook, 21 (7), Jul 1973, 472–475.

15 Johnson, W. L. Admission of men and ethnic minorities to schools of nursing, 1971–1972. Nursing Outlook, 22 (1), Jan 1974, 45–49.

16 Kovacs, A. R. Recruitment is everyone's job. International Nursing Review, 19 (2), 1972, 150–155.

17 Miller, M. H. On blacks entering nursing. Nursing Forum, 11 (3), 1972, 248–263.

18 Monaghan, G. Nurses and the myth of full employment. [Technological changes resulting in some posts becoming obsolete and the need for intensive retraining programs for new skills.] Canadian Nurse, 71 (9), Sep 1975, 21–22.

19 New Zealand Survey of nurses qualifications and practice. [Results of a 1974 Government survey to estimate recruitment needs.] New Zealand Nursing Journal, 69 (6), Jun 1975, 16–17.

20 Nursing Mirror Policing the wards? A pilot project in New York City which aims to train suitable retired policemen and firemen as nurses. Nursing Mirror, 138, 29 Mar 1974, 66–67.

21 Nursing Mirror South coast recruitment drive. Turning holidaymakers into nurses. Nursing Mirror, 135, 15 Sep 1972, 10–11.

22 Nursing Times The Midlands. Tapping the resources. [Supply of nurses.] Nursing Times, 70, 12 Sep 1974, 1436–1437.

23 Nursing Times University survey reveals ignorance. Nursing unattractive to students. Nursing Times, 69, 15 Nov 1973, 1507.

24 O'Connor, V. Careers extraordinary. Professional promoter. [Nursing recruitment officer at King's College Hospital.] Nursing Times, 68, 18 May 1972, 597–599.

25 Recruitment Services Planned, professional approach needed for nurse recruitment: seminar examines methods used by hospitals in Canada and United States to recruit, retrain and retain their nursing personnel. Hospital Administration in Canada, 17 (4), Apr 1975, 63–64.

26 RN Magazine Fourth annual guide to finding the right position for senior nursing students. RN Magazine, 36 (12), Dec 1973, G1–G7.

27 Robinson, A. M. Black nurses tell you: why so few blacks in nursing. RN Magazine, 35 (7), Jul 1972, 35–41, 73–74.

28 Schatz, P. S. Tom Gun in coming. [A successful campaign to recruit nurses for a new hospital.] Hospitals, 48, 1 Jan 1974, 74, 76–77.

29 Sczekan, M. and Betz, M. Effect of values, social support and academic performance in stabilizing occupational choice. [Study of pre-nursing students.] Nursing Research, 22 (4), Jul/Aug 1973, 339–343.

30 Sharp, T. Health occupations education at the secondary level. [In schools as a means of meeting the growing demand for trained assistants.] Hospital Progress, 53 (9), Sep 1972, 94.

31 Winder, A. E. Why young black women don't enter nursing. Nursing Forum, 10 (1), 1971, 56–63.

d RETURN TO NURSING

1 Back to nursing [A brief account of a refresher course for former nurses.] SA Nursing Journal, 38 (7), Jul 1971, 17.

2 Barnett, E. A story of 'talents' given wisely. [Westville Voluntary Nursing Service, a team of married ex-nurses.] SA Nursing Journal, 39 (11), Nov 1972, 25.

3 Brady, P. Carry on nursing – if you can. [A married nurse's experiences of returning to nursing.] Nursing Mirror, 139, 19 Dec 1974, 54.

4 Bramwell, Mrs Picking up the threads. [Return to nursing.] NATNews, 8 (1), Spring 1971, 23.

5 Brophy, S. F. The R.N. problem: returning to active practice. [Courses to keep non-practising nurses up-to-date.] Journal of Nursing Administration, 4 (5), Sep/Oct 1974, 45–47.

6 Bryson, M. G. Keep in touch with nursing. [Course run by Nottingham City Hospital for non-working mothers.] Nursing Mirror, 136, 11 May 1973, 28–29.

7 Buchanan, D. I. The bank is open. [St. Helier group of hospitals.] Nursing Times, 70, 17 Oct 1974, 1634–1635.

8 Carruthers, L. J. Back to nursing at Guy's. [Outline of the course planned for those joining the Guy's nursing bank.] Nursing Mirror, 141, 4 Sep 1975, 69.

9 Cooper, S. S. From retired to rehired. Journal of Nursing Administration, 1 (1), Jan 1971, 24–28.

10 Crews, J. D. Problems of a return. [To nursing.] New Zealand Nursing Journal, 65 (5), May 1972, 21.

11 Davies, E. M. East Birmingham nurse bank. Nursing Mirror, 136, 29 Jun 1973, 30–32.

12 Dunn, A. Liverpool's nurse bank. Nursing Times, 70, 21 Mar 1974, 416–417.

13 Gaspardy, B. Using permanent part-time nursing personnel effectively. One hospital's answer to the nursing shortage. [Use of relief staff.] Hospital Administration in Canada, 17 (8), Aug 1975, 50–52.

14 Hauer, R. M. and others Coming of age of a refresher program. [Professional Nurse Refresher Program at Beth Israel Medical Center, New York.] American Journal of Nursing, 75 (1), Jan 1975, 88–91.

15 Morgan, B. In touch with nursing. [A six week course at St. Martin's Hospital, Bath, aimed at trained nurses who have left nursing.] Nursing Mirror, 139, 28 Nov 1974, 73.

16 New Zealand Nursing Journal Farewell personal touch. [Changes in the hospital scene noted by a nurse returning to nursing after some years.] New Zealand Nursing Journal, 64 (9), Sep 1971, 26–27.

17 Niles, A. M. and Lutze, R. S. A clinical conference for inactive nurses. [Organized by the University of Wisconsin to help inactive nurses keep professionally in touch.] Supervisor Nurse, 6 (10), Oct 1975, 51–53.

18 Nursing Mirror A retainer scheme for nurses? Nursing Mirror, 140, 6 Mar 1975, 33.

19 Nursing Times Nurse bank in Cornwall. Nursing Times, 69, 1 Nov 1973, 1433.

20 Nursing Times Where have all the nurses gone? A collection of papers about nursing recruitment of both student and trained staff which first appeared as Occasional papers, 1970–1973. Macmillan Journals, 1974.

21 Nursing Times The Wordsley Hospital nurse bank. Nursing Times, 70, 31 Jan 1974, 133.

22 Nursing Week A list of hospitals running nurse banks. Nursing Week, 11/18, 1974, 8.

23 Office of Population Censuses and Surveys. Social Survey Division Reserves of nurses: an enquiry carried out on behalf of the Department of Health by Judy Sadler and Tony Whitworth. HMSO, 1975. Comment in Nursing Times, 71, 29 May 1975, 832.

24 Rose, V. 'Nurse bank' at Edgware General Hospital. Nursing Week, no. 19, 28 Feb 1974, 8.

25 Stewart, E. G. Part-time nurses: employment conditions. American Journal of Nursing, 71 (10), Oct 1971, 1957.

26 Walker-Smith, A. Night school for nurses. [Back to nursing course run by United Liverpool Hospitals.] Nursing Times, 71, 3 Jul 1975, 1065–1067.

27 Webb, B. B. Community nurse reserve bank. [Leicestershire.] Queen's Nursing Journal, 17 (3), Jun 1974, 60–61.

28 Wilcox, R. J. E. and others Where have all the nurses gone? A survey of reserve trained nurses spon-

sored jointly by King Edward's Hospital Fund and the Welsh Hospital Board. Nursing Times, 69, 8 Mar 1973, 37–40. Interview with Mr. Wilcox about the survey, Nursing Times, 69, 1 Mar 1973, 275–277.

29 Woollings, B. A. Keeping in touch. [Back to nursing courses at Basildon Hospital.] Nursing Mirror, 136, 2 Feb 1973, 13.

e WASTAGE AND TURNOVER

1 Armiger, B. Nursing shortage or unemployment? Nursing Outlook, 21 (5), May 1973, 312–316.

2 Baker, E. J. Associate degree nursing students: nonintellective differences between dropouts and graduates. Nursing Research, 24 (1), Jan/Feb 1975, 42–44.

3 Birch, J. To nurse or not to nurse: an investigation into the causes of withdrawal during nurse training. Rcn, 1975 (Research series). Based on MEd thesis, Newcastle University 1972. Summary in Nursing Times 73, 16 Jun 1977, Occ. papers, 87–88.

4 Bowman, M. P. What a waste! [Of nurses in training.] Nursing Mirror, 134, 28 Jan 1972, 13–15.

5 Cohen, H. A. and Gesner, F. P. Dropouts and failures: a preventive program. [Factors in students' withdrawal.] Nursing Outlook, 20 (11), Nov 1972, 723–725.

6 Dunkerley, D. and Mercer, G. Wastage among student and trained nurses. Nursing Times, 71, 30 Jan 1975, 194–195.

7 Dunkerley, D. and Mercer, G. Why nurses leave hospitals: some preliminary observations. [A study of labour turnover among British nurses.] Health and Social Service Journal, 84, 12 Oct 1974, 2362.

8 Hegarty, W. H. Organizational and sociological factors affecting attrition in collegiate schools of nursing. [Study by questionnaire sent to 150 American schools.] International Journal of Nursing Studies, 12 (4), 1975, 217–222.

9 Hutcheson, J. D. and others Toward reducing attrition in baccalaureate degree nursing programs: an exploratory study. Nursing Research, 22 (6), Nov/Dec 1973, 530–533.

10 Jones, C. W. Why associate degree nursing students persist. Nursing Research, 24 (1), Jan/Feb 1975, 57–59.

11 Lee, H. and Farrell, P. Mental health practitioner? [Problems of wastage among mental handicap nurses and a possible solution.] Nursing Times, 71, 6 Nov 1975, 1789–1790.

12 McCloskey, J. Influence of rewards and incentives on staff nurse turnover rate. Nursing Research, 23 (3), May/Jun 1974, 239–247.

13 Marshall, R. D. and Spencer, R. I. A more efficient use of hospital beds? [Closure of some acute beds in an attempt to reduce nurse wastage – experiment at Northampton General Hospital.] British Medical Journal, 3, 6 Jul 1974, 27–30.

14 Miller, M. H. A follow-up of first-year nursing student dropouts. Nursing Forum, 13 (1), 1974, 32–47.

15 Pecarchik, R. and Nelson, B. H. Employee turnover in nursing homes. American Journal of Nursing, 73 (2), Feb 1973, 289–290.

16 Ride, T. Why have all the nurses gone? [Wastage rate in the nursing profession.] Nursing Times, 70, 30 May 1974, 820–821.

17 Rogers, M. E. Nursing: to be or not to be? [The position of nurses who leave nursing to enter one of the paramedical professions, such as physician's assistants.] Nursing Outlook, 20 (1), Jan 1972, 42–46.

18 Singh, A. and Smith, J. Retention and withdrawal of student nurses. [Report of an on-going research project carried out by the GNC Research Unit.] International Journal of Nursing Studies, 12 (1), Mar 1975, 43–56.

19 : Watkin, B. Management topics: labour turnover. Nursing Mirror, 138, 10 May 1974, 84–85.

f AGENCY NURSES

1 Adams, M. The agency nurse. Nursing Times, 67, 25 Nov 1971, 1465–1467.

2 Agency nurses hit again [in an addendum to DHSS circular HSC (1S) 164]. Nursing Mirror, 141, 18 Sep 1975, 34. Further comment, 141, 9 Oct 1975, 34.

3 Alexander, F. W. A national nursing agency? Nursing Times, 67, 15 Jul 1971, 876–977.

4 Ball, D. Agency nursed. [From the point of view of a nurse who runs the office of a Nursing Agency.] New Society, 20, 4 May 1972, 235–236.

5 Boorer, D. Why agencies flourish. Nursing Times, 69, 16 Aug 1973, 1062–1063.

6 Cropper, D. J. Agency nurses. [Letter commenting on the DHSS circular.] British Medical Journal, 3, 19 Jul 1975, 158.

7 Cropper, D. 'It's a politically motivated scheme.' Agencies reply to government plans. [Comment on the government circular.] Nursing Times, 71, 3 Jul 1975, 1031.

8 Department of Health and Social Security Nurses agencies. Circular HSC (1S) 164. The Department, Jun 1975.

9 Dicker, K. Open forum. Agency nursing – such a bad thing? Nursing Mirror, 135, 21 Jul 1972, 25.

10 Federation of Personnel Services of Great Britain Survey into the motivation, attitudes and costs of employing temporary nursing staff. The Federation, 1974.

11 Federation of Personnel Services of Great Britain Survey on agency nurses in the NHS. The Federation, 1975.

12 Hansard. House of Commons Future of agency nurses within NHS. Adjournment debate. 28 Jul 1975, col 1456–1466. Government policy on reduction of agency nurses within NHS. Question 8 Jul 1975, col 306–397. Report of debate. Nursing Mirror, 141, 7 Aug 1975, 40.

13 Health and Social Service Journal Agency nurses are increasing. [Leading article.] Health and Social Service Journal, 85, 25 Jan 1975, 165–166.

14 Hospital Agency nurses. [Leading article.] Hospital, 68 (4), Apr 1972, 110–111.

15 Joyson, G. and Kent, R. J. Agency nurses. British Hospital Journal and Social Service Review, 81, 29 May 1971, 1047–1048.

16 Kavalier, F. Are agencies for you? Nursing Times, 69, 23 Aug 1973, 1102–1103.

17 Kavalier, F. SRN will lead new jobs group. London hospitals to set up agency. Nursing Times, 69, 17 May 1973, 622.

18 Luneski, I. D. Temporary nursing: is it for you? RN Magazine, 36 (9), Sep 1973, 46–50.

19 Nursing Times Editorial and other comment on government policy on agencies. Nursing Times, 71, 26 Jun 1975, 990; 3 Jul 1975, 1029; 18 Sep 1975, 1478; 2 Oct 1975, 1556.

20 Pacey, N. Nursing employment bureau. [Hospital and Community Nursing Bureau, North-west Herts

Health District.] Nursing Times, 71, 5 Jun 1975, 902–903.

21 Pasker, P. and others The boom in agency nursing – problem or promise for the NHS? Nursing Times, 68, 13 Jan 1972, Occ. papers, 5–8.

22 Royal College of Nursing Report of a working party on agency nurses. Rcn, 1972.

23 Royal College of Nursing Nursing Agencies Administrators Group. Recommended code of practice. Rcn, 1971.

24 Stover, W. R. Temporary nurse service. [Agency nursing service in Rochester, New York.] American Journal of Nursing, 75 (11), Nov 1975, 1998–1999.

25 Trenchard, H. Call for policy on agency nurses. Nursing Mirror, 140, 10 Apr 1975, 34. Nursing Times, 71, 19 Apr 1975, 554.

26 Watkin, B. Persecution of the agencies. Nursing Mirror, 141, 10 Jul 1975, 39.

27 Young, P. Agency nursing – a cause for concern. Nursing Mirror, 138, 22 Mar 1974, 42–43.

g AUXILIARIES

1 Barrowclough, F. Nursing auxiliaries training in geriatric hospitals. [In-service training programme.] Nursing Mirror, 141, 17 Jul 1975, 70–71.

2 Boughton, J. Report on a pilot study using a sample of nurse aides to investigate a staff selection technique. Australian Nurses' Journal, 3 (9), Apr 1974, 23–25.

3 Dane, J. H. Study explores hospital turnover. [With particular reference to role perception of orderlies and nurses' aides.] Hospital Topics, 49 (8), Aug 1971, 49–53, 55–56, 64.

4 Fretwell, J. E. Care enough to act. [Unqualified personnel in charge of patients.] Nursing Times, 70, 30 May 1974, 843.

5 Gale, C. B. Walking in the aide's shoes. [A nurse works as an aide in order to understand the aide's feelings and experiences.] American Journal of Nursing, 73 (4), Apr 1973, 628–631.

6 Hutton, S. W. Basic nursing care: a guide for nursing auxiliaries. Baillière Tindall, 1974.

7 Jani, S. M. The plight of auxiliary nurses. Nursing Journal of India, 63 (9), Sep 1972, 299.

8 Kankalil, M. The woman in white. [Auxiliary nurse midwives.] Nursing Journal of India, 66 (4), Jun 1975, 123–125.

9 Murphy, J. C. Setting the stage for teaching ancillary personnel. Journal of Nursing Administration, 1 (6), Nov/Dec 1971, 51–52.

10 Rose, V. The role of the nursing auxiliary. Health Services, 26, Apr 1973, 68–69.

11 Wright, M. Why the 'nursing assistant'? SA Nursing Journal, 42 (5), May 1975, 9.

h GRADUATES

1 Association of Integrated and Degree Courses in Nursing The graduate's contribution to nursing: report of the first open conference, University of Edinburgh, 13–15 July 1973. The Association, 1973.

2 Bendall, E. The nurse graduate in the United Kingdom: career motivation. International Nursing Review, 19 (1), 1972, 53–91.

3 Chapman, C. N. The graduate in nursing. Nursing Times, 71, 17 Apr 1975, 615–617.

4 Hayter, J. Follow-up study of graduates of the

University of Kentucky, College of Nursing, 1964–1969. Nursing Research, 20 (1), Jan/Feb 1971, 55–60.

5 Jackson, I. J. Registered nurses with degrees. [A list of names of nurses with degrees.] Nursing Times, 67, 30 Sep 1971, Occ. papers, 155–156.

6 Kramer, M. and others Self-actualization and role adaption of baccalaureate degree nurses. Nursing Research, 21 (2), Mar/Apr 1972, 111–123.

7 Kratz, C. R. and others The degree nurse – advanced nursing students' views. Nursing Times, 71, 20 Feb 1975, 290–295.

8 MacGuire, J. M. and Jackson, I. J. The graduate/nurse expansion. Nursing Times, 69, 25 Jan 1973, Occ. papers, 13–15.

9 MacGuire, J. M. The nurse/graduate in the United Kingdom – career paths. International Nursing Review, 18 (4), 1971, 367–378.

10 Morrison, A. T. and Tsekouras, M. P. Graduate recruitment to nursing: a survey of the information and opinions of undergraduates in three Scottish universities on nursing and nursing as a career for graduates. Dundee: Eastern Regional Hospital Board, 1973. Summary in British Journal of Medical Education, 7 (4), Dec 1973, 271–277; Nursing Times, 69, 15 Nov 1973, 1507.

11 Peplau, H. E. An open letter to a new graduate. [Responsibility of the new graduate in the nursing profession.] Nursing Digest, 3 (2), Mar/Apr 1975, 36–37.

12 Pitel, M. and Vian, J. Analysis of nurse-doctorates. Data collected for the International Directory of Nurses with doctoral degrees. Nursing Research, 24 (5), Sep/Oct 1975, 340–351.

13 Smith, E. A. RN graduates: where do they go? A survey of senior nursing students. Hospitals, 46 (3), 1 Feb 1972, 136–137, 140, 142.

14 Smith, J. P. Conference report. Graduates in nursing. [Association of Integrated and Degree Courses in Nursing (AIDCN) Conference, the graduate's contribution to nursing.] Nursing Times, 69, 26 Jul 1973, 951.

15 Smith, P. A. Graduate nurses and their problems of adjustment. Nursing Times, 68, 30 Mar 1972, 386–387.

16 Taylor, S. D. and others. Nurses with earned doctoral degrees: an analysis of information collected for the American Nurses' Foundation's Directory. Nursing Research, 20 (5), Sep/Oct 1971, 415–427.

17 Vian, J. Nurse-doctorate analysis revised to include new data. Nursing Research Report, 7 (2), Jun 1972, 1, 3–7.

i LICENSED PRACTICAL NURSES (US)

1 Anderson, M. The LPN – a unique commodity. Bedside Nurse, 4 (10), Oct 1971, 29–32.

2 Hampton, P. J. Why do they care? [Licensed practical nurses.] Bedside Nurse, 5 (7), Jul 1972, 12–17.

3 Hoffman, C. A. LP/VN: potential unlimited. Journal of Practical Nursing, 22 (7), Jul 1972, 16–17.

4 Journal of Practical Nursing The licensed practical/vocational nurse. A profile. Journal of Practical Nursing, 21 (7), Jul 1971, 13.

5 Knopf, L. Practical nurses in the health labor force. [National League for Nursing survey of employment.] Nursing Care, 8 (3), Mar 1975, 24–25, 27.

6 Lathan, B. Lead the way. [The expanding role of

the licensed practical/vocational nurse.] Journal of Practical Nursing, 24 (11), Nov 1974, 35.

7 Light, I. How can our licensing processes be improved? Journal of Practical Nursing, 22 (2), Feb 1972, 24–26, 30–31, 34.

8 McTernan, E. J. Today's trends – tomorrow's traditions. [NAPNES Conference lecture.] Journal of Practical Nursing, 23 (6), Jun 1973, 16–17, 39–40.

9 Martin, R. G. How to ease the nursing shortage. [In New York City by recruiting LPNs.] Journal of Practical Nursing, 24 (4), Apr 1971, 25, 29.

10 Mason, M. LPN as head of central service. Journal of Practical Nursing, 21 (1), Jan 1971, 35–37.

11 Parkhurst, R. The new nurse. [Role of the LPN and LVN.] Nursing Care, 7 (11), Nov 1974, 19–21.

12 RN Magazine Growth of the paraprofessionals: nursing in transition. [Increasing numbers of LPNs and technicians.] RN Magazine, 37 (7), Jul 1974, 38–39.

13 Sharp, D. and Hass, D. Profile of the LPN. A view from Kansas. Nursing Care, 7 (7), Jul 1974, 16–18.

14 Torrop, H. M. A true fairy tale. [History and development of NAPNES.] Journal of Practical Nursing, 23 (6), Jun 1973, 18–21.

16 Tucker, G. L. The licensed practical nurse in today's setting or the licensed practical solution. Journal of Practical Nursing, 22 (8), Aug 1972, 24–26, 34.

16 Wysocki, H. E. Historical perspective: the LPN in Veterans Administration Nursing Service. Nursing Care, 6 (7), Jul 1973, 15–19.

j MALE NURSES

1 Baripaul, J. Male nurses. Nursing Journal of India, 63 (9), Sep 1972, 300.

2 Bedside Nurse Men in nursing. Bedside Nurse, 5 (1), Jan 1972, 29–31.

3 Brown, R. G. S. Male nurses. 1. Patterns of success and wastage. [Findings of a research team at the University of Hull.] Nursing Times, 70, 10 Jan 1974, 58–61.

4 Brown, R. G. S. Male nurses. 2. After registration. Nursing Times, 70, 17 Jan 1974, 89–91.

5 Brown, R. G. S. Male nurses. 3. The enrolled nurse. Nursing Times, 70, 24 Jan 1974, 125–128.

6 Brown, R. G. S. Male nurses' careers. 1. After registration. [Final phase of the University of Hull research project showing causes of wastage and post registration career patterns of 372 male nurses.] Nursing Times, 71, 18 Sep 1975, Occ. papers, 93–95.

7 Brown, R. G. S. Male nurses' careers. 2. Post-registration training. Nursing Times, 71, 25 Sep 1975, Occ. papers, 97–99.

8 Brown, R. G. S. and Stones, R. W. H. The decision to nurse: a study of male recruits. Nursing Times, 67, 25 Mar 1971, Occ. papers, 45–48.

9 Brown, R. G. S. and Stones, R. W. H. The decision to nurse: the image of nursing – nursing seen through men's eyes. Nursing Times, 67, 1 Apr 1971, Occ. papers, 49–52.

10 Brown, R. G. S. and Stones, R. W. H. The decision to nurse: the career intentions of male nurses. Nursing Times, 67, 8 Apr 1971, Occ. papers 53–56.

11 Brown, R. G. S. and Stones, R. W. E. The male nurse. Bell, 1973. (Occasional papers on social administration no. 52.)

12 Brown, R. G. S. and Stones, R. W. H. Personality and intelligence characteristics of male

nurses. International Journal of Nursing Studies, 9 (3), Aug 1972, 167–176.

13 Colledge, M. Men in nursing. British Hospital Journal and Social Service Review, 80, 26 Dec 1970, 2593.

14 Crotty, J. J. Barrier nursing? [A male nurse's view of prejudices he has encountered.] Nursing Times, 71, 16 Oct 1975, 1645.

15 Dias, M. Male nurses in Ceylon: a study of the career problems of male nurses in the Ceylon health service, 1972. MPhil thesis, York University, 1973.

16 Dingwall, R. Nursing: towards a male dominated occupation? Nursing Times, 68, 12 Oct 1972, 1294–1295.

17 Greenberg, E. and Levine, B. Role strain in men nurses. Nursing Forum, 10 (4), 1971, 416–430.

18 Hunter, D. G. Gender discrimination in the health care delivery system: men in nursing. Hospital Administration in Canada, 16 (3), Mar 1974, 33–36.

19 Hunter, D. G. Men in nursing. Canadian Journal of Psychiatric Nursing, 15 (4), Jul/Aug 1974, 12–14.

20 Jenny, J. The masculine minority. Canadian Nurse, 71 (12), Dec 1975, 21–22.

21 Lancet Male nurses. [Review of study by R. G. S. Brown and R. W. H. Stones.] Lancet, 2, 15 Dec 1973, 1400.

22 Morrison, I. 'Yes but you're a man'. Nursing Mirror, 140, 23 Jan 1975, 74.

23 Nafziger, J. Men in nursing: more is expected from them. Bedside Nurse, 4 (7), Jul 1971, 27.

24 Nursing Times The men at number 10. [Editorial on ratio of men to women in chief nursing officer posts.] Nursing Times, 69, 16 Aug 1973, 1043.

25 O'Connell, D. Careful – nurses integrating. [In mental health nursing.] Nursing Mirror, 134, 14 Jan 1972, 8.

26 Ogundeji, M. O. Men and the nursing profession in Nigeria. Nigerian Nurse, 7 (1), Jan/Mar 1975, 6–8.

27 Robinson, A. M. Men in nursing: their career goals and image are changing. RN Magazine, 36, Aug 1973, 36–41.

28 Rosen, J. G. Male nurses in general nursing: a study in male emancipation. MPhil thesis, York University, 1971.

29 Rosen, J. G. and Jones, K. The male nurse. New Society, 19, 9 Mar 1972, 493–494.

30 Rosen, J. G. and Jones, K. Profile of the male nurse: a reseach report. In McLachlan, G., editor. Problems and progress on medical care. Seventh series. Oxford University Press for Nuffield Provincial Hospitals Trust, 1972, 83–92.

31 Shaw, J. S. A man's place: at the bedside? [Male nurses.] Modern Healthcare, 2 (1), Jul 1974, 66–67.

32 Stephens, I. Why not more male nurses. Nursing Journal of India, 64 (2), Feb 1973, 59.

33 Watson, F. Nehi Tane [male nurse]. [Male nurses in New Zealand.] New Zealand Nursing Journal, 67 (4), Apr 1974, 10–11.

34 Whitworth, P. A. What is a male nurse. Nursing Mirror, 133, Aug 1971, 35.

35 Whyte, S. B. Sex and our profession. [Men in nursing.] Nursing Mirror, 141, 23 Oct 1975, 75.

36 Williams, A. Characteristics of male baccalaureate students who selected nursing as a career. Nursing Research, 22 (6), Nov/Dec 1973, 520–525.

37 Wilson, T. G. Men in nursing. New Zealand Nursing Journal, 65 (11), Nov 1972, 6–7.

k OVERSEAS NURSES IN BRITAIN

1 Akinsanya, J. A. Qualified Nigerian nurses in Britain. Nigerian Nurse, 7 (3), Jul/Sep 1975, 40–42.

2 Bosanquet, N. Immigrants and the NHS. [Examination of overseas doctors and the pattern of recruitment of nurses.] New Society, 33, 17 Jul 1975, 130–132.

3 Bristow, S. The West African student in Great Britain: a report of a seminar held at the University of Ibadan, Nigeria, organized by the Commonwealth Students Children Society. Nursing Mirror, 140, 12 Jun 1975, 62.

4 Clarke, M. Social relationships between British and overseas nurses. MPhil thesis, Department of Psychology, Surrey University, 1975.

5 Cox, M. Problems of overseas nurses training in Britain. [Research undertaken by Dr. Sen.] International Nursing Review, 19 (2), 1972, 157–165.

6 Dunn, A. Entering the British way of life. [The King's Fund report on 'The language barrier and the overseas nurse trainee.'] Nursing Times, 70, 21 Nov 1974, 1798.

7 Kendall, M. N. Overseas Nursing students in Britain. [A survey of recruitment trends.] International Nursing Review, 19 (3), 1972, 246–259. Shortened version in New Society, 21, 3 Aug 1972, 239–240.

8 King's Fund Centre The language barrier and the overseas nurse trainee: report of a working party set up to discuss the problems of orientation for overseas nurse trainees. The Centre, 1974. (Project paper no 8.)

9 Longhorn, E. Lesson one: welcome to the British way of life. [Orientation course for overseas nurses at Claybury Hospital.] Nursing Times, 69, 13 Sep 1973, 1195–1196.

10 McCarrick, H. If you can wait and not be tired by waiting. [Delay in recognizing the qualifications of overseas nurses who come to work in this country.] Nursing Times, 69, 5 Apr 1973, 446–448.

11 Myers, G. A model orientation course. [Course for overseas learners at Mount Vernon Hospital, Northwood, Middlesex.] Nursing Times, 68, 12 Oct 1972, 1275–1278.

12 Nursing Times Overseas trainees. [Editorial.] Nursing Times, 70, 21 Nov 1974, 1791.

13 Nursing Times Seeking a better deal for overseas students. [Joint Rcn/UKCOSA workshop.] Nursing Times, 71, 13 Nov 1975, 1802–1803.

14 Roland, N. Planning an orientation course [for overseas nurses at Brompton Hospital]. Nursing Mirror, 140, 12 Jun 1975, 63–65.

15 Scottish Home and Health Department Nurses and midwives: orientation of nursing and midwifery trainees from abroad. Edinburgh: The Department, 1972. (Scottish hospital memorandum 42/1972.)

16 Stones, R. W. H. Overseas nurses in Britain: a study of male recruits. Nursing Times, 68, 7 Sep 1972, Occ. papers, 141–144.

17 Thomas, M. and Williams, J. M. Overseas nurses in Britain: a PEP survey for the United Kingdom Council for Overseas Student Affairs. Political and Economic Planning, 1972. (Broadsheet 539.)

18 Thompson, S. Overseas nurses deserve better protection. [Problems faced by overseas nurses working in Britain and the steps being taken to help them.] New Psychiatry, 1 (1), 19 Sep 1974, 22–23.

19 United Kingdom Council for Overseas Student Affairs Overseas nursing students in Britain: evidence to the Committee on Nursing. The Council, 1971.

20 Yates, A., editor Students from overseas. National Foundation for Educational Research in England and Wales, 1971. (Exploring education.) Summary of Sen, A. Problems of overseas students and nurses. NFER, 1970.

l STATE ENROLLED NURSES

1 Bridges, A. SEN in the team. [In a group practice.] District Nursing, 15 (3), Jun 1972, 56.

2 Central Health Services Council. Subcommittee of the Standing Nursing Advisory Committee The state enrolled nurse. HMSO, 1971.

3 Hadley, R. D. and others The SEN in the psychiatric hospital. Nursing Mirror, 139, 30 Aug 1974, 65–68.

4 Hockey, L. Use or abuse? [A summary of a study of the state enrolled nurse in the local authority nursing services.] District Nursing, 15 (3), Jun 1972, 54–55.

5 Linday, L. H. Group attachment and the SEN in Birmingham. District Nursing, 15 (3), Jun 1972, 57–58.

6 Makin, J. S. 'Action' project. [Project carried out by an experienced SEN as part of a pilot scheme in clinical management organized by the Sheffield Regional Hospital Board.] Nursing Mirror, 136, 19 Jan 1973, 31–32.

7 Manduku, S. B. Enrolled nurses programme at Machakos General Hospital School of Nursing. Kenya Nursing Journal, 1 (1), Jun 1972, 14–15.

8 Proudfoot, S. E. Only the SEN? Think again. [Hospital management course for SENs at the Regional Staff College, Monsall, Manchester.] Nursing Times, 68, 5 Oct 1972, 1266–1267.

9 Rae, A. V. Clinical management for SENs; a recent pilot scheme undertaken by Sheffield Regional Hospital Board. Nursing Mirror, 136, 19 Jan 1973, 29–30.

10 Royal College of Nursing Enrolled nursing – new thoughts. [Report of Rcn study day.] Nursing Times, 69, 18 Oct 1973, 1375.

11 Royal College of Nursing Opportunities for enrolled nurses. 6th ed. Rcn, 1972.

10 MANAGEMENT

a GENERAL

1 Babajide, L. O. The place of management in nursing profession. Nigerian Nurse, 6 (2), Jan/Mar 1974, 38, 40–42.

2 Bowman, M. P. Management. 1. Individual and personality growth. Nursing Times, 71, 26 Jun 1975, 1022–1023.

3 Bowman, M. P. Management. 2. Work. Nursing Times, 71, 3 Jul 1975, 1060–1061.

4 Bowman, M. P. Management. 5. Practical application of management as an aid to nursing. Nursing Times, 71, 24 Jul 1975, 1175–1177.

5 Christie, L. S. Management philosophy. Nursing Mirror, 132, 14 May 1971, 36–37; 21 May 1971, 30–31.

6 Davenport, P. Nurses are learning to 'manage' in large hospitals. Australian Nurses' Journal, 1 (7), Jan 1972, 20–21.

7 Dooley, E. The nurse administrator at regional and national level. World of Irish Nursing, 3 (8), Aug 1974, 141–143.

8 Erickson, E. H. Are nurses needed for admin-

istration or management in hospitals. Journal of Nursing Administration, 4 (4), Jul/Aug 1974, 20–21.

9 Galloway, B. T. The nurse as a professional manager. [Participants in a management training workshop define the role of the nurse in professional management.] Hospitals, 48, 1 Nov 1974, 89, 92, 94.

10 Germaine, A. Developing a nursing service department. Hospital Administration in Canada, 17 (11/12), Nov/Dec 1975, 46, 48.

11 Graves, H. H. Can nursing shed bureaucracy? American Journal of Nursing, 71 (3), Mar 1971, 491–494.

12 Harrison, F. P. Today's administrator wears many hats. Canadian Nurse, 71 (7), Jul 1975, 15.

13 Haywood, S. and Dellar, H. The nursing view of management. [Research project at Hull University into problems of nurses who become purely administrators.] British Hospital Journal and Social Service Review, 81, 30 Jan 1971, 223–224.

14 Highman, A. A management information system for the nursing department. Hospital Administration in Canada, 13 (10), Oct 1971, 54, 56.

15 Kings Fund Centre The 120-bed nursing unit. [Conference on a Wessex experiment.] Nursing Times, 67, 11 Nov 1971, 1421. Hospital, 67 (12), Dec 1971, 434–435.

16 Lambertsen, E. C. A greater voice for nursing service administrators. Hospitals, 46, 16 Apr 1972, 101, 104, 108.

17 Lemin, B. Organizations and their processes. Nursing Times, 69, 14 Jun 1973, Occ. papers, 93–96.

18 Mellish, J. M. Current problems in nursing service administration. SA Nursing Journal, 41 (4), Apr 1974, 17–20; (5), May 1974, 14–15.

19 Nelson, J. Fugitives from the wards. [Problems of administrators out of the ward situation.] Nursing Mirror, 140, 10 Apr 1975, 75.

20 New Zealand Nurses' Association Guidelines for nurses. New Zealand Nursing Journal, 65 (10), Oct 1972, 14–15.

21 Offhouse, C. D. Nursing administration in extended care. Journal of Nursing Administration, 11 (5), Sep/Oct 1972, 39–42.

22 Orr, E. P. The matron as a phenomenon. [Problems of nurse administration in a period of marked change.] Australian Nurses' Journal, 4 (8), Mar 1975, 36–38.

23 Quinn, S. Centre lunch talk. Nurses, patients, and management. [Reported by L. Paine.] British Hospital Journal and Social Service Review, 82, 25 Mar 1972, 654.

24 Robb, J. H. Nurses and administration. New Zealand Nursing Journal, 68 (7), Jul 1974, 4, 6–7, 9, 16.

25 Schurr, M. C. Nurses and management: what is it all about? English UP, 1975.

26 Sheahan, D. The game of the name: nurse professional and nurse technician. Nursing Outlook, 20 (7), Jul 1972, 440–444.

27 Sheahan, D. Short shrift for hospital nursing. [Examination of the assumption that the head of nursing in a hospital can serve the best interests of nursing whilst acting as a bureaucrat in the hospital organization.] American Journal of Nursing, 73 (3), Mar 1973, 485–490.

28 Smith, D. Organizational theory and the hospital. Journal of Nursing Administration, 11 (3), May/Jun 1972, 19–24.

29 Smith, J. P. On being a district nursing officer. Queen's Nursing Journal, 17 (6), Sep 1974, 124–125, 127.

30 Stevens, B. J. The problem in nursing's middle management. Journal of Nursing Administration, 11 (5), Sep/Oct 1972, 35–38.

31 Sukaimi, M. Issues on management development in the nursing service. Nursing Journal of Singapore, 13 (2), Nov 1973, 95–98.

32 Taaffe, P. Planning nursing services. World of Irish Nursing, 3 (8), Aug 1974, 129–130.

33 Watkin, B. Do we manage to care? [Nursing Mirror Forum '75.] Nursing Mirror, 141, 2 Oct 1975, 48–50.

34 Watkin, B. Management topics. Series of articles. Nursing Mirror, 139, Jul/Sep 1974.

35 Watkin, B. Management topics. Books on management. Nursing Mirror, 139, 12 Sep 1974, 54–55.

36 Watkin, B. Use of management and administrative technique in nursing. In Ferrer, H. P. editor. The health services – administration, research and management. Butterworths, 1972, 65–96.

37 Weiss, O. Is your administrative gap showing? Australian Nurses' Journal, 3 (3), Sep 1973, 18–19, 45.

38 World Health Organization Report of the Inter-Regional Seminar on the application of the planning process to nursing for nurse administrators at national level. Geneva: WHO, 1972.

39 Young, P. Scottish nurse administrators meet in Melrose. Nursing Mirror, 139, 31 Oct 1974, 37–38.

b TECHNIQUES AND TEXTBOOKS

1 Alexander, E. L. Nursing administration in the hospital health care system. St. Louis: Mosby, 1972.

2 American Hospital Association Practical approaches to effective functioning of the department of nursing service: a guide for administrators of nursing service. Chicago: The Association, 1972.

3 Archer, S. E. PERT: a tool for nurse administrators. [Program Evaluation Review Technique.] Journal of Nursing Administration, 4 (5), Sep/Oct 1974, 26–32.

4 Arnot, C. and Huckabay, L. M. D. Nursing administration: theory for practice with a systems approach. St. Louis: Mosby, 1975.

5 Bailey, J. T. and Claus, K. E. Decision making in nursing: tools for change. St. Louis: Mosby, 1975.

6 Bermosk, L. S. and Corsini, R. J. editors Critical incidents in nursing. Philadelphia: Saunders, 1973.

7 Beyers, M. and Philips, C. Nursing management for patient care. Boston: Little Brown, 1971.

8 Conway, M. E. Management effectiveness and the role making process. Journal of Nursing Administration, 4 (6), Nov/Dec 1974, 25–28.

9 Cortazzi, D. and Roote, S. Don't talk – draw! [The use of illustrations in learning from critical incidents in patient care.] Nursing Times, 69, 30 Aug 1973, 1134–1136.

10 Cullinan, J. Sister's foot in the CNO's door. [Management audit at Doncaster Royal Infirmary.] Nursing Times, 69, 29 Mar 1973, 411–413.

11 Daniel, W. W. and Longest, B. B. Some practical statistical procedures [for the nurse administrator]. Journal of Nursing Administration, 5 (1), Jan 1975, 23–27.

12 Dickens, S. and Stansbie, P. Management by ob- .

jectives in nursing. Nursing Mirror, 136, 8 Jun 1973, 28–30.

13 Divincenti, M. Administering nursing service. Boston: Little Brown, 1972.

14 Doncaster Hospital Group Management Audit Panel Management audit for the nursing services. Nursing Times, 69, 29 Mar 1973, Occ. Papers, 49–52; 5 Apr 1973, Occ. papers. 53–55.

15 Donovan, H. M. Nursing service administration: managing the enterprise. St. Louis: Mosby, 1975.

16 Ganong, W. L. and Ganong, J. M. Good advice. ABP for nursing administration. [Annual business plan]. Journal of Nursing Administration, 3 (3), May/Jun 1973, 6–7, 60–61.

17 Ganong, W. L. and Ganong, M. J. Reducing organizational conflict through working committees. Journal of Nursing Administration, 11 (1), Jan/Feb 1972, 12–19.

18 Geach, B. The problem-solving technique: is it relevant to practice? Canadian Nurse, 70 (1), Jan 1974, 21–22.

19 Gelder, J. E. The 'flow chart' assists nursing. Canadian Hospital, 48 (10), Oct 1971, 81, 83.

20 Germaine, A. The annual report: an effective management tool in the nursing department. Hospital Administration in Canada, 16 (6), Jun 1974, 60, 62.

21 Germaine, A. Nursing administration. How well do we manage our time? Hospital Administration in Canada, 16 (11), Nov 1974, 47–48.

22 Germaine, A. Nursing manuals: an element of effective management. Hospital Administration in Canada, 15 (3), Mar 1973, 64, 66, 68.

23 Germaine, A. and Penwarden, G. H. Management by objectives in the nursing department. Hospital Administration in Canada, 14 (4), Apr 1972, 34–36.

24 Journal of Nursing Administration Organization of nursing care. Wakefield, Massachusetts: Contemporary Publishing, 1975.

25 Journal of Nursing Administration The technique of nursing management: a reader. Wakefield, Massachusetts: Contemporary Publishing, 1975.

26 Joyson, G. Nurses and hospital finance. British Hospital Journal and Social Service Review, 81, 27 Mar 1971, 557–558.

27 Palmer, J. Management by objectives. Journal of Nursing Administration, 1 (1), Jan 1971, 17–23; 3 (5), Sep/Oct 1973, 55–60.

28 Pan, L. Planned program budgeting: a workshop report. Nursing Outlook, 19 (1), Oct 1971, 656–658.

29 Price, M. and others Nursing management: a programmed text. New York: Springer, 1974.

30 Prouty, M. P. Making an organizational chart. Journal of Nursing Administration, 4 (1), Jan/Feb 1974, 32–35.

31 Smith, B. J. Management audit for the nursing services. Doncaster Hospital Management Committee, 1972.

32 Stevens, B. J. Nursing division budget: generation and control. Journal of Nursing Administration, 4 (6), Nov/Dec 1974, 16–20.

33 Stevens, B. The Playscript method of developing administrative procedures. Supervisor Nurse, 6 (6), Jun 1975, 40–42, 44–45.

34 Stevens, B. J. Use of groups for management: the organization of committees in a nursing division. Journal of Nursing Administration, 5 (1), Jan 1975, 14–22.

35 Stubbs, V. Delegation [in nursing administration]. District Nursing, 15 (6), Sep 1972, 117, 119.

36 Sylvester, M. J. Management games: a useful link between theory and practice. Journal of Nursing Administration, 4 (4), Jul/Aug 1974, 28–32.

37 Thomson, W. Management for nurses. 1. Keeping up to date. Nursing Mirror, 134, 14 Apr 1972, 16–17.

38 Thomson, W. Management for nurses. 2. Sitting on a committee. Nursing Mirror, 134, 21 Apr 1972, 47–48.

39 Thomson, W. Management for nurses. 3. Holding a conversation. Nursing Mirror, 134, 28 Apr 1972, 40–41.

40 Thomson, W. Management for nurses. 6. The problem of priorities. Nursing Mirror, 134, 19 May 1972, 50–51.

41 Veninga, R. Interpersonal feedback: a cost-benefit analysis. Journal of Nursing Administration, 5 (2), Feb 1975, 40–43.

42 Warstler, M. E. Some management techniques for nursing service administrators. Journal of Nursing Administration, 11 (6), Nov/Dec 1972, 25–34.

43 Watkin, B. Management topics. Budgets. Nursing Mirror, 139, 26 Jul 1974, 62.

44 Watkin, B. Management topics. Cost benefit analysis. Nursing Mirror, 139, 19 Jul 1974, 58.

45 Watkin, B. Management topics. Delegation. Nursing Mirror, 138, 7 Jun 1974, 75.

46 Watkin, B. Management topics. Objectives. Nursing Mirror, 138, 29 Mar 1974, 49.

c COMPUTERS AND AUTOMATION

1 Ashcroft, J. M. and Berry, J. L. Computers or nurses? [Letter written in the light of experiences in the cardiothoracic department, Wythenshawe Hospital, Manchester.] Lancet, 2, 30 Nov 1974, 1321.

2 Automation at St. Elizabeth More care, fewer people, less paperwork, lower cost. [Administrative communications control centres replace nurses' stations.] Modern Hospital, 118 (3), Mar 1972, 93–96.

3 Barker, M. The era of the computer and its impact on nursing. Supervisor Nurse, 2 (8), Aug 1971, 26, 30–31, 33–36.

4 Barlow, A. J. Nurse allocation by computer. Nursing Mirror, 134 (4), 28 Jan 1972, 43–45.

5 Birckhead, L. M. Automation of the health care system: implications for nursing. 1. Dangers to nursing practice in the automation of the health care system. International Nursing Review, 22 (1), Jan/Feb 1975, 28–31.

6 Butler, E. A. Computers in the ward situation. [Computer projects in the USA.] Nursing Times, 69, 25 Jan 1973, 119–121.

7 Cornell, S. A. and Brush, F. Systems approach to nursing care plans. [Using computers.] American Journal of Nursing, 71 (7), Jul 1971, 1376–1378.

8 Cornell, S. A. and Carrick, A. G. Computerized schedules and care plans. Nursing Outlook, 21 (12), Dec 1973, 781–784.

9 Crooks, J. Drug administration. 2. The contribution of the computer. Nursing Mirror, 142, 1 Apr 1975, 55–57.

10 Farlee, C. and Goldstein, B. A role for nurses in implementing computerized hospital information systems. Nursing Forum, 10 (4), 1971, 339–357.

11 Goldstein, B. and Farlee, C. Characteristics of nursing units and accommodation to technological change. [Including the use of a hospital computer information system.] Nursing Research, 21 (1), Jan/Feb 1972, 63–68.

12 Goodwin, J. O. and others Developing a computer program to assist the nursing process. Nursing Research, 24 (4), Jul/Aug 1975, 299–305.

13 Goshen, C. E. Your automated future. [Technology and nursing.] American Journal of Nursing, 72 (1), Jan 1972, 62–67.

14 Jelinek, R. C. and others Tell the computer how sick the patients are and it will tell how many nurses they need. [In the hospital data centre, computer operators calculate the number of nursing personnel needed on the units.] Modern Hospital, 121 (6), Dec 1973, 81–85.

15 Keliher, P. The standardized form: a seven part computer form reprinted and prepared by the data processing can eliminate much of the repetitive writing of patient data. Supervisor Nurse, 6 (11), Nov 1975, 40–41, 44–45.

16 Knight, J. E. and Streeter, J. The computer as an aid to nursing records. [Work being done at King's College Hospital Computer Unit.] Nursing Times, 66, 19 Feb 1970, 233–235.

17 Mather, B. S. An automated ward census and reporting system: nursing staff attitudes. Australian Nurses' Journal, 3 (1), Jul 1973, 20–22.

18 Mershimer, R. and others. Automating the paperwork. American Journal of Nursing, 71 (6), Jun 1971, 1164–1167.

19 Meyer, D. R. What we need today is a data processing system for nursing. New York: National League for Nursing, 1973. (Publication 46.53.)

20 Murray, D. J. Computer makes the schedules for nurses. Modern Hospital, 117 (6), Dec 1971, 104–105.

21 Randall, C. E. Unusual incident? Tell the computer: a computerized tabulation of unusual incident reports. Hospitals, 46 (23), 1 Dec 1972, 56–57, 100.

22 Somers, J. B. A computerized nursing care system. [For formulating nursing care plans and keeping them up to date.] Hospitals, 45 (8), 16 Apr 1971, 93–100.

23 Tate, S. P. Automation of the health care system: implications for nursing. 2. Change strategies for nurses. International Nursing Review, 22 (2), Mar/Apr 1975, 39–42.

24 Tomasovic, E. R. 'Turning nurses on' to automation. Hospitals, 46 (9), 1 May 1972, 80, 84, 86.

25 Thomson, M. E. An automated ward census and reporting system: how computers help nurses. Australian Nurses Journal, 3 (1), Jul 1973, 16–19, 22.

26 Wesseling, E. Automating the nursing history and care plan: computerization of an admission questionnaire. Journal of Nursing Administration, 11 (3), May/Jun 1972, 34–38.

27 Willer, B. and Stasiak, E. Automated nursing notes in a psychiatric institution. Journal of Psychiatric Nursing, 11 (2), Mar/Apr 1973, 27–29.

28 Zielstoriff, R. D. The planning and evaluation of automated systems: a nurse's point of view. Journal of Nursing Administration, 5 (6), Jul/Aug 1975, 22–25.

d LEADERSHIP AND SUPERVISION

1 Alexander, C. J. Leaders influence, guide nursing by specific action. AORN Journal, 21 (2), Feb 1975, 195–196, 198.

2 Bell, J. Leadership and responsibility. [Higher Institute of Nursing, Alexandria.] Nursing Times, 69, 15 Nov 1973, 1542–1543.

3 Ciancutti, A. R. and others Creating harmony between supervisor and nurse. Supervisor Nurse, 6 (8), Aug 1975, 35, 38, 40–41.

4 Douglass, L. M. and Bevis, E. O. Nursing leadership in action; principles and application to staff situations. 2nd ed. St. Louis: Mosby, 1974.

5 Feeley, E. and Tarr, J. Alternative leadership experiences for senior students in an acute care setting. Journal of Nursing Education, 18 (2), Feb 1979, 25–28.

6 Francis, H. T. A. Leadership experience for ADN students. American Journal of Nursing, 72 (7), Jul 1972, 1264–1265.

7 Guan, H. K. Creative leadership in supervision: the effects on students' behaviour and performance. Nursing Journal of Singapore, 12 (2), Nov 1972, 99–101.

8 Hughes, R. Styles of leadership among nurses. Nursing Times, 70, 22 Aug 1974, Occ. papers, 57–59.

9 Ingmire, A. E. The effectiveness of a leadership programme in nursing. International Journal of Nursing Studies, 10 (1), Jan 1973, 3–17.

10 Jain, P. An experience for leadership. [Colleges of Nursing in India.] Nursing Journal of India, 63 (3), Mar 1972, 77.

11 James, J. Re: Challenge in leadership for nursing administration from the point of view of the director of nursing. Lamp, 31 (9), Sep 1974, 9, 11, 13, 15.

12 Jones, M. C. Leadership experiences for senior students. Nursing Outlook, 22 (6), Jun 1974, 394–397.

13 Kelly, W. L. Psychological prediction of leadership in nursing. Nursing Research, 23 (1), Jan/Feb 1974, 38–42.

14 Kovacs, A. R. Preparation for leadership: a philosophy [for nursing education]. International Nursing Review, 21 (5), Sep/Oct 1974, 145–146.

15 Kron, T. The management of patient care: putting leadership skills to work. Philadelphia: Saunders, 1971.

16 Kruse, L. C. and Stogdill, R. M. The leadership role of the nurse: a report submitted to US Department of Health, Education and Welfare. Ohio State University Research Foundation, 1973.

17 Lasca, L. Motivation, evaluation and leadership. [Industrial methods applied to nursing.] Journal of Nursing Administration, 11 (5), Sep/Oct 1972, 17–21.

18 Leininger, M. The leadership crisis in nursing: a critical problem and challenge. Journal of Nursing Administration, 4 (2), Mar/Apr 1974, 28–34.

19 Levenstein, A. Art and science of supervision: your leadership role. Supervisor Nurse, 6 (8), Aug 1975, 42–44.

20 McLaughlin, F. E. Personality changes through alternate group leadership. Nursing Research, 20 (2), Mar/Apr 1971, 123–130.

21 McLaughlin, F. E. and White, E. Small group functioning under six different leadership formats. Nursing Research, 22 (1), Jan/Feb 1973, 37–54.

22 McLaughlin, F. E. and others Effects of three types of group leadership structure on the self-perceptions of undergraduate nursing students. [At the University of California.] Nursing Research, 21 (3), May/Jun 1972, 244–257.

23 Nelson, P. Instantaneous leadership. Supervisor Nurse, 6 (3), Mar 1975, 34–35, 39.

24 Nicholas, A. D. Rational decision making as an

attribute of nursing leadership. Jamaican Nurse, 12 (2), Aug 1972, 15–17.

25 Nouri, C. J. and Rainville, C. Supervisory development for nursing leaders. Journal of Nursing Administration, 11 (2), Mar/Apr 1972, 52–59.

26 O'Donovan, T. R. Leadership dynamics. Journal of Nursing Administration, 5 (7), Sep 1975, 32–35.

27 Pyrer, M. W. and Distefano, M. K. Perceptions of leadership, behaviour, job satisfaction, and internal–external control across three nursing levels. Nursing Research, 20 (6), Nov/Dec 1971, 534–537.

28 Ramadas, P. Leadership role of the nursing officer. Nursing Journal of Singapore, 15 (2), Nov 1975, 100–101.

29 RN Magazine We need leadership courses, but —. RN Magazine, 34 (9), Sep 1971, 34–37.

30 Smith, B. J. How well does a nurse supervisor know her nurses? Australian Nurses' Journal, 3 (10), May 1974, 29–30.

31 Watkin, B. Management topics. Leadership. Nursing Mirror, 138, 22 Mar 1974, 62.

32 Watts, S. M. Leadership education for all. New Zealand Nurses Journal, 65 (7), Jul 1972, 8–9.

33 We need leadership courses, but —. RN Magazine, 34 (9), Sep 1971, 34–37.

33 Wengerd, J. S. and others Leadership development at the clinical unit level: workshops and individual guidance. Journal of Nursing Administration, 4 (5), Sep/Oct 1974, 19–25.

34 White, H. C. Perceptions of leadership styles by nurses in supervisor positions. Journal of Nursing Administration, 1 (2), Mar/Apr 1971, 44–51.

35 Wiles, V. The challenge in leadership for nursing administration from the point of view of a charge sister. Lamp, 32 (6), Jun 1975, 29–33.

36 Yale University School of Nursing Leadership. [Report of a three-day conference sponsored by the Yale University School of Nursing.] American Journal of Nursing, 72 (8), Aug 1972, 1445–1456.

e MANAGEMENT TRAINING

1 Charleton, J. W. Partnership in management development. 2. (First line management course.) Nursing Times, 71, 21 Aug 1975, Occ. papers, 85–88.

2 Collis, R. and Knight, F. Tropical encounter. [First line course in management at University Hospital of the West Indies.] Jamaican Nurse, 12 (2), Aug 1972, 8–10, 24–26.

3 Conton, J. Middle management course. [At the Regional Technical College, Dundalk.] World of Irish Nursing Journal, 1 (9), Sep 1972, 181. See also, Irish Nurses Journal, 4 (10), Nov 1971, 5–6.

4 Cossey, M. Introduction to management: study days for trained nurses. Nursing Times, 66, 26 Nov 1970, Occ. papers, 177–178.

5 Danks, P. M. Sisters in the role of manager. [Training student nurses as managers at Sydney Hospital.] Australian Nurses' Journal, 1 (4), Oct 1971, 28–29.

6 Danks, P. M. Sydney Hospital training programme. [In management.] Lamp, 28 (9), Sep 1971, 7, 9, 11.

7 Davies, J. An evaluation of first-line management training courses for ward sisters in the Manchester region: a study of management training in its organizational context. Manchester Centre for Business Research, Manchester Business School, 1971.

8 Davies, G. W. Management training – where

now? 1. [Conclusions of a research project to evaluate first line management training.] Nursing Mirror, 141, 10 Jul 1975, 63–64.

9 Davies, G. W. Management training – where now? 2. [Proposed training scheme developed in Gwent College of Higher Education.] Nursing Mirror, 141, 17 Jul 1975, 68–69.

10 Del Bueno, D. J. and others Leadership courses in action. 1. For head nurses in a large hospital, by D. J. del Bueno. 2. An each-one-teach-the-others approach, by C. Isler. 3. WICHE, the two-year seminar programme, by C. Isler. RN Magazine, 34 (9), Sep 1971, 38–47.

11 Department of Health and Social Security. National Staff Committee Management development of nurses and midwives: a progress report 1969–1971. The Department, 1971.

12 Fautrel, F. Training for ward management. [Project at St. Bernard Hospital, Middlesex whereby third year student nurses took charge of wards for two separate days.] Nursing Mirror, 133, 19 Nov 1971, 33–37.

13 Gourlay, D. H. F. Development of courses for nurses. [4-week courses in middle management at Robert Gordon's Institute of Technology, Aberdeen.] British Hospital Journal and Social Service Review, 82, 2 Dec 1972, 2690.

14 Holden, W. M. and others Can management aid our patient care? [In service management training in the Central Wirral Group.] Nursing Mirror, 138, 19 Apr 1974, 76–78.

15 Lemin, B. Management for the senior state enrolled nurses. [An experimental course held at William Rathbone Staff College.] Nursing Times, 67, 8 July 1971, Occ. papers, 107–108.

16 McCullagh, M. and others The effects of role exchange. [Charge nurses at John Connolly Hospital, Birmingham 'acting up' as an opportunity of developing their managerial skills.] Nursing Times, 70, 22 Aug 1974, 1318–1321.

17 Macmillan, P. Case studies for nursing management courses. Pitman, 1975.

18 MacPherson, M. E. Management training for ward sisters: inferences from the Hornsby Hospital Study. Lamp, 29 (9), Sep 1972, 23–25.

19 Magner, M. A management course revisited. Supervisor Nurse, 6 (3), Mar 1975, 19, 21–22.

20 Miles, I. M. Diploma in nursing administration course 1973. An experiment in post-basic nursing education. 1. SA Nursing Journal, 41 (1), Jan 1974, 11–15.

21 Neuman, M. M. Developing a nurses' ability to manage; a program design. Journal of Continuing Education in Nursing, 4 (6), Nov/Dec 1973, 28–33.

22 Nuallain, C. O. Training for multi-management. [Includes a summary of a paper by Professor Searle on the training of nurses for management.] British Hospital Journal and Social Service Review, 81, 25 Sep 1971, 1971–1972.

23 Pritchard, R. E. A philosophy of teaching applied to administration. Journal of Nursing Administration, 5 (7), Sep 1975, 38–40.

24 Sartain, B. The benefits of multidisciplinary management courses. District Nursing, 15 (1), Apr 1972, 11–12.

25 Schurr, M. C. Learning together. 1. Management training for ward sisters. Nursing Times, 69, 22 Nov 1973, 1582–1584.

26 Stubbs, V. Modular training. [Inservice management courses.] Queen's Nursing Journal, 17 (3), Jun 1974, 57, 61.

27 Sukaimi, M. Issues on management development in the nursing service. Nursing Journal of Singapore, 13 (2), Nov 1973, 95–98.

28 Thomas, B. Prediction of success in a graduate nursing service administration program: a study of the effectiveness of student selection practices from 1967–1971. Nursing Research, 23 (2), Mar/Apr 1974, 156–159.

29 Thomas, B. and others Survey of nursing service administration graduates. Nursing Outlook, 22 (7), Jul 1974, 457–459.

30 Veith, S. and others Teaching nursing management by programmed instruction. Journal of Nursing Education, 14 (2), Apr 1975, 25–29.

31 Westbrook, K. Management courses – are they a waste of time? Nursing Times, 71, 30 Jan 1975, 190–191.

32 White, D. Business management for administrators: benefits for the NHS. [A summary of the gains made by 19 hospitals and nursing officers attending management courses.] Health and Social Service Journal, 84, 2 Nov 1974, 2535–2536.

33 White, D. Learning together. 2. [Evaluation of first-line management course for ward sisters.] Nursing Times, 69, 29 Nov 1973, 1623–1625.

34 White, D. and Frawley, A. Partnership in management development. [Evaluation of a first-line management course held at the United Manchester Hospital.] Nursing Times, 71, 14 Aug 1975, Occ. papers, 81–84.

f NON-NURSING DUTIES

1 Collier, G. L. Food for thought. Non nursing duties – line of demarcation. [Implications for medical record officers of relieving nurses of clerical duties.] Medical Record, 16 (2), 1975, 53–54.

2 Duke, M. G. Non-clinical tasks: a review of non-clinical duties performed by nurses and a planned transfer of tasks to related areas. New Zealand Nursing Journal, 66 (1), Jan 1973, 4–5.

3 Horne, D. Decision making 'near the bed'. [Proposals for the removal of non-nursing duties to a central service department and the management training of ward staff.] New Zealand Nursing Journal, 69 (10), Oct 1975, 25–29.

4 Meates, M. The diminishing island of nursing duties. [Increasing number of non nursing duties.] Nursing Times, 68, 26 Oct 1972, 1348.

5 Nicholas, M. L. The Hospitals Commission of New South Wales. Increasing demands on nursing staff. [Nursing and non-nursing duties.] Lamp, 29 (11), Nov 1972, 7, 9.

6 Page, B. M. Housekeeping at the Royal Gwent. Introducing housekeeping teams to relieve nurses of non-nursing duties. Nursing Times, 67, 2 Dec 1971, 1512–1513.

7 Scottish Home and Health Department Non-nursing duties. Edinburgh: The Department, 1972.

8 Swaffield, L. The domestic issue: can there ever be a clear dividing line between nursing and non-nursing duties? [Conference report.] Nursing Times, 70, 28 Nov 1974, 1838–1839.

g NURSING OFFICER

1 Charleton, J. W. Developing the role of the nursing officer. Nursing Times, 70, 25 Jul 1974, 1171.

2 Cheadle, J. The work of a nursing officer. [Research project at St. Wulstan's Hospital, Malvern.] Nursing Mirror, 135, 18 Aug 1972, 34–37.

3 Fenn, M. and others Developing the role of the unit nursing officer: a report on the work of the Fulbourn nursing administration study group. Nursing Times, 71, 13 Feb 1975, 262–264.

4 Holden, W. M. and others Nursing officer – has she a role and function? Nursing Times, 68, 26 Oct 1972, 1361–1362.

5 Kenny, G. The unit nursing officer. World of Irish Nursing, 2 (5), May 1973, 87, 89–90.

6 Kings Fund Centre Nursing Officers (No. 6 and 7) Salmon structure: report of meetings held on 22 November 1971, 15 and 19 May 1972. The Centre, 1972. (THC reprint nos 626, 685.)

7 McCarrick, H. Linkman . . . or stepping stone? The role of the number seven. Nursing Times, 70, 17 Jan 1974, 68–69.

8 O'Toole, R. Where should the NO's office be? [Whether it should be in the individual unit or centrally situated, with particular reference to subnormality hospitals.] Nursing Mirror, 133, 3 Dec 1971, 17–18.

9 Roberts, G. A year in post. [Role of the nursing officer.] Nursing Mirror, 137, 28 Sep 1973, 38–40.

10 Taylor, V. R. E. In-service training: preparation of the nursing officer. Nursing Mirror, 136, 25 May 1973, 41–42.

11 Wilson-Barnett, J. A description of the working environment and work of the unit nursing officer. [Research study.] International Journal of Nursing Studies, 10 (3), Aug 1973, 185–192.

12 Wilson-Barnett, J. An enquiry into the job of the unit nursing officer in the Scottish Hospital Service. MSc (Soc.Sc.) thesis, Edinburgh University, 1972.

13 Wilson-Barnett, J. The work of the unit nursing officer. Nursing Times, 69, 21 Jun 1973, Occ. papers, 97–99; 28 Jun 1973, Occ. papers, 101–103.

h POLICY AND PLANNING

1 Asprec, E. S. The process of change: supervisors and managers can learn to minimize resistance and maximize cooperation. Supervisor Nurse, 6 (10), Oct 1975, 15–16, 18–24.

2 Brunner, L. S. A guide to writing your policy manual. RN Magazine, 37 (4), Apr 1974, OR1, OR4, OR6.

3 Colledge, M. Policy making and management. Nursing Times, 69, 15 Mar 1973, Occ. papers, 41–43.

4 Colls, J. Future shock invades nursing. [Coping with stress produced by rapid organizational change.] Journal of Nursing Administration, 5 (3), Mar/Apr 1975, 27–28.

5 Frey, M. Administration in nursing service – the stimulus for change. International Nursing Review, 22 (2), Mar/Apr 1975, 50–53.

6 Haiman-Elkind, H. Changing the structure of nursing services. [Experimentation at the 700 bed hospital of the Hadassah Hebrew University Medical Centre in Jerusalem.] Nursing Times, 70, 31 Oct 1974, 1712–1713.

7 Labovitz, G. H. How to improve your management effectiveness in coping with change. Hospital Topics, 52 (7), Jul/Aug 1974, 24–27, 36, 40–41.

8 May, K. Optimizing nurse effectiveness: nursing reorganization at Borgess Hospital, Kalamazoo, Michigan Hospital Progress, 55 (5), May 1974, 38, 40.

9 Moore, M. Standard 3. Policies . . . guidelines for action. Journal of Nursing Administration, 11 (3), May/Jun 1972, 29–33.

10 Morrison, I. L. Planning an effective nursing service. Nigerian Nurse, 4 (1), Jan/Mar 1972, 28–30.

11 Mussallem, H. K. The nurse's role in policy making and planning. International Nursing Review, 20 (1), Jan/Feb 1973, 9–11.

12 National League for Nursing Division of Community Planning Developing strategies to effect change: presentations at the 1973 forum for nursing service administrators in the West. New York: The League, 1974.

13 Nehls, D. and others Planned change: a quest for nursing autonomy. [Reorganization of the nursing department in a large university hospital in the USA.] Journal of Nursing Administration, 4 (1), Jan/Feb 1974, 23–27.

14 Poulin, M. A. Nursing service: change or managerial obsolescence. [Future demands on the administrator of nursing services.] Journal of Nursing Administration, 4 (4), Jul/Aug 1974, 40–43.

15 Ramphal, M. Clinical and administrative judgment. American Journal of Nursing, 72 (9), Sep 1972, 1606–1611.

16 Seivwright, M. J. The nurses' participation in policy making. Jamaican Nurse, 12 (2), Aug 1972, 12–14.

17 Seivwright, M. J. A nurse's role in policy making and planning. Jamaican Nurse, 13 (3), Dec 1973/Jan 1974, 10, 23.

18 Stevens, B. J. Effecting change. [Procedures for the nurse administrator.] Journal of Nursing Administration, 5 (2), Feb 1975, 23–26.

19 Thomson, W. Management for nurses. 4 and 5. The planning team. Nursing Mirror 134, 5 May 1972, 38–39; 12 May 1972, 44–45.

20 Watkin, B. Management topics. Change. Nursing Mirror, 139, 9 Aug 1974, 54.

21 World Health Organization Planning and programming for nursing services. Geneva: WHO, 1971. (Public health papers no. 44.)

i SALMON REPORT

1 Bagley, C. Nursing the Salmon Way. Health and Social Service Journal, 84, 16 Feb 1974, 359–360.

2 Boorer, D. and Boorer, J. Lines of communication. [Salmon in Cornwall.] Nursing Times, 69, 25 Oct 1973, 1397–1399.

3 Brain, M. A. 'Salmon'. Midwives Chronicle, 86, Mar 1972, 80–81.

4 British Medical Journal Practicalities of nursing. [Leading article on the effects of the Salmon report.] British Medical Journal, 3, 4 Sep 1971, 545–546. Correspondence from I. G. Bryce, M. M. Collidge, 20 Oct 1971, 50; 23 Oct 1971, 237.

5 British Medical Journal Salmon – a two-pronged trident? [Criticism of the report and comment on DHSS 'Progress on Salmon'.] British Medical Journal, 4, 21 Oct 1972, 125–126.

6 Carr, A. Salmon – a leap into the future. Nursing Times, 67, 15 Apr 1971, 454–456.

7 Cormack, D. Salmon – for and against. 1. Management – for nurses? Nursing Mirror, 133, 10 Dec 1971, 25–26.

8 Dee, J. A tale of modern medicine. [A matron's experiences after Salmon reorganization.] New Statesman, 84, 15 Sep 1972, 353.

9 Department of Health and Social Security and Welsh Office Progress on Salmon: a report. The Department, 1972.

10 Emery, J. J. Open forum – what price Salmon now? Nursing Mirror, 134, 19 May 1972, 13.

11 MEvans, E. 'Salmon'. Midwives Chronicle, 86, Apr 1972, 118–119.

12 Garrett, S. Salmon – blueprint to reality. Nursing Times, 68, 27 Jan 1972, Occ. papers, 13–16.

13 Goodland, N. L. Some views on the Salmon structure. Nursing Mirror, 133, 30 Jul 1971, 9–10.

14 Hamilton, D. Salmon and Salmonitis: an attempt at clarification. [Comment from a clinical psychologist, 472.] Occupational Therapy, 25 (7), Jul 1972, 485–486.

15 Haslock, I. Personal view. [The Salmon report seen by a medical research fellow.] British Medical Journal, 4, 14 Oct 1972, 106.

16 Hatton, D. An over 40's view of 'Salmon'. Nursing Times, 68, 20 Jan 1972, 93.

17 Hickey, N. M. 'Salmon'. Midwives Chronicle, 86, Feb 1972, 50–51.

18 Hospital and Health Services Review Organization of nursing. [Progress on Salmon and nurses in an integrated health service.] Hospital and Health Services Review, 68 (11), Nov 1972, 389–392.

19 IHA East of Scotland Branch Study Group Report Implementation of Salmon. Hospital, 65 (5), May 1970, 174–176.

20 Imrie, V. J. Salmon – for and against. 2. Leave it to the administrator. Nursing Mirror, 133, 10 Dec 1971, 26–27, 31.

21 Jacobson, B. Nursing by numbers. [Criticism of the Salmon structure.] World Medicine, 9, 5 Jun 1974, 46, 48, 51–52, 54.

22 Jarrett, R. The Salmon structure. [Comments of an outside observer.] Nursing Mirror, 134, 16 Jun 1972, 17.

23 Jefferies, P. M. Personal view. [Salmon scheme and the ward sister.] British Medical Journal, 3, 7 Aug 1971, 367.

24 Kavalier, F. How many chiefs is too many chiefs? [The Salmon report and it implementation and the work of consultants in Australia.] Nursing Times, 69, 4 Jan 1973, 17–19.

25 King's Fund Centre Meetings on the Salmon structure, 1971–1972. The Centre, 1971–1972. (THC reprints 540, 623, 685, 699, 748.)

26 Kings Fund Centre No. 9 – jam in the sandwich? [Meeting of Principal Nursing Officers.] Nursing Mirror, 132, 12 Feb 1971, 14–15.

27 Lee, B. F. Think again on Salmon. [Letter.] British Medical Journal, 1, 2 Feb 1974, 202.

28 Lyall, A. The ward sister. [Letter concerning BMA policy on the Salmon report and its implementation.] British Medical Journal, 3, 28 Aug 1971, 534.

29 McCarrick, H. Salmon versus the doctors. [Debate held by the Medical Journalists' Association on Feb 15 when speakers included Brian Salmon and Dame Muriel Powell.] Nursing Times, 70, 28 Feb 1974, 296–297.

30 Marne, C. The road back. [A nurse's experiences of the problems of Salmon reorganization.] Nursing Mirror, 141, 17 Jul 1975, 64.

31 Paulley, J. W. Is it too late to scrap Salmon – a charter for incompetents? Nursing Times, 67, 18 Feb 1971, 212–213.

32 Pembrey, S. The Salmon report: effect on organization and recruitment of nurses. Nightingale Fellowship Journal, 84, Jan 1971, 177–180.

33 Royal College of Nursing Salmon under scrutiny.

Report of a conference held at Towers Hospital, Leicester, September 1970. Nursing Mirror, 131, 25 Sep 1970, 15–18.

34 Scottish Home and Health Department Review of the senior nursing staff structure. (Salmon Report). Edinburgh: The Department, 1974.

35 Subiar, J. J. What Salmon did. [Conversation between two tutors which concludes that the Salmon report created a sterile career structure.] Nursing Times, 68, 5 Oct 1972, 1268–1269.

36 Temple, L. J. Think again on Salmon. [Letter.] British Medical Journal, 4, 29 Dec 1973, 786.

37 Wall, T. and Hespe, G. The attitudes of nurses towards the Salmon report. Nursing Times, 68, 6 Jul 1972, Occ. papers, 105–108.

38 Wherry, C. E. B. Open forum – Hello Salmon! Nursing Mirror, 132, 15 Jan 1971, 17.

j WARD MANAGEMENT

1 Ajadi, T. A. Improved nursing care of patients: a ward sister's responsibility. Nigerian Nurse, 5 (2), Apr/Jun 1973, 37–38.

2 Brinham, R. O. J. Looking at ward activity. Nursing Times, 68, 14 Sep 1972, 1154–1155.

3 Clissold, B. G. Ward Eight – Bevendean Hospital. Nursing Times, 68, 30 Nov 1972, 1524–1525.

4 Dann, N. Ward sisters discuss the process of administration and its application to promote quality patient care. Jamaican Nurse, 15 (1), May 1975, 7, 9.

5 En, M. C. K. The threefold role of the ward sister as a nurse, an administrator and a teacher. Nursing Journal of Singapore, 12 (2), Nov 1972, 103–105.

6 Frost, M. New ward sisters – and old ward sisters. Nursing Times, 67, 18 Feb 1971, 216–217.

7 Harvey, F. M. and Girling-Butcher, A. We uncovered treasure: an experiment in ward management at Cook Hospital, Gisborne. New Zealand Nursing Journal, 66 (10), Oct 1973, 26–27.

8 Hunter, B. The administration of hospital wards: factors influencing length of stay in hospital. Manchester: Manchester University Press, 1972. (Studies in social administration.)

9 Manchester Regional Hospital Board A handbook of ward management. Manchester, The Board, 1971.

10 Murphy, J. The role of the ward sister. Nursing Mirror, 140, 13 Feb 1975, 71–72.

11 Redgard, J. A day in the life of a ward sister. Health, 8 (2), Summer 1971, 37–38.

12 Rosaire, M. The ward sister as an ideal evaluator. Australian Nurses' Journal, 2 (5), Nov 1972, 32–33.

13 Swaffield, L. Teamtalk. [Experiments at West Middlesex Hospital in ward teamwork involving multi-disciplinary meetings.] Nursing Times, 71, 3 Jul 1975, 1036.

k UNIT MANAGEMENT AND HEAD NURSE (US)

1 Aydelotte, M. K. Administration and directors of nursing. Hospitals, 48, 16 Dec 1974, 61–63.

2 Barrett, J. and others The head nurse: her leadership role. New York: Appleton-Century-Crofts, 1975.

3 Behrens, A. D. The pleasures and problems of the director of nursing in a small hospital. Journal of Nursing Administration, 5 (2), Feb 1975, 31–34.

4 Ganong, J. and Ganong, W. Are head nurses obsolete? Journal of Nursing Administration, 5 (7), Sep 1975, 16–18.

5 Ganong, J. W. and Ganong, W. Help for the head nurse: a management guide. 2nd ed. Chapel Hill: W. L. Ganong, 1974.

6 Garfield, S. R. An ideal nursing unit. Hospitals, 45 (12), 16 Jun 1971, 80–82, 84–86.

7 Germaine, A. Who should manage the patient unit? Hospital Administration in Canada, 13 (3), Mar 1971, 76, 78.

8 Germaine, A. Why not a unit service co-ordinator? Hospital Administration in Canada, 14, 6, Jun 1972, 56, 62.

9 Hilgar, E. E. Unit management systems. Journal of Nursing Administration, 11 (1), Jan/Feb 1972, 43–49.

10 Hospitals A profile of the nursing service administrator. Hospitals, 48 (9), May 1974, 65–66, 68, 114.

11 Marcinszyn, C. Decentralization of nursing service. Journal of Nursing Administration, 1 (4), Jul/Aug 1971, 17–24.

12 Marylander, S. J. The dual role of the director of nursing. Hospitals, 48, 1 Jul 1974, 119–120, 124.

13 Peterson, G. G. The director of nursing should be a nurse. American Journal of Nursing, 73 (11), Nov 1973, 1902–1904.

14 Stevens, B. J. The head nurse as manager. Journal of Nursing Administration, 4 (1), Jan/Feb 1974, 36–40.

15 Tamez, E. G. How does the unit manager system affect the head nurse? Supervisor Nurse, 6 (9), Sep 1975, 34–40.

11 STAFFING

a GENERAL

1 Aydelotte, M. K. Nurse staffing methodology: a review and critique of selected literature. Washington: Department of Health, Education and Welfare, 1973.

2 Aydelotte, M. K. Standard 1. Staffing for quality care. Journal of Nursing Administration, 3 (2), Mar/Apr 1973, 33–36.

3 Borgmeyer, W. A. E. Charting manpower. [Techniques of manpower planning for nursing administrators.] Health and Social Service Journal, 85, 20/27 Dec 1975, 2788.

4 Cobb, P. W. and Warner, D. M. Task substitution among skill classes of nursing personnel. Nursing Research, 22 (2), Mar/Apr 1973, 130–137.

5 Germaine, A. Staffing patterns and mobility of nursing personnel. Hospital Administration in Canada, 17 (5), May 1975, 46, 48, 50.

6 O'Dwyer, E. Staffing structures within the hospitals' service. World of Irish Nursing, 3 (8), Aug 1974, 143–144.

7 Price, E. M. Staffing: the most basic nursing service problem. Supervisor Nurse, 6 (7), Jul 1975, 26–31.

8 Revans, R. W. and Cortazzi, D. Psychosocial factors in hospitals and nurse staffing. [Human problems in hospitals.] International Journal of Nursing Studies, 10 (3), Aug 1973, 149–158.

9 Warstler, M. E. compiler Staffing: a 'Journal of Nursing Administration' reader. Wakefield, Massachusetts: Wafefield Publishing, 1974.

b INTERPROFESSIONAL RELATIONSHIPS

1 Aradine, C. R. and Pridham, K. F. Model for collaboration. [Joint problem-solving for nurses and physicians.] Nursing Outlook, 21 (10), Oct 1973, 655–657.

2 Bergman, R. and others Opinion on nursing. [Survey among nurses, doctors and medical students in an attempt to examine ways to improve nurse/doctor co-operation.] International Nursing Review, 18 (3), 1971, 195–227.

3 Brink, P. J. Natural triad in health care. [Doctor-nurse-patient-relationship.] American Journal of Nursing, 72 (5), May 1972, 897–899.

4 Coleman, V. Nurses' little red book? [A doctor's view of nursing protocol and attitudes.] Nursing Times, 67, 27 May 1971, 652.

5 Cross, Y. Rogue nurses. The day of 'Sir' is over. [Relations between nurses and doctors discussed.] Nursing Mirror, 134, 24 Mar 1972, 16–17.

6 Davidson, G. E. Collaborating with the medical staff in developing standards of care. Nursing Clinics of North America, 8 (2), Jun 1973, 219–225.

7 Frank, R. K. Societal and educational challenges to health care personnel in the United States. [The combination of good relations between the health professions in an effective health service.] International Nursing Review, 19 (2), 1972, 180–185.

8 Graf, R. The nurse–doctor relationship: a doctor's view. [Difficulties of a houseman.] Nursing Times, 70, 31 Jan 1974, 151.

9 Health and Social Service Journal Administration. Nurse's working relationships with health service administrators. [Leading article.] Health and Social Service Journal, 84, 2 Nov 1974, 2530.

10 Hoekelman, R. A. Nurse–physician relationships. American Journal of Nursing, 75 (7), Jul 1975, 1150–1152.

11 Joint Symposium on Nursing and the Medical Profession [Report of conference organised by the Royal College of Nursing and other Royal Colleges.] British Medical Journal, 4, 7 Dec 1974, 550–551; Nursing Mirror, 139, 5 Dec 1974, Nursing Times, 70, 5 Dec 1974, 1875.

12 Kahn, J. H. Team work: theoretical and practical issues. [Collaboration between different professions.] Medical Officer, 125, 8 Jan 1971, 25–26.

13 Kalisch, B. J. Of half gods and mortals: aesculapian authority. [The authoritarian relationship of the doctor to the patient and the implications for the nurse.] Nursing Outlook, 23 (1), Jan 1975, 22–28; Canadian Nurse, 71 (6), Jun 1975, 20–26.

14 Lee, S. A. and Likeman, C. A. Open forum. [Problems of communication between doctor, patient and nurse.] Nursing Mirror, 133, 15 Oct 1971, 24–26.

15 Lewis, H. L. Nurses: how much like doctors? [Problems of nursing staff-hospital management relations in the United States.] Modern Healthcare, 3 (6), Jun 1975, 45–49.

16 Lynaugh, J. E. and Bates, B. The two languages of nursing and medicine. American Journal of Nursing, 73 (1), Jan 1973, 68–69.

17 Metcalf, W. K. and others Doctor and nurse. [Letter.] Lancet, 1, 23 Jan 1971, 184.

18 Occupational Therapy Salmon and Salmonitis. [Relation between the work of nurses and occupational therapists under Salmon.] Occupational Therapy, 35 (4), Apr 1972, 225–226.

19 Parry-Jones, W. Ll. Human relations training in the general hospital. International Journal of Nursing Studies, 8 (3), Aug 1971, 153–160.

20 Pearse, F. Doctor nurse relationship: past, present and future. Nigerian Nurse, 7 (1), Jan/Mar 1975, 50–52.

21 Pluckan, M.L. Professional territoriality. 2. Problems affecting the delivery of health care. Nursing Forum, 11 (3), 1972, 300–310.

22 Powell, M. Nurses – Doctors: can they work in harmony? [Salmon and Cogwheel.] Nursing Times, 66, 10 Dec 1970, 1594–1596.

23 Raven, K. A. Doctors and nurses: a deteriorating relationship? [Report of a meeting between nurses and doctors.] Nursing Times, 68, 17 Feb 1972, 222.

24 Royal College of Nursing and British Medical Association Partners in patient care. Rcn/BMA conference. Nursing Times, 67, 9 Dec 1971, 1543–1545; British Medical Journal, 4, 4 Dec 1971, 616–618. mon.] Occupational Therapy, 35 (4), Apr 1972, 225–226.

25 Searle, D. J. Nurses and doctors – can they work in harmony? Rcn/BMA conference on Harmony in management – Salmon and Cogwheel. Nursing Mirror, 131, 11 Dec 1970, 13–14; 18 Dec 1970, 17–18.

26 Smoyak, S. A. The confrontation process. [Regarded as a means of restoring autonomy to the nurse in relation to other professionals such as doctors.] American Journal of Nursing, 74 (9), Sep 1974, 1632–1635.

27 Stubbs, V. and Rathbone, W. Social skills at work. [Human relationships in the work situation.] Nursing Mirror, 139, 12 Dec 1974, 43–46.

28 Subiar, J. J. So Ko Lo but Sob. [Nurses' difficulty in interpreting doctors' notes.] Nursing Mirror, 136, 22 Jun 1973, 45–46.

29 Trop, J. L. Consultation to groups in conflict: some aspects of group design. [Solving the problem of conflict between a ward sister and her staff nurses.] Journal of Psychiatric Nursing and Mental Health Services, 13 (6), Nov/Dec 1975, 11–15.

30 Varga The nurse–doctor relationship. Nursing Times, 70, 10 Jan 1974, 44–48.

31 Veninga, R. The management of conflict [in hospital staff relationships]. Journal of Nursing Administration, 3 (4), Jul/Aug 1973, 13–16.

32 Young, P. Nursing and the medical profession – a discussion of mutual problems. [Report of a joint conference between the Royal College of Nursing, Midwives, Surgeons, Physicians, Obstetricians and Gynaecologists.] Nursing Mirror, 139, 5 Dec 1974, 36–37.

c JOB DESCRIPTIONS AND JOB EVALUATION

1 Carr, A. Writing a job description. Nursing Times, 67, 10 Jun 1971, Occ. papers, 89–92.

2 Germaine, A. Job descriptions for RNs. Hospital Administration in Canada, 14 (11), Nov 1972, 61–62, 64.

3 Hamilton, D. Job descriptions and their use in nursing. Nursing Times, 67, 27 May 1971, Occ. papers, 81–82.

4 Hanrahan, K. A. Are job descriptions necessary in Irish nursing? World of Irish Nursing, 3 (2), Feb 1974, 29; (3), Mar 1974, 44–45.

5 New York State Nurses Association. Council on Nursing Practice New position descriptions in nursing. Journal of Nursing Administration, 3 (6), Nov/Dec 1973, 17–20.

6 Roberts, T. How good are job descriptions? British Hospital Journal and Social Service Review, 81, 17 Apr 1971, 717–718.

7 Steel, B. W. A systematic analysis of job descriptions for nursing management: how to produce them (and) how to use them. Watford: Paul Hill, 1971.

8 Stevens, B. J. A second look at 'New position descriptions in nursing.' [Produced by the New York State Nurses Association.] Journal of Nursing Administration, 3 (6), Nov/Dec 1973, 21–23.

9 Watkin, B. Management topics. Job descriptions. Nursing Mirror, 138, 26 Apr 1974, 81.

10 Watkin, B. Management topics. Job evaluation. Nursing Mirror, 138, 24 May 1974, 60.

d JOB SATISFACTION

1 Benton, D. A. and White, H. C. Satisfaction of job factors for registered nurses. Journal of Nursing Administration, 11 (6), Nov/Dec 1972, 55–63.

2 Carey, R. G. Measuring organizational climate. [A survey to measure effective performance and job satisfaction and to identify problem areas.] Hospital Progress, 56 (2), Feb 1975, 53–57.

3 Frost, M. Job satisfaction. [The disappointments and gratifications of a nursing career.] Nursing Mirror, 137, 2 Nov 1973, 9.

4 Gaynor, A. K. and Berry, R. K. Observations of a staff nurse: an organizational analysis [of patterns of work and interpersonal relations in an attempt to reduce nursing turnover]. Journal of Nursing Administration, 3 (3), May/Jun 1973, 43–49.

5 Hines, G. H. Motivational influences in job satisfaction [in full and part time nurses.] New Zealand Nursing Journal, 68 (6), Jun 1974, 18–20.

6 Hurka, S. J. Organizational environment and work satisfaction. [Survey among nurses in Saskatchewan.] Dimensions in Health Service, 51 (1), Jan 1974, 41–43.

7 Jehring, J. J. Motivational problems in the modern hospital. Journal of Nursing Administration, 11 (6), Nov/Dec 1972, 35–41.

8 Levenstein, A. Job satisfaction and hospital loyalty. Supervisor Nurse, 6 (6), Jun 1975, 8–9, 12.

9 Longest, B. B. Job satisfaction for registered nurses in the hospital setting. Journal of Nursing Administration, 4 (3), May/Jun 1974, 46–52.

10 Lysaught, J. P. No carrots, no sticks: motivation in nursing. Journal of Nursing Administration, 11 (5), Sep/Oct 1972, 43–50.

11 McCloskey, J. C. What rewards will keep nurses on the job? [A study by questionnaire to examine job satisfaction.] American Journal of Nursing, 75 (4), Apr 1975, 600–602.

12 MacDonald, M. R. Matching personalities with position: a study of job satisfaction. [A study of 14 nurses at middle management level.] Supervisor Nurse, 6 (4), Apr 1975, 43–45, 47, 50.

13 Munson, F. C. and Heda, S. S. An instrument for measuring nursing satisfaction. Nursing Research, 23 (2), Mar/Apr 1974, 159–166.

14 Slocum, J. W. and others An analysis of need satisfaction and job performance among professional and paraprofessional hospital personnel. Nursing Research, 21 (4), Jul/Aug 1972, 338–342.

15 Taylor, M. Motivation at all levels. Australian Nurses' Journal, 2 (8), Feb 1973, 28–31.

16 Thomas, B. Job satisfaction and float assignments. Journal of Nursing Administration, 11 (5), Sep/Oct 1972, 51–59.

17 Watkin, B. Management topics. Attitude surveys. Nursing Mirror, 138, 14 Jun 1974, 55.

18 Watkin, B. Management topics. Motivation. Nursing Mirror, 138, 5 Apr 1974, 75.

19 White, C. H. and Maquire, M. C. Job satisfaction and dissatisfaction among hospital nursing supervisors: the applicability of Herzberg's theory. Nursing Research, 22 (1), Jan/Feb 1973, 25–30.

e STAFF APPRAISAL

1 Albrecht, S. Reappraisal of conventional performance appraisal systems. Journal of Nursing Administration, 11 (2), Mar/Apr 1972, 29–35.

2 Bernhardt, J. and Schuette, L. PET A method of evaluating professional nurse performance. [Point Evaluation Tool developed at the University of Michigan, Ann Arbor.] Journal of Nursing Administration, 5 (8), Oct 1975, 18–21.

3 Blackstock, B. Staff appraisal. [Scheme of the Preston and Chorley Hospital Management Committee.] Nursing Mirror, 136, 4 May 1973, 45.

4 Blenkinsop, D. Nursing staff appraisal in the Durham group of hospitals. Nursing Times, 69, 5 Jul 1973, Occ papers, 105–108.

5 Bowman, M. P. I'm all right Jack: the art of effective appraisal. Nursing Mirror, 136, 15 Jun 1973, 14–15.

6 Caple, J. Job performance review scheme. 1. [The aims and procedures of a scheme developed for district nurses at Waltham Forest.] Nursing Times, 71, 13 Mar 1975, Occ. papers, 17–20.

7 Department of Health and Social Security. National Nursing Staff Committee Staff appraisal in the hospital nursing service: explanatory notes. DHSS, 1971.

8 Dyer, E. D. and others Can job performance be predicted from biographical, personality and administrative climate inventories? Nursing Research, 21 (4), Jul/Aug 1972, 294–304.

9 Foulds, J. How am I doing? [Staff appraisal schemes in the community nursing services.] Health Visitor, 47 (3), Mar 1974, 70–71.

10 Ganong, J., Ganong, W. and Huenefeld, J. Motive force: a key to evaluating nurse managers. Journal of Nursing Administration, 4 (4), Jul/Aug 1974, 17–19.

11 Ho, K. G. A study of work performance. Nursing Journal of Singapore, 15 (1), May 1975, 25–27.

12 Howarth, J. and others Staff appraisal – a participative approach. Hospital and Health Service Review, 70 (9), Sep 1974, 311–314.

13 Kimball, S. J. and others Evaluation of staff performance. American Journal of Nursing, 71 (9), Sep 1971, 1744–1746.

14 Lemin, B. Staff appraisal. Nursing Times, 67, 22 Apr 1971, Occ. papers, 61–64.

15 McCarville, M. Performance appraisals work. [For operating room staff.] Dimensions in Health Service, 52 (2), Feb 1975, 51.

16 Maisey, P. W. People processing. [Criticism of National Nursing Staff Committee booklet on staff appraisal.] Nursing Times, 68, 16 Nov 1972, 1462–1464.

17 Pankratz, D. Effects of coaching nursing service personnel. [On performance.] Nursing Research, 20 (6), Nov/Dec 1971, 517–521.

18 Saffer, J. B. and Saffer, L. D. Academic record

as a predictor of future job performance of nurses. Nursing Research, 21 (5), Sep/Oct 1972, 457–462.

19 Stubbs, V. Staff appraisal for community nursing staff. Queen's Nursing Journal, 16 (9), Dec 1973, 205–206, 208–209.

20 Taylor, J. W. Outcome criteria as a measurement of nurse performance. [Reprinted from the Journal of the New York State Nurses' Association.] Nursing Digest, 3 (5), Sep/Oct 1975, 41–45.

21 Verralls, S. Understanding staff appraisal. [A two-day training course in appraisal techniques by North West Metropolitan Regional Hospital Board.] Nursing Times, 68, 9 Nov 1972, 1424–1429.

22 Watkin, B. Management topics. Staff appraisal. Nursing Mirror, 138, 31 May 1974, 53.

23 Welches, L. J. and others Typological prediction of staff nurse performance rating. [A study of 650 staff nurses from 15 hospitals in San Francisco.] Nursing Research, 23 (5), Sep/Oct 1974, 402–409.

f STAFF SELECTION AND DEVELOPMENT

1 Anderson, M. I. and Denyes, M. J. A ladder for clinical advancement in nursing practice: implementation. [Operation of the system at University of Wisconsin which reallocated nurses to advanced clinical staff nurse level.] Journal of Nursing Administration, 5 (2), Feb 1975, 16–22.

2 Bigham, G. D. Developing staff and records where traditional roles are changing. Journal of Nursing Administration, 3 (1), Jan/Feb 1973, 36–48.

3 Bowman, M. P. Is interviewing enough? [Staff selection in nursing.] Nursing Times, 67, 14 Oct 1971, 1275.

4 Carr, A. J. Check list for appointment of nursing staff. Nursing Times, 68, 1 Jun 1972, Occ. papers, 85–87.

5 Casey, B. J. What is the head nurse's key role in effective staff development? Hospital Topics, 53 (6), Nov/Dec 1975, 24.

6 Christie, L. S. Preparation for promotion. Nursing Mirror, 134, 2 Jun 1972, 23–24.

7 Cicatiello, J. S. A. The personal development interview. Supervisor Nurse, 6 (11), Nov 1975, 15–17, 21–24.

8 Gough, C. The nurse in personnel. World of Irish Nursing, 4 (5), May 1975, 6.

9 Hope, R. M. A study of the factors influencing the career decisions of the newly qualified staff nurse and their implications for staff development. MSc thesis Bath University, 1975.

10 Kowalski, K. E. Job interviewing: an effective tool for hiring staff nurses. Journal of Nursing Administration, 5 (1), Jan 1975, 28–32.

11 McClelland, M. Personnel department and nursing management. [Ipswich.] Nursing Times, 70, 25 Jul 1974, Occ. papers, 45–46.

12 Miller, M. H. and Bigler, H. F. Nurses beware: the Peter Principle may be upon you. [The concept that every employee tends to rise to his level of incompetence, as applied to nursing.] Journal of Nursing Administration, 4 (3), May/Jun 1974, 32–33.

13 Miller, R. Career ladder program: a problem solving device. Journal of Nursing Administration, 5 (5), Jun 1975, 27–29.

14 Reres, M. E. Personnel management: tapping human resources. Journal of Nursing Administration, 5 (6), Jul/Aug 1975, 18–19.

15 Reid, M. F. and Mutton, C. J. How to get the job you want. [Job applications and interviews.] Nursing Times, 70, 20 Jun 1974, 970–971.

16 Williams, R. C. and Giles, A. I. Team work at Sully. [Staff selection.] Nursing Times, 67, 1 Apr 1971, 396–397.

17 Tan, K. H. Personnel management and the nursing service. Nursing Journal of Singapore, 15 (1), May 1975, 50–52.

18 Watkin, B. Management topics. Development. Nursing Mirror, 139, 30 Aug 1974, 69.

19 Watkin, B. Management topics. Employment interviewing. Nursing Mirror, 138, 19 Apr 1974, 51.

20 Watkin, B. Management topics. Staff selection. Nursing Mirror, 138, 12 Apr 1974, 69.

g WORKLOAD, ESTABLISHMENT AND PATIENT DEPENDENCY

1 Auld, M. G. A method of estimating the requisite nursing establishment for a hospital. M. Phil thesis, Edinburgh University, 1974. (Published as 'How many nurses?' Rcn, 1976; Research series.)

2 Aydelotte, M. K. Staffing for high-quality care. How can we staff for high-quality care when we don't really know what quality is? Hospitals, 47 (2), 16 Jan 1973, 58, 60, 65.

3 Barr, A. and others A review of the various methods of measuring the dependency of patients on nursing staff. International Journal of Nursing Studies, 10 (3), Aug 1973, 195–208.

4 Boxall, S. F. Staff establishment: the unavoidable key. [Tools to analyze nursing care must now be used to predict staffing accurately.] Australian Nurses' Journal, 4 (6), Dec/Jan 1975, 34–37.

5 Bryant, Y. M. and Heron, K. Monitoring patient–nurse dependency. [Computer system designed to monitor short term variations in ward workloads.] Nursing Times, 70, 9 May 1974, Occ. papers, 1–4; 16 May 1974, Occ. papers, 5–7.

6 Calder, J. Measuring nursing workload. 1. A summary of the Rhys-Hearn method of assessing nursing workload based on nurse patient dependency studies. North West Thames Nursing Research Bulletin, 1, Feb 1974, 13–17.

7 Cochran, J. and Derr, D. Patient acuity system for nurse staffing. [Staffing method based on the time required to care for various types of patients.] Hospital Progress, 56 (11), Nov 1975, 51–54.

8 Ferres, S. B. Loeb Center and its philosophy of nursing. [The use of high quality nursing care at the post acute stages results in shorter hospitalization.] American Journal of Nursing, 75 (5), May 1975, 810–815.

9 Fine, R. B. Controlling nurses' workloads. American Journal of Nursing, 74 (12), Dec 1974, 2206–2207.

10 Gelder, R. Work sampling or utilization studies – a management tool for nursing administration. Canadian Hospital, 48 (2), Feb 1971, 44–45.

11 Gordon, I. Measuring nursing workload. 2. Nurse–patient dependency studies undertaken in the North West Metropolitan Region, based on the Rhys-Hearn method. North West Thames Nursing Research Bulletin, 1, Feb 1974, 18–22.

12 Gray, J. Nurse staffing in a teaching hospital: a study in measurement. MPhil thesis, Department of Sociology and Social Administration, Southampton University, 1974.

13 **Halter, H. H. L. E.** Nursing staff and work load. [Letter advocating adjustment of the workload to fit the staff available in an attempt to reduce nurse wastage.] British Medical Journal, 3, 31 Aug 1974, 580.

14 **Hassell, D.** Patient dependency related to nurse staffing in a MS hospital. Nursing Times, 67, 20 May 1971, Occ. papers, 77–80; 27 May 1971, Occ. papers, 83–84.

15 **Hockey, L.** Applying an economic model to nursing management. [Decisions on the appropriate combination of different grades of staff in a particular situation.] Nursing Times, 68, 27 Jul 1972, 946–948.

16 **Hope, M.** Nurse utilization study. [Use of the American Resource Monitoring System for assessing staffing requirements in three Sydney hospitals.] Lamp, 32 (12), Dec 1975, 14–17, 28.

17 **Howarth, M. H.** Report on a study of nursing workload and staff deployment in Manchester Royal Eye Hospital, 1969–1972. The author, 1972.

18 **King's Fund Centre** Nurse–patient dependency studies: report on a seminar. The Centre, 1972 (THC reprint 654.)

19 **Laberge-Nadeau, C. and Feuvrier, M.** A simulation study of nursing staff utilization. Canadian Hospital, 49 (5), May 1972, 54–57.

20 **Laberge-Nadeau, C. and Feuvrier, M.** Utilization of a MEDSIM program in a task study of nursing staff. Canadian Hospital, 49 (5), May 1972, 58, 60, 62–64.

21 **Lebourdais, E.** Patient classification does not work. [Staffing arrangements advocated by Dr. Elmina Price.] Dimensions in Health Service, 51 (5), May 1974, 50–51.

22 **Lippert, S.** Nurses' travel. [A method to reduce the distance covered by nursing staff in the course of their work.] Journal of Nursing Administration, 11 (2), Mar/Apr 1972, 36–41.

23 **Lockett, R. W.** Assessment of patients' dependency in relation to nurse staffing levels in a hospital group caring for the mentally handicapped. Nursing Times, 68, 13 Apr 1972, Occ. papers, 57–60.

24 **McCormick, P. and others** Predicting nurse staffing. At Washington Hospital Center a system for predicting nurse staffing takes into account patients' direct and indirect care needs. Hospitals, 47 (9), 1 May 1973, 68, 73–74, 77–79.

25 **MacGuire, J.** Nurse-patient dependency measures: a management tool. King's Fund Centre, 1973 (KFC reprint 776.)

26 **McPhail, A.** The meaning of patient classification. [For assessing nursing needs.] Dimensions in Nursing Service, 52 (6), Jun 1975, 30–31, 39.

27 **Minetti, R. and Hutchinson, J.** System achieves optimal staffing. [A patient classification system results in distribution of nursing staff according to requirements.] Hospitals, 49 (9), 1 May 1975, 61–62, 64.

28 **Mulligan, B.** How many nurses equal enough? [Measurement of patient dependency and workload index using Barr method.] Nursing Times, 68, 13 Apr 1972, 428–430.

29 **Mulligan, B.** Measurement of patient–nurse dependency and work load index: an explanatory booklet demonstrating two practical applications of patient–nurse dependency classification in controlling work load for wards and nursing units. King's Fund Centre, 1974. (Project paper 2.)

30 **Murray, F. A. and others** Nurses and their workload. [A study carried out at St. Mary's Hospital, Portsmouth.] Health and Social Service Journal, 84, 23 Nov 1974, 2723–2724.

31 **Nield, M.** Developing a projected nurse staff program. [To determine the personnel required.] Supervisor Nurse, 6 (7), Jul 1975, 17–18, 20–24.

32 **Norwich, H. S. and Senior, O. E.** Determining nursing establishment. [Based on Barr method.] Nursing Times, 67, 4 Feb 1971, Occ. papers, 17–20.

33 **Porcheron, Y.** An approach to patient care classification. Hospital Administration in Canada, 15 (4), Apr 1973, 26, 28.

34 **Price, J.** Patient care classification system. Nursing Outlook, 20 (7), Jul 1972, 445–448.

35 **Rhys Hearn, C.** Evaluating patients' nursing needs: an assessment of nursing workload based on nurse patient dependency studies leading to prediction of staffing requirements. Nursing Times, 68, 27 Apr 1972, Occ. papers, 65–68.

36 **Rhys Hearn, C.** Evaluation of patients' nursing needs: a prediction of staffing. In McLachlan, G. editor. Problems and progress in medical care: essays on current research. Ninth series. Oxford University Press for Nuffield Provincial Hospitals Trust, 1973. Reprinted in Nursing Times, 70, 19 Sep 1974; 26 Sep 1974; 3 Oct 1974; 10 Oct 1974, Occ. papers, 69–75, 77–84.

37 **Rhys Hearn, C.** How many high-care patients? 1. How Birmingham tackles the problem. [Method of collecting information on patient care requirements in order to assess nursing workload.] Nursing Times, 68, 20 Apr 1972, 472–474.

38 **Rhys Hearn, C.** How many high-care patients? 2. Deployment of nursing staff. Nursing Times, 68, 27 Apr 1972, 504–505.

39 **Rhys Hearn, C.** West Midlands nursing resource study. [Assessment of nursing needs and their relationship to nurse staffing requirements.] North West Thames Nursing Research Bulletin, 3, Spring 1975, 24–29.

40 **Ryan, T. and others** A system for determining appropriate nurse staffing. [By assessment of patient's needs and flexibility of staff allocation.] Journal of Nursing Administration, 5 (5), Jun 1975, 30–38.

41 **Sax, S. and Johnson, S.** Nursing in general hospital wards. [Most effective methods of utilizing available manpower. The findings of a New South Wales report.] Lamp, 29 (8), Aug 1972, 35–43.

42 **Sheppard, R.** Nurses help conduct time study [to facilitate the calculation of a workload index]. Hospital Topics, 53 (3), May/Jun 1975, 4–5.

43 **Sullivan, M. T. and Boyle, M. A.** Establishment setting and control in small hospitals. Nursing Times, 67, 15 Jul 1971, Occ. papers, 109–111.

44 **Trivedi, V. M. and Hancock, W. M.** Measurement of nursing workload using head nurses' perceptions. Nursing Research, 24 (5), Sep/Oct 1975, 371–376.

45 **Wagner, K.** Work study from a nurse's point of view. SA Nursing Journal, 40 (12), Dec 1973, 15, 17, 39.

46 **Wandel, S.E. and Hershey, J. C.** Quantitative procedures for nurse staffing management: a survey. Stanford: Stanford University School of Medicine, 1975.

NURSE AND PATIENT

12 PATIENT CARE

a GENERAL

1 Copp, L. A. Improvement of care through evaluation. Change of shift report. Bedside Nurse, 5 (2), Feb 1972, 19–23.

2 Copp, L. A. Improving nursing care through evaluation. 2. As you make nursing rounds. Bedside Nurse, 5 (6), Jun 1972, 25–28.

3 Copp, L. A. Improved patient care through evaluation. 3. Your plan of nursing care. Bedside Nurse, 5 (9), Sep 1972, 25–29.

4 Cowper-Smith, F. Nurse caring: lessons to be learned today. Nursing Mirror Forum '75. Nursing Mirror, 141, 2 Oct 1975, 35.

5 Dodge, R. H. and Nadler, G. A descriptive model of patient care. Hospital Management, Jun 1971, 14–20.

6 Eckelberry, G. K. Administration of comprehensive nursing care: the nature of professional practice. New York: Appleton-Century-Crofts, 1971.

7 Germaine, A. What method of nursing is best for you? [Discussion of the concepts of case, functional and team methods.] Hospital Administration in Canada, 17 (3), Mar 1975, 34–36.

8 Goodwin, P. The need for compassion. [A personal view of the deterioration in nursing care.] Nursing Mirror, 141, 11 Dec 1975, 71.

9 Joy, P. M. Maintaining continuity of care during shift change. Journal of Nursing Administration, 5 (9), Nov/Dec 1975, 28–29.

10 Kraegel, J. M. and others Patient care systems. Philadelphia: Lippincott, 1974.

11 Linn, L. S. A survey of the 'Care-Cure' attitudes of physicians, nurses and their students. [An analysis of answers to ten statements about patient care.] Nursing Forum, 14 (2), 1975, 145–159.

12 McCarthy, R. T. A practice theory of nursing care. Nursing Research, 21 (5), Sep/Oct 1972, 406–410.

13 McFarlane, J. K. A charter for caring. [Nursing Lecture 1975.] Nursing Mirror, 141, 4 Dec 1975, 40–42.

14 Mary, J. An approach to general nursing care. World of Irish Nursing, 4 (7), Jul 1975, 7.

15 Mogli, G. D. and Andre, J. S. Organization of patient care in the ward. Nursing Journal of India, 62 (9), Sep 1971, 293–294, 302.

16 Nursing Clinics of North America Symposium on a systems approach to nursing. Nursing Clinics of North America, 6 (3), Sep 1971, 383–462.

17 Nursing Clinics of North America Symposium on the management and supervision of patient care. Nursing Clinics of North America, 8 (2), Jun 1973, 203–373.

18 Nursing Clinics of North America Symposium on nursing leaders look at clinical nursing. Nursing Clinics of North America, 6 (2), Jun 1971, 215–269.

19 Parsons, R. A study of nursing in general hospital wards. Lamp, 28 (8), Aug 1971, 21–26.

20 Shout, M. G. Do we learn to care? [Nursing Mirror Forum '75.] Nursing Mirror, 141, 2 Oct 1975, 50–51.

21 Taylor, A. J. W. A therapeutic community. [Adaptation of the therapeutic community in a general hospital to improve patient care.] New Zealand Nursing Journal, 68 (5), May 1975, 24–26.

22 Verhonick, P. J. Clinical studies in nursing: models, methods and madness. Nursing Research, 21 (6), Nov/Dec 1972, 490–493.

b NURSING PROCESS

1 Browning, M. H., compiler The nursing process in practice. New York: American Journal of Nursing, 1974. (Contemporary nursing series.)

2 Daubenmire, M. J. and King, I. M. Nursing process models: a systems approach. [In nurse education.] Nursing Outlook, 21 (8), Aug 1973, 512–517.

3 Deininger, J. M. The nursing process implementation and evaluation. Journal of Practical Nursing, 25 (12), Dec 1975, 18, 32.

4 Goodwin, J. O. and Edwards, B. S. Developing a computer program to assist the nursing process; Phase 1. From systems analysis to an expanding program. [A program to collect data and formulate diagnosis.] Nursing Research, 24 (4), Jul/Aug 1975, 299–305.

5 Hargreaves, I. The nursing process: the key to individualized care. [How nursing care as taught in schools of nursing, can be achieved in practice, with a brief review of the literature.] Nursing Times, 71, 28 Aug 1975, Occ. papers, 89–92.

6 Judy, M. G. Continuing education for the nursing process skills. Occupational Health Nursing, 23 (5), May 1975, 18, 40.

7 McFarlane, J. K. What do we mean by care? [Nursing Mirror Forum '75. Includes description of nursing process.] Nursing Mirror, 141, 2 Oct 1975, 47–48.

8 Marriner, A. The nursing process: a scientific approach to nursing care. St. Louis: Mosby, 1975.

9 Mauksch, I. G. and David, M. L. Prescription for survival. [The nursing process.] American Journal of Nursing, 72 (12), Dec 1972, 2189–2193.

10 Orlando, I. J. The discipline and teaching of nursing process: an evaluative study. New York: Putman, 1972.

11 Schaefer, J. The interrelatedness of decision making and the nursing process. [Decision making and the care plan must be involved with the patient who becomes a connecting link.] American Journal of Nursing, 74 (10), Oct 1974, 1852–1855.

c EVALUATION AND STANDARDS

1 American Nurses' Association and American Hospital Association Quality assurance for nursing care: proceedings of an Institute, October 29–31, 1973. Kansas City: The Association, 1974.

2 Bailit, H. and others Assessing the quality of care: an overview of recent developments and ultimate goals in the quality of care assessment, with special reference to the nurse practitioner. Nursing Outlook, 23 (3), Mar 1975, 153–159.

3 Barnett, D. Standards of nursing care – why are they falling? Nursing Mirror, 140, 26 Jun 1975, 58–60.

4 Bidwell, C. M. and Froebe, D. J. Development of an instrument for evaluating hospital nursing performance. Journal of Nursing Administration, 1 (5), Sep/Oct 1971, 10–15.

5 Bloch, D. Evaluation of nursing care in terms of process and outcome: issues in research and quality assurance. Nursing Research, 24 (4), Jul/Aug 1975, 256–263.

6 Caribbean Nurses Seminar Nursing care standards in the hospital area. Jamaican Nurse, 15 (1), May 1975, 24–25.

7 Carter, J. H. and others Standards of nursing care: a guide for evaluation. New York: Springer, 1972.

8 Cornell, S. A. Development of an instrument for measuring the quality of nursing care: a two-dimension Q instrument. [Spinal cord injured patients.] Nursing Research, 23 (2), Mar/Apr 1974, 108–117.

9 Curtis, J. and others A practical evaluation of nursing care as part of the nursing process. Journal of Nursing Education, 13 (3), Aug 1974, 11, 13–15.

10 Dyer, E. D. and others Increasing the quality of patient care through performance counseling and written goal setting. Nursing Research, 24 (2), Mar/Apr 1975, 139–144.

11 Frevert, E. I. and Galligan, K. A. Evaluation of nursing care: a primary nursing project. 2. Experiences of non-participant nurse observers. Supervisor Nurse, 6 (1), Jan 1975, 40–43.

12 Germaine, A. How do we assess the quality of care? Hospital Administration in Canada, 26 (9), Sep 1974, 42–44.

13 Gerson, L. W. Variation in the quantity of direct nursing care: results of a four-month study in three Newfoundland hospitals. Hospital Administration in Canada, 16 (4), Apr 1974, 36–38.

14 Gonnella, J. S. and Zeleznik, C. Factors involved in comprehensive patient care evaluation. Medical Care, 12 (11), Nov 1974, 928–934.

15 Hegyvary, S. T. and Haussmann, R. K. D. Monitoring nursing care quality. [New methodology focusing on the delivery of nursing care.] Journal of Nursing Administration, 5 (5), Jun 1975, 17–26.

16 Highman, A. Quality control in patient care. Hospital Administration in Canada, 13 (8), Aug 1971, 45–48.

17 Holdgate, E. Emphasis on quality. New Zealand Nurses Journal, 65 (7), Jul 1972, 5–7.

18 Jelinek, R. and others A methodology for monitoring quality of nursing care. Washington: US Department of Health, Education and Welfare, Division of Nursing, 1974.

19 Jenkinson, V. M. Select the right yard stick to measure nursing quality. Dimensions in Health Service, 52 (5), May 1975, 40–41.

20 Keane, M. C. Standards of nursing care. [Shown in a survey by the Irish Nurses Organization.] World of Irish Nursing, 4 (7), Jul 1975, 1–3.

21 Kelly, R. L. Evaluation is more than measurement. American Journal of Nursing, 73 (1), Jan 1973, 114–116.

22 Miller, M. B. A physician views skilled nursing care. Journal of Nursing Administration, 3 (1), Jan/Feb 1973, 20–21.

23 Moore, M. A. The Joint Commission on Accreditation of Hospitals – standards for nursing services. Journal of Nursing Administration, 11 (2), Mar/Apr 1972, 12–17, 20–24.

24 Nicholls, M. E. Quality control in patient care. American Journal of Nursing, 74 (3), Mar 1974, 456–459.

25 Nursing Clinics of North America Symposium on quality assurance. Nursing Clinics of North America, 9 (2), Jun 1974, 303–379.

26 Nursing Mirror Standards of care. A question of care. [Papers from Nursing Mirror Forum '75.] Nursing Mirror, 141, 2 Oct 1975, 47–51; 9 Oct 1975, 41–42.

27 O'Malley, N. C. JCAH accreditation. Supervisor Nurse, 6 (3), Mar 1975, 12–14, 18; (4), Apr 1975, 20–22, 27–30, 35.

28 Orme, J. Y. and Lindbeck, R. S. Nurse participation in medical peer review. Nursing Outlook, 22 (1), Jan 1974, 27–30.

29 Pardee, G. and others Patient care evaluation is every nurses' job. American Journal of Nursing, 71 (10), Oct 1971, 1958–1960.

30 Pearson, B. D. A model for clinical evaluation. Nursing Outlook, 23 (4), Apr 1975, 232–235.

31 Phaneuf, M. C. Quality assurance: a nursing view. [Measuring the quality of nursing care by various systems, including nursing audit.] Hospitals, 47 (20), 16 Oct 1973, 62, 64, 66–68.

32 Phaneuf, M. C. and Wandelt, M. A. Quality assurance in nursing. Nursing Forum, 13 (4), 1971, 328–345.

33 Ramey, I. G. Setting nursing standards and evaluating care. Journal of Nursing Administration, 3 (3), May/Jun 1973, 27–35.

34 Ramphal, M. Peer review. [The measurement of quality of nursing care by nurses.] American Journal of Nursing, 74 (1), Jan 1974, 63–67.

35 Risser, N. L. Development of an instrument to measure patient satisfaction with nurses and nursing care in primary care settings. Nursing Research, 24 (1), Jan/Feb 1975, 45–52.

36 Shetland, M. L. On nursing standards [in the context of social change]. New Zealand Nursing Journal, 68 (12), Dec 1975, 11–14.

37 Smith, M. C. Perceptions of head nurses, clinical nurse specialists, nursing educators, and nursing office personnel regarding performance of selected nursing activities. Nursing Research, 23 (6), Nov/Dec 1974, 505–510.

38 Stevens, B. J. Analysis of trends in nursing care management. [Quality control systems.] Journal of Nursing Administration, 11 (6), Nov/Dec 1972, 12–17.

39 Stevens, B. J. ANA's standards of nursing practice: what they tell us about the state of the art. Journal of Nursing Administration, 4 (5), Sep/Oct 1974, 16–18.

40 Tucker, S. M. and others Patient care standards. St. Louis: Mosby, 1975.

41 Wandelt, M. A. and Ager, J. W. Quality patient care scale. New York: Appleton-Century-Crofts, 1974.

42 Wandelt, M. A. and Phaneuf, M. C. Three instruments for measuring the quality of nursing care. [Slater Nursing Competencies Rating Scale; Quality Patient Care Scale; Nursing Audit.] Hospital Topics, 50 (8), Aug 1972, 20–23, 29.

43 Wandelt, M. A. and Stewart, D. S. Slater nursing competencies rating scale. New York: Appleton-Century-Crofts, 1975.

44 Williams, L. B. Evaluation of nursing care: a primary nursing project. 1. Report of the controlled study. Supervisor Nurse, 6 (1), Jan 1975, 32, 35–36, 38–39.

45 Zimmer, M. J. A model for evaluating nursing care. Hospitals, 48, 1 Mar 1974, 91–95, 131.

d NURSING AUDIT

1 Berg, H. V. Nursing audit and outcome criteria. Nursing Clinics of North America, 9 (2), Jun 1974, 331–335.

2 Eddy, L. and Westbrook, L. Multidisciplinary retrospective patient care audit. [Audit tool developed by the Joint Commission of Accreditation of Hospitals.] American Journal of Nursing, 75 (6), Jun 1975, 961–963.

3 Germaine, A. Having problems with the nursing audits? Hospital Administration in Canada, 16 (7), Jul 1974, 45–47.

4 Isler, C. Nursing audit: new yardstick for patient care. RN Magazine, 37 (12), Dec 1974, 31–35.

5 Morgan, D. M. Evaluation by audit: a check system for nursing care. Dimensions in Health Service, 51 (4), Mar 1974, 10–12.

6 National League for Nursing. Council of Hospital and Related Institutional Nursing Services The nursing audit . . . a necessity – how shall it be done? New York: The League, 1973.

7 Pelley, G. One step toward quality assurance. [Nursing audit at an Illinois hospital.] Hospitals, 49, 16 Apr 1975, 77–78, 82.

8 Ramirez, M. S. Auditing of nursing care plans. [Method used at St. Luke's Hospital, New York.] Supervisor Nurse, 6 (6), Jun 1975, 29, 32, 34–35, 37–38.

9 Rinaldi, L. A. and Rubin, C. P. Adding retrospective audit. [A method of auditing nursing care by outcomes which also provides feedback.] American Journal of Nursing, 75 (2), Feb 1975, 265–269.

10 Rubin, C. F. and others Nursing audit-nurses evaluating nursing. [Scrutiny of nurses' notes, nursing care plans and patients' records.] American Journal of Nursing, 72 (5), May 1972, 916–921.

11 Trout, F. Three methods of nursing audit. Dimensions in Health Service, 51 (9), Sep 1974, 38–40, 43–44.

e NURSING CARE PLAN

1 Bower, F. L. The process of planning nursing care: a theoretical model. St. Louis: Mosby, 1972.

2 Carlson, S. A practical approach to the nursing process. [Recording the nursing care plan.] American Journal of Nursing, 72 (9), Sep 1972, 1589–1591.

3 Ciuca, R. L. Over the years with the nursing care plan. [Review of the literature over the past 30 years and a comparison with actual practice.] Nursing Outlook, 20 (11), Nov 1972, 706–711.

4 Collingwood, M. P. The nursing care plan as a basis for an information system based upon individualized patient care. [Using a card which supplements the Kardex.] Nursing Times, 71, 20 Mar 1975, Occ. papers, 21–22.

5 Cornell, S. A. and Brush, F. Systems approach to nursing care plans. [Using computers.] American Journal of Nursing, 71, Jul 1971, 1376–1378.

6 Garant, C. A basis for care. [Patient records and nursing care plans.] American Journal of Nursing, 72 (4), Apr 1972, 699–701.

7 Grant, N. The nursing care plan. 2. [Data collected used as basis for information system.] Nursing Times, 71, 27 Mar 1975, Occ. papers, 25–28.

8 Heath, J. K. and Griffith, E. W. An experience in role implementation. [To develop a systematic plan of care based on an assessment of the patient's nursing needs.] Journal of Nursing Education, 11 (2), Apr 1972, 13–20.

9 Hefferin, E. A. and Hunter, R. E. Nursing assessment and care plan statements. [An investigation of scope, specificity and interrelatedness of patient problem and nursing intervention.] Nursing Research, 24 (5), Sep/Oct 1975, 360–366.

10 Henderson, V. On nursing care plans and their history. Nursing Outlook, 21 (6), Jun 1973, 378–379.

11 Kramer, M. Standard 4. Nursing care plans . . .power to the patient. Journal of Nursing Administration, 2 (5), Sep/Oct 1972, 29–34.

12 Little, D. and Carnevali, D. The nursing care planning system. Nursing Outlook, 19 (3), Mar 1971, 164–167.

13 McCloskey, J. C. The nursing care plan, past, present and uncertain future – a review of the literature. Nursing Forum, 14 (4), 1975, 364–382.

14 McCloskey, J. C. The problem-oriented record vs the nursing care plan: a proposal. Nursing Outlook, 23 (8), Aug 1975, 492–495.

15 McKechnie, A. M. and Miller, N. R. The nursing care plan. [Developed by tutors of the Auckland School of Nursing.] New Zealand Nursing Journal, 64 (12), Dec 1971, 10–12.

16 Mayers, M. G. A systematic approach to the nursing care plan. New York: Appleton-Century-Crofts, 1972.

17 Neal, M. C. Workshops offer nurses opportunity to learn to write nursing-care plans. Hospital Topics, 49 (9), Sep 1971, 29–31.

18 Palisin, H. E. Nursing care plans are a snare and a delusion. American Journal of Nursing, 71 (1), Jan 1971, 63–66.

19 Palmer, M. E. The nursing care plan: a tool for staff development. Journal of Nursing Administration, 4 (3), May/Jun 1974, 42–45.

20 Ryan, B. J. Nursing care plans: a systems approach to developing criteria for planning and evaluation. Journal of Nursing Administration, 3 (3), May/Jun 1973, 50–58.

21 Saxton, D. F. and Hyland, P. F. Planning and implementing nursing intervention. St. Louis: Mosby, 1975.

22 Smith, D. M. Writing objectives as a nursing practice skill. American Journal of Nursing, 71 (2), Feb 1971, 319–320.

23 Stevens, B. J. Why won't nurses write nursing care plans? Journal of Nursing Administration, 11 (6), Nov/Dec 1972, 6–7, 91.

f NURSING RECORDS

1 Cates, M. E. How to write easy, efficient and excellent nurses' notes. Journal of Practical Nursing, 22 (6), Jun 1972, 24–25.

2 Cohn, S. and others Reliability study of a nursing flow sheet. Journal of Nursing Administration, 5 (9), Nov–Dec 1975, 30–33.

3 Davis, B. C. and others Implementation of problem oriented charting in a large regional community hospital. [Monitoring patient care.] Journal of Nursing Administration, 4 (6), Nov/Dec 1974, 33–41.

4 Frost, M. Ward reports – sense or nonsense? Nursing Mirror, 140, 1 May 1975, 67.

5 Howard, F. and Jessop, P. I. Problem oriented charting – a nursing viewpoint. Canadian Nurse, 69 (8), Aug 1973, 34–37.

6 Linkert, M. Nurses can improve data collection. [Basic points for record system.] Dimensions in Health Service, 52 (9), Sep 1975, 32, 34.

7 Marshall, B. Medical records and the patient. [With reference to Florence Nightingale's 'Notes on Nursing'.] Medical Record, 14 (1), Feb 1973, 11–20.

8 Mitchell, P. H. A systematic nursing progress record: the problem-oriented approach. Nursing Forum, 12 (2), 1973, 187–210.

9 Mitchell, P. H. and Atwood, J. Problem-oriented recording as a teaching-learning tool: use in critical thinking and identification of patient problems. Nursing Research, 24 (2), Mar/Apr 1975, 99–103.

10 Murray, F. A. and Topley, L. Patients as record holders. [Experiment at St. Mary's Maternity Hospital, Portsmouth.] Health and Social Service Journal, 84, 27 Jul 1974, 1675.

11 Nathanson, C. A. and Becker, M. H. Doctors, nurses and clinical records. Medical Care, 11 (3), May/Jun 1973, 214–223.

12 Nursing Clinics of North America Symposium on the problem-oriented record. Nursing Clinics of North America, 9 (2), Jun 1974, 215–302.

13 Roberts, G. Patient reporting. [At Clatterbridge Hospital.] Nursing Mirror, 140, 23 Jan 1975, 68–69.

14 Roper, N. Collecting patient data. [Development of a data collecting instrument as a research tool, based on Kardex.] Nursing Mirror, 141, 11 Dec 1975, 72–74.

15 Rosenfield, V. L. A chronological team-oriented patient record. Hospital Administration in Canada, 16 (6), Jun 1974, 36–40.

16 Rozovsky, L. E. Unwritten medical orders. [Advocates written communication between doctors and nurses.] Dimensions in Health Service, 5 (1), Jan 1975, 8–9.

17 Rubin, C. and others Auditing the POMR system. Supervisor Nurse, 6 (9), Sep 1975, 23, 25, 27–31.

18 Schell, P. L. and Campbell, A. T. POMR – not just another way to chart. Nursing Outlook, 20 (8), Aug 1972, 510–514.

19 Thoma, D. and Pittman, K. Evaluation of problem-oriented nursing notes. Journal of Nursing Administration, 11 (3), May/Jun 1972, 50–58.

20 Van Meter, M. J. and Scott, L. K. An experience with problem-oriented nursing notes. Journal of Neurosurgical Nursing, 7 (1), Jul 1975, 42–56.

21 Woody, M. and Mallison, M. The problem-oriented system for patient-centred care. American Journal of Nursing, 73 (7), Jul 1973, 1168–1175.

22 Yarnall, S. R. and Atwood, J. Problem-oriented practice for nurses and physicians. Nursing Clinics of North America, 9 (2), Jun 1974, 215–228.

g NURSING DIAGNOSIS

1 American Journal of Nursing Patient assessment: taking a patient's history. Programmed instruction. American Journal of Nursing, 74 (2), Feb 1974, 293–324.

2 Aspinall, M. J. Development of a patient-completed admission questionnaire and its comparison with the nursing interview. Nursing Research, 24 (5), Sep/Oct 1975, 377–381.

3 Bircher, A. U. On the development and classification of diagnoses. Nursing Forum, 14 (1), 1975, 10–29.

4 Brown, M. M. The epidemiologic approach to the study of clinical nursing diagnosis. Nursing Forum, 13 (4), 1974, 346–359.

5 Fowkes, W. C. and Hunn, V. K. Clinical assessment for the nurse practitioner. St. Louis: Mosby, 1973.

6 Froemming, P. and Quiring, J. Teaching health history and physical examination. Nursing Research, 22 (5), Sep/Oct 1973, 432–434.

7 Fry, J. and Majumdar, B. Basic physical assessment [and data collection for nurses]. Canadian Nurse, 70 (5), May 1974, 17–22.

8 Gebbie, K. and Lavin, M. A. Classifying nursing diagnoses. [Work of the First National Conference.] American Journal of Nursing, 74 (2), Feb 1974, 250–253.

9 Hagopian, G. and Kilpack, V. Baccalaureate students learn assessment skills. [Physical assessment of the patient.] Nursing Outlook, 22 (7), Jul 1974, 454–456.

10 Hobson, L. B. Examination of the patient: a text for nursing and allied health personnel. New York: McGraw-Hill, 1975.

11 Langner, S. R. The nursing process and the interview. [Patient assessment.] Occupational Health Nursing, 21 (12), Dec 1973, 19–23.

12 Lynaugh, J. E. and Bates, B. Physical diagnosis: a skill for all nurses? American Journal of Nursing, 74 (1), Jan 1974, 58–59.

13 McPhetridge, L. M. Relationship of patients responses to nursing history questions and selected factors. Preliminary study. Nursing Research, 22 (4), Jul/Aug 1973, 310–320.

14 Mansell, E. and others Patient assessment: examination of the abdomen. Programmed instruction. American Journal of Nursing, 74 (9), Sep 1974, 1679–1702.

15 Mundinger, M. O. and Jauron, G. D. Developing a nursing diagnosis. Nursing Outlook, 23 (2), Feb 1975, 94–98.

16 Myers, N. Nursing diagnosis. Nursing Times, 69, 20 Sep 1973, 1229–1230.

17 Nursing Clinics of North America Symposium on assessment as part of the nursing process. Nursing Clinics of North America, 6 (1), Mar 1971, 113–200.

18 Roy, C. The impact of nursing diagnosis. AORN Journal, 21 (6), May 1975, 1023–1030.

19 Sana, J. M. and Judge, R. D., editors Physical appraisal methods in nursing practice. Boston: Little Brown, 1975.

20 Seedor, M. M. The physical assessment: a programmed unit of study for nurses. New York: Teachers College Press, 1974.

21 Sherman, J. L. and Fields, S. K. Guide to patient evaluation: history taking, physical examination, the problem oriented method. H. K. Lewis, 1974.

h PATIENT ASSIGNMENT

1 Bird, K. Working with patient assignment. [Total patient care.] Australian Nurses' Journal, 3 (10), May 1974, 35–36.

2 Higham, E. M. Patient allocation (plus good planning) works wonders. Australian Nurses' Journal, 1 (11), May 1972, 33–34.

3 Kenny, D. Patient assignment. Lamp, 30 (1), Jan 1973, 17–18.

4 Matthews, A. Patient allocation – a review. Nursing Times, 71, 10 Jul 1975, Occ. papers, 65–68; 17 Jul 1975, Occ. papers 69–72.

5 Pembrey, S. From work routines to patient assignment: an experiment in ward organization. [A change from task to patient assignment.] Nursing Times, 71, 6 Nov 1975, 1768–1772.

6 Peterson, C. G. What head nurses look for when evaluating assignments. [Patient care assignments.] American Journal of Nursing, 73 (4), Apr 1973, 641–644.

7 Scheideman, J. M. Chronicity: a key to learning. [Assigning students to chronically ill patients to improve nursing care.] American Journal of Nursing, 75 (3), Mar 1975, 446–447.

i PATIENT CENTRED CARE

1 Brinham, R. O. J. Learning while caring. [Ward teaching by patient centred care at Elizabeth Garrett Anderson Hospital.] Nursing Mirror, 140, 22/29 May 1975, 81–82.

2 Holloway, A. J. Patient centred nursing care. [A case study.] New Zealand Nursing Journal, 68 (9), Sep 1974, 14–16.

3 Kraegel, J. M. and others A system of patient care based on patient needs. Nursing Outlook, 20 (4), Apr 1972, 257–264.

4 Lay, J. Patient-centred care. Australian Nurses' Journal, 2 (6), Dec 1972, 30–32, 35.

5 McDonnell, C. and others What would you do? [Conflict between two different approaches to patient care – one being based on the standardized methods of the institution, the other on the needs of the individual patient.] American Journal of Nursing, 72 (2), Feb 1972, 296–301.

6 McKay, L. Do you practice what is taught? [Patient-centred care.] New Zealand Nursing Journal, 69 (7), Jul 1975, 4–5.

7 Porter, K. W. Change – for patients' sake. [Bringing the nurse back to the patient's bedside.] Hospitals, 46 (19), 1 Oct 1972, 78, 80, 85–86, 88, 90; Journal of Nursing Administration, 3 (2), Mar/Apr 1973, 37–42.

8 Richards, A. C. Toward more person centered care. AORN Journal, 22 (5), Nov 1975, 782–785.

9 Santorum, C. D. and Sell, V. M. A patient-centered nursing service. Journal of Nursing Administration, 3 (4), Jul/Aug 1973, 32–40.

10 Trent, M. and Kramer, M. The question behind the question. [Climate of nursing care which gives priority to the patient.] Journal of Nursing Administration, 11 (1), Jan/Feb 1972, 20–27.

11 Woody, M. and Mallison, M. The problem-oriented system for patient-centered care. American Journal of Nursing, 73, Jul 1973, 1168–1175.

j TEAM NURSING

1 Baumgart, A. J. Are nurses ready for teamwork? Canadian Nurse, 68 (7), Jul 1972, 19–20.

2 College of Nursing, Australia The case of team nursing. [Symposium.] Australian Nurses' Journal, 1 (10), Apr 1972, 38–40.

3 Douglass, L. M. Review of team nursing. St. Louis: Mosby, 1973.

4 Forrest, A. Modified team nursing. Nursing Journal of India, 44 (8), Aug 1973, 260, 263.

5 Froebe, D. Scheduling: by team or individually. [Team nursing.] Journal of Nursing Administration, 4 (3), May/Jun 1974, 34–36.

6 Germaine, A. Applying the concept of team nursing. Hospital Administration in Canada, 13 (5), May 1971, 58, 62–64.

7 Germaine, A. What makes team nursing tick. Journal of Nursing Administration, 1 (4), Jul/Aug 1971, 46–49.

8 Haren, M. The practical experience of team nursing at St. Vincent's Hospital. Lamp, 28 (11), Oct 1971, 7, 9, 11, 13, 15.

9 Kramer, M. Team nursing – a means or an end? Nursing Outlook, 19 (10), Oct 1971, 648–652.

10 Kron, T. Team nursing – how viable is it today? Journal of Nursing Administration, 1 (6), Nov/Dec 1971, 19–22.

11 Lamp Seminar held at St. Vincent's Hospital. [Papers on team nursing.] Lamp, 30 (1), Jan 1973, 7, 9, 11–16.

12 Lawson, O. Functional approach versus team nursing. Nigerian Nurse, 7 (3), Jul/Sep 1975, 10–14.

13 Lio, A. M. Leadership and responsibility in team nursing. Nursing Clinics of North America, 8 (2), Jun 1973, 267–281.

14 Nelson, M. C. Team nursing – what does it mean? Lamp, 29 (9), Sep 1972, 15, 17, 19–20.

15 Newcomb, D. P. and Swansburg, R. C. The team plan: a manual for nursing service administrators. 2nd ed. New York: Putnam, 1971.

16 O'Brien, R. A. Team nursing: an essential ingredient for success. Australian Nurses' Journal, 5 (1), Jul 1975, 39–40.

17 RN Magazine Speciality nursing teams in a small hospital? RN Magazine, 37 (2), Feb 1974, 34–35, 62, 64.

18 Schultz, L. and Yaremchuk, M. 'Think-in' at St. Paul's Hospital: an annual workshop to revitalize team nursing. Canadian Hospital, 49 (3), Mar 1972, 34–35.

19 Stubber, B. F. Team nursing – why? Australian Nurses' Journal, 4 (9), Apr 1975, 34–35; Reprinted in Nursing Mirror, 141, 11 Sep 1975, 72–73.

20 Theis, G. A change from team nursing. [System that combines the best of traditional district and team

nursing.] Nursing Outlook, 22 (4), Apr 1974, 258–259.

k TOTAL PATIENT CARE (Primary nursing)

1 Bakke, K. Primary nursing: perceptions of a staff nurse. [Day to day duties of a nurse giving total patient care]. American Journal of Nursing, 74 (8), Aug 1974, 1432–1434.

2 Brainerd, S. M. and LaMonica, E. L. A creative approach to individualized nursing care. Nursing Forum, 14 (2), 1975, 188–193.

3 Ciske, K. L. Primary nursing: evaluation. [A nurse clinician evaluates the effect of total patient care on nurse job satisfaction and turnover rates, and also the patients' responses.] American Journal of Nursing, 84 (8), Aug 1974, 1436–1438.

4 Ciske, K. L. Primary nursing: an organization that promotes professional practice. Journal of Nursing Administration, 4 (1), Jan/Feb 1974, 28–31.

5 Daeffler, R. J. Patients' perception of care under team and primary nursing. [Study of 82 patients on medical-surgical units which showed more satisfaction with primary nursing.] Journal of Nursing Administration, 5 (3), Mar/Apr 1975, 20–26; Comments from A. M. Putt, 5 (6), Jul/Aug 1975, 7, 11–12.

6 Davies, M. J. Total patient care assessments of students and pupil nurses during the community care option. Nursing Mirror, 140 (6), 6 Feb 1975, 64–65.

7 Felton, G. Increasing the quality of nursing care by introducing the concept of primary nursing: a model project. Nursing Research, 24 (1), Jan/Feb 1975, 27–32.

8 Fleming, J. The secret of total patient care. Nursing Mirror, 136, 5 Jan 1973, 37.

9 Johnston, D. F. Total patient care: foundations and practice. 3rd ed. St. Louis: Mosby, 1972.

10 Keane, V. R. What are the challenges – the major elements of primary nursing care? Hospital Topics, 52 (9), Nov/Dec 1974, 43–46.

11 Manthey, M. Primary nursing is alive and well in the hospital. American Journal of Nursing, 73 (1), Jan 1973, 83–87.

12 Marram, G. D. and others Primary nursing: a model for individualized care. St. Louis: Mosby, 1974.

13 Martin, N. M. and others Nurses who nurse. [Project to establish comprehensive care.] American Journal of Nursing, 73 (8), Aug 1973, 1383–1385.

14 Matthews, A. Total patient care in the ward. Nursing Mirror, 134, 11 Feb 1972, 29–31.

15 Mundinger, M. O. Primary nurse – role evolution. Nursing Outlook, 21 (10), Oct 1973, 642–645.

16 Neuman, B. M. and Young, R. J. A model for teaching total person approach to patient problems. Nursing Research, 21 (3), May/Jun 1972, 264–269.

17 Page, M. Primary nursing: perceptions of a head nurse. American Journal of Nursing, 74 (8), Aug 1974, 1435–1436.

18 Race, G. A. TPC A plan with R N's at the center. [Total patient care.] RN Magazine, 37 (4), Apr 1974, 34–35.

17 Robinson, A. M. Primary-care nursing at two teaching hospitals. RN Magazine, 47 (4), Apr 1974, 31–34.

20 Slater, P. V. Nursing the whole patient. Australian Nurses' Journal, 2 (6) Dec 1972, 25–29.

21 Warrier, P. 'Don't be 10 years behind.' [Conference on total patient care.] Nursing Mirror, 134, 4 Feb 1972, 12.

l LONG TERM CARE

1 Bystran, S. F. and others An evaluation of nurse practitioners in chronic care clinics. International Journal of Nursing Studies, 11 (3), Sep 1974, 185–193.

2 Isler, C. Day hospitals for the chronically ill? RN Magazine, 37 (4), Apr 1974, 36–39.

3 King, R. T. Nursing notes on long-stay care. Nursing Mirror, 132, 15 Jan 1971, 38–39.

4 Mellor, H. W. Health Services in the dark. [Supportive services for those caring for invalids at home.] British Hospital Journal and Social Service Review, 81, 20 Feb 1971, 333–334.

5 Rawlinson, H. L. Planning home care services. Hospitals 49 (12), 16 Jun 1975, 66–71.

6 Rioux, C. Health and social services under the same roof. [Home care program at Edmonton.] Canadian Nurse, 71 (5), May 1975, 24–26.

7 Steen, J. Liaison nurse: ombudsman for the chronically ill. American Journal of Nursing, 73 (12), Dec 1973, 2102–2104.

8 Trager B. Home care: providing the right to stay home. Hospitals, 49 (20), 16 Oct 1975, 93–96, 98.

9 Wilson, G. The chronically sick in hospital. [Comment on possible future improvements in care.] British Hospital Journal and Social Service Review 81, 24 Apr 1971, 765.

13 NURSING PRACTICE

a TEXTBOOKS

1 Broome, M. E. and Ogden, E. Tables, charts and diagrams for nurses. Butterworth, 1971.

2 Brown, M. M. and Fowler, G. R. Psychodynamic nursing. 4th ed. Philadelphia: Saunders, 1971.

3 Clarke, M. Practical nursing. 11th ed. Baillière Tindall, 1971. (Nurses' aids series.)

4 Darwin, J. and others Bedside nursing: an introduction. 3rd ed. Heinemann, 1972.

5 Dison, N. G. An atlas of nursing technique. 2nd ed. St. Louis: Mosby 1971.

6 Fream, W. C. Notes on medical nursing. Churchill Livingstone, 1971.

7 Houghton, M. and Chapman, C. M. Medical nursing. 8th ed. Baillière Tindall, 1972. (Nurses' aids series.)

8 Kelly, L. Y. Dimensions of professional nursing. 3rd ed. New York: Collier Macmillan, 1975.

9 Morgan, W. and Whyte, B. Pupil nurse's workbook, McGraw-Hill, 1975.

10 Pearce, E. C. A general textbook of nursing. 19th ed. Faber, 1975.

11 Roper, N. Principles of nursing. 2nd ed. Churchill Livingstone, 1973.

12 Spencer, M. and Tait, K. M. Introduction to nursing. 3rd ed. Oxford: Blackwell, 1973.

13 Welsh, E. M. and others An outline to basic nursing care. Heinemann, 1971. (Modern practical nursing series, parent volume.)

14 West, N. C. A handbook for nurses: common medical and surgical conditions. 2nd ed. English University Press, 1975.

b PROCEDURES

1 Andrews, I. D. Observations. Nursing Times, 70, 7 Mar 1974, 341–342.

2 **Betson, C.** The nurse's role in blood gas monitoring. Cardio-Vascular Nursing, 7 (6), Nov/Dec 1971, 83–86.

3 **Brown, J.** Defibrillation by nursing staff in general medical wards. Nursing Times 71, 2 Oct 1975, 1572–1573.

4 **Coleman, V.** The history of the syringe. Nursing Mirror, 139, 5 Dec 1974, 57.

5 **Crane, G.** New bath system saves man-hours. Nursing Times, 68, 18 May 1972, 618–619. [Reprinted from British Hospital Journal and Social Service Review 81, 28 Aug 1971.]

6 **Daniels, S.** What are nursing duties? Nursing Times, 68, 27 Jan 1972, 121.

7 **del Bueno, D. J.** Making effective use of blood gas determinations. RN Magazine, 37 (4), Apr 1974, 40–43.

8 **Hardy, J.** Bathing patients without soap and water. Nursing Care 7 (2), Feb 1974, 25–27.

9 **Hatcher, J.** The 'English Syringe'. [Higginson's enema syringe.] Nursing Times, 69, 7 Jun 1973, 740.

10 **Hatcher, J.** Evolution of the hypodermic. Midwives Chronicle, 87, Feb 1974, 64.

11 **Hatcher, J.** Specimen identification. Nursing Mirror, 133, 23 July 1971, 26.

12 **Hayes, B. A.** Helping to meet the patients needs for basic nursing care. UNA Nursing Journal, 71, Jan/Feb 1973, 27–32.

13 **Hays, D.** Do it yourself the Z-track way. [Technique for intra-muscular injections.] American Journal of Nursing, 74 (6), Jun 1974, 1070–1071.

14 **LeCompte, W. F. and others** Effects of training on behavioral observations by nurses. Nursing Research, 21 (5), Sep/Oct 1972, 448–452.

15 **Massachusetts General Hospital. Department of Nursing** Manual of nursing procedures. Boston: Little Brown, 1975.

16 **Moore, J. and Weinberg, M.** The case of the warm moist compress. [A study comparing two methods of preparing compresses.] Canadian Nurse, 71 (3), Mar 1975, 19–21.

17 **Noone, A. and Levins, M.** Nursing observations: a ward based nursing project. [To discover the correlation of agreement (COA).] Nursing Mirror, 138, 10 May 1974, 59–62.

18 **Petrello, J. M.** Temperature maintenance of hot moist compresses. American Journal of Nursing, 73, (6), Jun 1973, 1050–1051.

19 **Pitel, M.** The subcutaneous injection. American Journal of Nursing, 71, (1), Jan 1971, 76–79; Canadian Nurse, 67, (5), May, 54–57.

20 **Quiring, J.** The autotutorial approach: the effect of timing of videotape feedback on nursing students' achievement of skill in giving subcutaneous injections. Nursing Research, 21, (4), Jul/Aug 1972, 332–337.

21 **St. John's Hospital for Diseases of the Skin, London** Procedure book. The Hospital, 1973.

22 **St. Joseph Hospital Medical Center** Nursing service procedure manual. St. Louis: Catholic Hospital Association, 1971.

23 **St. Thomas Hospital, Nashville, Tennessee** Patient care services policy manual for the Nursing Department, compiled by Sister Leone Douville. St. Louis: Catholic Hospital Association, 1974.

24 **White, M. B.** Importance of selected nursing activities. [Study of fifty activities.] Nursing Research, 21, (1), Jan/Feb 1972, 4–14.

c LIFTING PATIENTS

1 **Hollis, M. and Waddington, P. J.** Lifting patients. 1. Nursing Mirror, 140, 23 Jan 1975, 45–47.

2 **Hollis, M. and Waddington, P. J.** Lifting patients. 2. The shoulder (Australian) lift. Nursing mirror, 140, 30 Jan 1975, 60–62.

3 **Hollis, M. and Waddington, P. J.** Lifting patients. 3. The through-arm lift. Nursing Mirror, 140, 6 Feb 1975, 69–70.

4 **Hollis, M. and Waddington, P. J.** Lifting patients. 4. The three or two person total lift. Nursing Mirror, 140, 13 Feb 1975, 58–59.

5 **Hollis, M. and Waddington, P. J.** Lifting patients. 5. Rocking and auxillary lift. Nursing Mirror, 140, 20 Feb 1975, 63–65.

6 **Hollis, M. and Waddington, P. J.** Lifting patients. 6. The elbow lift. Nursing Mirror, 140, 27 Feb 1975, 52–53.

7 **Hollis, M. and Waddington, P. J.** Lifting patients. 7. Getting out of bed. Nursing Mirror, 140, 6 Mar 1975, 66–67.

8 **Hollis, M. and Waddington, P. J.** Lifting patients. 8. Standing up and sitting down – balance and support for walking. Nursing Mirror, 140, 13 Mar 1975, 58–59.

9 **Hollis, M. and Waddington, P. J.** Lifting patients. 9. Walking with crutches and sticks. Nursing Mirror, 140, 20 Mar 1975, 70–72.

10 **Hollis, M. and Waddington, P. J.** Lifting patients. 10. The hemiplegic patient. Nursing Mirror, 140, 27 Mar 1975, 66–68.

11 **Kennedy, P.** Posture and lifting. Queen's Nursing Journal, 16 (7), Oct 1973, 155–157.

12 **King's Fund Centre** Stop think – then lift. [Description of a training package for teaching good lifting techniques, produced by Heinemann and The King's Fund.] Nursing Mirror, 134, 23 Jun 1972, 9–11.

13 **Works, R. F.** Hints on lifting and pulling. American Journal of Nursing, 72, Feb 1972, 260–261.

d TEMPERATURES

1 **American Journal of Nursing** Taking adult temperatures. New York: American Journal of Nursing Company, 1972.

2 **Blainey, C. G.** Site selection in taking body temperature. American Journal of Nursing, 74 (10), Oct 1974, 1859–1861.

3 **Burnley School of Nursing** Temperatures and their accuracy. [Student investigation of minimum time necessary to ensure accurate temperature readings.] Nursing Times, 67, 16 Sep 1971, 1139.

4 **Dorgu, M. P.** Temperature variation and nursing care. Butterworth, 1971. (Nursing in depth series.)

5 **Ferguson, G. T. and others** The advantages of the electronic thermometer. Hospitals, 45, (15), 1 Aug 1971, 62–63.

6 **Graas, S.** Thermometer sites and oxygen. Study challenges the routine practice of taking rectal temperatures when a patient is receiving oxygen by nasal cannula. American Journal of Nursing, 74, (10), Oct 1974, 1862–1863.

7 **Hatcher, J.** The clinical thermometer. Midwives Chronicle, 86, Feb 1973, 46.

8 **Ketefian, S.** Application of selected nursing research findings into nursing practice: a pilot study. [Application of oral mode of temperature determination based on research findings by Nichols and colleagues.] Nursing Research, 24, (2), Mar/Apr 1975, 89–92.

9 **Lee, R. V. and Atkins, E.** Spurious fever. [Patients' ways of faking a high temperature and methods of prevention.] American Journal of Nursing, 72, (6), Jun 1972, 1094–1095.

10 **Morrison, M. and Moore, R. V.** Single-use clinical thermometer. [A study of its advantages carried out by student nurses at the South Edinburgh School of Nursing.] Nursing Mirror, 141, 4 Sep 1975, 67–68.

11 **Nichols, G. A.** Time analysis of afebrile and febrile temperature readings. Nursing Research, 21, (5), Sep/Oct 1972, 463–464.

12 **Nichols, G. A. and Kucha, D. H.** Taking adult temperatures. Oral measurements. American Journal of Nursing, 72, (6), Jun 1972, 1090–1092.

13 **Nichols, G. A. and others** Rectal thermometer placement times for febrile adults. Nursing Research, 21, (1), Jan/Feb 1972, 76–77.

14 **Schmidt, A. J.** TPR: an old habit or a significant routine? Nursing staff questions its procedure for routine temperature checks. Hospitals, 46, (24), 16 Dec 1972, 57–58, 60.

15 **Soo, B.** Temperatures and their accuracy. Nursing Journal of Singapore, 12, (1), May 1972, 48–49.

14 CLINICAL NURSE SPECIALIST

a GENERAL (See also under speciality)

1 **American Hospital Association** The clinical nurse specialist. [Report of conference organized jointly by American Hospital Association and American Nurses' Association.] Hospitals, 47, 1 Feb 1973, 135, 138–141.

2 **Anders, R. L.** Matrix organization: an alternative for clinical specialists. [Team of diverse specialists working on specific projects.] Journal of Nursing Administration, 5 (5), Jun 1975, 11–14.

3 **Aradine, C. R.** The challenge of clinical nursing practice in an interdisciplinary office setting. Nursing Forum, 12 (3), 1973, 290–302.

4 **Aradine, C.R. and Denyes, M. J.** Activities and pressures of clinical nurse specialists. Nursing Research, 21 (5), Sep/Oct 1972, 411–418.

5 **Ashworth, P. M.** The clinical nurse consultant. Nursing Times, 71, 10 Apr 1975, 574–577.

6 **Ayers, R.** The clinical nurse specialist: an experiment in role effectiveness and role development: final project report. Duarte, California: City of Hope National Medical Center, Division of Nursing, 1972.

7 **Barnett, J. G.** In pursuit of clinical excellence. Nursing Times, 67, 19 Aug 1971, 1030–1032.

8 **Barrett, J.** Administrative factors in development of new nursing practice roles. [Clinical nurse specialist.] Journal of Nursing Administration, 1 (4), Jul/Aug 1971, 25–29.

9 **Brazley, M.** Public participation in nursing. [Reorganization of nursing services and establishment of a career structure to allow nurses to remain in the clinical field.] New Zealand Nursing Journal, 69 (10), Oct 1975, 13–15.

10 **Burnside, H.** Perceived need for technical specialists in nursing care of hospitalized patients. New York: National League for Nursing, 1974.

11 **Campbell, E. B.** The nurse specialist: catalyst for reuniting service and education. Hospital Progress, 52 (11), Nov 1971, 86–90.

12 **Canadian Nurses' Association** Specialization in

nursing – where? when? how? Canadian Nurse, 68 (5), May 1972, 39–42.

13 Castronovo, F. The effective use of the clinical specialist. Supervisor Nurse, 6 (5), May 1975, 49, 51–52, 56.

14 Cleland, V. Implementation of change in health care systems. [The role of the nurse clinician.] Journal of Nursing Administration, 11 (6), Nov/Dec 1972, 64–69.

15 Colavecchio, R. and others A clinical ladder for nursing practice. Journal of Nursing Administration, 4 (5), Sep/Oct 1974, 54–58.

16 Cronk, H. M. Doing one's own thing. [Clinical nurse consultant.] Nursing Times, 69, 29 Mar 1973, 422.

17 D'Addio, D. L. and others The clinical co-ordinator: a multifaceted role. Nursing Clinics of North America, 8 (2), Jun 1973, 257–265.

18 DeMeyer, J. A. A nurse consultant in action. Journal of Nursing Administration, 11 (2), Mar/Apr 1972, 42–45.

19 Dolan, M. M. The clinical specialist as director of nursing services. Nursing Clinics of North America, 6 (6), 1971, 237–245.

20 Dworkin, C. Spotlight on the clinical nurse specialist. Canadian Nurse, 69 (9), Sep 1973, 40–42; New Zealand Nursing Journal, 67 (3), Mar 1974, 10–11.

21 Edwards, J. Clinical specialists are not effective – why? Supervisor Nurse, 2 (8), 1971, 38–41.

22 Flynn, B. C. Study documents reactions to nurses in expanded roles. [Study of the reactions of non-nursing personnel and patients to the care provided by four nurse clinicians.] Hospitals, 49 (21), 1 Nov 1975, 81–83.

23 Georgopoulos, B. S. and Sana, J. M. Clinical nursing specialization and intershift report behavior. American Journal of Nursing, 71 (3), Mar 1971, 538–545.

24 Germaine, A. Hello, nurse clinician – and what's your job? Hospital Administration in Canada, 15 (5), May 1973, 64, 66.

25 Gold, H. and others Peer review: a working experiment. [Evaluation of clinical nursing specialist program at University Hospital, Ann Arbor, Michigan.] Nursing Outlook, 21 (10), Oct 1973, 634–636.

26 Hellman, C. The making of a clinical specialist. Nursing Outlook, 22 (3), Mar 1974, 165–167.

27 Jackson, M. M., editor Clinical nurse specialist symposium, 1972. Papers presented at the University of Michigan Medical Center. . . April 28–29, 1972. Ann Arbor, Michigan: The University, 1973.

28 Jacox, A. Job description for clinical specialist. Supervisor Nurse, 2 (8), Aug 1971, 47.

29 Jollands, E. J. The clinical specialist: improving patient care. A report on a six-month trial at Wellington Hospital. New Zealand Nursing Journal, 67 (3), Mar 1974, 11–14; 69 (10), Oct 1975, 23–24.

30 Kerrane, T. A. The clinical nurse specialist. [Report of a study tour in America to examine the relevance for the UK.] Nursing Mirror, 140, 30 Jan 1975, 63–65.

31 Kerrane, T. A. The clinical nurse specialist: one answer to our problems? A report of the seminar on 'The clinical nurse specialist' organized recently by the Rcn [at Leeds Castle]. Nursing Mirror, 141, 30 Oct 1975, 41–42.

32 Kinsella, C. R. Who is the clinical nurse specialist? Hospitals, 47 (11), 1 Jun 1973, 72, 74, 76, 78, 80.

33 Kirkman, R. H. and Miller, M. E. The clinical specialist in a community hospital. Journal of Nursing Administration, 11 (1), Jan/Feb 1972, 30–33.

34 Knecht, A. A. Evaluation of a nursing consultant. Journal of Nursing Administration, 11 (2), Mar/Apr 1972, 46–51.

35 McCallum, J. and Carey, S. Case for clinical nursing. [The clinical nurse specialist.] New Zealand Nursing Journal, 67 (3), Mar 1974, 8–10.

36 McGann, M. R. The clinical specialist: from hospital to clinic, to community. [A personal view of the role.] Journal of Nursing Administration, 5 (3), Mar–Apr 1975, 33–36.

37 McGee, J. Development of clinical nursing. [Including the work of the Clinical Nurse Specialists' Association in New South Wales.] Lamp, 31 (11), Nov 1974, 11, 13.

38 MacPhail, J. Reasonable expectations for the nurse clinician. Journal of Nursing Administration, 1 (5), Sep/Oct 1971, 16–18.

39 Moon, S. T. Clinical nurse specialist – in name only. American Journal of Nursing, 71 (3), Mar 1971, 546–548.

40 Murray, V. V. Clinical specialization in nursing and the hospital administration. Hospital Administration in Canada, 13 (2), Feb 1971, 21–22, 24–26.

41 Nursing Clinics of North America Symposium on the clinical specialist in action. Nursing Clinics of North America, 8 (4), Dec 1973, 683–764.

42 Padilla, G. V. The bases of the clinical nurse specialists' influence. Hospital Progress, 53 (4), Apr 1972, 29–31.

43 Parkis, E. W. The management role of the clinical specialist. Supervisor Nurse, 5 (9), Oct 1974, 44–46; 6 (10), Sep 1974, 24–27.

44 Pearson, L. E. The clinical specialist as role model or motivator? Nursing Forum, 11 (1), 1972, 71–77.

45 Riehl, J. P. and McVay, J. W., editors The clinical nurse specialist: interpretations. New York: Appleton-Century-Crofts, 1973.

46 Riehl, J. P. and McVay, J. W. The emerging role of the clinical nurse specialist. New York: Appleton-Century-Crofts, 1972.

47 Rogers, C. G. Conceptual models as guides to clinical nursing specialization. Journal of Nursing Education, 12 (4), Nov 1973, 2–6.

48 Sedgwick, R. The role of the process consultant. Nursing Outlook, 21, 12 Dec 1973, 773–775.

49 Shaefer, J. A. The satisfied clinician: administrative support makes the difference. [Job satisfaction of the clinical nurse specialist.] Journal of Nursing Administration, 3 (4), Jul/Aug 1973, 17–20.

50 Shepherd, E. W. Is Salmon a scapegoat? [Letter discussing the specialist nurse after a conference held at the Royal College of Physicians.] British Medical Journal, 4, 21 Dec 1974, 716.

51 Smith, A. P. A day in my double life. [Clinical nurse specialist.] American Journal of Nursing, 71 (1), Jan 1971, 84–85.

52 Smith, J. P. Clinical nurse consultants: a case for caution? Nursing Times, 67, 24 Jun 1971, 779–780.

53 Smith, M. C. The clinical specialist: her role in staff development. Journal of Nursing Administration, 1 (1), Jan 1971, 33–36.

54 Tierney, B. A new nursing structure. [Involving senior nurse clinicians.] World of Irish Nursing, 1 (4), Apr 1972, 80–81.

55 Unangst, C. Clinician's use of nursing rounds. [A medical-surgical nursing clinician describes the weekly rounds she has been making with team leaders since 1967.] American Journal of Nursing, 71 (8), Aug 1971, 1566–1567.

56 Whitehead, J. A. and Fannon, D. A clinical role for senior nurses. [An experiment at St. Francis Hospital, Hove.] Lancet, 2, 2 Oct 1971, 756–758.

57 Wiles, V. A. The practice of nursing: clinical specialization. [Implications of the Australian 'Goals in nursing education' Report for the clinical practitioner.] Australian Nurses' Journal, 5 (3), Sep 1975, 6–9.

58 Woodrow, M. and Bell, J. A. Clinical specialization: conflict between reality and theory. Journal of Nursing Administration, 1 (6), Nov/Dec 1971, 23–28.

59 Zimmer, M. J. Rationale for a ladder for clinical advancement in nursing practice. Journal of Nursing Administration, 11 (6), Nov/Dec 1972, 18–24.

b NURSE PRACTITIONERS

1 Anderson, A. and others The expanded role of the nurse: independent practitioner or physician's assistant? Canadian Nurse 71 (9), Sep 1975, 34–35.

2 Anderson, E. M. and others Epigenesis of the nurse practitioner role. [University of Minnesota.] American Journal of Nursing, 74 (10), Oct 1974, 1812–1816.

3 Barrett, J. The nurse specialist practitioner: a study. Nursing Outlook, 20 (8), Aug 1972, 524–527.

4 Bullough, B. Is the nurse practitioner role a source of increased work satisfaction? [Results of questionnaire measuring job satisfaction in nurses.] Nursing Research, 23 (1), Jan/Feb 1974, 14–19.

5 Canada. Committee on Nurse Practitioners Report to the Department of National Health and Welfare, Canada. Ottawa: The Department, 1972.

6 Canada. Health and Welfare Department. Health Manpower Directorate Report of cross Canada survey to examine the emergence of the nurse practitioner, prepared by H. R. Imai. Ottawa: The Department, 1974. (Health manpower report no. 6–74).

7 Cassidy, J. T. The advanced nursing practitioner: a dilemma for supervisors. Journal of Nursing Administration, 5 (6), Jul/Aug, 40–42.

8 Ford, L. and others The nurse practitioner question. American Journal of Nursing, 74 (12), Dec 1974, 2188–2191.

9 Good, J. L. Current personnel development and the nurse practitioner. Occupational Health Nursing, 23 (7), Jul 1975, 7–9.

10 Hurd, J. L. Directional signals for nursing's expanding role. [As 'practitioner associate'.] Canadian Nurse, 68 (1), Jan 1972, 21–25.

11 Lewis, E. P. Nurse practitioner: the way to go? [Editorial.] Nursing Outlook, 23 (3), Mar 1975, 147.

12 Linn, L. S. Care vs cure: how the nurse practitioner views the patient. Nursing Outlook, 22 (10), Oct 1974, 641–644.

13 Linn, L. S. Expectation vs realization in the nurse practitioner role. Nursing Outlook, 23 (3), Mar 1975, 166–171.

14 McAtee, P. R. and Silver, H. K. What about a national nurse-practitioner program? [Proposals for training nurse practitioners.] RN Magazine, 38 (12), Dec 1975, 22–26.

15 Malkemes, L. C. Resocialization: a model for nurse practitioner preparation. [Attitude and role change in nursing education.] Nursing Outlook, 22 (2), Feb 1974, 90–94.

16 Mauksch, I. G. and Rogers, M. E. Nursing is coming of age. . .through the practitioner movement. American Journal of Nursing, 75 (10), Oct 1975, 1834–1843.

17 Moore, A. C. Nurse practitioner: reflections on the role. Nursing Outlook, 22 (2), Feb 1974, 124–127.

18 National League for Nursing Department of Baccalaureate and Higher Degree Programs Who is the nurse practitioner? New York: The League, 1975.

19 Pohl, M. The teaching function of the nurse practitioner. 2nd ed. Dubuque, Iowa: Brown, (Foundations in nursing series.)

20 Popiel, E.S. Nurse practitioner: a new program in continuing education. Journal of Nursing Education, 12 (1), Jan 1974, 29, 31–36.

21 Robinson, A. M. The nurse practitioner: expanding your limits. RN Magazine, 36 (11), Nov 1973, 27–34.

22 Taller, S. L. and Feldman, R. The training and utilization of nurse practitioners in adult health appraisal. Medical Care, 12 (1), Jan 1974, 40–48.

23 Weston, J. L. Whither the 'nurse' in nurse practitioner. Nursing Outlook, 71 (3), Mar 1975, 148–152.

24 White, M. S. Psychological characteristics of the nurse practitioner. [The need for research.] Nursing Outlook, 23 (3), Mar 1975, 160–166.

25 Wood, L. A. A career model for nurse practitioners. Los Angeles: Allied Health Professions Project Division of Vocational Education, University of California, 1972.

c PHYSICIAN'S ASSISTANTS

1 Andreoli, K. G. A look at the physician's assistant. American Journal of Nursing, 72 (4), Apr 1972, 710–713.

2 Bergman, A. B. Two views on the latest health manpower issue. Physician's assistants belong in the nursing profession. American Journal of Nursing, 71 (5), May 1971, 975–977.

3 Bicknell, W. J. and others Substantial or decorative? Physicians' assistants and nurse practitioners in the United States. Lancet, 2, 23 Nov 1974, 1241–1244.

4 Biggs, B. Nurse-clinician-practitioner-assistant-associate. American Journal of Nursing, 71 (10), Oct 1971, 1936–1937.

5 Coe, R. M. and Fichtenbaum, L. Utilization of physician assistants: some implications for medical practice. Medical Care, 10 (6), Nov/Dec 1972, 497–504.

6 David, H. P. Training and utilization of feldshers in the USSR. From a WHO Expert Committee Report. Journal of Psychiatric Nursing, 11 (1), Jan/Feb 1973, 32–34.

7 DuGas, B. M. The need for a health worker to assist the physician. [Nurses as physician's assistants or associates.] Canadian Hospital, 49 (5), May 1972, 67–71.

8 Dunkley, P. Physician assistant – why not? [Use in United States.] New Zealand Nursing Journal, 68 (4), Apr 1975, 8–12.

9 Ferguson, M. Nurse or feldsher? A crisis of identity. [USSR.] Nursing Times, 69, 25 Oct 1973, 1410–1412.

10 Gardziella, W. A. The training of medical assistants in Rhodesia today? Rhodesian Nurse, 5 (4), Dec 1972, 1, 3.

11 Hospitals The physician's assistant: exploration of the concept. Hospitals, 45 (11), 1 Jun 1971, 42–50.

12 King, P. E. Nursing at cross roads. A world wide perspective. [Development of physicians' assistants and their relationship to the nurse.] Nursing Journal of India, 66 (2), Feb 1975, 27, 30–31.

13 Lambertsen, E. C. Perspective on the physician's assistant. Nursing Outlook, 20 (1), Jan 1972, 32–36.

14 Mellish, J. M. The threat of the physician's assistant: implications of nursing education. SA Nursing Journal, 40 (9), Sep 1973, 21–22.

15 National Commission for the Study of Nursing and Nursing Education Assistance for the physician: nurse clinician or physician assistant. Journal of Nursing Administration, 1 (6), Nov/Dec 1971, 10–11; Occupational Health Nursing, 19 (11), Nov 1971, 28–29.

16 Rothberg, J. S. Nurse and physician's assistant: issues and relationships. Nursing Outlook, 21 (3), Mar 1973, 154–158.

17 Searle, C. The second class doctor and the medical assistant in South Africa. [Further training for nurses to enable them to act as health assistants in the absence of doctors.] SA Nursing Journal, 40 (7), Jul 1973, 12–13, 15, 17.

18 Scheffler, R. M. and Stinson, O. D. Characteristics of physician's assistants: a focus on specialty. Medical Care, 12 (12), Dec 1974, 1019–1030.

19 World Health What's in a name. Issue devoted to the role of the medical assistant within the health service. World Health, Jun 1972, 2–33.

20 Young, L. S. Physician's assistants and the law. Nursing Outlook, 20 (1), Jan 1972, 36–41.

15 NURSE AND PATIENT

a NURSE/PATIENT RELATIONSHIP

1 Aiken, L. and Aiken, J. L. A systematic approach to the evaluation of interpersonal relationships. American Journal of Nursing, 73 (5), May 1973, 863–867.

2 Altman, N. W. Understanding your patient's emotional responses. Journal of Practical Nursing, 22 (10), Oct 1972, 22–25.

3 Bowman, M. P. Management. 4. The nurse and the patient. Nursing Times, 71, 17 Jul 1975, 1147–1148.

4 Condell, P. The patient. World of Irish Nursing, 1 (7), July 1972, 146–147.

5 Copp, L. A. Illness-sustaining role prescriptions. [Nurse-patient relationships.] Nursing Forum, 10 (1), 1971, 37–48.

6 Copp, L. A. A projective cartoon investigation of nurse-patient psychodramatic role perception and expectation. Nursing Research, 20 (2), Mar/Apr 1971, 100–112.

7 Copp, L. A. The psychology of patient satisfaction: understanding the patient's changes and needs. Bedside Nurse, 4 (3), Mar 1971, 23–26.

8 Davitz, L. J. and Davitz, J. R. How do nurses feel when patients suffer? [Interviews with 200 nurses.] American Journal of Nursing, 75 (9), Sep 1975, 1505–1510.

9 Davitz, L. J. and Davitz, J. R. How nurses view patient suffering. [A research project.] RN Magazine, 38 (10), Oct 1975, 69–72, 74.

10 Deutch, E. B. A stereotype – or an individual? Nursing Outlook, 19 (2), Feb 1971, 106–108.

11 Dillon, K. M. A patient-structured relationship. Lamp, 29 (7), Jul 1972, 38–41.

12 Epstein, C. Effective interaction in contemporary nursing. Englewoof Cliffs, New Jersey: Prentice-Hall, 1974.

13 Florer, R. M. Nurse patient relationships in general nursing. Nursing Mirror, 136, 23 Mar 1973, 42–43.

14 Foster, B. and Foster, F. Nursing students' reaction to the crying patient. Nursing Research, 20 (3), May/Jun 1971, 265–268.

15 Gardner, S. and Boorer, D. Involvement: one nurse's view on the importance of caring. Nursing Times, 67, 18 Feb 1971, 214–215.

16 Goodall, J. Only connect. (Nurse patient relationship.] Nursing Mirror, 140, 23 Jan 1975, 58.

17 Hampton, P. J. The bedside manner: the dual role of the nurse as mother surrogate and healer. Bedside Nurse, 4 (4), Apr 1971, 9–13.

18 Holder, S. Rediscovering the patient. Nursing Times, 69, 4 Oct 1973, 1275–1277.

19 Huber, C. J. and Hanson, S. Sensitivity training: a step toward involvement with patients. [Provision of individualized care.] Nursing Forum, 14 (2), 1975, 175–187.

20 Jacobson, Z. A. Counter aggression toward patients: the hidden enemy. Supervisor Nurse, 6 (4), Apr 1975, 36–38.

21 Kalisch, B. J. Strategies for developing nurse empathy. Nursing Outlook, 19 (11), Nov 1971, 714–718.

22 Mercer, L. S. and O'Connor, P. Fundamental skills in the nurse-patient relationship: a programmed text. 2nd ed. Philadelphia: Saunders, 1974.

23 Parkhurst, R. A bedside manner: do we have it? Nursing Care, 6 (3), Mar 1973, 16–20.

24 Parkinson, M. H. Is it. . . or isn't it? [An account of a nurse-patient relationship.] New Zealand Nursing Journal, 65 (10), Oct 1972, 10–11.

25 Purtilo, R. The allied health professional and the patient: techniques of effective interaction. Philadelphia: Saunders, 1973.

26 Rickards, M. Coping with the problem of the grateful patient syndrome. Nursing Mirror, 134, 10 Mar 1972, 20–22.

27 Rickelman, B. L. Bio-psycho-social linguistics: a conceptual approach to nurse-patient interaction. Nursing Research, 20 (5), Sep/Oct 1971, 398–403.

28 RN Magazine Handling the difficult patient. [Three case histories.] RN Magazine, 38 (5), May 1975, 41–47.

29 Robinson, A. M. Keys to understanding the patient. Journal of Practical Nursing, 21 (3), Mar 1971, 24, 50; (4) Apr 1971, 18, 20, 40, 42.

30 Robinson, L. Liaison nursing: psychological approach to patient care. Philadelphia: Davis, 1974.

31 Robinson, L. Pyschological aspects of the care of the hospitalized patient. 2nd ed. Philadelphia: Davis, 1972.

32 Royal, M. L. The nurse-patient relationship. Jamaican Nurse, 12 (1), Apr 1972, 26–27.

33 Salawu, R. A. Pyschosocial aspects of the nursing care of patients. Nigerian Nurse, 7 (1), Jan/Mar 1975, 18–21.

34 Schrock, R. A. Basic interpersonal nursing skills. [How to reassure the anxious patient.] Nursing Mirror, 133, 17 Sep 1971, 40–43.

35 Schwartz, L. H. and Schwartz, J. L. The psychodynamics of patient care. New Jersey: Prentice-Hall, 1972.

36 Stockwell, P. The unpopular patient. Rcn, 1972. (Study of Nursing Care project, series 1, no. 2.)

37 Ujhely, G. B. The patient as an equal partner. Canadian Nurse, 69 (6), Jun 1973, 21–23.

38 Wallston, K. A. and others Development of a scale to measure nurses' trust of patients: a preliminary report. Nursing Research, 22 (3), May/Jun 1973, 232–235.

39 Wylie, N. Nurse-patient relationships in chronic illness. Nursing Journal of Singapore, 15 (2), Nov 1975, 93–95.

b COMMUNICATION AND COUNSELLING

1 Hambling, E. How do you feel? [Report of the first course in counselling for nurses at William Rathbone Staff College.] Nursing Times, 71, 19 Jun 1975, 986–987.

2 Haggerty, V. C. Listening: an experiment in nursing. Nursing Forum, 10 (4), 1971, 383–391.

3 Hardiman, M. A. Interviewing? Or social chitchat? American Journal of Nursing, 71 (7), July 1971, 1379–1381.

4 Hein, E. C. Communication in nursing practice. Boston: Little Brown, 1973.

5 Hill, A. Sit down and listen. [Tape recordings of patients talking about their conditions.] Nursing Times, 67, 4 Nov 1971, 1377–1378.

6 Jesudoss, M. J. Communication in patient care. Nursing Journal of India, 65 (8), Aug 1974, 209–211, 216.

7 Kopacz, M. S. and O'Connor, C. M. Through a glass darkly. [Techniques for nurses counselling patients.] American Journal of Nursing, 75 (12), Dec 1975, 2159–2160.

8 Kron, T. Communications in nursing. 2nd ed. Philadelphia: Saunders, 1972.

9 Langlois, P. and Teramoto, V. Helping patients cope with hospitalization. [Group therapy by nurses.] Nursing Outlook, 19 (5), May 1971, 334–336.

10 Lewis, F. The role of the nurse counsellor. UNA Nursing Journal, 71, May/Jun 1973, 14–15, 17.

11 Lewis, G. K. Nurse-patient communications. 2nd ed. Dubuque, Iowa, 1973.

12 Loesch, L. C. and Loesch, N. A. What do you say after you say Mm – hmm? [Client centred counselling of patients.] American Journal of Nursing, 75 (5), May 1975, 807–809.

13 Meir, E. Nursing is. . . 1. Talking. 2. Listening. Nursing Mirror, 135, 14 Jul 1972, 12–13; 21 Jul 1972, 24.

14 Nurse, G. Counselling and the nurse: an introduction. Aylesbury: H. M. and M. Publishers, 1975. (Topics in community health series.)

15 Peitchinis, J. A. Therapeutic effectiveness of counselling by nursing personnel: review of the literature. Nursing Research, 21 (2), Mar/Apr 1972, 138–148.

16 Rodmell, J. C. Better nursing communication: by-product of improving patient care. [Reprinted from Australian Nurses' Journal, March 1973.] Nursing Times, 69, 10 May 1973, 608–611.

17 Schumacher, M. E. 'Nursing communication act' is the core of nursing. Canadian Nurse, 67 (2), Feb 1971, 40–41.

18 Sharp, C. First or last name? [For addressing patients.] American Journal of Nursing, 71 (5), May 1971, 958–959.

19 Smiley, O. G. and Smiley, C. W. Interviewing techniques for nurses. [Talking to the patient.] Community Health, 6 (2), Sep/Oct 1974, 102–105.

20 Smith, E. Reassure the patient. Nursing Times, 68, 19 Oct 1972, 1334–1335.

21 Stewart, W. Nursing and counselling – a conflict of roles? Nursing Mirror, 140, 6 Feb 1975, 71–73.

22 Teo, A. S. and Chua, P. C. Patient orientation. [Study to evaluate the effectiveness of an orientation programme.] Nursing Journal of Singapore, 15 (1), May 1975, 18–21.

23 Thomas, P. A. Coping with emotions. [Communicating with patients to allay their fears.] Nursing Times, 71, 9 Jan 1975, 80–81.

24 Underwood, P. R. Communication through role playing. American Journal of Nursing, 71 (6), Jun 1971, 1184–1186.

25 Veninga, R. Communications: a patient's eye view. American Journal of Nursing, 73 (2), Feb 1973, 320–322.

26 Wallston, K. A. and Wallston, B. S. Nurses' decisions to listen to patients: a role-playing simulation approach toward studying. Nursing Research, 24 (1), Jan/Feb 1975, 16–22.

c PATIENT TEACHING

1 Briant, N. When you make your own tape. . . [For teaching patients.] Canadian Nurse, 70 (12), Dec 1974, 38–39.

2 Copp, L. A. The waiting room – a health teaching site. [Nurses should use patients waiting time for health care instruction.] Nursing Outlook, 19 (7), Jul 1971, 481–483.

3 Dodge, J. S. What patients should be told [about their condition]: patients' and nurses' beliefs. American Journal of Nursing, 72 (10), Oct 1972, 1852–1854.

4 Lindeman, C. A. Audiovisuals orient patients: sound-on-slide programs prepared for individual instruction at the bedside. Hospitals, 47 (5), 1 Mar 1973, 129–130.

5 Pearson, B. Learning tool selection. [Teaching materials for patient teaching.] Supervisor Nurse, 6 (3), Mar 1975, 30–31.

6 Reader, G. G. and Schwartz, D. Developing patients' knowledge of health. Hospitals, 47 (5), 1 Mar 1973, 111–112, 114.

7 Redman, B. K. Guidelines for quality of care in patient education. Canadian Nurse, 71 (2), Feb 1975, 19–21.

8 Redman, B. K. The process of patient teaching in nursing. 2nd ed. St. Louis: Mosby, 1972.

9 Schweer, S. F. and Dayani, E. C. The extended role of professional nursing – patient education. International Nursing Review, 20 (6), Nov/Dec 1973, 174–175, 180.

10 Sharp, A. E. Four steps to better patient-teaching. RN Magazine, 37 (5), May 1974, 62–63.

11 Shaw, J. S. New hospital commitment: teaching patients how to live with illness and injury. [Multidisciplinary patient education.] Modern Hospital, 121 (4), Oct 1973, 99–102.

12 Storlie, F. A philosophy of patient teaching. Nursing Outlook, 19 (6), Jun 1971, 387–389.

13 Welford, W. Closing the communications gap. [Use of cassette tapes of doctors' advice.] Nursing Times, 71, 16 Jan 1975, 114–117.

d THERAPEUTIC TOUCH

1 Amacher, N. J. Touch is a way of caring and a way of communicating with an aphasic patient. American Journal of Nursing, 73 (5), May 1973, 852–854.

2 Barnett, K. A survey of the current utilization of touch by health team personnel with hospitalized patients. International Journal of Nursing Studies, 9 (4), Nov 1972, 195–208.

3 Barnett, K. A theoretical construct of the concepts of touch as they relate to nursing. Nursing Research, 21 (2), Mar/Apr 1972, 102–110.

4 Burnside, I. M. Touching is talking. [With elderly psychiatric patients.] American Journal of Nursing, 73 (12), Dec 1973, 2060–2063.

5 Dominian, J. The psychological significance of touch. Nursing Times, 67, 22 Jul 1971, 896–898.

6 Durr, C. A. Hands that help. . . but how? [Effects of physical contact between nurse and patient.] Nursing Forum, 10 (4), 1971, 392–400.

7 Hardy, J. The importance of touch: patient and nurse. Journal of Practical Nursing, 25 (6), Jun 1975, 26–27.

8 Johnson and Johnson Nursing survey reveals vital role of touch in patient care. Journal of Psychiatric Nursing and Mental Health Services, 12 (6), Nov/Dec 1974, 52.

9 Krieger, D. Therapeutic touch: the imprimatur of nursing. [Research.] American Journal of Nursing, 75 (5), May 1975, 784–787.

10 Kron, T. How we communicate nonverbally with patients. [The importance of 'bedside manners'.] Canadian Nurse, 68 (11), Nov 1972, 21–23.

11 McCorkle, R. Effects of touch on seriously ill patients. Nursing Research, 23 (2), Mar/Apr 1974, 125–132.

12 Unger, B. Please touch. Journal of Practical Nursing, 24 (12), Dec 1974, 29, 38.

16 PATIENT

a PATIENT PSYCHOLOGY

1 Allekian, C. I. Intrusions of territory and personal space: an anxiety-inducing factor for hospitalized persons – an exploratory study. Nursing Research, 22 (3), May/Jun 1973, 236–241.

2 Anderson, M. and Mottram, K. It's our problem too. [Group techniques to encourage greater awareness of psychological processes in nurses and patients.] International Journal of Nursing Studies, 10 (2), May 1973, 81–84.

3 Bhatia, A. K. Patient perception of needs and problems in the hospital set-up. [In a New Delhi hospital.] International Journal of Health Education, 14 (3), 1971, 145–150.

4 Brown, B. G. The language of space: a silent component of the therapeutic process. [Importance of patient's personal space.] Nursing Papers, 4 (1), Jul 1972, 29–35.

5 Connolly, M. P. Social roles and their implications. [The role of the patient as an area of potential role conflict.] Nursing Mirror, 141, 4 Dec 1975, 71–72.

6 Deliege, D. The sociological framework surrounding inpatients. [Sources of conflict in hospitals, including problems of communication, authority and function.] International Nursing Review, 21 (1), Jan/Feb 1974, 16–20.

7 Edelstein, R. R. G. The time factor in relation to illness as a fertile nursing research area: review of the literature. Nursing Research, 21 (1), Jan/Feb 1972, 72–76.

8 Foster, S. B. An adrenal measure for evaluating nursing effectiveness. [Physiological measurement of stress in patients before and after nursing intervention.] Nursing Research, 23 (2), Mar/Apr 1974, 118–124.

9 Franklin, B. L. Patient anxiety on admission to hospital. Royal College of Nursing and National Council of the United Kingdom, 1974. (Study of nursing care project series 1, no. 5.)

10 Gannon, B. Psychology and the nurse. 1. Who's afraid of psychology? 2. Perception. Nursing Mirror, 134, 3 Mar 1972, 42–43.

11 Gillis, L. Human behavior in illness: psychology and interpersonal relationships. 2nd ed. Faber, 1972.

12 Houston, C. S. and Pasanen, W. E. Patients' perceptions of hospital care. Hospitals, 46 (8), 16 Apr 1972, 70–74.

13 Johnson, J. E. Effects of structuring patients' expectations on their reactions to threatening events. Nursing Research, 21 (6', Nov/Dec 1972, 499–504.

14 Lagina, S. M. A computer program to diagnose anxiety levels. Nursing Research, 20 (6), Nov/Dec 1971, 484–492.

15 Levitt, R. Becoming a patient. [An analysis of the process of becoming a patient with a view to developing an understanding of patient needs.] Community Health, 6 (3), Nov/Dec 1974, 138–141.

16 Lorber, J. Good patients and problem patients: conformity and deviance in a general hospital. [Study investigating attitudes and behaviour.] Journal of Health and Social Behaviour, 16 (2), 1975, 213–225.

17 Mikulic, M. A. Reinforcement of independent and dependent patient behaviors by nursing personnel: an exploratory study. Nursing Research, 20 (2), Mar/Apr 1971, 162–165.

18 Munday, A. Physiological measures of anxiety in hospital patients. Rcn, 1973. (Study of nursing care research project series 2, no. 3.)

19 Murray, R. Illness as a crisis: nursing care for the patient in crisis. Journal of Practical Nursing, 23 (4), Apr 1973, 20–23.

20 The Nursing Clinics of North America Symposium on the concept of body image. Nursing Clinics of North America, 7 (4), Dec 1972, 593–707.

21 Pasquali, E. A. Personification: patient and nurse problem. [Helping patients to express emotions without relying on personification.] Perspectives in Psychiatric Care, 8 (2), Apr/Jun 1975, 58–61.

22 Peterson, M. H. Understanding defense mechanisms. Programmed instruction. American Journal of Nursing, 72 (9), Sep 1972, 1651–1672.

23 Polenz, J. M. Pyschological aspects of patient care. Nursing Care, 8 (10), Oct 1975, 16–20.

24 Radtke, M. and Wilson, A. Team conferences that work. [Nursing care meetings attended by a clinical psychologist and the patient concerned.] American Journal of Nursing, 73 (3), Mar 1973, 506–508.

25 Rao, S. K. R. Nurses' participation in patients' psychological problems. Nursing Journal of India, 66 (6), Jun 1975, 141–142.

26 Rice, P. L. Involvement: from the classroom to the community. [Nursing students' project to study behaviour as related to disfigurement.] Journal of Nursing Education, 12 (4), Nov 1973, 23, 25–28.

27 Rosenbaum, V. How to handle psychological regression in patients. Nursing Care, 8 (7), Jul 1973, 20–21.

28 Ryder, R. D. Attitudes and feelings in physical illness. District Nursing, 14 (6), Sep 1971, 116–117; Reprinted in Nursing Mirror, 135, 18 Aug 1972, 20–23.

29 Shontz, F. C. The psychological aspects of physical illness and disability. Collier Macmillan, 1975.

30 Skowronski, S. M. Proxemics and nursing care. [The structuring of personal and social space in interpersonal contacts.] Hospital Progress, 53 (8), Aug 1972, 72–77.

31 Smith, E. Only seeking attention. [Theories to explain behaviour.] Nursing Mirror, 136, 15 Jun 1973, 42–43.

32 Stevens, P. F. Adjusting to illness. Nursing Mirror, 134, 17 Mar 1972, 37–38.

33 Strong, P. G. Aggression in the general hospital. [Disturbed behaviour in patients.] Nursing Times, 69, 8 Feb 1973, Occ. papers, 21–24.

34 Thorpe, E. The meaning of illness: a social psychological perspective. Midwife and Health Visitor, 9 (7), Jul 1973, 222–224.

35 Volicer, B. J. and Bohannon, M. W. A hospital stress rating scale. [261 medical and surgical patients rank 49 events related to hospitalization in order of stress.] Nursing Research, 24 (5), Sep/Oct 1975, 352–359.

36 Volicer, B. J. Patients' perceptions of stressful events associated with hospitalization. Nursing Research, 23 (3), May/Jun 1974, 235–238.

37 Volicer, B. J. Perceived stress levels of events associated with the experience of hospitalization: development and testing of a measurement tool. Nursing Research, 22 (6), Nov/Dec 1973, 491–497.

38 United States. Department of Health, Education and Welfare. Nursing Department A new dimension in the care of hospital patients under stress: a multidisciplinary patient care study. Washington: The Department, 1974.

39 Vincent, P. Factors influencing patient noncompliance: a theoretical approach. Nursing Research, 20 (6), Nov/Dec 1971, 509–516.

40 Vincent P. The sick role in patient care. [A concept of patient behaviour which presents a basis for improving care.] American Journal of Nursing, 75 (7), Jul 1975, 1172–1173.

41 Wacker, M. S. Analogy: weapon against denial. [Of serious illness.] American Journal of Nursing, 74 (1), Jan 1974, 71–73.

42 Wells, R. W. Body image and surgical alterations. AORN Journal, 21 (5), Apr 1975, 812–815.

b SENSORY DEPRIVATION

1 Alderson, M. J. Effect of increased body temperature on the perception of time. Nursing Research, 23 (1), Jan/Feb 1974, 42–49.

2 Bolin, R. H. Sensory deprivation: an overview. A theoretical framework. . .[of] the concepts of sensory deprivation. . .[and] nursing implications. Nursing Forum, 13 (3), 1974, 240–258.

3 Cameron, C. F. and others When sensory deprivation occurs. [Nurses should provide patients with sensory stimulation.] Canadian Nurse, 68 (11), Nov 1972, 32–34.

4 Downs, F. S. Bed rest and sensory disturbances. [An experiment in sensory deprivation.] American Journal of Nursing, 74 (3), Mar 1974, 434–438.

5 Gimbel, L. The pathology of boredom and sensory deprivation. [Implications for nursing care particularly with geriatric patients.] Canadian Journal of Psychiatric Nursing, 16 (5), Sep/Oct 1975, 12–13.

6 Jackson, C. W. and Ellis, R. Sensory deprivation as a field of study. [In hospitalized patients.] Nursing Research, 20 (1), Jan/Feb 1971, 46–54.

7 Smith, M. J. Changes in judgment of duration with different patterns of auditory information for individuals confined to bed. [To investigate passage of time.] Nursing Research, 24 (2), Mar/Apr 1975, 93–98.

8 Thomson, L. R. Sensory deprivation: a personal experience. [Nurse's reactions as a patient on an intensive care unit.] American Journal of Nursing, 73 (2), Feb 1973, 266–268.

c PATIENTS' VIEWS

1 Daniel, D. What the patient thinks. [A senior nursing officer, reports on visits to over 300 ex-patients to collect their opinions of hospital life and procedures.] Nursing Mirror, 141, 4 Dec 1975, 73.

2 Eardley, A. and Wakefield, J. What patients think about the Christie Hospital: a report on 500 interviews. Manchester: Christie Hospital, 1973.

3 Farthing, D. My thoughts as a patient. Physiotherapy, 59 (12), Dec 1973, 393–394.

4 Germaine, A. Expectations and realities. Of patients and staff in the hospital community.] Hospital Administration in Canada, 16 (12), Dec 1974, 20, 22.

5 Hospitals Consumer views: respect is first demand: summary of surveys of patients' attitudes toward hospitals. Hospitals, 48, 16 Aug 1974, 57–58, 59–61.

6 Levitt, R. Attitudes of hospital patients. [Communication with staff. A study at Charing Cross Hospital.] Nursing Times, 71, 27 Mar 1975, 497–499.

7 Marram, G. D. Patients' evaluation of their care: importance to the nurse. Nursing Outlook, 21 (5), May 1973, 322–324.

8 Marram, G. D. Patients' evaluation of nursing performance. Nursing Outlook, 22 (2), Mar/Apr 1973, 153–157.

9 Moore, D. S. and Cook-Hubbard, K. Comparison of methods for evaluating patient response to nursing care. [Study of obstetric patients.] Nursing Research, 24 (3), May/Jun 1975, 202–204.

10 Nehring, V. and Geach, B. Patients' evaluation of their care: why they don't complain. Nursing Outlook, 21 (5), May 1973, 317–321.

11 Nemo Tender loving care. [A day in the life of a dissatisfied patient in a London teaching hospital.] Nursing Times, 69, 5 Jul 1973, 876–877.

12 Novak, B. J. and Cohn, R. E. It's often little details that make the most difference. . . From the patient's point of view. Nursing Care, 8 (6), Jun 1975, 28–29.

13 Pablo, R. Y. Assessing patient satisfaction in long-term care institutions. [Results of data collected by questionnaire from patients at Parkwood Hospital, London, Ontario.] Hospital Administration in Canada, 17 (3), Mar 1975, 22–23, 26–29, 31–32.

14 Phillips, D. The patient is a person. [A patient's view of his treatment received in hospital.] Nursing Mirror, 141, 24 Jul 1975, 64–65.

15 Pike, N. In hospital. 1. The adult patient's view. Nursing Mirror, 140, 24 Apr 1975, 67–69.

16 Pike, N. In hospital. 2. The outpatient's view. Nursing Mirror, 140, 1 May 1975, 51.

17 Pike, N. In hospital. 4. The senior citizen's view. Nursing Mirror, 140, 22/29 May 1975, 77–78.

18 Pollert, I. E. Expectations and discrepancies with hospital conditions as they actually exist. International Journal of Nursing Studies, 8 (3), Aug 1971, 135–143.

19 Raphael, W. Patients and their hospitals: a survey of patients' views of life in hospital. King Edwards Hospital Fund for London, 1973.

20 Rix, A. T. Monitoring system for patients. [Sample survey of standards of care.] Health and Social Service Journal, 83, 28 Jul 1973, 1694.

21 Tuckwell, P. The patient's point of view. [Inconveniences to patients on a small ward restricted to a minimum.] Nursing Mirror, 139, 26 Sep 1974, 69.

22 Wolfe, K. M. The strong and the weak. [The effect of his hospital stay on the author.] Nursing Times, 67, 16 Sep 1971, 1152–1154.

23 Wriglesworth, J. M. and Williams, J. T. The construction of an objective test to measure patient satisfaction. [Survey by questionnaire to patients in two male surgical wards at Wythenshawe Hospital, Manchester.] International Journal of Nursing Studies, 12 (3), 1975, 123–132.

d PATIENT WELFARE

1 American Nurses' Foundation Effects of family goals on performance of tasks and use of resources during acute illness. Nursing Research Report, 6 (1), Mar 1971, 1, 4, 6–7.

2 Bearden, F. C. An interactional approach to hospital visiting. Journal of Psychiatric Nursing, 10 (4), Jul/Aug 1972, 16–17.

3 Cameron, J. Patients must come first. Conference report. [Association of Nurse Administrators conference held at Swansea.] Nursing Mirror, 140, 17 Apr 1975, 35.

4 Catholic Hospital Association Visiting patients: hints on what to say and do. St Louis: The Association, 1972.

5 Cockburn, E. Relative helpers in the ward. Nursing Times, 71, 13 Nov 1975, 1833.

6 Corbus, H. F. and Connell, R. W. The patient's needs – does anyone care? Patient care committee for the human as well as the clinical needs of hospital patients. Hospitals, 48 (2), 16 Jan 1974, 46–49.

7 Cunningham, C. Traditional nursing – a harsh regime? [For the patient.] Nursing Mirror, 132, 4 Jun 1971, 38–39.

8 Davis, D. E. Visiting groups: blessing or curse? [A survey to discover the attitudes of patients and staff to such visits.] Nursing Times, 71, 30 Jan 1975, Occ. papers, 5–7.

9 Diers, D. Research for nursing. [Measurement of patient welfare.] Journal of Nursing Administration, 3 (1), Jan/Feb 1973, 8, 11.

10 Dolan, P. O. and Flumere, J. A. Patients' coffee hour: a means of increasing socialization. American Journal of Nursing, 74 (3), Mar 1974, 479–480.

11 Frost, M. Talking and listening to relatives. Nursing Times, 66, 3 Sep 1970, Occ. papers, 129–132.

12 Hare, F. The value of a co-ordinator of hospital visitors. [With particular reference to the Bethlem Royal and Maudsley Hospitals.] World Hospitals, 10 (4), Autumn 1974, 202–206.

13 Hodgson, H. Patients and privacy. Hospital and Health Services Review, 71 (2), Feb 1975, 44–46.

14 Langrehr, A. A. Social stimulation. [For patients in hospital by means of social gatherings.] American Journal of Nursing, 74 (7), Jul 1974, 1300–1301.

15 Leonard, M. and Leitch, M. The sister and the MSW. Nursing Times, 69, 5 Apr 1973, 437–438.

16 MacDonald, F. G. Longer visiting hours? Nursing Times, 66, 4 Jun 1970, 730.

17 McKeown, T. and others Influence of hospital siting on patient visiting. Lancet, 2, 13 Nov 1971, 1082–1086.

18 Mancino, D. J. and Harmon, V. Visiting trends and gift giving: some observations of differences between two racial groups. Nursing Forum, 11 (3), 1972, 264–272.

19 Portman, R. Who cares for the relatives? Nursing Times, 70, 18 Jul 1974, 1125.

20 Priestley, R. J. Social work in hospital – a look at the future: changes at St. James' Hospital, Balham. Hospital and Health Service Review, 70 (8), Aug 1974, 267–268.

21 Priestley, R. J. and Watkins, K. M. Social work in hospitals – a look at the future. An analysis of a case study at St. James' Hospital, Balham. Hospital and Health Services Review, 69 (7), Jul 1973, 250–253.

22 Rawcliffe, A. and Taylor, J. E. Visiting panels: a forerunner of community health councils? Hospital and Health Services Review, 68 (3), Mar 1972, 88–91.

23 Red Cross beauty care. Health and Social Service Journal, 83, 18 Aug 1973, 1861.

24 Roberts, H. Talking to relatives. Nursing Times, 67, 15 Jul 1971, 860–861.

25 Rose, G. and Udechuku, J. C. Cigarette smoking by hospital patients. British Journal of Preventive & Social Medicine, 25 (3), Aug 1971, 160–161.

26 Rudd, T. N. Improving the quality of life in hospital. [An outline of policies which might be adopted.] Nursing Mirror, 139, 5 Dec 1974, 53–54.

27 Schuster, E. A. Privacy and hospitalization: subject of nurse's investigation. Nursing Research Report, 8 (3), Oct 1973, 1, 3, 5, 8.

28 Smith, C. R. Social workers in hospitals: misplaced intruders or essential experts? British Medical Journal, 3, 25 Aug 1973, 443–446.

29 Speakman, J. Hospital visitors – a curse or a blessing? [Volunteers in long stay hospitals.] Nursing Times, 71, 13 Feb 1975, 274–275.

30 Speck, P. W. The hospital visitor. Nursing Times, 69, 5 Jul 1973, 878–879.

31 Standon–Batt, M. I. Hospital visiting: a survey at the maternity unit, Royal Berkshire Hospital, Reading. Midwives Chronicle, 86, Sep 1972, 284–286.

32 Westbrook, K. Coping with relatives. Nursing Mirror, 134, 2 Jun 1972, 38–39.

33 Williamson, E. A. The gentle art of visiting. Nursing Times, 67, 16 Dec 1971, 1565–1566.

e CULTURAL DIFFERENCES

1 Caudle, P. Found: one person. When a white nurse and a black patient began to know each other, they learned to trust. American Journal of Nursing, 73 (2), Feb 1973, 310–313.

2 Chandra, F. Hindu patients in hospital. Nursing Times, 70, 11 Apr 1974, 562–563.

3 Pasquali, E. East meets west: a transcultural aspect of the nurse-patient relationship. [Japanese-American patient.] Journal of Psychiatric Nursing and Mental Health Services, 12 (5), Sep/Oct 1974, 20–22.

4 Piero, P. Black white crisis. [Race relations between patients and nurses.] American Journal of Nursing, 74 (2), Feb 1974, 280–281.

5 Weinberg, H. Staff overcomes barriers to care. [The problems of dealing with ethnic groups seen at a New York hospital serving an Albanian population.] Hospitals, 49, 16 Aug 1975, 60–62.

6 White, E. H. Health and the black person: an annotated bibliography. American Journal of Nursing, 74 (10), Oct 1974, 1839–1841.

7 Wicker, I. B. Overcoming cultural barriers: an inservice education program can help to overcome barriers to understanding between nurses and minority group patients. Hospitals, 45, 16 Oct 1971, 77–78, 80.

17 INTENSIVE CARE

a GENERAL

1 Ashworth, P. Ethics in the intensive care therapy unit. Nursing Mirror, 139, 14 Nov 1974, 57–60, 63.

2 Ashworth, P and others Intensive therapy 1960–1973 – the development of a unit. [Broadgreen Hospital, Liverpool.] Nursing Times, 69, 6 Sep 1973, 1164–1166.

3 Bell, J. A. and others Six years of multidisciplinary intensive care. [At St. Thomas's Hospital.] British Medical Journal, 2, 1 Jun 1974, 483–488.

4 Blackburn Intensive care unit for Blackburn. Nursing Times, 68, 27 Jul 1972, 949; Nursing Mirror, 135, 28 Jul 1972, 27.

5 Clark, T. J. H. and others A review of experience operating a general medical intensive care unit. British Medical Journal, 1, 16 Jan 1971, 158–161.

6 Health and Social Service Journal and Hospital International Intensive care. The Journal, 1974. (British health care and technology series).

7 Johnson-Cadwell, E. Intensive care congress. [World Congress on Intensive Care, Imperial College, London.] Nursing Times, 70, 18 Jul 1974, 1121.

8 Klein, R. Intensive care. [Changing pattern of hospital use 1959–1973.] New Society, 32, 22 May 1975, 478.

9 Mercer, B. Intensive care units at Wellington. New Zealand Nursing Journal, 64 (8), Aug 1971, 21–22.

10 Morley, K. B. Impressions on a world tour, with particular reference to intensive care. Physiotherapy, 57 (7), 10 Jul 1971, 309–313.

11 Robinson, A. M. ICUs and CCUs: not even half a century. RN Magazine, 37 (2), Feb 1973, ICU 1, 4.

12 Robinson, A. M. Intensive care today – and tomorrow: a summing-up. RN Magazine, 35 (9), Sep 1972, 56–60.

13 Walker, W. F. and Taylor, D. E., editors Intensive care: proceedings of the 8th Pfizer International Symposium held in Edinburgh from 15–16 October, 1973. Edinburgh: Churchill Livingstone, 1975.

14 World Congress on Intensive Care 1st. London, 1974. Scientific abstracts, edited and compiled by I. Ledingham. Intensive Care Society, 1974.

b EQUIPMENT AND MONITORING

1 Ashcroft, J. Computers in intensive care units. Nursing Mirror, 138, 28 Jun 1974, 5–52.

2 Collins, J. V. and others Basic equipment for medical intensive-care units. Lancet, 1, 6 Feb 1971, 285–287.

3 Doyle, A. J. A study of nurses' attitudes towards the introduction of patient-monitoring equipment into hospitals. MPhil thesis, Birkbeck College, London University, 1971.

4 Freyer, R. and others Patient-information system for intensive care. Lancet, 2, 15 Jul 1972, 119–120.

5 Green, H. L. Hazards of electronic equipment in critical care areas: a research approach. Cardiovascular Nursing, 9 (2), Mar/Apr 1973, 7–12.

6 Green, H. L. Monitoring equipment for IC Units. British Hospital Journal and Social Service Review, 82, 29 Jul 1972, 1679–1680.

7 Hornaday, L. and Satterthwaite, M. ICU procedure assignment aided by use of magnetized panels. [Method of checking if nursing procedures completed.] Hospital Topics, 49 (6), Jun 1971, 41, 44.

8 Lancet Computers or nurses? [Editorial on the use of computers to assist nurses with particular reference to monitoring the patient in intensive care units.] Lancet, 2, 12 Oct 1974, 877–878; Correspondence 2 Nov 1974, 1081–1082.

9 Morrison, S. N. J. Electronics in nursing: biomedical applications of space related technology. [Monitoring of physiological functions in intensive care nursing.] New Zealand Nursing Journal, 65 (6), Jun 1972, 12–16.

10 Tinker, J. Information for intensive care. [Use of a computer system.] Nursing Mirror, 136, 6 Apr 1973, 34–37.

11 Walleck, C. The neurosurgical nurse and computer work together. [Use of computers in intensive care.] Journal of Neurosurgical Nursing, 7 (2), Dec 1975, 102–106.

12 Williams, M. A. Why the maze of monitors? [Types of equipment for different conditions in the intensive care unit.] SA Nursing Journal, 52 (12), Dec 1975, 17, 20–21.

c MANAGEMENT AND PLANNING AND STAFFING

1 Bobrow, M. L. and Craft, N. B. Planning – ICU and CCU facilities. Hospitals, 45, 16 May 1971, 47–51.

2 Browne, D. R. G. and others The Royal Free Hospital. 2. A mobile intensive care service. Nursing Times, 70, 10 Oct 1974, 1580–1582.

3 Cady, L. D. and others Optimizing the use of critical care beds: a new concentrated care unit provides buffer between intensive care and general care units. Hospitals, 46, 16 Feb 1972, 58–60.

4 Department of Health and Society Security and Welsh Office Intensive therapy unit. Rev. ed. HMSO 1974. [Hospital building note, 27.)

5 Hanson, G. C. Intensive therapy: staffing and management. Health and Social Service Journal, 84, 3 Aug 1974, 1738–1739.

6 Hanson, G. C. Organization and planning of an intensive therapy unit. Nutrition, 28 (5), 1974, 335–337.

7 Kinney, J. M. ICU organization, goals, growth, cost spotlighted at conference. Hospital Topics, 49 (9), Sep 1971, 22–24, 26–28, 31.

8 MacKenzie, S. Planning intensive therapy units. British Hospital Journal and Social Service Review, 81, 18 Sep 1971, 1911–1913, 1915.

9 Martin, L. E. Cost and management: problems of intensive care units. Modern Hospital, 118 (1), Jan 1972, 97–99.

10 Mitchell, T. N. and Groves, W. H. Two-part design for intensive ward. [Broadgreen Hospital, Liver-

pool.] British Hospital Journal and Social Service Review, 81, 18 Sep 1971, 1916–1918.

11 Modern Hospital At French Hospital the ICU and CCU share the space and the nurses. [Joint organization and equipment.] Modern Hospital, 119 (4), Oct 1972, 110–111.

12 Modern Hospital Feature on special care units. Modern Hospital, 118 (1), Jan 1972, 81–102. Includes: Standards for special care units: guidelines for organization, staffing and costs. 83–86.

13 Modern Hospital Special care units have special design requirements. Modern Hospital, 118 (3), Mar 1972, 105–108.

14 Morgan, D. M. Guidelines for the construction of an IC unit. Canadian Hospital, 48 (8), Aug 1971, 30, 32, 33, 36.

15 Morgan, D. M. The planning and operation of intensive care units. Canadian Hospital, 48 (8), Aug 1971, 28–30.

16 Purushotham, D. and others Team approach to intensive care? The ICU nurse: the medical director; the respiratory technologist. Hospital Administration in Canada, 15 (4), Apr 1973, 47–48, 50–51, 53.

17 Robinson, A. M. The nurse/doctor game (new style). Professional conflict in the ICU/CCU. RN Magazine, 35 (5), May 1972, 40–45, 101.

18 Rockwell, S. M. Conflicting orders in the ICU? Try the team captain idea. RN Magazine, 35 (9), Sep 1972, ICU 1, 4.

19 Tanser, A. R. and Wetten, B. G. Multipurpose intensive care unit in a district general hospital. [St. Martin's Hospital, Bath.] British Medical Journal, 3, 28 Jul 1973, 227–229.

20 Waddell, G. Movement of critically ill patients within hospital. [Study of movement to and from the intensive care unit at the Western Infirmary, Glasgow.] British Medical Journal, 2, 24 May 1975, 417–419.

21 Waddell, G. Moving the critically ill. [Five month survey of 55 patients admitted to an intensive care unit.] Nursing Times, 71, 4 Dec 1975, 1937–1939.

22 Wilson, P. Stock control in an intensive therapy unit. Nursing Times, 70, 14 Nov 1974, 1785–1787.

23 Wylie, D. M. Designing an Intensive Care Unit. Hospital Administration in Canada, 14 (5), May 1972, 68–69, 71.

d NURSING

1 Benner, P. and Kramer, M. Role conceptions and integrative role behaviour of nurses in special care and regular hospital nursing units. Nursing Research, 21 (1), Jan/Feb 1972, 20–29.

2 Burrell, Z. L. and Burrell, L. O. Intensive care nursing. 2nd ed. St. Louis: Mosby, 1973.

3 Charter, D. A nurse talks about intensive care. Canadian Hospital, 48 (8), Aug 1971, 45.

4 Clarke, D. B. and Barnes, A. D., editors Intensive care for nurses. 2nd ed. Blackwell, 1975.

5 Emery, E. R. J. and others Principles of intensive care. English Universities Press, 1973. (Modern nursing series.)

6 Finn, R. and Drury, P. M. A guide to the intensive therapy unit. Butterworth, 1974.

7 Froelich, R. Making rotation work. [Nursing staff rotation between the recovery room, intensive care and coronary care units and emergency departments.] RN Magazine, 35 (10), Oct 1972, 44–47.

8 Gerson, G., editor Intensive care. Heinemann Medical, 1973.

9 Harris, E. A. and others Intensive care of the heart and lungs: a text for nurses. 2nd ed. Blackwell Scientific, 1973.

10 Hudak, C. M. and others Critical care nursing. Philadelphia: Lippincott, 1973.

11 Kilgour, D. Y. Do special units need 'special nurses'? [Report of a research project to discover what qualities made nurses suitable for intensive therapy work.] Nursing Mirror, 133, 15 Oct 1971, 27–30.

12 Kilgour, D. Y. An investigation into the attitudes of nurses who work in intensive therapy units. MSc thesis, Edinburgh University, 1970.

13 Kilgour, D. Y. In intensive therapy units, are nurses more concerned with machines than with patients? [Report study.] Health Bulletin, 30 (1), Jan 1972, 23–25; Nursing Times, 68, 4 May 1972, 529–530.

14 Kirk, G. M. A matter of perspective. [The art of nursing in the technological situation of the intensive care unit.] Nursing Times, 68, 5 Oct 1972, 1242–1243.

15 Main, M. In intensive care units. Flexibility – the key to critical care nursing. Dimensions in Health Service, 51 (8), Aug 1974, 49–50.

16 Missen, J. Principles of intensive care for nurses. Heinemann, 1975.

17 Morgan, D. M. Nursing staff requirements for special care units. Canadian Hospital, 48 (8), Aug 1971, 46.

18 Nursing Clinics of North America Symposium on units for special care. Nursing Clinics of North America, 7 (2), Jun 1972, 311–406.

19 Pahwa, S. D. Intensive nursing care. Nursing Journal of India, 64 (11), Mar 1974, 377–378.

20 Purushotham, D. The challenge of ICU nursing. [The need for highly developed clinical skills and sensitivity to the patient's needs.] Hospital Administration in Canada, 14 (8), Aug 1972, 32–34.

21 Purushotham, D. Nursing the critically-ill patient. Hospital Administration in Canada, 16 (5), May 1974, 38–40.

22 Rains, A. J. H. Intensive care – background to relationships and responsibility. Nursing Mirror, 139, 14 Nov 1974, 78–80.

23 RN Magazine Overview: new challenge for with-it nurses. [RN survey of intensive care in 4 hospitals.] RN Magazine, 35 (1), Jan 1972, 32–39; (3), Mar 1972, 47–51.

24 Royal College of Nursing ITU nurses 'must look confident'. [Report of meeting of Rcn Intensive Therapy Group in Cardiff.] Nursing Times, 71, 2 Jan 1975, 6.

25 Royal College of Nursing Rcn's first symposium on intensive care. 'Keep the patient in focus.' [Report of the meeting.] Nursing Times, 70, 4 Jul 1974, 1014–1015.

26 Skillman, J. J. Intensive care. Boston: Little, Brown, 1975.

27 Stoddart, J. C. Intensive therapy. Blackwell, 1975.

28 Wahlin, A. and others Intensive care nursing continuing education review: 403 essay questions and referenced answers. Flushing: Medical Examination Publishing Co., 1974.

29 World Health Organization Regional Office for Europe Nursing in intensive care. Report on a Seminar convened by the Regional Office for Europe. . . Copenhagen, 10–14 November, 1969. Copenhagen: WHO, 1971.

e NURSING: EDUCATION AND TRAINING

1 Butterfield, S. Chandris scholar. [Report of a study tour in Europe and the USA to gain clinical experience in intensive care and to study teaching methods in special units.] New Zealand Nursing Journal, 68 (10), Oct 1974, 18–20.

2 Finn, B. Special training for intensive care. Courses approved by the Joint Board of Clinical Nursing Studies.] Nursing Times, 70, 28 Nov 1974, 1868–1869.

3 LaFontan, L. An approach to ICU nurse education in a small rural community hospital. Journal of Continuing Education in Nursing, 2 (5), Sep/Oct 1971, 32–37.

4 Lancour, J. and Reinders, A. A. A pilot project in continuing education for critical care nursing. Journal of Nursing Administration, 5 (8), Oct 1975, 38–41.

5 Lingley-Savas, C. Don't let the machines turn you off! [Orientation in the ICU Brookdale Hospital, Brooklyn.] RN Magazine, 38 (11), Nov 1975, ICU 1, 4, 8.

6 Mathie, J. R. Management research. Intensive care course: planning, progress and evaluation. [Course at Whiston Hospital, Lancs.] Nursing Times, 70, 29 Aug 1974, 1358–1359.

f PSYCHOLOGICAL ASPECTS
(Staff and patients)

1 Baxter, S. Pyschological problems of intensive care. [Part 2 includes coronary care. Reprinted from the British Journal of Hospital Medicine.] Nursing Times, 71, 2 Jan 1975, 22–23; 9 Jan 1975, 63–65.

2 Downey, G. W. Special care unit. ICU patients and staff are subject to emotional stress. Modern Hospital, 118 (1), Jan 1972, 88–91.

3 Freebury, D. R. The long arm of research. [Research project in an intensive care unit to determine if the setting contributed to psychiatric disorder.] Canadian Nurse, 68 (10), Oct 1972, 40–45.

4 Hutchinson, S. Some psychological aspects of CCU nursing. [Psychological care of an anxious patient and his relatives.] RN Magazine, 36 (6), Jun 1973, ICU 1, 4, 9.

5 Kahn, A. Stranger in the world of ICU. [Patients' psychosocial needs in the intensive care unit.] American Journal of Nursing, 75 (11), Nov 1975, 2022–2025.

6 Murray, R. L. E. Assessment of psychologic status in the surgical ICU patient. Nursing Clinics of North America, 10 (1), Mar 1975, 69–81.

7 Nursing Times Psychological apsects of intensive care. Nursing Times, 70, 6 Jun 1974, 883.

8 Rauen, K. Patients' view of an ICU. RN Magazine, 35 (9), Sep 1972, ICU 7–8.

9 Sullon, G. What happened to Mrs. Brown? – a study of acute psychotic reactions in patients nursed in intensive care units. Lamp, 32 (12), Dec 1975, 26–27.

10 Taylor, D. E. M. Problems of patients in an intensive care unit: the aetiology and prevention of the intensive care syndrome. International Journal of Nursing Studies, 8 (1), Feb 1971, 47–59.

11 Wallace, P. Relatives should be told about intensive care – but how much and by whom? Canadian Nurse, 67 (6), Jun 1971, 33–34.

12 West, N. D. Stresses associated with ICUs affect patients, families, staff. Hospitals, 49, 16 Dec 1975, 62–63.

13 Woods, N. F. and Falk, S. A. Noise stimuli in the acute care area. Nursing Research, 23 (2), Mar/Apr 1974, 144–150.

18 SPIRITUAL CARE

a NURSING

1 Christopher, W. I. Apostolic effectiveness of the hospital sister. Hospital Progress, 53 (2), Feb 1972, 44–46.

2 Dickinson, C. The search for spiritual meaning. [The nurse's role in spiritual care.] American Journal of Nursing, 75 (10), Oct 1975, 1789–1793.

3 Griffiths, Rev. J. W. Challenge to the nurse's faith. Nursing Mirror, 132, 26 Feb 1971, 39–41.

4 Griffiths, Rev. J. W. Emergency baptisms in hospitals. Nursing Mirror, 132, 19 Feb 1971, 40–41.

5 Griffiths, Rev. J. W. The patient and Holy Communion. Nursing Mirror, 132, 12 Feb 1971, 17–19.

6 Jell, F. E. Prayers of a nurse. Nursing Mirror, 141, 10 Jul 1975, 58; 28 Aug 1975, 48; 25 Sep 1975, 49.

7 Kelly, E. M. Shrine of hope. [Lourdes.] Nursing Times, 71, 5 Jun 1975, 895–897.

8 Morris, K. L. and Foerster, J. D. Team work: nurse and chaplain. American Journal of Nursing, 72 (12), Dec 1972, 2197–2199.

9 Porath, T. Humanizing the Sacrament of the Sick. Hospital Progress, 53 (7), Jul 1972, 44–47.

10 Raciappa, J. D. A total ministry: a priest of 15 years' standing goes to nursing school. American Journal of Nursing, 73 (4), Apr 1973, 645.

11 Simone, M. Demands on the Christian nurse. Hospital Progress, 52 (8), Aug 1971, 43–44, 46.

12 Toohey, T. J. The challenge of the new rite of anointing. Hospital Progress, 55 (5), May 1974, 60–63, 88.

13 Wheelock, R. D. Unmet patient needs. [Spiritual and emotional needs.] Hospital Progress, 55 (7), Jul 1974, 60–64, 68.

14 Zefron, L. J. The history of the laying on of hands in nursing. Nursing Forum, 14 (4), 1975, 350–363.

b HOSPITAL CHAPLAINS

1 Carey, R. G. Chaplaincy: component of total patient care? Hospitals, 47 (14), 16 Jul 1973, 166, 168, 170, 172.

2 Gruendemann, B. J. Hospital chaplain: the 'now' member of the health team. RN Magazine, 36 (10), Oct 1973, 38–40, 42, 46, 48, 52.

3 Hallman, H. W. Consider the poor pastor. Bedside Nurse, 4 (2), Feb 1971, 28–29.

4 Hofmann, P. B. Who refers chaplains to patients? Hospitals, 48 (1), 1 Jan 1974, 102–104.

5 Kuby, A. M. and Begole, C. M. AHA surveys chaplaincy programs. Hospitals, 48 (1), 1 Jan 1974, 98–102.

6 Long, Rev. R. J. TV Chapel reaches more patients. Hospitals, 47 (1), Jan 1973, 96–97.

7 McKeever, D. A. Ministry to staff aids quality control. [Hospital service chaplaincy alleviates employees' stress.] Hospitals, 49 (14), 16 Jul 1975, 181, 184.

8 McPhee, Rev. D. The hospital chaplain and the patient's family. Hospital Progress, 53 (10), Oct 1972, 55–57.

9 Nursing Times A selection of recently published literature 1970–1971. Relevant to the Ministry of the hospital chaplain. Nursing Times, 67, 11 Nov 1971, Occ. papers, 180, 18 Nov 1971, Occ. papers, 184.

10 O'Meara, Rev. T. F. Christian ministry and health service. Hospital Progress, 54 (1), Jan 1973, 89–92, 94.

11 Pett, Rev. D. The hospital chaplain: instances in which his services can prove invaluable. Nursing Times, 69, 13 Dec 1973, 1678–1682.

12 Phillips, A. K. The chaplain's role in a nursing home. Hospital Progress, 54 (6), Jun 1973, 75–78.

13 Smith, Rev. W. J. Hospital chaplains: areas for further professional education. Hospital Progress, 54 (4), Apr 1973, 62–64, 66.

14 Swafford, Rev. J. N. Planning a chapel and its services. Hospitals, 47 (1), Jan 1973, 98–99.

15 Weiler, C. Developing department of pastoral care. Hospital Progress, 54 (12), Dec 1973, 42–44.

16 Weiler, C. Patients evaluate pastoral care. [Results of a questionnaire.] Hospital Progress, 56 (4), Apr 1975, 34–35, 38.

17 Wheelock, Rev. R. D. Evaluating pastoral care. Hospital Progress, 54 (9), Sep 1973, 18, 20.

19 TERMINAL CARE AND DEATH

a DEATH AND DYING

1 Armstrong, M. E. Dying and death – and life experiences of loss and gain: a proposed theory. Nursing Forum, 14 (1), 1975, 95–104.

2 Benson, G. Death and dying – a psychoanalytic perspective. Hospital Progress, 53 (3), Mar 1972, 52–59, 74.

3 Cotter, Z. M. On not getting better. Hospital Progress, 53 (3), Mar 1972, 60–63.

4 Frost, M. Death. Nursing Mirror, 132, 29 Jan 1971, 41–42.

5 Gresham, G. A. Post-mortem examination. Nursing Times, 69, 7 Jun 1973, 726–729.

6 Gullo, S. V. Thanatology: the study of death and the care of the dying. Bedside Nurse, 5 (5), May 1972, 11–14.

7 Hinton, J. Dying. 2nd ed. Harmondsworth, Penguin, 1972.

8 Kosnik, A. R. Theological reflections on criteria for defining the moment of death. Hospital Progress, 54 (12), Dec 1973, 64–69.

9 Mead, J. M. It comes to us all. Nursing Mirror, 132, 29 Jan 1971, 40.

10 Rees, W. D. The distress of dying. Nursing Times, 68, 23 Nov 1972, 1479–1480.

11 Shusterman, L. R. Death and dying: a critical review of the literature. Nursing Outlook, 21 (7), Jul 1973, 465–471.

12 Simpson, M. A. Teaching about death and dying. Nursing Times, 69, 5 Apr 1973, 442–443.

13 Simpson, M. A. What is dying like? Nursing Times, 69, 29 Mar 1973, 405–406.

14 Speer, G. M. Learning about death. Perspectives in Psychiatric Care, 12 (2), Apr/Jun 1974, 70–73.

15 West, T. S. Approach to death. Nursing Mirror, 139, 10 Oct 1974, 56–59.

16 **Wise, D. J.** Learning about dying. Nursing Outlook, 22 (1), Jan 1974, 42–44.

b BEREAVEMENT

1 **Alfred Hospital, Melbourne – Medical Social Work Department** Learning to live with death and grieving. UNA Nursing Journal, 69, Apr 1971, 9–17.

2 **Bowen, A.** The psychiatric aspects of bereavement. Practitioner, 210, Jan 1973, 127–134.

3 **Brandon, S.** Grief. Practitioner, 212, Jun 1974, 867–875.

4 **Burnside, I. M.** 'You will cope, of course. . .' [A widow's reactions to her husband's death.] American Journal of Nursing, 71 (12), Dec 1971, 2354–2357.

5 **Caughill, R. E.** Outpatient care. Emergency after death. [Support to relatives and ED staff after death in ED.] Hospital Topics, 51 (6), Jun 1973, 37–41, 74.

6 **Deeble, K. A. K.** A chance to care. [Dealing with bereaved relatives.] Nursing Mirror, 140, 17 Apr 1975, 59–61.

7 **Dunlop, M.** Grief and mourning. Australian Nurses' Journal, 1 (6), Dec 1971, 22–24.

8 **Furman, F.** A child's parent dies: studies in childhood bereavement. New Haven: Yale University Press, 1974.

9 **Gibson, R.** Caring for the bereaved. Nursing Mirror, 139, 10 Oct 1974, 65–66.

10 **Hampe, S. O.** Needs of the grieving spouse in a hospital setting: study of 27 spouses before and after death of mates due to terminal illness. Nursing Research, 24 (2), Mar/Apr 1975, 113–120.

11 **Human, M. E.** Death of a neighbour. American Journal of Nursing, 73 (11), Nov 1973, 1914–1916.

12 **Leared, J.** The Camden Bereavement Project. Midwife and Health Visitor, 10 (1), Jan 1974, 15–16.

13 **Melville, J.** Talking out your grief. [Camden Bereavement Project.] New Society, 26, 8 Nov 1973, 327.

14 **Morris, S.** Grief and how to live with it. Allen and Unwin, 1971.

15 **Parkes, C. M.** Bereavement: studies of grief in adult life. Tavistock, 1972.

16 **Rees, W. D.** The hallucinations of widowhood. British Medical Journal, 4, 20 Oct 1971, 37–41.

17 **Rincar, E. E.** The nurse's challenge when death is unexpected. [Advice on how to help relatives after a sudden death.] RN Magazine, 38 (12), Dec 1975, 50–55.

18 **Robinson, A. M.** Keys to understanding the patient. Loss and grief. Journal of Practical Nursing, 21 (5), May 1971, 18–19, 34, 36–38.

19 **Rogers, J. and Vachon, M. L. S.** Nurses can help the bereaved. Canadian Nurse, 71 (6), Jun 1975, 16–19.

20 **Stephens, S.** Bereavement and the care of the bereaved. Midwife and Health Visitor, 8 (3), Mar 1972, 89, 91–94.

21 **Weller, M. F.** Bereavement. Health Visitor, 48 (5), May 1975, 155–156.

22 **Wilson, F. G.** Social isolation and bereavement. Nursing Times, 67, 4 Mar 1971, 269–270.

c EUTHANASIA

1 **Beauchamp, J. M.** Euthanasia and the nurse practitioner. Nursing Forum, 14 (1), 1975, 56–73.

2 **Berry, R.** Is death our failure? [The problem of euthanasia.] Journal of Practical Nursing, 24 (11), Nov 1974, 30, 37.

3 **Brown, N. K. and others** How do nurses feel about euthanasia and abortion? American Journal of Nursing, 71 (7), Jul 1971, 1413–1416.

4 **Fletcher, J.** Ethics and euthanasia. American Journal of Nursing, 73 (4), Apr 1973, 670–675.

5 **Galbally, B. P.** Resuscitation and euthanasia. Australian Nurses' Journal, 2 (12), Jun 1973, 26–29.

6 **Johnson, A. G.** The right to live or the right to die? Nursing Times, 67, 13 May 1971, 575–577.

7 **Lamerton, R.** Euthanasia. 'Is there an appropriate moment for death?' Nursing Times, 70, 21 Feb 1974, 260.

8 **Lant, A.** Euthanasia – a patient's point of view. Nursing Mirror, 140, 6 Feb 1975, 73.

9 **Smith, R.** The right to live or die. [A nurse's view on euthanasia.] Nursing Mirror, 140, 1 May 1975, 64.

10 **Vickery, K. O. Λ.** Euthanasia. (a) Medicated survival – the press, the public, the professions, and the patient. Royal Society of Health Journal, 94 (3), Jun 1974, 118–124.

11 **Webber, L. J.** Ethics and euthanasia: another view. American Journal of Nursing, 73 (7), Jul 1973, 1228–1231.

d HOSPICE CARE

1 **Craven, J. and Wald, F. S.** Hospice care for dying patients. [New Haven Region.] American Journal of Nursing, 75 (10), Oct 1975, 1816–1822.

2 **Downie, P. A.** Havens of peace. [Hostel of God, St. Joseph's Hospice, Marie Curie Memorial Foundation, St. Christopher's Hospice, St. Luke's Nursing Home, Sheffield.] Nursing Times, 69, 16 Aug 1973, 1069–1070.

3 **Hostel of God** [Home for the terminally ill at The Chase, Clapham Common.] Nursing Mirror, 139, 10 Oct 1974, 66–68.

4 **Ingles, T.** St. Christopher's Hospice. Nursing Outlook, 22 (12), Dec 1974, 759–763.

5 **Lamerton, R. C.** The need for hospices. [To provide terminal care.] Nursing Times, 71, 23 Jan 1975, 155–157.

6 **Moore, W. R.** A first glance at terminal care. [St. Christopher's Hospice.] Journal of the Royal College of General Practitioners, 21, Jul 1971, 387–392.

7 **Reading Department of Health Services** Total care of the terminally ill. [Report of a conference, including care at St Christopher's hospice.] District Nursing, 14 (5), Aug 1971, 103–104.

8 **Ward, A. W. M.** Terminal care homes. [Historical development of hospitals for the dying.] Hospital and Health Services Review, 71 (7), Jul 1975, 233–236.

9 **Wilmers, M. K.** A very nice place. [St Christopher's Hospice, Sydenham for chronically ill and dying patients.] New Society, 40, 12 Dec 1974, 669–670.

e NURSING

1 **American Journal of Nursing** Experiences with dying patients. [By various authors.] American Journal of Nursing, 73 (6), Jun 1973, 1058–1064.

2 **Anderson, E.** Experience in depth: care of the dying. S. A. Nursing Journal, 38 (6), Jun 1971, 28.

3 **Burkhalter, P. K.** Fostering staff sensitivity to the dying patient. Supervisor Nurse, 6 (4), Apr 1975, 55–59.

4 **Carrington, M.** Nursing care study. Henry – a case for spiritual healing. Nursing Times, 69, 29 Nov 1973, 1599–1600.

5 **Carson, J.** Learning from a dying patient. American Journal of Nursing, 71 (2), Feb 1971, 333–334.

6 **Corder, M. P. and Anders, R. L.** Death and dying – oncology discussion group. Journal of Psychiatric Nursing and Mental Health Services, 12 (4), Jul/Aug 1974, 10–14.

7 **Davidson, J. R.** Patient care in a district general hospital. [Research study of nursing care of the dying.] Nursing Mirror, 141, 24 Jul 1975, 55–56.

8 **Epstein, C.** Nursing the dying patient: learning processes for interaction. Reston, Virginia: Reston Publishing Co, 1975.

9 **Fleming, R. P.** Good physical care, priority for the dying. RN Magazine, 37 (4), Apr 1974, 46–48, 50, 53.

10 **Heusinkveld, K. B.** Cues to communications with the terminal cancer patient. [About dying.] Nursing Forum 11 (1), 1972, 105–113.

11 **Heymann, D. A.** Discussions meet needs of dying patients. [Group discussions with staff and terminally ill patients.] Hospitals, 48 (14), 6 Jul 1974, 57–58, 60, 62.

12 **Hoevet, M.** Dying is also living. [Care of the dying patient.] Nursing Care, 7 (7), Jul 1974, 12–15.

13 **Hoffman, E.** 'Don't give up on me!' [Nurse's account of a patient's death and her reactions.] American Journal of Nursing, 71 (1), Jan 1971, 60–62.

14 **Holford, J. M.** Terminal care. Nursing Times, 69, 25 Jun 1973, 113–115.

15 **Lamerton, R.** Care of the dying. 3. The right time to die. Nursing Times, 68, 14 Dec 1972, 1578.

16 **Lamerton, R.** Care of the dying. 4. Teamwork. Nursing Times, 68, 28 Dec 1972, 1642–1643.

17 **Lamerton, R.** Care of the dying. 5. Listening to the dying. Nursing Times, 69, 4 Jan 1973, 16.

18 **Lamerton, R.** Care of the dying. 6. The pains of death. Nursing Times, 69, 11 Jan 1973, 56–57.

19 **Lamerton, R.** Care of the dying. 7. Religion and the care of the dying. Nursing Times, 69, 18 Jan 1973, 88–89.

20 **Lamerton, R.** Ethical questions in the care of the dying. Nursing Mirror, 139, 10 Oct 1974, 61–63.

21 **MacMillan, S.** Nursing care study. Margaret. A study in perception. [Care of a dying patient.] Nursing Times, 68, 28 Dec 1972, 1644–1646.

22 **McNulty, B.** Care of the dying. Nursing Times, 68, 30 Nov 1972, 1505–1506.

23 **McNulty, B. J.** The nurse's contribution to terminal care. Nursing Mirror, 139, 10 Oct 1974, 59–61.

24 **Mervyn, F.** The plight of dying patients in hospitals. American Journal of Nursing, 71 (10), Oct 1971, 1988–1990.

25 **Moran, M. C.** Grief and dying: a student nurse's experiences with a terminal patient. Hospital Progress, 55 (5), May 1974, 76, 78, 80, 82.

26 **Nursing Times** Terminal care: a series of papers. Macmillan Journals, 1973.

27 **Padilla, G. V. and others** Interacting with dying patients: an inter-hospital nursing research and nursing education project. Duarto: City of Hope National Medical Center, 1975.

28 **Pett, D.** Caring for the fatally ill: a practical guide for those who work with dying persons. Guild of St. Raphael, 1975.

29 Rees, W. D. The distress of dying. [Describes a method of assessing the distress of dying patients by nurses.] British Medical Journal, 3, 8 Jul 1972, 105–107.

30 RN Magazine Four distinctive views of the dying patient. RN Magazine, 38 (4), Apr 1975, 33–38.

31 Sanford, N. and Deloughery, G. L. Teaching nurses to care for the dying patient. Journal of Psychiatric Nursing, 11 (1), Jan/Feb 1973, 24–26.

32 Starr, S. 'I'm going to die. . .' [Nurse's part in dealing with dying patients.] Nursing Times, 71, 1 May 1975, 706–707.

33 Thomas, C. H. Last offices – a reassessment. [Revised procedure for nursing staff at Plymouth General Hospital.] Nursing Mirror, 132, 9 Apr 1971, 30.

34 Unwin, D. But what kind of life? [Effective ways of helping dying patients.] New Zealand Nursing Journal, 68 (3), Mar 1975, 19–21.

35 Whitman, H. H. and Lukes, S. J. Behaviour modification for terminally ill patients. American Journal of Nursing, 75 (1), Jan 1975, 98–101.

36 Wilkes, E. Terminal care and the special nursing unit. Nursing Times, 71, 9 Jan 1974, 57–59.

f NURSING ATTITUDES

1 Barnsteiner, J. H. Death and dying: anxieties, needs and responsibilities of the nurse. Journal of Practical Nursing, 24 (6), Jun 1974, 28–30.

2 Breitung, J. Attitudes toward the dying patient. [Questionnaire survey of nurses, attendants and relatives.] Nursing Care 8 (6), Jun 1975, 34.

3 Bryne, D. P. 'He died.' [Nurse's thoughts on her first experience of laying out a patient.] Lamp, 31 (5), May 1974, 17.

4 Elder, R. Dying in the USA [General discussion on attitudes.] International Journal of Nursing Studies, 10 (3), Aug 1973, 171–184.

5 Golub, S. and Reznikoff, M. Attitudes toward death: a comparison of nursing students and graduate nurses. Nursing Research, 20 (6), Nov/Dec 1971, 503–508.

6 Lamerton, R. Care of the dying. 2. Attitudes to deathbed nursing. Nursing Times, 68, 7 Dec 1972, 1544–1545.

7 Lester, D. and others Attitudes of nursing students and nursing faculty toward death. Nursing Research, 23 (1), Jan/Feb 1974, 50–53.

8 Martin, L. B. and Collier, P. A. Attitudes toward death: a survey of nursing students. [Survey in a Catholic Education College with suggestions for curriculum development and research.] Journal of Nursing Education, 14 (1), Jan 1975, 28–35.

9 Robinson, L. 'We have no dying patients.' Some vicissitudes encountered in teaching nursing students about death. Nursing Outlook, 22 (10), Oct 1974, 651–653.

10 Snyder, M. and others Changes in nursing students' attitudes toward death and dying: a measurement of curriculum integration effectiveness. International Journal of Social Psychiatry, 19 (3/4), Autumn/Winter 1973.

11 Yeaworth, R. C. and others Attitudes of nursing students toward the dying patient. Nursing Research, 23 (1), Jan/Feb 1974, 20–24.

g PATIENT AND FAMILY

1 Aquilera, D. C. Crisis: moment of truth. [Dying patients.] Journal of Psychiatric Nursing, 9 (3), May/Jun 1971, 23–25.

2 Annas, G. J. Rights of the terminally ill patient. Journal of Nursing Administration, 4 (2), Mar/Apr 1974, 40–44.

3 British Medical Journal Talking about death. [Whether or not the doctor should inform the terminal patient of the truth about his condition.] British Medical Journal, 2, 20 Apr 1974, 131–132.

4 Carey, R. G. Living until death. [Research project into factors related to emotional adjustment of patients aware of their terminal illnesses.] Hospital Progress, 55 (2), Feb 1974, 82–87.

5 Hinton, J. Talking with people about to die. [Research study with terminal cancer cases to evaluate what they were told by staff about their illness.] British Medical Journal, 3, 6 Jul 1974, 25–27.

6 Kubler-Ross, D. Dying with dignity. Canadian Nurse, 67 (10), Oct 1971, 31–35. Reprinted in New Zealand Nursing Journal, 66 (11), Nov 1973, 8–12.

7 Kubler-Ross, E. What is it like to be dying? [Need for nurses to understand stages of acceptance which patients go through.] American Journal of Nursing, 71 (1), Jan 1971, 54–61.

8 Nursing Outlook Notes of a dying professor. Nursing Outlook, 20 (8), Aug 1972, 502–506.

9 Raven, R.W., editor The dying patient. Pitman, 1975.

10 Robinson, W. The dying patient and his relatives. [Royal Society of Health Conference.] Nursing Times, 69, 17 May 1973, 651.

11 Scottish Hospital Centre Preparing the way: problems faced by patients, relatives. . .and others in and after the period of terminal illness. Edinburgh: The Centre, 1973.

12 Twycross, R. G. The dying patient. Christian Medical Fellowship, 1975.

13 Webster, F. Perspectives on death and the dying patient. Hospital Progress, 54 (12), Dec 1973, 32–34.

14 Wilkes, E. The management of the family in fatal illness. Queen's Nursing Journal, 16 (7), Oct 1973, 150–151.

15 Wilkes, E. Relatives, professional care, and the dying patient. Nursing Mirror, 139, 10 Oct 1974, 53–56.

16 Wilson, J. M. Communicating with the dying. [With a commentary by C. M. Fletcher.] Journal of Medical Ethics, 1 (1), Apr 1975, 18–22.

17 Witzel, L. Behaviour of the dying patient. [Study of 110 patients during the 24 hours before death and 250 patients during the weeks before death.] British Medical Journal, 2, 12 Apr 1975, 81–82.

h PROLONGATION OF LIFE

1 Andrews, L. The last night. [Case study of a deliberate failure to resuscitate a patient dying of cancer of the lung.] American Journal of Nursing, 74 (7), Jul 1974, 1305–1306.

2 Bothamley, V. A. Prolonging life by mechanical means – the role of the nurse. Nursing Times, 70, 31 Oct 1974, 1702–1704.

3 Griffin, J. J. Family decision: a crucial factor in terminating life – support measures. [A case study.] American Journal of Nursing, 75 (5), May 1975, 795–796.

4 Hershey, N. On the question of prolonging life. American Journal of Nursing, 71 (3), Mar 1971, 521–522.

5 Hiscoe, S. The awesome decision: a nurse's honest answers to questions helped a family arrive at a decision to discontinue the machine which kept the patient breathing. American Journal of Nursing, 73 (2), Feb 1973, 291–293.

6 Nicholson, R. Should the patient be allowed to die? Journal of Medical Ethics, 1 (1), Apr 1975, 5–9.

7 Patey, E. H. Matters of life and death. To care or to kill? [Comments on the Church of England report 'On dying well'.] Nursing Mirror, 141, 2 Oct 1975, 40–41.

8 Pells, J. Prolonging life. 1. The pressures of progress. Two cases in which medical staff used every device at their disposal to save life. Nursing Times, 70, 21 Feb 1974, 258–259.

9 Pells, J. Prolonging life. 2. Transplant and pulling the switch. Nursing Times, 70, 28 Feb 1974, 320–321.

10 Pells, J. Prolonging life. 3. The hope in experiment. [Dangers in experimental surgery, abortion and euthanasia.] Nursing Times, 70, 7 Mar 1974, 352–353.

11 Pells, J. Prolonging life. 5. Opinions and guidance. Nursing Times, 70, 21 Mar 1974, 440–441.

12 Pells, J. Prolonging life. 6. Death and beyond. Nursing Times, 70, 28 Mar 1974, 481–482.

13 Skillman, J. J. Ethical dilemmas in the care of the critically ill. [Decisions concerning discontinuation of care.] Lancet, 2, 14 Sep 1974, 634–637.

i TERMINAL CARE

1 Agate, J. Care of the dying in geriatric departments. Lancet, 1, 17 Feb 1973, 364–366.

2 Cartwright, A. and Anderson, J. L. Help for the dying. New Society, 24, 21 Jun 1973, 679–681.

3 Cartwright, A. and others Life before death. Routledge and Kegan Paul. (Social studies in medical care.) 1973.

4 Cramond, W. A. The psychological care of patients with terminal illness. [Reprinted from the Journal of the Royal College of General Practitioners, October 1972.] Nursing Times, 69, 15 Mar 1973, 339–343.

5 Department of Health and Social Security Care of the dying: proceedings of a national symposium held on 29 November 1972. HMSO, 1973. (Reports on health and social subjects, no. 5.); British Medical Journal, 1, 6 Jan 1973, 29–41.

6 Downie, P. A. A personal commentary on the care of the dying on the North American continent. Nursing Mirror, 139, 10 Oct 1974, 68–70.

7 Downie, P. A. Physiotherapy and the care of the progressively ill patient. 1. The role of the physiotherapist. [Care of the dying patient.] Nursing Times, 69, 12 Jul 1973, 892–893.

8 Holford, J. M. Hospital care of the dying. [Introductory paper at DHSS symposium.] British Hospital Journal and Social Service Review, 82, 16 Dec 1972, 2804.

9 Holford, J. M. Terminal care. [Facilities.] Nursing Times, 69, 25 Jan 1973, 113–115.

10 Lack, S. and Lamerton, R., editors The hour of our death: a record of the conference on the care of the dying, held in London, 1973. Chapman, 1974.

11 Laister, P. The priest's care of the terminally sick. Nursing Mirror, 139, 10 Oct 1974, 63–65.

12 Lamerton, R. Care of the dying. Priory Press, 1973.

13 Lancet Care of the dying. Lancet 2, 2 Oct 1971, 753–754.

14 Morton, B. G. Caring for the dying. Physiotherapy, 58 (4), Apr 1972, 124–125.

15 Paine, L. Centre lunch talk. Care for a dying patient. [Based on experience at St. Christopher's Hospice.] Health and Social Service Journal, 83, 20 Jan 1973, 137.

16 Pett, D. Caring for the fatally ill: a practical guide for those who work with dying persons. Guild of St. Raphael, 1975.

17 Phillips, D. F. The hospital and the dying patient. Hospitals, 46 (4), 16 Feb 1972, 68, 72–75.

18 Schoenberg, B. B. and others, editors Psychosocial aspects of terminal care. New York: Columbia University Press, 1972.

19 Spoor, J. M. Terminal illness: some facts and feelings. [The psychological effect on patient, family and professionals with a description of hospital services available.] Social Work Today, 5, 20 Feb 1975, 702–707.

20 Winner, A. Care for a dying patient. Physiotherapy, 59 (2), Feb 1973, 59.

j TERMINAL CARE AT HOME

1 Canvin, R. W. and Newell, J. M. Care of the dying in Exeter. [An investigation into the adequacy of the home nursing service.] Nursing Times, 71, 12 Jun 1975, 942–943.

2 Gilmore, A. J. J. The care and management of the dying patient in general practice. Practitioner, 213, Dec 1974, 833–842.

3 Keywood, O. Care of the dying in their own home. Nursing Times, 70, 26 Sept 1974, 1516–1517.

4 Kobrzycki, P. Dying with dignity at home. Despite the need for complicated care, a young man and his family were taught what was necessary to allow him to die at home. American Journal of Nursing, 75 (8), Aug 1975, 1312–1313.

5 McNulty, B. J. Domiciliary care of the dying – some problems encountered. [Home care service organized by St. Christopher's Hospice.] Nursing Mirror, 136, 18 May 1973, 29–30.

6 McNulty, B. J. St. Christopher's outpatients. [Home care organized by hospice.] American Journal of Nursing, 71 (12), Dec 1971, 2328–2330.

7 Mitchell, W. Domiciliary care of the terminally ill and their relatives. Midwife and Health Visitor, 9 (11), Nov 1973, 366–367.

8 Murray, J. T. and others A study of the contribution of the health visitor to the support and care of terminally ill patients and their relatives. [Carried out in Edinburgh.] Health Bulletin, 32 (6), Nov 1974, 250–252.

EDUCATION AND RESEARCH

20 NURSING EDUCATION

a GENERAL

1 Abdel-Al, H. An approach to nurse education. [The relatedness of theory to practice in nurse education. Study of the Registered General Nurse training programme in Scotland.] Nursing Mirror, 139, 26 Jul 1974, 68–71.

2 Association of Integrated and Degree Courses in Nursing Higher education in nursing: report of the second open conference, Penarth, 12–14 July 1974. The Association, 1975.

3 Backlund, M. A category system for nursing education. [To be used in planning courses and programmes for students from developing countries.] International Nursing Review, 20 (5), Sep/Oct 1973, 137–139, 152.

4 Barritt, E. R. Florence Nightingale's values and modern nursing education. Nursing Forum, 12 (1), 1973, 6–47.

5 Bendall, E. A nursing dilemma. [Best kind of education for a nurse and problems involved.] Nursing Times, 67, 18 Mar 1971, Occ. papers, 41–44.

6 Collins, S. Briggs. Educating the nurse and midwife of the future. [Text of an address given at the Rcn conference on the Briggs Report.] Nursing Times, 68, 14 Dec 1972, 1592–1595.

7 Daniells, N. C., compiler Directory of nursing scholarships, bursaries and grants. Royal College of Nursing, 1974.

8 Godfrey, J. Value orientation: a problem for nursing education. International Nursing Review, 18 (2), 1971, 167–180.

9 Grady, T. E. Nurse training and education – history and hopes. Nursing Times, 68, 11 May 1972, 585–586.

10 Gray, M. Teaching or non teaching – who cares? [Advantages and disadvantages of training for registration in a teaching or non teaching hospital.] Nursing Times, 68, 3 Aug 1972, 973–974.

11 Harding, B. An OND for nurses? [Possibility of Ordinary National Diploma obtained in a Technical College.] Nursing Times, 67, 1 Jul 1971, 807–808.

12 Institute of Religion and Medicine A consultation on wider issues in nursing education: papers given at the Queen's College, Birmingham, 4–6 January, 1974. The Institute, 1974.

13 James, D. Trends in nurse education. Nursing Times, 68, 24 Feb 1972, Occ. papers 29–31.

14 Jupp, V. Professionalization and new forms of nursing education. [Looks at the status of the profession in the light of new education courses.] International Journal of Nursing Studies, 9 (1), Mar 1972, 19–25.

15 Lamond, N. Becoming a nurse: the registered nurse's view of general nurse education. Rcn, 1974. Based on MLitt thesis, Aberdeen University, 1970.

16 Leach, D. Why educate nurses? How Briggs missed the point. Nursing Times, 69, 19 Jul 1973, 939–940.

17 Lysaught, J. P. Action in nursing: progress in professional purpose. New York: McGraw-Hill.

18 McCarthy, W. H. 'Egotistical specialists' and nursing eduction. Nursing Times, 68, 20 Jan 1972, 84–85

19 Manock, H. M. Skills necessary to nursing education. Australian Nurses' Journal, 2 (11), May 1973, 22–24.

20 O'Neill, J. Reorganisation or reshuffle? [Plan for reforming the health service with more emphasis on health education and community centred care, together with a suggested training programme of nurse training.] Health Visitor, 46 (3), Mar 1973, 76–81.

21 Pomeranz, R. The lady apprentices: a study of transition in nurse training. Bell, 1973. (Occasional papers on social administration no. 51.)

22 Pounds, W. and Askins, B.E. Criterion – referenced teaching and testing. [Providing continuity in nursing education.] AORN Journal 21 (5), Apr 1975, 862, 864, 866.

23 Raybould, E., editor A guide for teachers of nurses. Blackwell, 1975.

24 Rye, D. Can the register and the roll survive? [Suggests new form of two-year training with follow-up courses.] Nursing Times, 67, 22 Apr 1971, 491–493.

25 Smith, J. P. Which bandwagon for nursing education? [Schools of nursing vs. colleges of education.] Nursing Mirror, 132, 18 Jun 1971, 19.

26 Treece, E. W. The philosophical basis for nursing education. International Nursing Review, 21 (1), Jan/Feb 1974, 13–15.

b CURRICULUM: GENERAL

1 Bevis, E. O. Curriculum building in nursing: a process. St. Louis: Mosby, 1973.

2 Bruton, M. R. The process of curriculum revision. Nursing Outlook, 22 (5), May 1974, 310–314.

3 Chapman, C. M. Nursing education – curriculum content. Queen's Nursing Journal, 17 (7), Oct 1974, 149–152.

4 Chater, S. S. A conceptual framework for curriculum development. Nursing Outlook, 23 (7), Jul 1975, 428–433.

5 Dineen, M. A. The open curriculum: implications for further education. Nursing Outlook, 20 (12), Dec 1972, 770–774.

6 Fenner, K. Developing a conceptual framework. [Use of Orem's self-care theory as a base for curriculum development.] Nursing Outlook, 27 (2), Feb 1979, 122–126.

7 Gordon, M. and Anello, M. A systematic approach to curriculum revision. Nursing Outlook, 22 (5), May 1974, 306–310.

8 Green, J. L. and Stone, J. C. Developing and testing Q-cards and content analysis in group interviews. [The use of group interviews to evaluate a new curriculum.] Nursing Research, 21 (4), Jul/Aug 1972, 342–347.

9 Hezekiah, J. A. An experiment with the ladder concept. [An experiment with a core curriculum for students in the nursing diploma and nursing assistant programs.] Canadian Nurse, 71 (1), Jan 1975, 20–22.

10 Hodgman, E. C. A conceptual framework to guide nursing curriculum. Nursing Forum, 12 (2), 1973, 110–131.

11 Johnson, W. L. Status of the open curriculum in nursing. Nursing Outlook, 19 (12), Dec 1971, 779–782.

12 Kelly, L. Y. Open curriculum – what and why. American Journal of Nursing, 74 (12), Dec 1974, 2232–2238.

13 Ketefian, S. Trends in curricular innovations in nursing eduction. [Results of a survey undertaken in the United States, May/June 1971.] International Nursing Review, 21 (5), Sep/Oct 1974, 139–142.

14 Langford, T. and others Criteria for choosing textbooks for the nontraditional professional nursing curriculum. Journal of Nursing Education, 12 (3), Aug 1973, 3–8.

15 Laverdier, R. An accelerated nursing curriculum: ten years of experience with credit by examination, individual program planning and independent study to reduce the basic nursing curriculum to one year. Nursing Outlook, 21 (8), Aug 1973, 524–526.

16 Lenburg, C., editor Open learning and career mobility in nursing. St. Louis: Mosby, 1975.

17 Lenburg, C. and Johnson, W. Career mobility through nursing education. A report on NLN's open curriculum project. Nursing Outlook, 22 (4), Apr 1974, 265–269.

18 Longway, I. M. Curriculum concepts: an historical analysis. Nursing Outlook, 22 (2), Feb 1972, 116–120.

19 MacMillan, A. M. More problems than answers: curriculum planning in the light of Briggs. Nursing Times, 69, 18 Oct 1973, 1374–1375.

20 National League for Nursing Department of Baccalaureate and Higher Degree Programs. Conceptual framework – its meaning and function. (Faculty-curriculum development, Part 3.] New York: The League, 1975.

21 O'Driscoll, D. L. An ADN approach to the open curriculum. Journal of Nursing Education, 12 (3), Aug 1974, 27–31.

22 O'Kelly, L. E. and McKinney, G. A conceptual model for medical-surgical nursing. [Curriculum design.] Nursing Outlook, 19 (11), Nov 1971, 731–736.

23 Quenzer, R. The development of patient-centred behaviour patterns in nurse training. MEd thesis, Manchester University, Department of Adult Education, 1974.

24 Quiring, J. A model for curriculum development in nursing. Nursing Outlook, 21 (11), Nov 1973, 714–716.

25 Redman, B. K. Why develop a conceptual framework? [Designed for the undergraduate curriculum at the University of Minnesota School of Nursing.] Journal of Nursing Education, 13 (3), Aug 1974 2–10.

26 Reidy, M. The use and abuse of a curricular model; an evaluative study of one C.E.G.E.P's nursing programme in Quebec. [Roy's adaptation model.] Nursing Papers, 7 (1), Spring 1975, 4–14.

27 Reilly, D. E. Why a conceptual framework? [for the curriculum]. Nursing Outlook, 23 (9), Sep 1975, 566–569.

28 Roy, C. Adaptation: implications for curriculum change. Nursing Outlook, 21 (3), Mar 1973, 163–168.

29 Schoen, D. C. Comparing the body systems and conceptual approaches to nursing education. [Study of a three year diploma program in San Francisco to compare two different approaches to the curriculum.] Nursing Research, 24 (5), Sep/Oct 1975, 383–387.

30 Shields, M. A model apt for measurement: the true value of a curriculum model is determined by how the faculty use it to explain all they do in the name of education. Nursing Outlook, 19 (9), Sep 1971, 600–601.

31 Shields, M. A model for a curriculum goal. Using a three-dimensional model, faculty can catagorize the learner's problem-solving activities in terms of the patient's needs. Nursing Outlook, 20 (12), Dec 1972, 782–785.

32 Smith, K. M. Episodic and distributive nursing in an emergent curricular plan. Journal of Nursing Education, 11 (4), Nov 1972, 11–20.

33 Stevens, B. J. Analysis of structural forms used in nursing curricula. Nursing Research, 20 (5), Sep/Oct 1971, 388–397.

34 Uprichard, M. An experimental nursing curriculum [at the University of British Columbia.] Canadian Nurse, 70 (5), May 1974, 30–32.

35 Wolf, V. C. and Smith, C. M. Curriculum change: evolution of a dynamic structure. Nursing Outlook, 22 (5), May 1974, 315–320.

c CURRICULUM: SPECIAL SUBJECTS

1 Anderson, E. The student nurse meets a new science. [Sociology for nurses.] Australian Nurses' Journal, 2 (1), Jul 1972, 27–29.

2 Batstone, S. M. Teaching social work to nurses [at St. Helier Hospital, Carshalton.] Health and Social Service Journal, 84, 16 Mar 1974, 612.

3 British Psychological Society Teaching psychology to nurses. Bulletin of the British Psychological Society, 27, 1974, 272–283.

4 Connolly, P. Why should the nurse study sociology? Queen's Nursing Journal, 18 (7), Oct 1975, 201–202.

5 Dammann, G. L. A. Interprofessional aspects of nursing and social work curricula. Nursing Research, 21 (2), Mar/Apr 1972, 160–163.

6 Elisha, D. S. Integration of public health in the basic curriculum of nursing. Nursing Journal of India, 64 (6), Jun 1973, 197, 208–209.

7 Green, V. What is the relevance of sociology to nursing? Lamp, 30 (2), Feb 1973, 7, 9, 11, 13.

8 Gudmundsen, A. Teaching psychomotor skills. Journal of Nursing Education, 14 (1), Jan 1975, 23–27.

9 Hall, J. Teaching psychology to nurses. Nursing Times, 70, 21 Nov 1974, 1828–1829.

10 Nolan, R. J. The development of teaching methods in human biology within nurse training schools. MEd thesis, Manchester University, 1973.

11 Passos, J. Y. and Stallings, A.A. Introduction of concepts of measurement and statistics to sophomore nursing students. Nursing Research. 22 (3), May/Jun 1973, 248–253.

12 Ruffing, M. A. Literature by consumers for nursing. [Incorporation of non standard material into the curriculum to accentuate the humanistic foundations of nursing practice.] Nursing Forum, 14 (1), 1975, 87–94.

13 Strong, P. G. Liberal studies in nursing education. Nursing Times, 67, 15 Apr 1971, Occ. papers 57–59.

14 Weyman, A. J. Extra-curricular general studies for student nurses: a feasibility study carried out at Westminster Hospital. Nursing Times, 69, 12 Jul 1973, Occ. papers 109–111.

15 Wilson, H. S. A case for humanities in professional nursing education. Nursing Forum, 13 (4), 1974, 406–417.

d CURRICULUM: SEX EDUCATION

1 Lief, H. E. and Payne, T. Sexuality – knowledge and attitudes. [Of nursing students.] American Journal of Nursing, 75 (11), Nov 1975, 2026–2029.

2 Malo-Juvera, D. Seeing is believing. When students see replays of themselves in simulated parent education scenes, they gain some understanding about their own attitudes toward sex education. Nursing Outlook, 21 (9), Sep 1973, 583–585.

3 Mandetta, A. F. and Woods, N. F. Learning about human sexuality – a course model. Nursing Outlook, 22 (8), Aug 1974, 525–527.

4 Megenity, J. A plea for sex education in nursing curriculums. American Journal of Nursing, 75 (7), Jul 1975, 1171.

5 Mims, F. and others Effectiveness of an interdisciplinary course in human sexuality. Nursing Research, 23 (3) May/Jun 1974, 248–253.

6 Renshaw, D. C. Nurses need formal sex education. Journal of Nursing Education, 14 (4), Nov 1975, 18–19.

7 Walker, E. G. Study of sexuality in the nursing curriculum. Nursing Forum, 10 (1), 1971, 18–30.

8 Who Chronicle Education in human sexuality for health practitioners. WHO Chronicle, 29 (2), Feb 1975, 49–54.

9 Wilbur, C. and Aug, R. Sex education. American Journal of Nursing, 73 (1), Jan 1973, 88–91.

10 Woods, N. F. and Mandetta, A. Changes in students' knowledge and attitudes following a course in human sexuality. Report of a pilot study. Nursing Research, 24 (1), Jan/Feb 1975, 10–15.

e EDUCATION: PRACTICE AND SERVICE NEEDS

1 Abdel-Al, H. Relating education to practice within a nursing context. PhD thesis, Edinburgh University, 1975.

2 Aydelotte, M. K. Nursing education and practice: putting it all together. Journal of Nursing Education, 11 (4), Nov 1972, 21–27.

2 Christman, N. J. Clinical performance of baccalaureate graduates. Nursing Outlook, 19 (1), Jan 1971, 54–56.

3 Davis, B. G. Effect of levels of nursing education on patient care: a replication. To compare levels of performance on a specific task. Nursing Research, 23 (2), Mar/Apr 1974, 150–155.

4 Fagan, E. A. Cooperative planning for student learning [Co-operation between nursing education and nursing service administration.] Hospitals, 49, 16 Jan 1975, 77–80, 102.

5 Fawkes, B. Needs of education and training in nursing and the relationship with other health personnel. Nursing Times, 68, 4 May 1972, Occ. papers, 69–71. Reprinted in International Nursing Review, 19 (4), 1972, 361–368.

6 Heckinger, R. A nurse's plea for hospital-centered nursing education. [Extracted from 'It's time to amalgamate our educational systems'.] RN Magazine, 34, Aug. 1971, 42. Hospitals, 46, 1 Jan 1972, 61.

7 Keller, N. S. Head nurse and clinical teacher: a first hand account of a faculty member's experience in a combined education-service role on the direct patient care level. Nursing Outlook, 19 (9), Sept 1971, 596–599.

8 King's Fund Centre The future of nurse education: balancing service and training needs. [King's Fund Centre meeting.] Nursing Times, 71, 25 Dec 1975, 2043.

9 King's Fund Centre Lower intake of student nurses: education and service needs clash, conference reveals. [King's Fund conference on the future of nurse education.] Nursing Times, 71, 19 Jun 1975, 951.

10 Krueger, J. C. The education and utilization of nurses: a paradox. Nursing Outlook, 19 (10), Oct 1971, 676–679.

11 Lewis, E. P. The two worlds of nursing. [Gap between education and practice and relationship of nursing service and education.] Nursing Outlook, 23 (7), Jul 1975, 421.

12 Loomis, M. E. Collegiate nursing education: an ambivalent professionalism. [The traditional conservative outlook of nursing must change to meet modern health care needs.] Journal of Nursing Education, 13 (4), Nov 1974, 39–48.

13 McMullan, D. Accountability and nursing education. Nursing Outlook, 23 (8), Aug 1975, 501–503.

14 MacPhail, J. Promoting collaboration between education service. Canadian Nurse 71 (5), May 1975, 32–34.

15 Meleis, A. I. and Benner, P. Process or product evaluation? [Of education programmes.] Nursing Outlook, 23 (5), May 1975, 303–307.

16 Morton, B. F. Nursing service and education in a comprehensive health care center. Journal of Nursing Administration, 3 (3), May/Jun 1973, 23–26.

17 Murphy, J. S. The dilemma in nursing practice. [Relations between nursing service and nursing education.] Journal of Nursing Administration, 4 (1), Jan/Feb 1974, 16–18.

18 Murphy, J. The nub of the learning process. [Evaluation of nurse education through patients' reactions.] American Journal of Nursing, 71 (2), Feb 1971, 306–310.

19 **Packwood, G. F.** Education and service. Nursing Mirror, 133, 26 Nov 1971, 41–43.

20 **Paulson, V. W. and Others** Commitment to change in Colorado. [Nurse educators and administrators establish mutual support systems and plan for change.] American Journal of Nursing, 75 (4), Apr 1975, 636–637.

21 **Pierik, M. M.** Joint appointments: collaboration for better patient care. [Nurses who hold appointments to both school of nursing and hospital.] Nursing Outlook, 21 (9), Sep 1973, 576–579.

22 **Veith, S. and Barloon, I.** Cooperation for learning: students, staff and patients benefit when education and service personnel have a close, sharing relationship. American Journal of Nursing, 72 (12), Dec 1972, 2178–2179.

23 **Weyman, A.** The nurse and the system. [Problems arising from inadequate nurse training.] Health and Social Service Journal, 85, 20/27 Dec 1975, 2789.

24 **Wisser, S. H.** Those darned principles. [Discrepancies between classroom instruction and hospital practice.] Nursing Forum, 13 (4), 1974, 386–392.

f MODULAR SYSTEM

1 **Beyers, M. and others** Developing a modular curriculum. [Auto-tutorial study using mediated learning materials.] Nursing Outlook, 20 (10), Oct 1972, 643–647.

2 **Hitchings, C. R. and Smyth, M.** The Royal Free Hospital. 3. Modular training. Nursing Times, 70, 17 Oct 1974, 1621–1622.

3 **Jackson, B.** Camden's community care course option. [Part of the modular system of nurse training at University College Hospital.] Nursing Mirror, 139, 2 Aug 1974, 59–60.

4 **Kempster, R. F. and Warcaba, B.** A module system in nurse education. An outline of the experimental scheme in nurse education carried out at St. Crispin Hospital Education Centre, Northampton. Nursing Times, 69, 3 May 1973, Occ. papers, 69–72.

5 **Parnell, J. E.** Modular systems and allocation. In A guide for teachers of nursing. ed. Raybould, E. Oxford: Blackwell Scientific Publications, 1975.

6 **Weatherhead, R. G.** Bringing students in from the cold at Callan Park [using the modular system of nurse training.] Australian Nurses' Journal, 4 (6), Dec/Jan 1975, 31–33.

g OBJECTIVES

1 **Alexander, C. J. and others** How to write objectives for education programs. AORN Journal, 22 (5), Nov 1975, 693–694, 696–698.

2 **Attridge, C. B.** Behavioral objectives: some perspective, please! [Questions their use in nursing education.] Nursing Papers, 6 (1), Spring 1974, 11–22.

3 **Bieszad, J. M. and Lawlor, St. M. A.** The development and use of level objectives in a diploma program. Journal of Nursing Education, 12 (4), Nov 1973, 30–38.

4 **Bloom, R. S.** Stating educational objectives in behavioral terms. Nursing Forum, 14 (1), 1975, 30–42.

5 **Chapman, C. M.** Nurse education. [How objectives in nursing education may be achieved in relation to the problems of providing patient care and making the best use of teaching resources.] Nursing Times, 70, 2 May 1974, 660–662.

6 **Geissler, E. M.** Matching course objectives to course content. [A method to identify teaching objec-

tives and to evaluate their effectiveness.] Nursing Outlook, 22 (9), Sep 1974, 579–582.

7 **Kramer, M. A.** A nursing objectives bank – fantasy or good sense? [For schools of nursing.] Nursing Outlook, 22 (11), Nov 1974, 706–707.

8 **Reilly, D. E.** Behavioral objectives in nursing: evaluation of learner attainment. New York: Appleton-Century-Crofts, 1975.

9 **Styles, M. M.** Serendipity and objectivity. [Behavioural objectives in education.] Nursing Outlook, 23 (5), May 1975, 311–313.

10 **Wolf, V. C.** Educational objectives. Journal of American Association of Nurse Anesthetists, 40 (6), Dec 1972, 436–446.

11 **Wolf, V. C.** Suggestions for improving your curriculum by writing better objectives. Journal of the American Association of Nurse Anesthetists, 41 (6), Dec 1973, 531–540.

h PRE-NURSING COURSES

1 **Handley, K. A.** The case against cadets. Nursing Mirror, 141, 16 Oct 1975, 42.

2 **Jones, E.** Controversy corner. The case for cadets. Nursing Mirror, 141, 11 Sep 1975, 42.

3 **Kalisch, B. J. and Kalisch, P. A.** Cadet nurse. The girl with a future. In this documentary of the publicity campaign of the US Cadet Nurse Corps, the Cadet nurse was the 'girl with a future' who was urged to 'enlist in a proud profession'. Nursing Outlook, 21 (7), Jul 1973, 444–449.

4 **Malden, H.** Could vacation schools be an answer to – student nurse wastage. [Pre-nursing courses.] Australian Nurses' Journal, 3 (10), May 1974, 31–32.

5 **Potter, L.** A positive programme for pre-nurses. Lamp, 30 (1), Jan 1973, 25.

i SCHOOLS OF NURSING

1 **Bailey, R. E.** From semi-basement to Hampstead's heights. The new Royal Free Hospital School of Nursing. [Mainly illustrations.] Nursing Mirror, 139, 10 Oct 1974, 38–39.

2 **Barritt, E. R.** The art and science of being a Dean. Nursing Outlook, 22 (12), Dec 1974, 748–750.

3 **Batchelor, E. V.** The Teaching Centre, Norfolk and Norwich Hospital. [Integration of postgraduate medical and nursing education.] Health and Welfare Libraries Quarterly, 2 (2–4), Jun–Dec 1975, 35–40.

4 **Bronglais Hospital** broadens its scope. [Including nurse training unit and residential staff accommodation.] Nursing Mirror, 137, 28 Sep 1973, 34–36.

5 **Brook, P. and others** Educational centre for hospital professionals. [Multi-disciplinary education at Warley Hospital, Brentwood, in a purpose-built shared education centre.] Health and Social Service Journal, 84, 21/28 Dec 1974, 2932–2933.

6 **Gerhart, M. E.** Competencies of nursing directors in junior colleges. Journal of Nursing Education, 12 (2), Apr 1973, 2–5.

7 **Gross, I. N.** Hospital schools as vital as ever. [Prepare to reaffirm their position as vital contributors of health professionals.] Hospitals, 49, 1 Jan 1975, 69–71.

8 **Johnson, B. M.** Decision making, faculty satisfaction, and the power of the school of nursing in the university. [Amount of school of nursing autonomy in the university.] Nursing Research, 22 (2), Mar/Apr 1973, 100–107.

9 **King Edward's Hospital Fund for London** Schools of nursing directory. The Fund, 1972, 2nd ed. 1974.

10 **King's College Hospital**: the School of Nursing, Midwifery and Physiotherapy. Physiotherapy, 59 (2), Feb 1973, 61.

11 **Lawrence, E.** Administration in nursing practice: administering a school of nursing – June 1975. Jamaican Nurse, 5 (3), Dec 1975, 21–24.

12 **Mansfield** Developments at Mansfield. Postgraduate medical education centre. [Including a group school of nursing.] Nursing Mirror, 137, 31 Aug 1973, 34–37.

13 **Nightingale Fellowship Journal** Series of articles describing the new Nightingale School and Gassiot House. Nightingale Fellowship Journal, No. 88, Jan 1973, 423–435.

14 **Nursing Times** Wales. Transfer from St. Tydfil's. [New District hospital at Merthyr Tydfil and the Merthyr and Aberdare School of Nursing.] Nursing Times, 70, 21 Nov 1974, 1802–1803.

15 **Royal Salop Infirmary** Group school of nursing. Doubled in size. Nursing Mirror, 134, 24 Mar 1972, 46–48.

16 **Schaefer, M. J.** Educational administration. Managing complexity. Journal of Nursing Administration, 5 (9), Nov–Dec 1975, 13–16.

17 **Schmidt, M.** Planning the teaching staff for schools of nursing. Australian Nurses' Journal, 4 (11), Jun 1975, 34–36.

18 **Slater, M.** The combined training school at the University Hospital of Wales – a personal view. Hospital and Health Services Review, 70 (7), Jul 1974, 233–235.

19 **Snelgrove, F. W.** A school to be proud of. [Nurses Training School in Salisbury, Rhodesia.] International Nursing Review, 21 (1), Jan/Feb 1974, 9–12.

20 **Soo, B.** Human relations in nursing school administration. Nursing Journal of Singapore, 12 (2), Nov 1972, 107–110.

j NURSE TEACHERS

1 **Ahmed, R. and others** Listening can be learning and sharing can be studying. [Account of a study day for tutors at Cassel Hospital, Richmond, on the practical needs of 'learners'.] Nursing Mirror, 140, 30 Jan 1975, 69–70.

2 **Clarke, M. and Koo, W. T.** Techniques of teaching evaluation. [How an individual may evaluate his effectiveness as a teacher.] Nursing Times, 67, 17 Jun 1971, Occ. papers, 93–96.

3 **Department of Health and Social Security** Report of the nurse tutor working party. Nursing Times, 66, 25 Jun 1970; Occ. papers 89–92; 2 Jul 1970, Occ. papers 93–95.

4 **Dutton, E. A.** Recruitment of sister tutors in the nursing profession: a study of a role-choice and its determinants. PhD thesis, Department of Social Psychology, London School of Economics 1971.

5 **Fieldhouse, A.** Preparation of teachers. New Zealand Nursing Journal, 66 (2), Feb 1973, 28–29.

6 **Fry, M. S.** An analysis of the role of a nurse-educator. [In a university setting.] Journal of Nursing Education, 14 (1), Jan 1975, 5–10.

7 **General Nursing Council for England and Wales** Teachers of nursing. Reports 1 and 2. The Council, 1975. Summary in Nursing Times, 71, 17 Apr 1975, 596; Journal of Advanced Nursing 1 (5), Sep 1976, 377–389.

8 **Green, M. D.** Report on the enquiry amongst

those who obtained the sister tutor's diploma, 1966–1970. The author, 1973.

9 Hendryx, R. and Whittingham, D. An experience with part-time faculty. [Report of . . . a plan for acquiring an adequate teaching staff.] Nursing Outlook, 19 (7), Jul 1971, 484–486.

10 Horrobin, F. W. Training and environment. [Attitudes of teaching staff create a successful climate for students.] Nursing Mirror, 140, 3 Apr 1975, 66.

11 Lancaster, A. Nurse teachers: the report of an opinion survey. Livingstone, 1972. (University of Edinburgh Department of Nursing Studies, Monograph no. 2).

12 Leydon, I. Is it possible to look forward without looking back. [Report of the Tutor's annual general meeting.] World of Irish Nursing, 4 (6), Jun 1975, 1–2.

13 Leydon, I. Tutor's responsibility for quality patient care. World of Irish Nursing, 4 (4), Apr 1975, 1–2.

14 Mesolella, D. W. Caring begins in the teacher-student relationship. Canadian Nurse, 70 (12), Dec 1974, 15–16.

15 Perry, E. All nurses should be teachers. Paper delivered on 16th April 1975 at an Rcn Conference entitled 'All nurses are teachers'. Royal College of Nursing, 1975.

16 Roberts, M. W. and Dixon, K. A course in a college of education for nurses preparing to become tutors in England and Wales. [Bolton.] International Journal of Nursing Studies, 8 (3), Aug 1971, 207–216.

17 Royal College of Nursing 'All nurses are teachers?' [Conference report.] Nursing Mirror, 140, 24 Apr 1975, 36; Nursing Times, 71, 24 Apr 1975, 437.

18 Schaefer, M. J. Toward a full profession of nursing: the challenge of the educator's role. Journal of Nursing Education, 11 (4), Nov 1972, 39–45.

19 Schrock, R. A. Nurse tutor students' experiences in teaching practice. Nursing Times, 71, 20 Feb 1975, Occ. papers, 9–12; 27 Feb 1975, Occ. papers, 13–15.

20 Seyfried, S. H. and Franck, P. Factors influencing acceptance of appointment to College of Nursing Faculty. Journal of Nursing Education , 11 (2), Apr 1972, 25, 27–32.

21 Stenton, J. H. Learning how to teach. [Refresher course for sisters and charge nurses at Stanley Road Hospital, Wakefield.] Nursing Mirror, 136, 12 Jan 1973, 27–32.

21 TEACHING AND LEARNING

a GENERAL

1 Bendall, E. The learning process in student nurses. Some problems and variables. Findings of a research project. Nursing Times, 67, 4 Nov 1971, Occ. papers, 173–175.

2 Bendall, E. R. The learning process in student nurses: some problems and variables. MA thesis in Education (Psychology), Institute of Education, London University, 1971.

3 Bendall, E. R. The relationship between recall and application of learning in trainee nurses. PhD thesis in Education (Psychology) Institute of Education, London University, 1973.

4 Boguslawski, M. and Judkins, B. Contemporary guidelines in teaching. Journal of Nursing Education, 10 (1), Apr 1971, 3–11.

5 Chapman, R. W. Sociometry as an adjunct to nurse teaching. Nursing Times, 67, 4 Mar 1971, Occ. papers, 33–36.

6 Conklin, K. R. Foundations of education for students and teachers of nursing. Journal of Nursing Education, 13 (3), Aug 1974, 16–22.

7 Czmowski, M. Value teaching in nursing education. Nursing Forum, 13 (2), 1974, 192–206.

8 Daubenmire, M. J. and King, I. M. Nursing process models: a systems approach. [In nursing education.] Nursing Outlook, 21 (8), Aug 1973, 512–517.

9 De Tournay, R. Strategies of teaching nursing. New York: Wiley, 1971.

10 Ferguson, M. A new look at nursing education. [Concurrent teaching of theory and practice as seen in a course on 'Child development' at the Department of Advanced Nursing Studies, Cardiff.] International Journal of Nursing Studies, 12 (2), Jul 1975, 87–93.

11 Gebhardt, S. A. A new model for nursing education. [Based at Governors State University, Illinois.] Nursing Outlook, 21 (4), Apr 1973, 252–255.

12 Geissler, E. M. A new way of looking at old ideas. [The organization of learning experience.] International Nursing Review, 21 (6), Nov/Dec 1974, 169–171.

13 Hooper, J. Training of mature entrants. Nursing Times, 71, 16 Oct 1975, Occ. papers, 105–107.

14 Hunt, J. M. The teaching and practice of basic nursing procedures in three hospitals. MPhil thesis, Department of Biological Sciences, Surrey University, 1971.

15 Kissinger, J. F. and others Teaching medical-surgical nursing by concepts. Nursing Outlook, 22 (10), Oct 1974, 654–658.

16 Lancaster, A. The comparative method in nursing education. Nursing Times, 68, 24 Aug. 1972, Occ. papers, 133–135.

17 Marshall, I. A. Creating an environment for learning. Nursing Outlook, 22 (12), Dec 1974, 773–776.

18 Marson, S. N. What it's all about, or the art of developing effective instruction – with apologies to R. F. Mager. Health Visitor, 47 (5), May 1974, 134–138.

19 Martin, J. L. The scope for learning. [A framework within which the tutor may begin to exercise the key function of the teacher-manager . . . planning.] Nursing Times, 69, 19 Jul 1973, Occ. papers 113–116.

20 Rauen, K. and Waring, B. The teaching contract. [A signed contract between student and instructor encourages academic achievement.] Nursing Outlook, 20 (9), Sep 1972, 594–596.

21 Saunders, P. Concept teaching in nursing. [With pain as example.] Nursing Papers, 5 (2), Sep 1973, 29–34.

22 Shaffer, S. M. and others Teaching in schools of nursing. St. Louis: Mosby, 1972.

23 Silva, D. Program development in nursing: some theoretical questions. Nursing Research, 20 (6), Nov/Dec 1971, 530–533.

24 Smith, J. P. Teaching care: the perennial dilemma. Nursing Mirror, 133, 22 Oct 1971, 11–14.

25 Thompson, M. Learning: a comparison of traditional and autotutorial methods. Nursing Research, 21 (5), Sep/Oct 1972, 453–457.

26 Whyte, D. Nursing skills. 1. [A study to identify the problems of training in basic nursing skills with regard to communication and learning. It relates research undertaken in the study of skill in other fields

to nursing.] Nursing Times, 70, 31 Oct 1974, Occ. papers, 93–96.

27 Whyte, D. Nursing skills. 2. [Research findings on the factors influencing the acquisition of skill.] Nursing Times, 70, 7 Nov 1974, Occ. papers 97–99.

28 Whyte, D. Nursing skills. 3. [Skills analysis.] Nursing Times, 70, 14 Nov 1974, Occ. papers, 101–104.

29 Whyte, D. Nursing skills. 4. [Methods of teaching nursing skills, including a tape/slide experiment.] Nursing Times, 70, 21 Nov 1974, Occ. papers, 105–108.

b AUDIOVISUAL AND LEARNING RESOURCE CENTRES

1 Bancroft, J. A. and Collins, K. Instructional design team. [Team composed of experts in nursing, education, and media production.] Nursing Outlook, 22 (4), Apr 1974, 254–257.

2 Brown, R. A. and Townsend, I. Educational technology in the school of nursing. [Establishment of a learning resources centre.] Nursing Times, 71, 20 Feb 1975, 316–317.

3 Brylski, E. and Gillsen, J. Audiovisuals made to order. Nursing Outlook, 20 (6), Jun 1972, 385–387.

4 Davidson, J. M. Concept and utilization of a multimedia laboratory in a community college registered nursing program. Journal of Nursing Education, 11 (3) Aug 1972, 23–35.

5 Graves, J. The Medical Recording Service Foundation. Physiotherapy, 61 (12), Dec 1975, 370–371.

6 Hackshaw, S. M. Slide sequences as a teaching aid. [Illustrating procedures dealing with Australian antigen patients in the operating room.] Nursing Times, 71, 16 Oct 1975. NATN Supplement, ix–x.

7 Harris, J. A. and others Making a film loop. An exercise in education. [Subject of the loop is irrigating an eye.] Nursing Times, 68, 25 May 1972, 649–651.

8 Keppelman, L. C. Films in nursing education. [A survey to examine and why and how nurses use films with the relative advantages and disadvantages.] Nursing Outlook, 23 (1), Jan 1975, 35–37.

9 Koch, H. B. The instructional media: an overview. Nursing Outlook, 23 (1), Jan 1975, 29–32.

10 Koch, H. The media center. Film or television? Nursing Outlook, 23 (8), Aug 1975, 489.

11 Koch, H. B. The media center. In planning the center. . . . Nursing Outlook, 23 (3), Mar 1975, 145.

12 Koch, H. The media center. Production and technical standards. Nursing Outlook, 23 (5), May 1975, 287.

13 Koch, H. The media center. Selecting the software. Nursing Outlook, 23 (4), Apr 1975, 219.

14 Koch, H. The media center. The static visual media. Nursing Outlook, 23 (6), June 1975, 355.

15 Koch, H. B. Where do you start? [Behavioural objectives and audiovisual media.] Nursing Outlook, 23 (2), Feb 1975, 85.

16 Kubo, W. and others Creative examination: use of a film provides a simulated clinical nursing experience to measure students' perceptions of patient-care problems. Nursing Outlook, 19 (8), Aug 1971, 524–526.

17 Langhoff, H. F. Audiovisual equipment. [In nursing education.] American Journal of Nursing, 72 (11), Nov 1972, 2029–2031.

18 Lutz, E. M. and Berthold, J. S. Creating a climate for educational technology in nursing. Cleveland, Ohio: Case Western Reserve University, Frances Payne Bolton School of Nursing, 1971.

19 McGinn, H. F. A/V materials – where should they be kept? Nursing Outlook, 23 (1), Jan 1975, 38–39.

20 McGrane, H. F. Tape recorded evaluation: a method of teaching. Journal of Nursing Education, 14 (1), Jan 1975, 11–17.

21 Miles, I. M. A multimedia approach to education. [An analysis of the use of educational media in Holland.] SA Nursing Journal, 42 (8), Aug 1975, 14–15.

22 Miller, A. H. The learning experience guide: a better teaching tool. [Audio-visual aids.] Journal of Nursing Education, 11 (2), Apr 1972, 9–12.

23 Nicholas, S. C. Making a medical documentary. Nursing Times, 71, 20 Feb 1975, 286–288.

24 Nightingale School of Nursing Nightingale enterprises. [Learning resources centre, Nightingale School of Nursing, St. Thomas's Hospital.] Nursing Times, 71, 20 Feb 1975, 298–299.

25 Nursing Outlook Audiovisuals in nursing education. [A survey of nursing schools and hospitals to examine purchasing procedures.] Nursing Outlook, 23 (1), Jan 1975, 33–34.

26 Nursing Outlook The media center. Utilization techniques in the classroom. Nursing Outlook, 73 (9) Sep 1975, 549.

27 Nursing Outlook The media scene. Nursing Outlook, 23 (1) Jan 1975, 29–39.

28 Poshek, N. Multimedia approaches to teaching and learning in a baccalaureate nursing program. Journal of Nursing Education, 11 (3) Aug. 1972, 36–43.

29 Price, A. W. The effective use of the multimedia approach to staff development. [In continuing and in-service education programs.] Journal of Nursing Administration, 1 (4), Jul–Aug 1971, 38–45.

30 Smith, A. P. Audio-visual teaching in nurse education. Nursing Times, 67, 17 Jun 1971, 736–737.

31 Smylie, H. From nurse-teacher to audiovisual advisor. [At St. Joseph's School of Nursing, Toronto.] Canadian Nurse, 68 (10), Oct 1972, 29–31.

32 Stein, R. F. A multimedia independent approach to learning. [Study of 60 students at Indiana University School of Nursing following a one year trial using audiovisual aids.] International Journal of Nursing Studies, 12 (4), 1975, 185–196.

33 Stein, R. F. and others A multimedia independent approach, for improving the teaching-learning process in nursing. Nursing Research, 21 (5), Sep/Oct 1972, 436–447.

34 Townsend, I. Audio-visual aids to teaching. Nursing Mirror, 141, 4 Dec 1975, 66–67.

35 Townsend, I. NHS Learning Resources Unit. [Responsible for the production and promotion of educational resources within nurse education.] Nursing Mirror, 141, 20 Nov 1975, 72–73.

36 Tunstill, A. M. Machinery and the nurse. Nursing Times, 68, 9 Mar 1972, 296–297.

37 Wells, M. D. Educational technology for beginners. Nursing Times, 67, 30 Dec 1971, 1642–1643.

38 White, L. D. and Chavigny, K. H. Direct tape access as an adjunct to learning. [A comparison of examination scores after some students had been given 15 minute taped summaries of each lecture.] Nursing Research, 24 (4), Jul/Aug 1975, 295–298.

39 Wiener, M. M. and others Nurse training goes modern. [A multimedia instructional system.] Hospitals, 45, 1 Oct 1971, 74, 76, 78, 80.

40 Wittmeyer, A. Teaching by audiotape. Nursing Outlook, 19 (3), Mar 1971, 162–163.

41 World Health Organization The selection of teaching/learning material in health sciences education: report of a WHO study group. Geneva: WHO (Technical report series, no 538), 1974.

c AUDIOVISUAL: TELEVISION

1 Allen, M. The development of clinical nursing situations on videotape for use via closed-circuit TV in the teaching of nursing. [Research study.] Nursing Papers, 4 (2), Dec 1972, 23–33.

2 Barlow, D. J. and Bruhn, J. G. Role-plays on television – a new teaching technique. Nursing Outlook, 21 (4) Apr 1973, 242–244.

3 Croton, G. Television on nurses. 'Had you gone to St. X's. . . Nursing Times, 67, 13 May 1971, 563–565.

4 Davis, G. L. and Eaton, S. L. On the move with micro-teaching. [The use of videotape in an extension course for teachers of nursing.] American Journal of Nursing, 74 (7), Jul 1974, 1292–1293.

5 Fish, E. J. Video-tapes in schools of nursing. Nursing Mirror, 132, 26 Feb 1971, 18–20.

6 Hector, W. The mass media in nurse education. [How to use the BBC programmes to best advantage.] Nursing Times, 69, 1 Feb 1973, 160.

7 James, P. E. Studies in learning: with particular reference to learning from television. PhD thesis, Liverpool University, 1972.

8 Longley, C. Role of broadcasting in nurse education. Nursing Mirror, 133, 13 Aug 1971, 32–33.

9 Miles, I. M. A multimedia approach to education. [An analysis of investigations into the use of television outside South Africa.] SA Nursing Journal, 42 (7), Jul 1975, 13–15.

10 Minehan, P. L. Adaption to open-circuit television: a method for nursing education. Nursing Forum, 11 (3), 1972, 230–247.

11 Minehan, P. L. Cool: nursing – cool: television or McLuhanism applied. International Nursing Review, 18 (2), 1971, 149–153.

12 Mondfrans, A. P. V. and others Live or taped? [Successful use of videotapes.] Nursing Outlook, 20 (10), Oct 1972, 652–653.

13 Nursing Outlook Preparing a teleclass: a case study. [Preparing a 30 minute videotape class.] Nursing Outlook, 23 (11), Nov 1975, 681.

14 O'Neill, J. Videotape recording: a practical experiment [in nursing education]. Nursing Mirror, 139, 5 Jul 1974, 55–58.

15 Quiring, J. The autotutorial approach: the effect of timing of videotape feedback on sophomore nursing students' achievement of skill in giving subcutaneous injections. Nursing Research, 21 (4), Jul/Aug 1972, 332–337.

16 Roth, D. H. and Price, D. W. Instructional television: a method for teaching nursing. St. Louis: Mosby.

17 Roth, D. H. Television utilization in nursing practice. Journal of Nursing Administration, 1 (5), Sep/Oct 1971, 33–43.

18 Sadlick, M. and Penta, F. B. Changing student nurse attitudes towards quadriplegics by use of television. [University of Illinois School of Nursing.]

Medical and Biological Illustration, 23 (3), Aug 1975, 129–132.

19 Sanborn, D. E. and others Continuing education for nurses via interactive closed-circuit television: a pilot study. Nursing Research, 22 (5), Sep/Oct 1975, 448–451.

20 Sigafoos, T. and Jordan, J. Education. Staff development via videotape. Hospitals, 46 1 Dec 1972, 40–42.

21 Simpson, M. J. You're on. [Television debates by senior nursing students.] American Journal of Nursing, 71 (9), Sep 1971, 1760–1761.

22 Woodhouse, R. Smile – you're on TV. Videotape as a teaching aid. Nursing Times, 67, 6 May 1971, 541–543.

23 Woolley, A. S. Reaching and teaching the older student. Nursing Outlook, 21 (1), Jan 1973, 37–39.

24 Zurhellen, J. H. Individualization: a strategy to develop tomorrow's practitioners. Nursing Forum, 13 (1), 1974, 87–93.

d CLINICAL TEACHING

1 Babajide, O. Ward based teaching and assessment. Nigerian Nurse, 4 (4), Oct/Dec 1972, 21–22, 24.

2 Bates, B. and Lynaugh, J. Teaching physical assessment. Nursing Outlook, 23 (5), May 1975, 297–302.

3 Barnett, D. E. Ward teaching. A simple and interesting five-week programme. Nursing Times, 70, 4 Jul 1974, 1046–1047.

4 Bavin, C. J. Clinical teaching and the use of audiovisual aids: a scholarship tour of North America. Nursing Times, 69, 12 Jul 1973, 912–913.

5 Brinham, R. O. J. Learning while caring. [Ward teaching by patient centred care at Elizabeth Garrett Anderson Hospital.] Nursing Mirror, 140, 22/29 May 1975, 81–82.

6 Burch, M. Teaching in the ward environment. Nursing Mirror, 141, 31 Jul 1975, 59–61.

7 Carter, A. and Lewis, J. Mini-courses for clinical teaching. New Zealand Nursing Journal, 66 (7), Jul 1973, 13.

8 Crouch, B. Clinical teaching on night duty. Nursing Times, 68, 19 Oct 1972, 1320–1321.

9 Darcy, P. T. Dynamic aspects in clinical learning. [Scheme at Tyrone and Fermanagh Hospital, Omagh.] Nursing Mirror, 141, 24 Jul 1975, 59–60; 31 Jul 1975, 72; 7 Aug 1975, 69.

10 Da Silva, A. L. The clinical instructor. Nigerian Nurse, 4 (2), Apr/Jun 1972, 11–12.

11 Davis, B. G. Clinical expertise as a function of educational preparation. Nursing Research, 21 (6), Nov/Dec 1972, 530–534.

12 Hagopian, G. and Kilpack, V. Baccalaureate students learn assessment skills. [Physical assessment of the patient.] Nursing Outlook, 22 (7), Jul 1974, 454–456.

13 Hanrahan, K. A. A clinical teacher. World of Irish Nursing, 1 (2), Feb 1972, 40–41.

14 Hayter, J. An approach to laboratory evaluation. Journal of Nursing Education, 12 (4), Nov 1973, 17–22.

15 Howarth, B. How can the vision of Janus help professional nursing? Australian Nurses' Journal, 4 (11), Jun 1975, 31–33, 36.

16 Infante, M. S. The clinical laboratory in nursing education. New York: Wiley, 1973.

17 Ingram, A. G. The laboratory in the school of nursing. Nursing Times, 69, 28 Jun 1973, 837–840.

18 Jackson, B. S. Nursing decisions: Experiences in clinical problem solving. [Case study approach to decision making designed to teach and assess clinical judgement.] RN Magazine, 38 (9), Sep 1975, 57–62.

19 Lamp Creative use of the laboratory. Lamp, 32 (8) Aug 1975, 34–36.

20 Lamp Summary of clinical instructors discussion. Lamp, 29 (7), Jul 1972, 50–53.

21 Little, D. and Carnevali, D. Complexities of teaching in the clinical laboratory. Journal of Nursing Education, 11 (1), Jan 1972, 15–22.

22 Lynaugh, J. and Bates, B. Clinical practicum in ambulatory care. [Special problems in incorporation in a nurse practitioner program.] Nursing Outlook, 23 (7), Jul 1975, 444–448.

23 Mathieson, S. Students' views on clinical teaching. Nursing Times, 70, 13 Jun 1974, 924–925.

24 Miller, P. Clinical knowledge: a needed curriculum emphasis. Nursing Outlook, 23 (4), Apr 1975, 222–224.

25 Nelson, S.E. Grand rounds, student style. [Patient assessments, nursing diagnosis, and care plans through students' peer review of patient care during rounds.] Nursing Outlook, 21 (8), Aug 1973, 519.

26 New Zealand Nursing Journal Communication [of instruction in clinical work to the student.] New Zealand Nursing Journal, 66 (6), Jun 1973, 23–26.

27 Paduano, M. A. Evaluation in the nursing laboratory: an honest appraisal. [Use of a clinical laboratory which can offer predictable situations in which nursing skills can be performed, observed and evaluated.] Nursing Outlook, 22 (11), Nov 1974, 702–705.

28 Pearson, B. D. Issues of student clinical nursing. [Problems facing clinical teachers.] Journal of Nursing Education, 14 (4), Nov 1975, 20–25.

29 Perkins, E. Clinical teachers. [Letter explaining a system used at Stafford Infirmary to define relationships between ward sisters and clinical teachers.] Nursing Times, 70, 19/26 Dec 1974, 1980–1981.

30 Robbins, J. Teaching nursing. [Meeting between clinical nurse teachers and practical work instructors.] Nursing Times, 69, 22 Mar 1973, 389.

31 Royal Australian Nurses' Federation Education. Clinical Instructors. [Report of a meeting on the subject: Should we have a Clinical Instructor's Course?] Australian Nurses' Journal, 1 (7), Jan 1972, 7–8.

32 Schweer, J. E. Creative teaching in clinical nursing. 2nd ed. St. Louis: Mosby, 1972.

33 Sheahan, J. A silver milestone in clinical teaching. [A survey of the literature.] Nursing Times, 68, 10 Aug 1972. Occ. papers. 125–127.

e COMPUTER LEARNING

1 Bitzer, M. D. and Bitzer, D. L. Teaching nursing by computer; an evaluative study. Computers in Biology and Medicine, 3 (3), Oct 1973, 187–204.

2 Collart, M. E. Computer assisted instruction and the learning process. Nursing Outlook, 21 (8), Aug 1973, 527–532.

3 Dixon, J. M. and others A computerised education and training record. Journal of Continuing Nursing Education, 6 (4), Jul/Aug 1975, 20–23.

4 Ertel, P. C. and others Learning from the computer: what every health care administrator should know. Modern Hospital, 119 (5), Nov 1972, 103–106.

5 Gordon, M. S. Learning from a cardiology patient simulator. [Computer programmed animated manikins.] RN Magazine, 38 (8), Aug 1975, ICU1, 4, 6.

6 Hoffer, E. P. and others Use of computer-aided instruction in graduate nursing education: a controlled trial. Journal of Emergency Nursing, 1 (2), Mar/Apr 1975, 27–29.

7 Jenkinson, V. M. Student nurses and the computer: an experimental project. Nursing Times, 68, 2 Mar 1972, 254–255.

8 Levine, D. and Wiener, E. Let the computer teach it. American Journal of Nursing, 75 (8), Aug 1975, 1300–1302.

9 Lidz, C. G. Computer-managed instruction in nursing. New York: National League for Nursing, 1974.

10 Reed, F. C. and others Computer assisted instruction for continued learning. American Journal of Nursing, 72 (11), Nov 1972, 2035–2039.

11 Silva, M. C. Nursing education in the computer age. Nursing Outlook, 21 (2), Feb 1973, 94–98.

12 Sumida, S. W. A computerised test for clinical decision making. Clinical incidents can be programmed to permit students to decide how they would respond. Nursing Outlook, 20 (7), Jul 1972, 458–461.

13 Valish, A. U. and others The role of computer-assisted instruction in continuing education of registered nurses: an experimental study. Journal of Continuing Education in Nursing, 6 (1), Jan/Feb 1975, 13–32.

f GROUP METHODS

1 Delorey, P. E. Multiple assignment: rehearsal for practice [Team learning instructional method in which a group of students are assigned to one patient.] American Journal of Nursing, 72 (2), Feb 1972, 292–295.

2 Floyd, G. J. Team teaching: advantages and disadvantages to the student. [Results of a questionnaire.] Nursing Research, 24 (1), Jan/Feb 1975, 52–56.

3 George, J. A. and Gowell, E. C. Transactional analysis in sensitivity groups for students of nursing. Nursing Forum, 12 (1), 1973, 82–95.

4 Hutchinson, S. and Talley, N. The group supervisory conference [as a means of stimulating students' ideas]. Journal of Nursing Education, 13 (4), Nov 1974, 13–17.

5 Linthwaite, P. Group methods of teaching. [Developmental psychology and reactions to illness.] Nursing Mirror, 134, 9 Jun 1972, 14–15.

6 McLaughlin, F. E. and White, E. Small group functioning under six different leadership formats. Nursing Research, 22 (1), Jan/Feb 1973, 37–54.

7 Mims, F. H. Experiential learning in groups. Journal of Nursing Education, 13 (4), Nov 1974, 30–36.

8 Plummer, E. M. The clinical conference discussion leader. [Fruitful use of group discussion in nursing education.] Nursing Forum, 13 (1), 1974, 94–104.

9 RN Magazine Specialty nursing teams in a small hospital? RN Magazine, 37 (2), Feb 1974, 34–35, 62, 64.

10 Robbins, E. Proceed with caution. [Changes in nurse education as exemplified in a recent advertisement for a qualified tutor prepared to experiment with new and various informal teaching methods and case assignment team nursing.] Nursing Times, 67, 25 Nov 1971, 1478–1479.

11 Saxon, J. Multiple assignments – try them! [As-

signing 3 students to each patient with practitioner, researcher and observer roles.] American Journal of Nursing, 75 (12), Dec 1975, 2183–2184.

12 Veninga, R. and Fredlund, D. J. Teaching the group approach. Nursing Outlook, 22 (6), Jun 1974, 373–376.

g PROGRAMMED LEARNING

1 Hedley, E. A. and others Programmed learning for nurses. Nursing Times, 67, 2 Dec 1971, Occ. papers, 189–190.

2 Hegge, M. L. Independent study in community health nursing: learning 'packets' in specific areas give students a guided and supervised opportunity to extend their learning. Nursing Outlook, 21 (10), Oct 1973, 652–654.

3 Koch, H. B. The media center. Autotutorial instruction. Nursing Outlook, 23 (10), Oct 1975, 619.

4 Lange, C. M. Autotutorial techniques in nursing education. New Jersey: Prentice-Hall, 1972.

5 Layton, J. Instructional packaging [for individual learning.] Journal of Nursing Education, 14 (4), Nov 1975, 26–30.

6 Lipson, L. F. Creating a learning environment. [Individualized instruction and the use of programmed learning.] Journal of Nursing Education, 11 (3), Aug 1972, 4–9.

7 Lowe, J. Programme for success in Sheffield. [Programmed learning library loan service in the Sheffield Region.] Nursing Times, 70, 13 Jun 1974, 923.

8 Lumsden, D. B. Another look at programmed instruction in nursing education. International Nursing Review, 21 (6), Nov/Dec 1974, 183, 187.

9 Marson, S. N. Programmed instruction applied to nurse training: final report. Sheffield Programmed Instruction Centre for Industry, 1971.

10 Marson, S. N. Programmed instruction in the nurse training school: a survey of the opinions of 190 practising nurse tutors on the effectiveness of programmed instruction and its place in the nurse training school. Sheffield Polytechnic Learning Resources Unit, 1973.

11 Marson, S. N. Programmed instruction – panacea or passing gimmick? A report on the introduction of programmed instruction into Nurse Training Schools in the Sheffield region. International Nursing Review, 19 (2), 1972, 126–137.

12 Marson, S. Sixteen years after Skinner. [Programmed learning.] Midwives Chronicle, 86, Feb 1972, 37–42.

13 Marson, S. N. What happened to programmed learning? Nursing Times, 71, 4 Sep 1975, 1425–1427.

14 Muscroft, V. P. Teachers' page. 12. Programmed instruction. Midwives Chronicle, 88, Sep 1975, 310–312.

15 Nursing Times Sheffield – pioneers of programmed learning. Nursing Times, 67, 20 May 1971, 618.

16 O'Connor, H. E. and Jones, D. An innovative teaching strategy for nursing education. [Use of learning packages.] Journal of Nursing Education, 14 (4), Nov 1975, 9–15.

17 Peterson, M. H. Understanding defense mechanisms. [Programmed instruction.] American Journal of Nursing, 72 (9), Sep 1972, 1651–1672.

18 Riley, M. E. Teaching nursing referrals by programmed instruction. [Teaching importance of continuity of care.] RN Magazine, 36 (1), Jan 1973, 57–58, 60.

h SELF DIRECTED LEARNING

1 Bogner, J. and Spatz, A. Independent approach to learning [for practical nursing students]. Journal of Practical Nursing, 24 (5), May 1974, 22–23.

2 Coffey, L. Modules for independent-individual learning in nursing. Philadelphia: Davis, 1975.

3 Finch, A. J. For students only: a system of learning. [Conceptual approach to problem solving.] Nursing Outlook, 19 (5), May 1971, 332–333.

4 Josberger, M. C. Independent study considered and reconsidered. Journal of Nursing Education, 14 (1), Jan 1975, 18–22.

5 Langford, T. Self directed learning. Nursing Outlook, 20 (10), Oct 1972, 648–651.

6 Lionberger, H. The senior year preceptorship. [Independent learning in a baccalaureate degree program.] Nursing Outlook, 23 (5), May 1975, 320–322.

7 Narrow, B. W. Independent study: impossible dream or intriguing challenge? Journal of Nursing Education, 11 (3), Aug 1972, 11–22.

8 Rosendahl, P. Self-direction for learners: an andragogical approach to nursing education. Nursing Forum, 13 (2), 1974, 136–146.

9 Wittkopf, B. Self-instruction for student learning. American Journal of Nursing, 72 (11), Nov 1972, 2032–2034.

i OTHER METHODS

1 Aavedal, M. and others Developing student-professor contracts in the clinical area. International Nursing Review, 22 (4), Jul/Aug 1975, 105–108.

2 Anstice, E. Plastics for practice. [Plastic anatomical models]. Nursing Times, 67, 8 Jul 1971, 840–841.

3 Coleman, V. A. Academic gaming in nurse teaching. Nursing Times, 69, 21 Jun 1973, 808–809.

4 Cortazzi, D. Illuminative incident analysis. [Everyday incidents involving personal relationships, used as teaching material.] British Hospital Journal and Social Service Review, 82, 7 Oct 1972, 2241–2242.

5 Godejohn, C. J. and Others Effect of simulation gaming on attitudes toward mental illness. [An investigation of student nurses' attitudes.] Nursing Research, 24 (5), Sep–Oct 1975, 367–370.

6 Journal of Nursing Education An instructional simulation system offering practice in assessment of patient needs. Journal of Nursing Education, 11 (1), Jan 1972, 23–28.

7 Kramer, M. The concept of modelling as a teaching strategy. Nursing Forum, 11 (1), 1972, 48–70.

8 Lowe, J. Games and simulations in nurse education. Nursing Mirror, 141, 4 Dec 1975, 68–69.

9 McGinty, D. and Janoscrat, A. J. The homeostatic nursing care plan. [Used in the tutorial approach in nurse training.] Journal of Nursing Education, 12 (2), Apr 1973, 14–19.

10 Maisey, P. W. and Weddell, M. Learning by discovery. A report on the introduction of project work in a hospital group training school. Nursing Times, 68, 10 Feb 1972, Occ. papers, 21–22; 17 Feb 1972, Occ. papers, 25–28.

11 Malo-Juvera, D. Seeing is believing. Nursing Outlook, 21 (9), Sep 1973, 583–585.

12 Mesolella, D. W. Teaching by telephone. American Journal of Nursing, 71 (6), Jun 1971, 1144–1145.

13 Mitchell, P. H. and Atwood, J. Problem-oriented recording as a teaching-learning tool: use in critical thinking and identification of patient problems. Nursing Research, 24 (2), Mar–Apr 1975, 99–101, 103.

14 Parker, N. I. A study of error-modelling in skills learning. [Experimental study of educational value of demonstration of errors.] Nursing Papers, 6 (1), Spring 1974, 33.

15 Pearson, B. D. Simulation techniques for nursing education. International Nursing Review, 22 (5), Sep–Oct 1975, 144–146.

16 Perry, L. C. The use of simulation with students having a community health nursing experience. [Simulation of a home visit by means of role-playing, using film.] Journal of Nursing Education, 12 (2), Apr 1973, 20–25.

17 Quiring, J. D. Utilizing questioning strategies in nursing education. Journal of Nursing Education, 12 (3), Aug 1973, 21–27.

18 Rubin, F. and others The seminar process – an aid to learning. Nursing Outlook, 19 (1), Jan 1971, 37–39.

19 Scheideman, J. M. Chronicity: a key to learning. [Assigning students to chronically ill patients to improve nursing care.] American Journal of Nursing, 75 (3), Mar 1975, 446–447.

20 Scholdra, J. D. and Quiring, J. D. The level of questions posed by nursing educators. Journal of Nursing Education, 12 (3), Aug 1973, 15–20.

21 Veith, S. Disputation. Nursing Outlook, 22 (11), Nov 1974, 699–701.

22 SELECTION AND ASSESSMENT

a SELECTION AND PSYCHOLOGICAL TESTS

1 Bergman, R. and others Psychological tests: their use and validity in selecting candidates for schools of nursing in Israel. International Journal of Nursing Studies, 11 (2), Jul 1974, 85–109.

2 Boughton, J. Report on a pilot study using a sample of nurse aides to investigate a staff selection technique. Australian Nurses' Journal, 3 (9), Apr 1974, 23–25.

3 Bradshaw, C. E. What makes an open door policy work? [Scheme at Santa Fe Community College in which assessment tests decide which course the individual student is fitted for.] American Journal of Nursing, 73 (3), Mar 1973, 464–465.

4 Burgess, M. A. and others Two studies of prediction of success in a collegiate program of nursing. Nursing Research, 21 (4), Jul/Aug 1972 357–366.

5 Burton, D. A. The selection of nurses by discriminant analysis. [Scheme at the Towers Hospital, Leicester.] International Journal of Nursing Studies, 9 (2), Jun 1972, 77–83.

6 Cordiner, C. M. and Hall, D. J. The use of motivational analysis test in the selection of Scottish nursing students. Nursing Research, 20 (4), Jul–Aug 1971, 356–362.

7 Davies, M. E. and Khosla, T. Predictive value of two intelligence tests as criteria of success in a health visitor examination. Nursing Times, 70, 28 Nov 1974, Occ. papers 109–112.

8 De Frank, J. L. Rips: a remedial instruction program. An experience with educationally disadvantaged students who were ineligible for admission to nursing because of reading deficiencies. Nursing Outlook, 19 (3), Mar 1971, 180–181.

9 Franklin, D. R. Selective and non-selective admissions criteria in junior college nursing programs. New York: National League for Nursing, 1975.

10 Gannon, B. Predicting success in clinical teacher students. Nursing Times, 71, 17 Apr. 1975, Occ. papers, 33–35.

11 Gannon, B. The relationship between the performance of clinical nurse teachers in certain tests of intelligence, cognitive style, and personality and performance in their professional examination. MEd thesis, Liverpool University, 1974.

12 Hack, K. A. Predictors of success in health visiting. Nursing Times, 69, 12 Apr 1973, Occ. papers, 57–60.

13 Heins, M. and Davis, M. How do we help 'high risk' students? [Students with poor academic qualifications, but good personal qualities.] Nursing Outlook, 22 (2), Feb 1972, 121–123.

14 Henricks, M. J. Audio slides streamline interviews. [For admission of students to school for nursing assistants, Ottawa Civic Hospital.] The Canadian Nurse, 67, (8), Aug 1971, 35–36.

15 Killcross, M. C. and Bates, W. T. G. Typical selection studies and procedures: example 3. Selecting student nurses. In: Killcross, M. C., and Bates, W. T. G. Selecting the younger trainee. HMSO. 1975. [16–17.]

16 Levitt, E. E. and others An attempt to develop an objective test battery for the selection of nursing students. Nursing Research, 20 (3), May/Jun 1971, 255–258.

17 Liddle, L. R. and others Predicting baccalaureate degree attainment for nursing students: a theoretical study using the TAV selection system. Nursing Research, 20 (3), May–Jun 1971, 258–261.

18 McCluhan, J. D. and others AD challenge exams: two approaches. A four part examination. [Selection tests for partially qualified nurses.] Nursing Outlook, 22 (9), Sep 1974, 585–586.

19 May, A. E. and Chitty, E. Selecting candidates for pupil nurse training. Nursing Mirror, 133, 17 Dec 1971, 12–13.

20 Nightingale, L. 'Oh' levels. [And nurse training.] Nursing Times, 68, 3 Aug 1972, 974.

21 Nursing Outlook Let's examine. Cognitive abilities related to attrition in a collegiate nursing program. Nursing Outlook, 19 (12), Dec 1971, 807–808.

22 Nursing Outlook Let's examine. The predictive validity of two entrance examinations in a school of practical nursing. Nursing Outlook, 19 (9), Sept 1971, 611.

23 Palmer, P. E. and Brown, S. K. AD challenge exams: two approaches. Testing knowledge and skills. [Selection tests for the associate degree nursing program at Union University, Jackson, Tennessee.] Nursing Outlook, 22 (9), Sep 1974, 583–585.

24 Reavley, W. Reading comprehension test for personnel selection: some implications regarding pre-student nurse training. Nursing Times, 68, 23 Mar 1972, Occ. papers, 45–46.

25 Reavley, W. and Wilson, L. J. Selection or diagnosis? The use of psychometric tests with candidates for student nurse training. Nursing Times, 68, 16 Nov 1972, Occ. papers, 183–184.

26 Rowe, W. and others A fresh slant on the dropout. [A study to identify the relationship between reading skills and successful examination performance of 99 students in Sydney hospitals.] Australian Nurses' Journal, 5 (3), Sep 1975, 31–32.

27 Seager, J. H. C. Centralizing applications for

nurse training. Nursing Times, 70, 5 Sep 1974. Occ. papers, 61–64.

28 Seither, F. G. A predictive validity study of screening measures used to select practical nursing students. Nursing Research, 23 (1) Jan/Feb 1974, 60–63.

29 Singh, A. The predictive value of cognitive tests for selection of pupil nurses. Nursing Times, 68, 8 Jun 1972. Occ. papers 89–92.

30 Thomas, B. Prediction of success in a graduate nursing service administration program: a study of the effectiveness of student selection practices from 1967–1971. Nursing Research, 23 (2), Mar/Apr 1974, 156–159.

31 Willett, E. A. and others Selection and success of students in a hospital school of nursing. Canadian Nurse, 67 (1), Jan 1971, 41–45; Reprinted in Nursing Journal of India 72 (7), Jul 1971, 215–218, 231.

b ASSESSMENT

1 Bower, F. L. Normative – or criterion – referenced evaluation. [Student evaluation.] Nursing Outlook, 22 (8), Aug 1974, 499–502.

2 Brown, D. E. The concept of on-going assessment. [Of students in community health.] District Nursing, 15, Aug 1972, 99–100.

3 Central Treaty Organization Cento workshop on evaluation in nursing educational achievement: held in Istanbul, Turkey, December 4–9, 1972. Ankara: Central Treaty Organization, 1973.

4 Chisholm, L. Assessment – a step in the right direction. [Scheme in use at Law Hospital, Lanarkshire, of continuous teaching and assessment with pupil nurses.] Nursing Times, 68, 5 Oct 1972, Occ. papers, 157–160.

5 Christman, N. J. Clinical performance of baccalaureate graduates. Nursing Outlook, 19 (1), Jan 1971, 54–56.

6 Chuan, H. Evaluation by interview. [A structured questionnaire helps in assessing students' ability to relate theory to practice.] Nursing Outlook, 20 (1), Nov 1972, 726–727.

7 Collyer, L. H. Ward assessments. [Difference between assessment for students taking an integrated degree course and ordinary general training.] Nursing Times, 71, 30 Oct 1975, 1752.

8 Elliott, J. and others Ward-based practical examinations. [Seen from the students' point of view.] Nursing Times, 69, 7 Jun 1973, 744–745.

9 Fitzharris, J. Verbal and written. [Reports for ward based practical examinations.] Nursing Times, 68, 11 May 1972, 581.

10 Frejlach, G. and Corcoran, S. Measuring clinical performance. Nursing Outlook, 19 (4), Apr 1971, 270–271.

11 Ghany, R. A. Evaluation in nursing education. Jamaican Nurse, 15 (2), Aug 1975, 23–24.

12 Hampton, P. J. The practical nursing student: at the top of the class. [Results of the Borow Inventory of Academic Adjustment on a random sample of female practical nursing students.] Nursing Care, 7 (2), Feb 1974, 14–17.

13 Hine, G. C. Evaluation of student nurses. [System developed at the Waikato School of Nursing.] New Zealand Nursing Journal, 69 (7), Jul 1975, 9–11.

14 Johnson, D. M. and Wilhite, M. J. Reliability and validity of subjective evaluation of baccalaureate

program nursing students. Nursing Research, 22 (3), May/Jun 1973, 257–262.

15 Journal of Nursing Education Evaluation of faculty and students . . . a means towards fuller communication and greater productivity. Journal of Nursing Education, 13 (1) Jan 1974, 3–7.

16 Katzell, M. E. Evaluation for educational mobility. Nursing Outlook, 21 (7), Jul 1973, 453–456.

17 King's Fund Centre Assessment: a guide for the completion of progress reports on nurses in training. The Fund, 1972.

18 King's Fund Centre Nurses' attitude to patients and assessment of nurses in training: report of meetings. . . The Fund, 1972. (THC reprint nos. 673, 687, 694, 702, 719.)

19 Kramer, M. A. and Cowles, J. T. Weighting and distributing course grades. [Evaluation procedures.] Nursing Outlook, 22 (3), Mar 1974, 176–179.

20 Krumme, U. S. The case for criterion referenced measurement. [To evaluate clinical nursing performance.] Nursing Outlook, 23 (12), Dec 1975, 764–770.

21 Litwack, L. and others Counselling, evaluation and student development in nursing education. Philadelphia: Saunders, 1972.

22 Lloyd, V. A. Another view of student assessment. Nursing Mirror, 133, 10 Sep 1971, 17.

23 McIntyre, H. M. and others A simulated clinical nursing test: development and testing of an instrument. Nursing Research, 21 (5), Sep/Oct 1972, 429–435.

24 Nurses' Association of Jamaica Report of a seminar on the clinical evaluation of the student in a basic nursing programme. Jamaican Nurse, 14 (2), Aug 1974, 9, 27–28.

25 Pollert, I. E. Concepts of experience and evaluation as educative processes in Registered Nurse Baccalaureate School Program. [Self assessment by students.] International Journal of Nursing Studies, 12 (4), 1975, 205–210.

26 Reilly, D. E. Behavioral objectives in nursing: evaluation of learner attainment. New York: Appleton-Century-Crofts, 1975.

27 Smith, J. P. Planning for the new practical assessments. Nursing Mirror, 132, 4 Jun 1971, 32–33.

28 Tibbles, H. J. GNC practical examinations: Organization in the King's College Hospital Group. Nursing Times, 68, 18 May 1972, Occ. papers, 77–80.

29 Umuna, F. C. 'This I believe about student nurse evaluation.' [Procedures for evaluation.] Nigerian Nurse, 7 (1), Jan/Mar 1975, 29–30.

30 Watkins, C. student evaluation by computer. Nursing Outlook, 23 (7), Jul 1975, 449–452.

31 Wood, V. A problem that won't go away: evaluation of student nurse performance. International Nursing Review, 19 (4), 1972, 336–343.

c EXAMINATIONS

1 Bhattacharya, A. Psychological aspects of examining. Nursing Times, 70, 1 Aug 1974, 1205–1206.

2 Bloomfield, E. Getting to grips with exam nerves. Nursing Times, 68, 1 Jun 1972, 687–688.

3 Broadley, M. E. Why they fail: a retired tutor looks at state examination results. Nursing Times, 69, 4 Jan 1973, 33.

4 Darling, V. H. Problem of written examinations [and advantages of objective tests.] Nursing Times, 70, 7 Jun 1973, 744–745.

5 Dubs, R. Comparison of student achievement with performance ratings of graduates and state board examination scores. Nursing Research, 24 (1), Jan/Feb 1975, 59–62, 64.

6 Eggert, L. L. Challenge exam in interpersonal skills: [to test students' clinical proficiency in their counselling role.] Nursing Outlook, 23 (11), Nov. 1975, 707–710.

7 Hirskyj, L. Dangers of examination assessment. Nursing Mirror, 132, 5 Feb 1971, 17.

8 Layton, J. Students select their own grades. Nursing Outlook, 20 (5), May 1972, 327–329.

9 McVey, P. J. Examinations: the concept of objective testing. Nursing Mirror, 140, 16 Jan 1975, 68–70.

10 Malleson, N. Pre-examination strain: treatment of tension in the over-anxious student. Nursing Times, 70, 16 May 1974, 735–736.

11 Marriner, A. Student self-evaluation and the contracted grade. Nursing Forum, 13 (2), 1974, 130–135.

12 Reed, C. L. and Feldhusen, J. F. State board examination score prediction for associate degree nursing program graduates. Nursing Research, 21 (2), Mar/Apr 1972, 149–153.

13 Robbins, E. Against the clock. [Nursing examinations.] Nursing Times, 68, 27 Jul 1972, 939.

14 Robbins, E. Examining examinations. 1. Essay and structured questions. [Information derived from a study tour of the US.] Nursing Times, 71, 16 Oct 1975, 1674–1675.

15 Robbins, E. Examining examinations. 2. Objective tests. Nursing Times, 71, 23 Oct 1975, 1702.

16 Robbins, E. Examining examinations. 3. Completion and true/false items. Nursing Times, 71, 30 Oct 1975, 1751–1752.

17 Robbins, E. Examining examinations. 4. Analogy and matching items. Nursing Times, 71, 6 Nov 1975, 1787–1788.

18 Robbins, E. Examining examinations. 5. The grid. [Used to attain a balanced test content with appropriate weighting]. Nursing Times, 71, 13 Nov 1975, 1827.

19 Robbins, E. Examining examinations. 6. Multiple choice items. Nursing Times, 71, 20 Nov 1975, 1867–1868.

20 Robbins, E. Examining examinations. 7. The matrix. Nursing Times, 71, 27 Nov 1975, 1912–1913.

21 Robbins, E. Examining examinations. 8. Final preparations – layout of objective test papers. Nursing Times, 71, 4 Dec 1975, 1950–1951.

22 Robbins, E. Objective testing in nurse education. [An investigation undertaken by the author as a project while attending a middle management course.] Nursing Times, 69, 1 Feb 1973, Occ. papers, 17–20.

23 Rodway, A. C. Overseas nurses' guide to examination English. Nursing Mirror, 133, 5 Nov 1971, 35–37.

24 Ross, T. Examiners go to school. [City and Guilds of London Institute Certificate in Achievement Testing.] Nursing Mirror, 141, 16 Oct 1975, 71.

25 Tubi, A. Aims of examination and types of questions. Nigerian Nurse, 4 (4), Oct/Dec 1972, 25–28.

26 White, H. H. Final state practical examinations at Guy's Hospital. Nursing Times, 69, 8 Feb 1973, 188–191.

27 Whyte, B. B. Question and answer: some helpful hints at examination time. Nursing Mirror, 141, 28 Aug 1975, 45–46.

23 PRACTICAL EXPERIENCE

a GENERAL AND ALLOCATION

1 Aitken, J. and others Improving general nurse training by psychiatric secondment. Nursing Times, 70, 27 Jun 1974, Occ. papers, 29–32.

2 Banks, I. Nurse allocation. Heinemann Medical, 1972.

3 Canadian Hospital Association Study recommends extra clinical experience for nurses of two-year program. [Committee on nursing report.] Canadian Hospital, 49 (5), May 1972, 73–74.

4 Carter-Brown, R. Controlled clinical experience. [A brief period of experience for the student nurse, without the demands and responsibilities of belonging to the ward team.] Lamp, 31 (11), Nov 1974, 25–26.

5 Claypool, J. and Ferris, P. Students' experiences with the prenatal care of high-risk pregnant women. [In low social groups.] Journal of Nursing Education, 12 (4), Nov 1973, 7–15.

6 Cooke, S. A. Achieving a standard duty rota by staff participation. [In a group nurse training school.] Nursing Times, 69, 17 May 1973, 130–137.

7 Davis, B. G. Clinical expertise as a function of educational preparation. Nursing Research, 21 (6), Nov/Dec 1972, 530–534.

8 Geels, W. J. and others The ICU and collegiate nursing education. Journal of Nursing Education, 13 (1), Jan 1974, 15–20.

9 Glanville, C. L. Multiple student assignment as an approach to clinical teaching in pediatric nursing. Nursing Research, 20 (3), May–Jun 1971, 237–244.

10 Keller, M. J. Nursing education and the occupational health setting. [Learning opportunities for nursing students.] Occupational Health Nursing, 22 (1), Jan 1974, 14–18.

11 King Edward's Hospital Fund for London Allocation work book: guidelines for developing planned programmes of education and training for student and pupil nurses. The Fund, 1971.

12 Moores, B. and Thompson, A. Attitudes towards student nurses allocation programmes. [A research study by questionnaire of attitudes of ward sisters and student nurses.] International Journal of Nursing Studies, 12 (2), Jul 1975, 107–117.

13 O'Reilly, E. A comprehensive record. [Nurse education/ward allocation Kardex record system for student nurses.] Nursing Times, 68, 18 May 1972, 612–614.

14 Roper, N. Clinical experience in nurse education: a survey of the available nursing experience for general student nurses in a school of nursing in Scotland. MPhil thesis, Edinburgh University, 1975.

15 Safier, G. Nursing students and their learning experiences in geriatrics. [At the University of California, San Francisco.] Journal of Psychiatric Nursing and Mental Health Services, 10 (3), May/Jun 1974, 34–41.

16 Schrock, R. A. No rhyme or reason: a clinical area identification project. [Project to rationalize the allocation of student and pupil nurses to certain clinical areas in the course of their training.] International Journal of Nursing Studies, 10 (2), May 1973, 69–79.

b COMMUNITY

1 Boyle, M. T. and Kaufman, A. Strep screening to prevent rheumatic fever. [Health education program using student nurses needing clinical community experience.] American Journal of Nursing, 75 (9), Sep 1975, 1487–1488.

2 Brown, D. E. Community option. Survey after one year's activities in Newham. Nursing Times, 71, 13 Nov 1975, Occ. papers, 113–116; 20 Nov 1975, Occ. papers 117–120.

3 Callender, B. and others Students' comments. [On community care. Secondment undertaken in Berkshire by four second year student nurses from the Royal Free Hospital]. Nursing Times, 68, 20 Apr 1972, Occ. papers 64.

4 Clark, J. An evaluation of changes in the student. [After community care secondment in Berkshire of four second year student nurses from the Royal Free Hospital.] Nursing Times, 68, 20 Apr 1972, Occ. papers, 61.

5 Davies, M. J. Community care. 1. The present basic nurse education in the community. Nursing Times, 70, 17 Oct 1974, 1613–1633.

6 Davies, M. J. Community care. 2. The future basic nurse education in the community. Nursing Times, 70, 24 Oct 1974, 1669–1671.

7 Davies, M. J. Community option – an evaluation. [An analysis of the value of community nursing experience to nursing students.] Nursing Times, 70, 31 Jan 1974, 164–165.

8 Davies, M. J. The P.W.I. and the student nurse. [The practical work instructor and the community care option at Nottingham School of Nursing.] Queen's Nursing Journal, 16 (3), Jun 1973, 60–61.

9 Davies, M. J. Total patient care assessments of students and pupil nurses during the community care option. Nursing Mirror, 140, 6 Feb 1975, 64–65.

10 Eggebroten, E. F. Why not the laundromat? [Teaching and learning opportunities for student nurses in the community.] Nursing Outlook, 21 (12), Dec 1973, 758–762.

11 Evans, E. M. Dealing with patients as real people. [Community nursing secondment for student nurses.] Nursing Mirror, 134, 19 May 1972, 16–17.

12 Hassall, D. A home visit program for students: Visits to expectant parents. Nursing Outlook, 22 (8), Aug 1974, 522–524.

13 Hutt, A. Community care – the students' needs. District Nursing, 15 (2), May 1972, 39–40.

14 Hutt, A. Meeting new challenges. [Secondment of student nurses into the community.] Practice Team, no. 42/43, Nov/Dec 1974, 11, 12.

15 Hutt, A. and Wilson, J. Community care option. [Community care secondment undertaken in Berkshire by four second year student nurses from the Royal Free Hospital.] Nursing Times, 68, 20 Apr 1972. Occ. papers, 61–62.

16 Illing, M. Community care experience. To help with the teaching of the community option for student nurses a local technical college used its specialist staff in the department of applied social studies. Nursing Times, 70, 16 May 1974, 753–755.

17 Illing, M. The community care option – a survey of one year's experience in 10 centres. [Information collected from an exchange of ideas between ten local authority nursing officers.] Midwife, Health Visitor and Community Nurse, 11 (4), Apr 1975, 104–106.

18 Jackson, B. Camden's community care course option. [Part of the modular system of nurse training at University College Hospital.] Nursing Mirror, 139, 2 Aug 1974, 59–60.

19 Kennedy, W. E. and Gemmy, E. C. Aspects of community care. [Six-week secondment of two student nurses to Chesterfield Health Department.] Nursing Times, 69, 19 Apr 1973, 517–518.

20 Large, A. and Roberts, L. Attachment of ward sisters to the district. [In order to gain insight into the work in the community before their student nurses did their secondment.] District Nursing, 14 (11), Feb 1972, 226–228.

21 O'Connell, P. E. Community and hospital in university nurse education: the Southampton experience. PhD thesis, Department of Sociology and Social Administration, Southampton University 1975.

22 Perry, L. C. The use of simulation with students having a community health nursing experience. [Simulation of a home visit by means of role-playing, using film.] Journal of Nursing Education, 12 (2), Apr 1973, 20–25.

23 Peterson, P. Life on the district: a pupil nurse's impression of domiciliary nursing. Nursing Times, 68, 27 Jan 1972, 124–125; Journal of the Royal College of General Practitioners 21, Sep 1971, 559–560.

24 Redmond, B. M. Health visiting and interpersonal relationships. [Case structure of a student nurse taking a community care option in Berkshire.] Health Visitor, 47 (11), Nov 1974, 315–317.

25 Reissman, R. Towards better training. Nurses in training at Plumstead Hospital, Norwich, undertake a 12-week course in community care for the mentally subnormal. Nursing Times, 70, 17 Jan 1974, 92–93.

26 Slack, P. A. Six week community care programme for student nurses. [In the City of Westminster.] Health Visitor, 46 (4), Apr 1973, 117–118.

27 Smiley, O. R. Clinical experience at Moose Factory. [The experience of five third year nursing students and their professor in a small community in Northern Ontario.] International Journal of Nursing Studies, 11 (3), Sep 1974, 155–160.

28 Wong, D. M. Providing experience in physical assessment for students in basic programs. [Creation of a child health maintenance centre at a university.] American Journal of Nursing, 73 (6), Jun 1975, 974–975.

c THEATRE

1 Alexander, C. Rationale for student experience with the OR AORN Journal, 15 (6), Jun 1972, 23–26.

2 AORN Journal OR forum. [Series of seven articles giving views of nurse educators and OR nurses on whether OR experiences should be included in nurse education.] AORN Journal, 21 (4), Mar 1975, 621–641.

3 Brown, I. The role of the clinical teacher in the operating theatre. NATNews, 9 (2), Apr 1972, 8.

4 Greaves, D. M. Ward nurses in the operating theatre. [Student nurses accompanied patients into the theatre to gain insight into theatre procedures.] NATNews, 10 (3), Jun 1973, 21, 38.

5 Gruendemann, B. Student experience study: a cause for jubilation. AORN Journal, 18 (2), Aug 1973, 267–268.

6 Lay, J. Student nurses in the operating theatre. Australian Nurses' Journal, 2 (10), Apr 1973, 32–35.

7 MacClelland, D. Student reaction to OR experience. AORN Journal, 23 (3), Sep 1975, 440, 442, 444, 446.

8 NATNews Two weeks theatre experience. NATNews, 8 (1), Spring 1971, 20.

9 Olson, R. E. Cooperative approach to nursing education. [Cooperation between education and service in the operating room.] AORN Journal, 23 (3), Sep 1975, 448, 450, 452, 454.

10 Richardson, A. M. The two week student nurse in the operating theatre – and the clinical teacher. [Modular training at University College Hospital.] NATNews, 11 (5), Jul 1974, 17–18.

11 Robertson, P. A. OR nursing content in curriculum design. AORN Journal, 23 (3), Sep 1975, 429–432.

12 Wakeley, J. The need for a clinical teacher [in the operating department]. NATNews, 11 (3), Apr 1974, 20, 22.

24 DEGREE AND EXPERIMENTAL COURSES

a DEGREE COURSES

1 Armstrong-Esther, C. A. A new approach to education. [University degrees in nursing.] Nursing Times, 71, 3 Apr 1975, 549.

2 Clarke, M. A degree – linked nursing course. [Two articles.] Nursing Mirror, 133, 23 Jul 1971, 27–29; 133, 30 Jul, 37–39.

3 Colledge, M. M. Towards patient centred learning. [Objectives of a BA degree course in nursing at Newcastle centred round a team teaching plan.] Nursing Times, 71, 1 May 1975, 701–703.

4 Copp, L. A. Critical concerns and commitments of a new department of nursing. Inaugural Lecture, Department of Nursing, University of Manchester, October 8, 1973. International Journal of Nursing Studies, 2 (4), Dec 1974, 203–210.

5 Lancet Professor of nursing. Comment on the appointment of Jean McFarlane as Professor of Nursing at Manchester University. Lancet, 1, 22 Jun 1974, 1300.

6 Liddell, A. Learning to work effectively. [Experiences of a student studying for the Bachelor of Nursing degree at Manchester University.] Nursing Times, 71, 20 Feb 1975, 292–293.

7 McFarlane, J. K. 'A dramatic day for nursing': England's first nursing professor appointed. [Jean McFarlane.] Nursing Times, 70, 20 Jun 1974, 933.

8 McFarlane, J. K. Higher education in nursing. [WHO symposium on ways in which the resources of universities and higher education might be used to develop nursing leadership.] Nursing Times, 69, 12 Apr 1973, 481–482.

9 Pearson, J. Attitudes of undergraduates to their courses. [Obtained by visits to five universities in Britain by members of the GNC Research Unit.] Nursing Times, 71, 15 May 1975, 783–785.

10 Scott Wright, M. Nursing and the universities. [Abridged version of University of Edinburgh Chair of Nursing inaugural lecture.] Nursing Times, 69, 15 Feb 1973, 222–227.

11 Scott Wright, M. Unique occasion in Edinburgh. First inauguration of Chair of Nursing. [Inaugural lecture on nursing and the university.] Nursing Mirror, 136, 9 Feb 1973, 19–21; 16 Feb 1973, 12–14.

b DEGREE COURSES: OVERSEAS COUNTRIES

1 Aggarwal, K. C. There is a difference: [between diploma degree and post basic degree courses.] Nursing Journal of India, 46 (12), Dec 1975, 268, 279.

2 Aroskar, M. A. Change processes should involve baccalaureate nursing students. [Students as change

agents.] Journal of Nursing Education, 13 (1), Jan 1974, 26–30.

3 Bevil, C. W. The New York Regents external degree in nursing. Nursing Forum, 13 (3), 1974, 216–239.

4 Bullough, B. and Sparks, C. Baccalaureate vs Associate Degree nurses: the care-cure dichotomy. [Research study.] Nursing Outlook, 23 (11), Nov 1975, 688–692.

5 Canadian Nurse University schools of nursing in Canada. Each of Canada's twenty-two university schools of nursing describes the programs to be offered in the fall of 1973. Canadian Nurse, 69 (1), Jan 1973, 23–33.

6 Caulkwell, P. Nursing education within the university. New Zealand Nursing Journal, 64 (7), Jul 1971, 4–5.

7 Chater, S. S. COGEN: Cooperative graduate education in nursing. Nursing Outlook, 23 (10), Oct 1975, 630–632.

8 DeChow, G. H. The associate degree programs. RN Magazine, 34 (5), May 1971, 40–43, 66, 70, 72, 74, 76.

9 Donley, R. and others Graduate education for practice realities. Nursing Outlook, 21 (10), Oct 1973, 646–649.

10 Grossman, H. T. The diversity within graduate nursing education. [What part should research play in the curriculum of graduate study?] Nursing Outlook, 20 (7), Jul 1972, 464–467.

11 Harrison, P. Degree in nursing – University of Cape Town. S. A. Nursing Journal, 39 (3), Mar 1972, 13–12.

12 Hoexter, J. and McGriff, E. P. Why know how if you don't know what? [Graduate education in nursing.] Nursing Outlook, 19 (12), Dec 1971, 794–796.

13 Hover, J. Diploma vs degree nurses: are they alike? [Research study to investigate whether goals and attitudes about nursing differ because of the type of education experienced.] Nursing Outlook, 23 (11), Nov 1975, 684–687.

14 Hutcheson, J. D. and others Toward reducing attrition in baccalaureate degree nursing programs: an exploratory study. Nursing Research, 22 (6), Nov/Dec 1973, 530–533.

15 Joel, L. A. The preparation of the nurse in the university setting. Journal of Nursing Education, 11 (1), Jan 1972, 9–14.

16 Journal of Nursing Education Issue on associate-degree education in nursing. Journal of Nursing Education, 13 (2), Apr 1974, 2–31.

17 Kangori, S. W. University education for nurses at the University of Nairobi. Kenya Nursing Journal, 1 (1), Jun 1972, 42–43, 52.

18 Koffman, R. and Andruskiw, O. From Diploma or Associate degree to Bachelor's degree. American Journal of Nursing, 71 (11), Nov 1971, 2184–2186.

19 Lenburg, C. B. and Yeaworth, R. C. Who shall be admitted to graduate study? [A survey of admission to master's programs of nurses with non-nursing degrees.] Nursing Outlook, 23 (10), Oct 1975, 633–637.

20 Leveck, P. An extended Master's degree program. [University of California in San Francisco.] Nursing Outlook, 23 (10), Oct 1975, 646–649.

21 Love, I.D. Graduation – the end or the beginning? Australian Nurses' Journal, 4 (3), Sep 1974, 38–40.

22 Mereness, D. A. The baccalaureate and higher degree programs. RN Magazine, 34 (5), May 1971, 44–47, 80–82.

23 Mereness, D. A. Graduate education: as one Dean sees it. Nursing Outlook, 23 (10), Oct 1975, 638–641.

24 Ndlovu, R. The role of degree programmes in nursing education in Africa. International Nursing Review, 19 (4), 1972, 344–348.

25 Newman, M. A. The professional doctorate in nursing: a position paper. [Professional degrees as a means of improving the status of nursing.] Nursing Outlook, 23 (11), Nov 1975, 704–706.

26 Nyquist, E. B. The external degree program and nursing. Nursing Outlook, 21 (6), Jun 1973, 372–377.

27 Peterson, C. J. and others Theoretical framework for an associate degree curriculum. Nursing Outlook, 22 (5), May 1974, 321–324.

28 Platt, D. M. A preliminary study of nurses engaged in the profession of nursing in New South Wales who are working towards a University degree or have graduated from a University. Lamp, 29 (7), Jul 1972, 46–48.

29 Pretoria University Some points of interest in relation to the B. Cur (1 et A) Nursing Degree Course held at Pretoria University. Rhodesian Nurse, 5 (1), Mar 1972, 6–7.

30 Raderman, R. and Allen, D. V. Registered nurse students in a baccalaureate program. Factors associated with completion. [Survey of aptitude difference between students who completed the baccalaureate degree and those who did not.] Nursing Research, 23 (1), Jan/Feb 1974, 71–73.

31 Robinson, P. Trends in baccalaureate nursing education. Nursing Outlook, 20 (4), Apr 1972, 273–276.

32 Roods, J. The international dimension: how to implement an international dimension within an Associate Degree nursing programme in a community college. International Nursing Review, 20 (5), Sep/Oct 1973, 147–152.

33 Searle, C. Extra mural and external nursing degree courses: a query and an answer. [University of South Africa.] Rhodesian Nurse, 8 (4), Dec 1975, 15–23.

34 Selden, W. K. Are problems in graduate nursing education unique? [Master's degree programmes.] Nursing Outlook, 23 (10), Oct 1975, 622–624.

35 Simmons, S. A university extension program for RNs. [Michigan State University.] Nursing Outlook, 20 (12), Dec 1972, 798–801.

36 Stone, J. C. and Green, J. L. The impact of a professional baccalaureate degree program. [Results of a five-year investigation of a bachelors degree course at the University of San Francisco.] Nursing Research, 24 (4), Jul–Aug 1975, 287–292.

37 Waters, V. H. and others Technical and professional nursing: an exploratory study. [Associate degree nursing and baccalaureate nursing.] Nursing Research, 21 (2), Mar/Apr 1972, 124–131.

38 Williamson, S. B. The degree of Bachelor of Science in nursing at the University of the Witwatersrand. SA Nursing Journal, 61 (13), Jan 1973, 15.

39 Wilson, H. S. and Chater, S.S. Graduate education: challenge to the status quo. Nursing Outlook, 21 (7), Jul 1973, 440–443.

c EXPERIMENTAL AND INTERDISCIPLINARY EDUCATION

1 Association of Integrated and Degree Courses in Nursing Nursing: an education or training? Report of the third open conference, University of Surrey, 11–13 July, 1975. The Association, 1975.

2 Bohm, S. M. Colleges of health sciences. New Zealand Nursing Journal, 64 (9), Sep 1971, 23–25.

3 Corbett, D. Student nurses share in clinical learning: a program designed for student physicians has been adapted to include nursing students. [Clinical Learning Centre, Queen's University, Kingston.] Canadian Nurse, 69 (11), Nov 1973, 21.

4 Connelly, T. and Hoyle, J. D. Students learn about the health care system. [Teaching concepts of the health care team by means of multi-disciplinary education at the University of Kentucky.] Hospitals, 49 (8), 16 Apr 1975, 71–72, 74–75.

5 Ellis, F. Comprehensive nurse training in Scotland – a prelude to Briggs. [System followed at the College of Nursing, Ninewells.] Nursing Mirror, 140, 10 Apr 1975, 46–50.

6 Harding, E. H. and others A nursing course for medical students. [Students observe nurses at work and learn about patient care at University of California, San Francisco.] Nursing Outlook, 23 (4), Apr 1975, 240–242.

7 Hooper, J. E. Training for mature entrants: progress report on an experimental scheme. [Mature women's course at Portsmouth School of Nursing.] Nursing Times, 71, 9 Oct 1975, 16 Oct 1975, Occ. papers 101–108.

8 Hospitals Health care changes challenge educators. [Multi-disciplinary education.] Hospitals, 48 (18), 16 Sep 1974, 85–86, 90.

9 Jones, P. E. and Dunn, E. V. Education for the health team: a pilot project [in a joint educational experience involving work with a health team for seminar undergraduate students of medicine at the University of Toronto.] International Journal of Nursing Studies, 11 (1), Jun 1974, 61–69.

10 Kintgen, J. K. Health occupations education: will the profession respond? [Nursing education in relation to the education of other health workers.] American Journal of Nursing, 74 (9), Sep 1974, 1652–1654.

11 Lloyd, K. N. A combined training institute at the new University Hospital of Wales. Physiotherapy, 57 (2), Feb 1971, 73–75.

12 Martin, C. Milestone in education. [Establishment of a Nursing Department in the School of Health Sciences in a multi-disciplinary college – the Western Australian Institute of Technology.] Australian Nurses' Journal, 4 (7), Feb 1975, 16–18.

13 O'Neill, J. A planned programme – with Briggs in mind [Wythenshawe Hospital.] Nursing Times, 71, (8), 20 Feb 1975, 303–306.

14 Parkes, M. E. The importance of seeing the whole picture. [Use of inter-disciplinary educational programmes to promote understanding between professions.] Australian Nurses' Journal, 4 (11), Jun 1975, 20–23.

15 Rosenaur, J. A. and Fuller, D. J. Teaching strategies for interdisciplinary education. [Nursing and medical students.] Nursing Outlook, 21 (3), Mar 1973, 159–162.

16 Sawyer, M. B. and Serafini, P. Interdisciplinary education: is it valid? [Trial with senior nursing and medical students, at Boston University.] American Journal of Nursing, 75 (5), May 1975, 825.

17 Smith, J. Applications and admissions to experimental courses: a report on the 1969 intake. Nursing Times, 67, 7 Oct 1971, Occ. papers, 157–160.

18 Steel, M. Under one roof? The new multi-

disciplinary teaching centre at Norfolk and Norwich Hospital. Nursing Mirror, 139, 2 Aug 1974, 71–72.

19 Valberg, B. The nurse in a student physician's 'practice'. [Nurse-administrator provides student physicians with a learning experience in their medical studies.] Canadian Nurse, 69, Nov 1973, 17–20.

20 Warley Hospital A multi-disciplinary centre. Hospital and Health Services Review, 71 (4), Apr 1975, 138-139.

21 Yeaworth, R. and Mims, F. Interdisciplinary education as an influence system. Nursing Outlook, 21 (11), Nov 1973, 696–699.

25 NURSE LEARNERS

a GENERAL (Includes personality and characteristics)

1 Brattin, C. J. Diary of a student. [Excerpts from her diary following the student through her first semester in nursing.] American Journal of Nursing, 72 (7), Jul 1972, 1282–1285.

2 Fredericks, M. A. and others The nursing student: social background, attitudes and expressed willingness to work in poverty programs. Journal of Nursing Education, 12 (3), Aug 1973, 29–36.

3 Frerichs, M. Relationship of self-esteem and internal-external control to selected characteristics of associate degree nursing students. Nursing Research, 22 (4), Jul/Aug 1973, 350–353.

4 Gilbert, M. A. Personality profiles and leadership potential of medical-surgical and psychiatric nursing graduate students. Nursing Research, 24 (2) Mar/Apr 1975, 125–130.

5 Gilmour, M. and others The disadvantaged student in nursing education. [Defined as the student from a low-income family who has had poor academic preparation.] Journal of Nursing Education, 13 (4), Nov 1974, 2–12.

6 Hall, J. N. and Andrews, W. T. Apparent homogeneity of characteristics of student nurse groups. [Retrospective survey of students at a psychiatric hospital.] International Journal of Nursing Studies, 9 (2), Jun 1972, 103–108.

7 Krueger, C. S. Good girls – bad nurses. [Study of a group of rebels among the student nurses in a nursing school in the United States.] New Society, 19, 12 Jan 1972, 172–173.

8 Lamond, Prof. N. K. Nursing commitment and the student. SA Nursing Journal, 39 (11), Nov 1972, 30–33.

9 McCutchan, A. The student: a discoverer. New Zealand Nursing Journal, 64 (11), Nov 1971, 10–11.

10 Madden, B. P. Raising the consciousness of nursing students [to feminist issues in professional practice]. Nursing Outlook, 23 (5), May 1975, 292–296.

11 Martires, C. R. Socio-economic-psychological changes in society and the nurse. [With results of a research study in personality patterns of student nurses in the Philippines.] Philippine Journal of Nursing, 44 (1), Jan/Mar 1975, 36–40.

12 Mealey, A. R. and Peterson, T. L. Self-actualization of nursing students resulting from a course in psychiatric nursing. [Personality changes in psychiatric nursing students measured on the Personnel Orientation Inventory (POI).] Nursing Research, 23 (2), Mar/Apr 1974, 138–143.

13 Meleis, A. I. and Farrell, K. M. Operation con-

cern. A study of senior nursing students in three nursing programs. [To determine whether baccalaureate, associate degree and diploma programs present a different quality of nursing care.] Nursing Research, 23 (6), Nov/Dec 1974, 461–468.

14 Paduano, M. A. The greening of the classroom. [Course orientation for new students.] Journal of Nursing Education, 14 (2), Apr 1975, 20–23.

15 Parry-Jones, W. Ll. Roles in nursing. 1. The student. Nursing Times, 67, 7 Jan 1971, 30–31.

16 Paynich, M. L. Why do basic nursing students work in nursing? Nursing Outlook, 19 (4), Apr 1971, 242–245.

17 Pender, N. J. Students who choose nursing: are they success oriented? Nursing Forum, 10 (1), 1971, 65–71.

18 Reavley, W. and Wilson, L. J. Personality structure of general and psychiatric student nurses: a comparison. International Journal of Nursing Studies, 9 (4), Nov 1972, 225–232.

19 Richards, M. A. B. A study of differences in psychological characteristics of students graduating from three types of basic nursing programs. Nursing Research, 21 (3), May/Jun 1972, 258–261.

20 Richek, H. G. and Nichols, T. Personality and cognitive characteristics of prenursing majors. [University of Oklahoma.] Nursing Research, 22 (5), Sep/Oct 1973, 443–448.

21 Rosendahl, P. L. Effectiveness of empathy, non-possessive warmth, and genuineness of self-actualization of nursing students. Nursing Research, 22 (3), May/Jun 1973, 253–257.

22 Singh, A. Norms for first-year student nurses. General intelligence and personality. Nursing Times, 67, 29 Jul 1971 Occ. papers, 117–119.

23 Singh, A. Personality needs of an English sample of student nurses. Nursing Times, 68, 23 Mar 1972, Occ. papers, 47–48.

24 Singh, A. The student nurse on experimental courses 2. Personality patterns. International Journal of Nursing Studies, 8 (3), Aug 1971, 189–203.

25 Singh, A. The student nurse on experimental courses. 3. Basic values. International Journal of Nursing Studies, 8 (3), Aug 1971, 207–216.

26 Stevens, B. J. Adapting nursing education to today's student population. Journal of Nursing Education, 10 (1) Apr 1971, 15, 18–20.

27 Stewart, R. A. C. and Liddell, J. M. Where success lies: a comparison of personal characteristics of high and low ability students. [Study of 75 student nurses.] New Zealand Nursing Journal, 68 (3), Mar 1975, 13–14, 19.

28 Williams, A. Characteristics of male baccalaureate students who selected nursing as a career. Nursing Research, 22 (6), Nov/Dec 1973, 520–525.

29 Wren, G. R. Some characteristics of freshman students in baccalaureate, diploma and associate degree nursing programs. Nursing Research, 20 (2), Mar/Apr 1971, 167–172.

b ATTITUDES

1 Brown, J. S. and others Baccalaureate students' images of nursing: a replication. Nursing Research, 23 (1), Jan/Feb 1974, 53–59.

2 Griffiths, G. M. Nurse training – a moulding of attitudes. Nursing Times, 68, 3 Feb 1972, 152–154.

3 Hall, J. N. Nurses' attitudes and specialized treatment settings: an exploratory study. [Use of attitude scales to select students for work on a behaviour modification ward at Stanley Royal Hospital, Wakefield.] British Journal of Social and Clinical Psychology, 13 (3), Sep 1974, 333–334.

4 **Hess, G. and Stroud, F.** Racial tensions: barriers in delivery of nursing care. [Racial tensions among students in the University of California School of Nursing.] Journal of Nursing Administration, 11 (3), May/Jun 1972, 47–49.

5 **Humphrey, P.** Learning about poverty and health. Students who enter nursing usually have little understanding of what poverty means and how it affects health. This author describes a course designed to give them such insight. Nursing Outlook, 22 (7), Jul 1974, 441–443.

6 **Kalisch, B. J.** An experiment in the development of empathy in nursing students. Nursing Research, 20 (3), May–Jun 1971, 202–211.

7 **Linn, L. S.** A survey of the 'Care-Cure' attitudes of physicians, nurses, and their students. [An analysis of answers to ten statements about patient care.] Nursing Forum, 14 (2), 1975, 145–159.

8 **Moody, P. M.** Attitudes of cynicism and humanitarianism in nursing students and staff nurses. Journal of Nursing Education, 12 (3), Aug 1973, 9–13.

9 **O'Neill, M. F.** A study of baccalaureate nursing student values. Nursing Research, 22 (5), Sep/Oct 1973, 437–443.

10 **O'Neill, M. F.** A study of nursing student values. [A comparison of the values of nurses with other student groups.] International Journal of Nursing Studies, 12 (3), 1975, 175–181.

11 **Robbins, J.** Students' attitudes toward evening experience. Nursing Outlook, 21 (3), Mar 1973, 169–170.

12 **Singh, A.** The student nurse on experimental courses. 1 Attitudes towards nursing as a career. International Journal of Nursing Studies, 7 (4), Nov 1970, 201–221.

13 **Walsh, M.** Rcn student nurses share concern for quality of patient care. Nursing Mirror, 141, 25 Sep 1975, 35.

14 **Weber, J. P.** Nursing students' opinions about acupuncture and Chinese medicine. Nursing Research, 24 (3), May/Jun 1975, 205–206.

c EVALUATION OF TEACHERS AND COURSES

1 **Akinsanya, J. A.** Talking to the students. Nursing Times, 68, 13 Jul 1972, 882–883.

2 **Armington, C. L. and others** Student evaluation – threat or incentive? Nursing Outlook, 20 (12), Dec 1972, 789–792.

3 **Kiker, M.** Characteristics of the effective teacher. Undergraduate students in nursing and in education place professional competence of a teacher higher than the teacher's personal attributes, whereas graduate students rank creativity first. Nursing Outlook, 21 (11), Nov 1973, 721–723.

4 **Lowery, B. J. and others** Nursing students' and faculty opinion on student evaluation of teachers. Nursing Research, 20 (5), Sep/Oct 1971, 436–439.

5 **Mackie, J. B.** Comparison of student satisfaction with educational experiences in two teaching process models. Nursing Research, 22 (3), May/Jun 1973, 262–266.

6 **Mauksch, I. G.** Let's listen to the students. [Students' involvement in the educational process.] Nursing Outlook, 20 (2), Feb 1972, 103–107.

7 **Millard, R. M.** The new accountability. [The

rights of the student as a consumer.] Nursing Outlook, 23 (8), Aug 1975, 496–500.

8 **Nanson, J.** A students' view of education. New Zealand Nursing Journal, 67 (12), Dec 1974, 27–28.

9 **Schrock, R. A.** Student nurses' responses to a study block evaluation project. Nursing Times, 68, 13 Jul 1972, Occ. papers, 109–112.

10 **Singh, A.** Attitudes of students towards nursing education courses. International Journal of Nursing Studies, 9 (1), Mar 1972, 3–13, 17–18.

11 **Wood, V.** Student evaluation of their tutors in four schools of nursing. Nursing Times, 67, 24 Jun 1971, Occ. papers, 97–100; 67, 1 Jul, Occ papers, 101–104.

d STUDENT STATUS AND ORGANIZATIONS

1 **Bendall, E.** Report on the 4th international students meeting. Nursing Mirror, 139, 17 Oct 1974, 34–35.

2 **Byrne, M.** Once upon a time. Could the word 'student' be taken literally in nursing? [Experiences of a student nurse contrasted with those of a university student.] Nursing Times, 69, 8 Nov 1973, 1494–1495.

3 **Dunn, A.** The mistakes of fifty years. [Rcn student conference, Nottingham.] Nursing Times, 71, 25 Sep 1975, 1526–1527.

4 **Greenwood, V.** Student status for student nurses. [Reproduced from Health Team.] Nursing Mirror, 139, 23 Aug 1974, 57.

5 **Montag, M. C.** Nursing student – learner or worker. Lamp, 32 (12), Dec 1975, 31–34.

6 **Monteiro, S.** Student status in nursing. Nursing Journal of India, 65 (6), Jun 1974, 176.

7 **National Student Nurses' Association** At NSNA's convention. . . American Journal of Nursing, 72 (6), Jun 1972, 1131–1136.

8 **Royal College of Nursing** Student Section. Report of conference. Nursing Mirror, 139, 9 Aug 1974, 42–43.

26 CONTINUING EDUCATION

a GENERAL

1 **Coleman, V.A.** Teaching in a specialized unit. [Methods of teaching used in post-registration and post-enrolment course at Glasgow Ear, Nose and Throat Hospital.] Nursing Times, 69, 21 Jun 1973, 806–808.

2 **Hardy, G. and Lemin, B.** William Rathbone Staff College: past, present and future. District Nursing, 15 (6), Sep 1972, 120–121.

3 **Harrold, A. E.** Planning for Briggs 3. Post-certificate training. Nursing Times, 70, 6 Jun 1974, Occ. papers, 17–19.

4 **Jones, M.** The open university. Nursing Times, 70, 16 May 1974, 762–763.

5 **Judy, M. G.** The concept of the workshop method for a continuing education program. Occupational Health Nursing, 21 (9), Sep 1973, 19–22.

6 **Lego, S.** Continuing education by mail. American Journal of Nursing, 73 (5), May 1973, 840–841.

7 **Leichsenring, M.** Teaching seminars for new faculty. Nursing Outlook, 20 (8), Aug 1972, 528–531.

8 **Maillart, V.** Higher education in nursing. WHO Chronicle, 27 (6), Jun 1973, 242–244. [Reprinted in Journal of Psychiatric Nursing and Mental Health Services, 11 (6), Nov/Dec 1973, 42–45.]

9 **Mitsunage, B. K.** Evaluation in continuing education. Journal of Nursing Education, 12 (1), Jan 1973, 21, 23–28.

10 **Nursing Times** Open Univesity degrees for nurses? Working Party will sound out course possibilities. Nursing Times, 71, 25 Sep 1971, 1521.

11 **Pauline, M.** The questioning approach. [Continuing education in nursing.] Australian Nurses' Journal, 3 (3), Sep 1973, 30–32.

12 **Reed, F. C. and others** Computer assisted instruction for continued learning. American Journal of Nursing, 72 (11), Nov 1972, 2035–2039.

13 **Roehm, M. E.** The continuing education unit: a new concept of measurement. Journal of Nursing Administration, 4 (2), Mar/Apr 1974, 56–59.

14 **Schumacher, M. E.** Continuing education for nurses. [Paper given at ICN Congress, Mexico.] Hong Kong Nursing Journal, 16, May 1974, 41–45.

15 **Searle, C.** Nursing education – the future. An aspect for consideration. [Continuing education.] SA Nursing Journal, 42 (8), Aug 1975, 24–27.

16 **Shore, H. L.** Adopters and laggards. [Study to measure the adoption of nursing practices as a result of continuing education.] Canadian Nurse, 68 (7), Jul 1972, 36–39.

17 **William Rathbone Staff College** [Survey of work with reminiscences of former staff and students.] Queen's Nursing Journal, 18 (7), Oct 1975, 186–189, 191–192.

b MANDATORY OR VOLUNTARY

1 **Cooper, S. S.** Should continuing education be required for licensure renewal? Occupational Health Nursing, 22 (6), Jun 1974, 7–9.

2 **Cooper, S. S.** Steps in self development [as an alternative to mandatory continuing education.] Journal of Nursing Administration, 4 (3), May/Jun 1974, 53–56.

3 **Cooper, S. and Allison, E. W.** Should continuing education be mandatory? [Two authors put opposing views.] American Journal of Nursing, 73 (3), Mar 1973, 442–443.

4 **De Tournay, R.** Continuing education – professional responsibility or governmental regulation? Occupational Health Nursing, 23 (6), Jun 1975, 7–10.

5 **Flaherty, M. J.** Continuing education should be voluntary. Canadian Nurse, 71 (7), Jul 1975, 19–21.

6 **Hatfield, P.** Mandatory continuing education. Journal of Nursing Administration, 3 (6), Nov/Dec 1973, 35–40.

7 **McGriff, E. P.** A case for mandatory continuing education in nursing. Nursing Outlook, 20 (11), Nov 1972, 712–713.

8 **Mayberry, M. A.** Continuing education – mandatory vs voluntary. Journal of Practical Nursing, 24 (7), Jul 1974, 16–17; (8), Aug 1974, 21–23.

9 **Palmer, I. S.** Continuing education: professional responsibility or societal mandate? Nursing Forum, 13 (4), 1974, 402–405.

10 **Stevens, B. J.** Mandatory continuing education for professional nurse relicensure. What are the issues?

Journal of Nursing Administration, 3 (5), Sep/Oct 1973, 25–28.

11 Stinson, S. M. Frankly speaking about nursing education. Mandatory continuing education? Canadian Nurse, 71 (8), Aug 1975, 17.

12 Whitaker, J. G. The issue of mandatory continuing education. Nursing Clinics of North America, 9 (3), Sep 1974, 475–483.

c UNITED STATES

1 Alexander, C. J. Recent decisions affecting continuing education. AORN Journal, 20 (4), Oct 1974, 573–574, 576.

2 American Journal of Nursing Recognition for continuing education. [Report on the progress of state programs.] American Journal of Nursing, 74 (5), May 1974, 878–880.

3 Bevis, M. E. Role conception and the continuing learning activities of neophyte collegiate nurses. Nursing Research, 22 (3), May/Jun 1973, 207–216.

4 Blume, D. M. Continuing education in nursing: what it is – where it's going. The Catherine R. Dempsey lecture. Occupational Health Nursing, 22 (7), Jul 1974, 11–17.

5 Boback, P. Coming – emphasis on continuing rather than basic education. Hospital Topics, 53 (1), Jan/Feb 1975, 32–33.

6 Buckner, K. E. Continuing education for nurse faculty members. Nursing Forum, 13 (4), 1974, 393–401.

7 Cantor, M. M. Staff development. What about the CEU? [The need for continuing education.] Journal of Nursing Administration, 4 (5), Sep/Oct 1974, 8–9.

8 Cooper, S. S. A brief history of continuing education in nursing in the United States. Journal of Continuing Education in Nursing, 4 (3), May–Jun 1973, 5–14.

9 Cooper, S. S. This I believe . . . about continuing education in nursing. Nursing Outlook, 20 (9), Sep 1972, 579–583.

10 Cooper, S. S. Trends in continuing education in the United States. International Nursing Review, 22 (4), Jul/Aug 1975, 117–120.

11 Cooper, S. S. Why continuing education in nursing? Cardio Vascular Nursing, 8 (6), Nov/Dec 1972, 23–28.

12 Dake, M. A. CEU – a means to an end? [To achieve continuing competence in practice.] American Journal of Nursing, 74 (1), Jan 1974, 103–104.

13 Forni, P. R. Continuing education vs. continuing competence. Journal of Nursing Administration, 5 (9), Nov–Dec 1975, 34–38.

14 Gibbs, G. E. Will continuing education be required for license renewal? American Journal of Nursing, 71 (11), Nov 1971, 2175–2179.

15 Glancy, K. E. and Courtney, M. E. Making sense out of the CEU. RN Magazine, 37 (10), Oct 1974, 32–35.

16 Gwaltney, B. H. The continuing education unit. Nursing Outlook, 21 (8), Aug 1973, 500–503.

17 Hugue, H. Conceptual aspects of continuing education in nursing. Nursing Journal of India, 46 (11), Nov 1975, 252–253.

18 Lewis, F. M. Continuing education, a Service Agency's response. Journal of Nursing Administration, 4 (2), Mar/Apr 1974, 53–55.

19 McGriff, E. P. Continuing education in nursing. Nursing Clinics of North America, 8 (2), Jun 1973, 325–353.

20 Marriner, A. Continuing education in nursing. Supervisor Nurse, 6 (6), Jun 1975, 20, 22–23, 25–26, 28.

21 Marshall, K. Monitoring professional development. [Annual records of the time spent in continuing education at Belleville General Hospital.] Hospital Administration in Canada, 17 (7), Jul 1975, 31–32.

22 Medearis, N. D. You can help it happen. [Nurse participation in educational conferences.] Journal of Nursing Administration, 3 (1), Jan/Feb 1973, 12–13.

23 Popiel, E. S. Continuing education: provider and consumer. American Journal of Nursing, 71 (8), Aug 1971, 1586–1587.

24 Sanborn, D. E. and others Continuing education for nurses via interactive closed-circuit television: a pilot study. Nursing Research, 22 (5), Sep–Oct 1973, 448–451.

25 Schlotfeldt, R. M. Continuing education: no proof of competency. AORN Journal, 22 (5), Nov 1975, 770, 772, 774–775, 778, 780.

26 Schweer, J. E. Continuing education climatology. Journal of Nursing Administration, 1 (1), Jan 1971, 45–48.

27 Skipper, J. K. and King, J. A. Continuing education: feedback from the grass roots. Nursing Outlook, 22 (4), Apr 1974, 252–253.

28 Smalser, L. C. Continuing LP/VN education. Journal of Practical Nursing, 24 (5), May 1974, 18–20.

29 Taylor, C. R. Continuing education for nurses. [Provision in the USA with recommendations for improvement in England and Wales.] Nursing Times, 71, 10 Apr 1975, Occ. papers, 29–32.

30 Thomas, L. A. Prescriptive education. [Continuing education.] Nursing Outlook, 21 (7), Jul 1973, 450–452.

31 Trussel, P. M. and Tait, E. A. Private university contributes to community health through a continuing nursing education program. [St. Louis University.] International Nursing Review, 18 (1), 1971, 66–73.

32 Wood, L. A. A reality for LP/VNs: continuing education. Nursing Care, 7 (3), Mar 1974, 27–28.

d OTHER OVERSEAS COUNTRIES

1 Canadian Nurses' Association Specialization in nursing – where? when? how? Canadian Nurse, 68 (5), May 1972, 39–42.

2 Comerford, J. and Negus, N. Research to establish to what extent successful completion of a diploma course at the New South Wales College of Nursing relates to subsequent job satisfaction. Lamp, 29 (3), Mar 1972, 42–47.

3 De Sousa, M. D. D. Portugal's post basic nursing school: five years later. International Nursing Review, 21 (5), Sep/Oct 1974, 147–150, 152.

4 Dunstone, J. R. Canberra nursing science course. [Associate Diploma course in nursing science for post basic students.] Australian Nurses Journal, 4 (2), Aug 1974, 17–18, 20, 30.

5 Henderson, J. and Archibald, B. How CNF scholars are selected. Canadian Nurse, 69 (5), May 1973, 33–35.

6 Jibueze, M. W. Continuing education for nurses in Nigeria. Nigerian Nurse, 5 (2), Apr/Jun 1973, 39, 41.

7 Kroman, L. M. Continuing education in the non-university setting. Canadian Hospital, 49 (11), Nov 1972, 42–43, 46, 49.

8 Laboure, M. Post-basic courses. Australian Nurses' Journal, 2 (4), Oct 1972, 26–27.

9 Massey University proposes to offer from 1973, courses for registered nurses who wish to further their professional and general education. New Zealand Nursing Journal, 65 (8), Aug 1972, 25.

10 Miles, I. M. Some suggestions for progress toward continuing nursing education. SA Nursing Journal, 40 (2), Feb 1973, 7–8, 10–11, 30.

11 Moghadassy, M. and others Progress: post-basic nursing education in Iran. International Nursing Review, 19 (1), 1972, 3–10.

12 Morgan, D. M. Continuing education and staff development in hospitals. Canadian Hospital, 49 (11), Nov 1972, 35–36, 39–41.

13 Schumacher, M. E. Continuing education for nurses. Nigerian Nurse, 5 (4), Oct/Dec 1973, 6–9.

14 Seivwright, M. J. Up to date information about advanced nursing education at the University of the West Indies. Jamaican Nurse, 15 (2), Aug 1975, 12–14, 24.

15 Shore, H. L. Adopters and laggards. [Study to measure the adoption of nursing practices as a result of continuing education.] Canadian Nurse, 68 (7), Jul 1972, 36–39.

16 Warkentin, W. Continuing nursing education. Nursing Journal of India, 46 (11), Nov 1975, 247–248.

e INSERVICE EDUCATION

1 Blenkinsop, D. Durham advance. [Nursing staff meet regularly to hear of advances in medicine and nursing practices.] Nursing Times, 69, 11 Jan 1973, 61–62.

2 Bodington, M. Inservice training. [At Royal Hospital and Home for Incurables, Putney.] Nursing Mirror, 135, 14 Jul 1972, 31–33.

3 Boylan, A. An approach to nursing. 3. Clinical communication. [Continuing education in the ward situation as a part of clinical responsibility.] Nursing Times, 70, 28 Nov 1974, 1858–1859.

4 Coxon, W. E. Establishing a training department – changes, challenges, chances. [In-service training department within the Tunbridge Wells and Leybourne Group of Hospitals.] Nursing Mirror, 138, 31 May 1974, 47–51.

5 King's Fund Centre In-service training in hospitals. [Report of first King's Fund meeting.] Nursing Times, 67, 24 Jun 1971, 781.

6 Nash, P. Open forum. In touch. [In-service training has now become necessary to fulfil the caring role of the nurse adequately.] Nursing Mirror, 140, 30 Jan 1975, 74.

7 Palladino, E. Planning of inservice education. International Nursing Review, 20 (3), May–Jun 1973, 94–95.

8 Poole, D. L. and Wilson, F. Integrated 'teach-ins'. [Sessions on nursing topics held by and for nurses and other disciplines.] Nursing Times, 71, 14 Aug 1975, 1310–1311.

9 Taylor, V. R. E. In-service training: preparation of the nursing officer. Nursing Mirror, 136, 25 May 1973, 41–42.

f INSERVICE EDUCATION: OVERSEAS COUNTRIES

1 Adebo, E. O. In-service education in nursing: its

nature and uses in Nigeria. Nigerian Nurse, 6 (4), Oct/Dec 1974, 25–29, 31–34.

2 **Alexander, M. E. F.** In-service training education. SA Nursing Journal, 41 (11), Nov 1974, 6–9.

3 **Amundsen, M. A. and Appelbaum, J. J.** An in-service continuing education and expanded role program for occupational health nurses. Occupational Health Nursing, 23 (7), Jul 1975, 10–13.

4 **Arnold, P.** What is an inservice instructor? [Twenty-six facets of the job.] Supervisor Nurse, 6 (2), Feb 1975, 56–57, 59.

5 **Beekman, M. E. G. A.** The need for in-service education for nursing with suggestions for its organization. Lamp, 29 (2), Feb 1972, 20–33.

6 **Bennett, A. C.** How to plan an inservice education program by United Hospital Fund of New York Nursing Home Trainer Program. Journal of Nursing Administration, 4 (2), Mar–Apr 1974, 45–52.

7 **Bush, M. L.** Itinerant inservice educator. [For small nursing homes.] Nursing Outlook, 21 (1), Jan 1973, 25–27.

8 **Cantor, M.** Staff development: certifying competencies of personnel. [In-service training.] Journal of Nursing Administration, 5 (5), Jun 1975, 8–9.

9 **Cantor, M. M.** Staff development: what are the qualifications? [Criteria for selection of inservice training coordinators.] Journal of Nursing Administration, 5 (3), Mar–Apr 1975, 7, 9, 11.

10 **Cantor, M.** Standard 5. Education for quality care. [Inservice education.] Journal of Nursing Administration, 3 (1), Jan/Feb 1973, 49–54.

11 **Chatte, B. L.** What are the elements of development, responsibility, structuring programs? [Inservice education.] Hospital Topics, 53 (1), Jan–Feb 1975, 33.

12 **Convenuto, S.** Giving zest to inservice. [Inservice education transfers from the classroom to the nursing units at Ochsner Foundation Hospital, New Orleans.] American Journal of Nursing, 74 (10), Oct 1974, 1835.

13 **Forni, P. R. and Bolte, I. M.** Planning for continuing education in Kentucky. American Journal of Nursing, 73 (11), Nov 1973, 1912–1913.

14 **Germaine, A.** More on inservice education. Nursing education is not entirely dependent on doctors lecturing to nurses, but it is a responsibility that nursing departments should take on themselves. Hospital Administration in Canada, 14 (9), Sep 1972, 54, 58, 60.

15 **Grad, R. K.** Innovative continuing education in small hospitals. [In an in-service education program in Virginia, nursing specialists visit rural hospitals.] American Journal of Nursing, 75 (2), Feb 1975, 283.

16 **Hebestreit, L.** Inservice education. S. A. Nursing Journal, 38 (1), Jan 1971, 24–28, 38.

17 **Holle, M. L.** Staff education programs on a 'shoestring'. [Problems of in-service education programmes in small hospitals.] Supervisor Nurse, 6 (2), Feb 1975, 17–19.

18 **Keough, G.** Educational experiences for nursing service personnel in a Veterans Administration Hospital. [Inservice education and staff development.] Nursing Clinics of North America, 8 (2), Jun 1973, 337–347.

19 **Latta, D.** Thoughts on inservice education. New Zealand Nursing Journal, 65 (1), Jan 1972, 24–25.

20 **Maalouf, E.** Zaire: establishing an in-service education programme. International Nursing Review, 21 (5), Sep/Oct 1974, 143–144.

21 **MacDougall, M.** A diploma is not an oil painting.

[Importance of inservice education.] Canadian Nurse, 70 (2), Feb 1974, 19–21.

22 **Maher, E.** Stature not status. [Orientation and in-service training programmes in North America.] Nursing Mirror, 133, 31 Dec 1971, 6–7.

23 **Medearis, N. D. and Popiel, E. S.** Guidelines for organizing inservice education. Journal of Nursing Administration, 3 (6), Nov/Dec 1973, 52–58.

24 **Medearis, N. D. and Popiel, E. S.** Guides for organizing inservice education. Journal of Nursing Administration, 1 (4), Jul–Aug 1971, 30–37.

25 **Munroe, J.** In-service nursing education at UHWI. Jamaican Nurse, 12 (2), Aug 1972, 27.

26 **Nelson, M. C.** Education – grappling with a dragon. [In- service education programme at a Sydney hospital improves teaching role of the ward sister.] Australian Nurses' Journal, 4 (7), Feb 1975, 25–28.

27 **Nichols, J.** The need for inservice education for nursing with suggestions for its organisation. Lamp, 28 (12), Dec 1971, 31–44.

28 **Oatway, L.** Inservice education benefits all teachers. [The Hamilton and District School of Nursing.] Canadian Nurse, 67 (8), Aug 1971, 32–34.

29 **Practical Approaches to Nursing Service Administration** Nursing service staff development [through in-service education.] Practical Approaches to Nursing Service Administration, 13 (1), Winter 1974, 1–6.

30 **RN Magazine** Inservice education. how it really is. RN Magazine, 34 (2), Feb 1971, 36–41, 78.

31 **Robinson, A. M.** Ongoing inservice programs are a must. RN Magazine, 35 (7), Jul 1972, 50–56.

32 **Rockwell, S. M.** Inservice education. How to upgrade your program: a case history. RN Magazine, 34 (2), Feb 1971, 48–52.

33 **Rockwell, S. M.** Inservice education. What it ought to be: as the experts see it. RN Magazine, 34 (2), Feb 1971, 32–35.

34 **Rudnick, B. R. and Bolte, I. M.** The case for on-going inservice education. Journal of Nursing Administration, 1 (2), Mar–Apr 1971, 31–35.

35 **Tobin, H. M. and Wengerd, J. S.** What makes a staff development progam work? [Inservice training.] American Journal of Nursing, 71 (5), May 1971, 940–943.

g ORIENTATION

1 **Armstrong, M. L.** Bridging the gap between graduation and employment. [An orientation unit introduces the graduate to clinical nursing experience.] Journal of Nursing Administration, 4 (6), Nov/Dec 1974, 42–48.

2 **Crancer, J. and others** Clinical practicum before graduation. A culminating six-week experience eases the transition [from student to staff nurse]. Nursing Outlook, 23 (2), Feb 1975, 99–102.

3 **Fitzhugh, Z. A. and others** A patient centered orientation program, [for new staff nurses at University Hospital, Boston.] Hospitals, 48, 16 Jan 1974, 72, 74–75, 78.

4 **Fleming, B. W. and others** From student to staff nurse: a nurse internship program. [Program at Medical College of Virginia Hospitals for graduate nurses.] American Journal of Nursing, 75 (4), Apr 1975, 595–599.

5 **Frank, B. and Powell, B.** A skills check list for orientation of associate nurses. Supervisor Nurse, 6 (5), May 1975, 39, 42–43, 45.

6 **Golub, J. C.** A nurse-intership program: a pro-

gram for new nursing graduates helps to bridge the gap between the graduate's expectations and nursing service demands. Hospitals, 45 (17), 16 Aug 1971, 73, 76–78.

7 **Harris, S. W.** A model unit for baccalaureate RNs. [Decentralized unit permits bedside nursing care for recently qualified nurses in an attempt to reduce staff wastage.] Hospitals, 48 (6), 16 Mar 1974, 79–80, 82–84, 125.

8 **Kjolberg, G. L. and Glynn, K.** Orientation – would it work for you? Part 2. Recruiting for the Far North. [Six month orientation program to attract new graduate nurses.] Canadian Nurse, 71 (11), Nov 1975, 25–26.

9 **Martel, G. B. and Edmunds, M. W.** Nurse-internship program in Chicago. [To assist new graduates to bridge the gap between the status of student and that of independent practitioner.] American Journal of Nursing, 72 (5), May 1972, 940–943.

10 **Martin, L. and Paskowitz, J.** PACE Planned acquisition of clinical experience. [New graduates work with expert clinical nurses to bridge gap from student to nurse.] Supervisor Nurse, 6 (9), Sep 1975, 20–22.

11 **Nixon, K. and Russell, M.** Orientation – would it work for you? 1. Creating a learning environment. [Problems of new graduate nurses.] Canadian Nurse, 71 (11), Nov 1975, 24, 26.

12 **Nursing Times** Learning how to run a ward. [Course for newly qualified students at Calderdale AHA to help in coping with staff nurse status.] Nursing Times, 71, 4 Sep 1975, 1392.

13 **Reagan, P.** Orientation the off off Broadway Way. [Use of dramatized situations to orientate new staff.] American Journal of Nursing, 73 (7), Jul 1973, 1223–1227.

14 **Stopera, V. and Sully, D.** A staff development model. [Orientation of new nursing staff.] Nursing Outlook, 22 (6), Jun 1974, 390–393.

15 **Taylor, V.** In-service training orientation programmes. Nursing Times, 68, 1 Jun 1972, 691–692.

16 **Watkin, B.** Management topics – induction. Nursing Mirror, 138, 3 May 1974, 77.

h POST-BASIC CLINICAL COURSES (See also under special fields)

1 **Bendall, E.** Teach-in. Joint Board of Clinical Nursing Studies. 2. Curriculum planning. Nursing Times, 59, 19 Apr 1973, Occ. papers, 63–64; 69, 26 Apr, Occ. papers, 65–67.

2 **Cullinan, J.** Your specialist course. [Report of a teach-in organized by the Joint Board of Clinical Studies.] Nursing Times, 69, 19 Apr 1973, 505–507.

3 **Finn, B.** Curriculum planning: [of Joint Board of Clinical Studies courses.] Nursing Times, 71, 29 May 1975, 859.

4 **Finn, B.** Post-basic training in renal nursing. [JBCNS Course.] Nursing Times, 69, 28 Jun 1973, 833.

5 **Finn, B.** Special training for intensive care. [Paper presented at the First World Conference on Intensive Care, June 1974, describing courses approved by the Joint Board of Clinical Nursing Studies.] Nursing Times, 70, 28 Nov 1974, 1868–1869.

6 **Finn, B.** Training the stoma care nurse. [JBCNS Course]. Nursing Times, 70, 18 Apr 1974, 579.

7 **Gardener, M. G.** Teach-in. Joint Board of Clinical Nursing Studies. 1. The philosophy. Nursing Times, 69, 19 Apr 1973, Occ. papers, 61–63.

8 Joint Board of Clinical Nursing Studies Nursing Times, 70, 7 Nov 1974, 1746–1748.

9 Joint Board of Clinical Nursing Studies. Nursing Times, 68, 10 Aug 1972, 1006–1011.

10 Joint Board of Clinical Nursing Studies Series of outline curricula. The Board. Various dates.

11 Lancet Stomal-therapy specialists. [The training of nurses, JBCNS course.] Lancet, (1), 9 Feb 1974, 204.

12 Lancour, J. and Reinders, A. A. A pilot project in continuing education for critical care nursing. Journal of Nursing Administration, 5 (8), Oct 1975, 38–41.

13 Mathie, J. R. Management research. Intensive care course: planning, progress and evaluation. [How the course at Whiston Hospital, Lancs, was adjusted to meet the requirements of the JBCNS syllabus.] Nursing Times, 70, 29 Aug 1974, 1358–1359.

14 Parker, M. J. Infection control nursing education. [JBCNS course.] Nursing Times, 70, 29 Aug 1974, Supplement 3.

15 Purcell, R. One person's opinion. Specialist training in geriatric nursing? [JBCNS course]. Nursing Mirror, 141, 4 Dec 1975, 61.

16 Speight, I. Attitude change. [Teaching and measuring nurses' attitudes on post-basic courses run by the Joint Board of Clinical Nursing Studies.] Nursing Times, 70, 31 Jan 1974, 159–160.

17 Tiffany, R. Cancer education and training. [With special reference to the JBCNS course at the Royal Marsden Hospital and the concept of the clinical specialist.] Nursing Mirror, 141, 14 Aug 1975, 66–68.

27 NURSING RESEARCH

a UNITED KINGDOM

1 Boorer, D. Nursing. [Review of 'The proper study of the nurse, by Jean McFarlane.]

2 Chater, S. S. Understanding research in nursing. Geneva: WHO, 1975. (WHO offset publication, no. 14.)

3 Coleman, V. Controversy corner. Research. [Comment on the current "research trend."] Nursing Mirror 1141, 24 Jul 1975, 40.

4 Davies, M. How can research assist the nurse in the community? North West Thames Nursing Research Bulletin, 2, Autumn 1974, 13–16.

5 Department of Education and Science Research in British universities, colleges and polytechnics. HMSO. Issued annually.

6 Department of Health and Social Security Annual report on departmental research and development. HMSO. Includes nursing research.

7 Dingwall, R. Sociology and nursing research. Nursing Times, 25 Jul 1974, Occ. papers, 47–48.

8 Donaldson, R. J. Research in community care. Public Health, 88 (2), Jan 1974, 63–70.

9 Humphreys, D. Recipe for research. [Nursing research at the United Manchester Hospitals.] Nursing Times, 68, 6 Apr 1972, 397–399.

10 Inman, U. Nursing research – fact or fiction? Nursing Times, 68, 13 Jan 1972, 46.

11 Inman, U. Towards a theory of nursing care: an account of the Rcn/DHSS research project 'The study of nursing care.' Royal College of Nursing, 1975. (Study of nursing care project report series concluding

monograph.) Summary in Nursing Times, 72, 29 Apr 1976, 64.

12 Johnson, M. N. and Okunade, A. O. Roles that nurses in the community can play in nursing research. International Nursing Review, 22 (5), Sep/Oct 1975, 147–149; Nigerian Nurse, 7 (3), Jul/Sep 1975, 28–30.

13 Jones, D. Nursing research. Introduction to research. Nursing Times, 69, 13 Dec 1973, 1704–1705. Reprinted in Nursing Journal of India, 65 (6), Jun 1974, 170–172.

14 Lancaster, A. Research and nursing. North West Thames Nursing Research Bulletin no. 1, Feb 1974, 6–8.

15 McFarlane, J. K. The nature of nursing and the place of research. World of Irish Nursing, 1 (12), Dec 1972, 251, 253; 2 (1), Jan 1973, 8–9.

16 McFarlane, J. K. The proper study of the nurse: an account of the first two years of a research project "The study of nursing care", including a study of the relevant background literature. Royal College of Nursing, 1972.

17 McFarlane, J. K. Research – use and abuse. Jean McFarlane talks to Alison Dunn. Nursing Times, 70, 21 Mar 1974, 442–443.

18 Munday, A. M. Nursing Care. [Study of Nursing Care research project.] Nursing Times, 70, 4 Apr 1974, 520–521.

19 North West Thames Nursing Research Bulletin The Nursing Research Liaison Officer Project. North West Thames Nursing Research Bulletin no 1, Feb 1974, 2–3.

20 Norton, D. Discussion group. [Nursing Research Discussion Group.] Nursing Times, 70, 4 Apr 1974, 522.

21 Nursing Times Nursing and research in Scotland. [List of studies in progress, concluded or discontinued.] Nursing Times, 69, 15 Mar 1973, 356–357.

22 Nursing Times Research skills will make tomorrow's nurses. Nursing Times, 69, 14 Jun 1973, 778–779.

23 Scott Wright, M. Progress and prospects in nursing research. Nursing Times, 67, 21 Jan 1971, Occ. papers, p. 9–12.

24 Scott Wright, M. Research: the basis of professional practice. Royal College of Nursing and National Council of Nurses of the United Kingdom, 1973. (Rcn nursing lecture, 1973.)

25 Scott Wright, M. Three years on. [The work of the Nursing Research Unit, University of Edinburgh.] Nursing Times, 71, 23 Jan 1975, 130.

26 Scottish Health Service Centre The nurse and research. Meeting held on 29 Nov 1974 chaired by M. Scott-Wright. Edinburgh: The Centre, 1974.

27 Scottish Health Service Centre Research work by nurses. [Conference report on research in progress at Edinburgh University and Southern General Hospital, Glasgow.] Health and Social Service Journal, 85, 24 May 1975, 1138; Nursing Mirror, 141, 24 Jul 1975, 54–57

28 Scottish Hospital Centre The nurse and research. Edinburgh: The Centre, 1973.

29 Scottish Hospital Centre Nursing research progress report. [The activities of the Nursing Research Unit, University of Edinburgh, presented at a Scottish Hospital Centre conference.] Health and Social Service Journal, 84, 15 Jun 1974, 1340.

30 Simpson, H. M. Research in nursing – the first step. [Nursing Mirror Lecture.] Nursing Mirror, 132, 12 Mar 1971, 22–27; reprinted in International Nursing Review, 18 (3), 1972, 231–245.

31 Slide, G. M. Nursing research – is it not for nurses? Nursing Times, 68, 3 Feb 1972, 154.

b OVERSEAS COUNTRIES

1 Abdellah, F. G. Problems, issues, challenges of nursing research. Canadian Nurse, 67 (5), May 1971, 44–46.

2 Abdellah, F. G. United States National Center for Health Service Research and Development. Overview of nursing research, 1955–1968. Washington: US Department of Health, Education and Welfare, 1971.

3 Adebo, E. O. The role of the nurse in research. Kenya Nursing Journal, 2 (2), Dec 1973, 35–38.

4 American Nurses' Assocation Nursing research conference. [Eighth], Albuquerque, New Mexico, 1972. New York: The Association, 1972. Ninth, March 21–23, 1973, San Antonio, Texas. Kansas City: The Association, [1974.]

5 American Nurses' Association Council of Nurse Researchers Issues in research: social, professional, and methodological: Selected papers, Kansas City: A.N.A., 1974.

6 American Nurses' Foundation Nursing research – who cares? Panel focuses on problems of nurses in research. Nursing Research Report, 7 (3), Oct 1972, 1–5.

7 Batey, M. V. Values relative to research and to science in nursing as influenced by a sociological perspective. Nursing Research, 21 (6), Nov/Dec 1972, 504–508.

8 Beckingham, A. C. History, trends and planning for research in nursing. [Nursing research in Africa, especially Nigeria.] Nigerian Nurse, 6 (2), Apr/Jun 1974, 36–37, 39–40; (3), Jul/Sep 1974, 19–22.

9 Beekman, F. and others Nursing research. Lamp, 28 (7), Jul 1971, 21–36.

10 Berthold, J. S. Nursing research grant proposals: what influenced their approval or disapproval in two national granting agencies. Nursing Research, 22 (4), Jul/Aug 1973, 292–299.

11 Bourgeois, M. J. The special nurse research fellow: characteristics and recent trends. [Program of the Division of Nursing, Washington.] Nursing Research, 24 (3), May/Jun 1975, 184–188.

Brown, W. A. and others Staff attitudes toward research. Journal of Psychiatric Nursing and Mental Health Services, 9 (2), Mar/Apr 1971, 7–11.

13 Canadian Nurse National conference on research in nursing practice. Canadian Nurse, 67 (4), Apr 1971, 34–40.

14 Canadian Nurses' Association Index of Canadian nursing studies. Ottawa: The Association, 1974.

15 Carnegie, M. E. Financial assistance for nursing research – past and present. Nursing Research, 24 (3), May/Jun 1975, 163.

16 Carnegie, M. E. The journal's contribution to research in nursing. [Contribution of the American Journal of Nursing, 1900–1952.] Nursing Research, 24 (6), Nov/Dec 1975, 403.

17 Charter, D. Canada's first conference on research in nursing practice. Canadian Hospital, 48 (5), May 1971, 37–40.

18 Chater, S. S. Operation update: nurses eyeball current issues. [NLN conference report including a summary of recent research in the US.] Hospitals, 49 (13), 1 Jul 1975, 49–52.

19 Diers, D. Research for nursing. Journal of Nursing Administration, 11 (1), Jan/Feb 1972, 6–7, 62.

20 Dodge, G. H. Nurses reveal a restless attitude towards research. [Report from an ANA Convention.] AORN Journal, 20 (5), Nov 1974, 747–748, 751.

21 Downs, F. S. Research in nursing: the genie in Florence Nightingale's lamp. Nursing Forum, 12 (1), 1973, 48–57.

22 Downs, F. S. This I believe . . . about the dimensions of nursing research. Nursing Outlook, 19 (11), Nov 1971, 719–721.

23 Eisler, J. Research is fun! Nursing Forum, 11 (4), 1972, 385–394.

24 Gortner, S. R. Research in nursing: the federal interest and grant program. American Journal of Nursing, 73 (6), Jun 1973, 1052–1055.

25 Hayes, M. Canadian Nurse, 70 (10), Oct 1974.

26 McGill University. School of Nursing Research Proceedings of the colloquium on nursing research, March 28–30, 1973. Montreal: the University, 1973.

27 Medical College of Virginia. School of Nursing Proceedings [of the] Eastern Conference on Nursing Research, January 14–16, 1974. Williamsburg: The College, 1974.

28 National Conference on Nursing Research Development and use of indicators in nursing research: proceedings of the conference, Nov 3–5, 1975, Edmonton. Edmonton: University of Alberta School of Nursing, 1975.

29 New Zealand Nursing Journal Inquiry '74. Research and nursing. [Report of a seminar.] New Zealand Nursing Journal, 67 (12), Dec 1974, 17.

30 Notter, L. E. The case for nursing research. Nursing Outlook, 23(12),Ded 1975, 760–763.

31 Notter, E. and Spector, A. F. Nursing research in the South: a survey. Atlanta: Southern Regional Hospital Board, 1974.

32 Nuckolls, K. B. Nursing research – good for what? Nursing Forum, 11 (4), 1972, 374–384.

33 Nursing Research ANA's Ninth Nursing Research Conference. [Editorial]. Nursing Research, 22 (3), May/Jun 1973, 197.

34 Nursing Research Approaches to the study of nursing questions and the development of nursing science. [Introduction by Razella M.Schlotfeldt, 484–485.] Nursing Research, 21 (6), Nov/Dec 1972, 484–517.

35 Nursing Research The editor's report. [Editorial analysing trends in nursing research as reflected in recent articles in the journal.] Nursing Research, 24 (1), Jan/Feb 1975, 3; 25 (1), Jan/Feb 1976, 3; 27 (1), Jan/Feb 1978, 3.

36 Nursing Research Funding for nursing research. Nursing Research, 22 (2), Mar/Apr 1973, 99.

37 Pitel, M. An overview of ANF–supported research, 1955–1971. 1. The broad perspective. Nursing Research Report, 7 (1), Mar 1972, 3–4, 6.

38 Pitel, M. Private philanthropy and nursing research. Nursing Research Report, 8 Z(3), Oct 1973, 1–2, 4, 6.

39 Ramsay, J. Critique: nursing research is not every nurse's business. Rebuttal of article by M. Hayes, Canadian Nurse, Oct 1974. Canadian Nurse, 71(2),Feb 1975, 28–29.

40 Schlotfeldt, R. M. Cooperative nursing investigations: a role for everyone. [The need for research in the nursing profession.] Nursing Research, 23 (6), Nov/Dec 1974, 452–456.

41 Schlotfeldt, R. M. Creating a climate for nursing research. Cleveland: Case Western Reserve University, 1973.

42 Schlotfeldt, R. M. Research in nursing and research training for nurses: retrospect and prospect. Nursing Research, 24 (3), May/Jun 1975, 177–183.

43 Schlotfeldt, R. M. The significance of empirical research for nursing. Nursing Research, 20 (2), Mar/Apr 1971, 140–142.

44 Schlotfeldt, R. M., editor Symposium on approaches to the study of nursing questions and the development of nursing science. Nursing Research, 21 (6), Nov/Dec 1972, 484–517.

45 Soo, B. Towards research-mindedness. Nursing Journal of Singapore, 13 (1), May 1973, 40–41.

46 Taylor, H. D. The Canadian Nurses' Foundation is its members. [A Foundation to provide scholarships and grants for nursing research.] Canadian Nurse, 71 (3), Mar 1975, 22–23.

47 Taylor, S. D. Bibliography on nursing research 1950–1974. Nursing Research, 24 (3), May/Jun 1975, 207–225. Also published separately, New York: American Journal of Nursing Co., 1975.

48 Wallis, M. A. Chicken or the egg. [Nursing research.] New Zealand Nursing Journal, 66 (4), Apr 1973, 36–37.

49 Werley, H. H. and Shea, F. P. The first center for research in nursing: its development, accomplishments and problems. [Center for Nursing Research, Wayne State University College of Nursing.] Nursing Research, 22 (3), May/Jun 1973, 217–231; Research conducted at Wayne State University College of Nursing, 268–270.

c ETHICS

1 Allen, M. Ethics of nursing practice. [Problems reported by Canadian nurses engaged in nursing research.] Canadian Nurse, 70 (2), Feb 1974, 22–23.

2 American Nurses Association Human rights guidelines for nurses in clinical and other research. Kansas City: A.N.A., 1975.

3 Canadian Nurses' Association Special Committee on Research. Ethics of nursing research. [Paper accepted by the CNA directors June 24, 1972 as a guideline for nurses doing research.] Canadian Nurse, 68 (9), Sep 1972, 23–25.

4 MacKay, R. C. and Soule, J. A. Nurses as investigators: some ethical and legal issues. [Problems and hazards encountered in research.] Canadian Nurse, 71 (9), Sep 1975, 26–29.

5 Norton, D. Talking point. The research ethic. Nursing Times, 71, 25 Dec 1975, 2048–2049.

d METHODS

1 Batey, M.V. Conceptualizing the research process. Nursing Research, 20 (4), Jul/Aug 1971, 296–301.

2 Brewer, J. K. and Knowles, R. D. Some statistical considerations in nursing research. Nursing Research, 23 (1), Jan/Feb 1974, 68–70.

3 Christy, T. E. The methodology of historical research: a brief introduction. Nursing Research, 24 (3), May/Jun 1975, 189–192.

4 Dickoff, J. and others 8–4 research. 1. A stance for nursing research – tenacity or inquiry. 2. Designing nursing research – eight points of encounter. Nursing Research, 24 (2), Mar/Apr 1975, 84–88; (3), May/Jun 1975, 164–176.

5 Downs, F. S. and Newman, M. A. A source book of nursing research. Philadelphia: F. A. Davis, 1973.

6 Fleming, J. W. and Hayter, J. Reading research reports critically. Nursing Outlook, 22 (3), Mar 1974, 172–175.

7 Heidgerken, L. E. The research process. Canadian Nurse, 67 (5), May 1971, 40–43.

8 Jackson, B. S. An experience in participant observation. [As a research method.] Nursing Outlook, 23 (9), Sep 1975, 552–555.

9 Kalisch, B. Creativity and nursing research. Nursing Outlook, 23(5), May 1975, 314–319.

10 Kratz, C. R. Participant observation in dyadic and triadic situations. International Journal of Nursing Studies, 12 (2), 1975, 169–174.

11 Kratz, C. R. Two methodological problems. [Definition and classification in nursing research.] Nursing Times, 70, 15 Aug 1974, Occ. papers, 53–56.

12 Lancaster, A. Guidelines to research in nursing. 1. Nursing, nurses and research. Introductory paper. Nursing Times, 15 May 1975, Occ. papers, 42–44.

13 Lancaster, A. Guidelines to research in nursing. 2. An introduction to the research process. [An overview of the kind of activities involved.] Nursing Times, 71, 22 May 1975, Occ. papers, 45–47.

14 Lancaster, A. Guidelines to research in nursing. 3. Compiling references and bibliographies. [Includes the bibliography from 'The proper study of the nurse' by J. K. McFarlane.] Nursing Times, 71, 29 May 1975, Occ. papers, 49–51.

15 Lancaster, A. Guidelines to research in nursing. 5. An introduction to methods of data collection. Nursing Times, 71, 19 Jun 1975, Occ. papers, 57–60.

16 Lancaster, A. Reading a research report. Nursing Times, 71, 12 Jun 1975, Occ. papers, 56.

17 Notter, L. E. Essentials of nursing research. New York: Springer, 1974.

18 Nursing Research The case for historical research in nursing. Nursing Research, 21 (6), Nov/Dec 1972, 483.

19 Nursing Research Improving our skills in developing research protocols. [Editorial.] Nursing Research, 22(4), Jul/Aug 1973, 291.

20 Oyediran, A. B. O. O. The use of statistics in research. Nigerian Nurse, 7 (1), Jan/Mar 1975, 10–14.

21 Pierce, L. M. Usefulness of a systems approach for problem conceputalization and investigation. Nursing Research, 21 (6), Nov/Dec 1972, 509–513.

22 Resio, D. T. and Verhonick, P. J. On the measurement and analysis of clinical data in nursing. [Studies of low and high risk decubitus ulcer patients used as an example of data analysis.] Nursing Research, 22 (5), Sep/Oct 1973, 388–393.

23 Roper, N. Collecting patient data. [Development of a data collecting instrument as a research tool.] Nursing Mirror, 141, 11 Dec 1975, 72–74.

24 Spitzer, W. O. Ten tips on preparing research proposals. Canadian Nurse, 69 (3), Mar 1973, 30–33.

25 Taylor, S. D. Development of a classification for current nursing research. Nursing Research, 23 (1), Jan/Feb 1974, 63–68.

26 Treece, E. W. and Treece, J. W. Elements of research in nursing. St. Louis: Mosby, 1973.

27 Verhonick, P. J. Clinical studies in nursing: models, methods and madness. Nursing Research, 21 (6), Nov/Dec 1972, 490–493.

28 Verhonick, P. J., editor Nursing research. Boston: Little, Brown, 1975.

29 Wandelt, M. A. Guide for the beginning researcher. New York: Appleton-Century-Crofts, 1970.

30 Wilson, K. J. W. Guidelines to research in nursing. 4. An introduction to sampling and statistical concepts. Nursing Times, 71, 12 Jun 1975, Occ. papers, 53–55.

e EDUCATION

1 Burmester, D. Learning through counterpoint research. [The use of nursing research into the moods of hospitalised patients as an educational tool.] American Journal of Nursing, 72 (3), Mar 1972, 516–519.

2 Cleland, V. Nursing research and graduate education. [Integration into the program.] Nursing Outlook, 23 (10), Oct 1975, 642–645.

3 Grossman, H. T. The diversity within graduate nursing education. [What part should research play in the curriculum of graduate study?] Nursing Outlook, 20 (7), Jul 1972, 464–467.

4 Jacox, A. The research component in the nursing service administration master's program. Journal of Nursing Administration, 4(2), Mar/Apr 1974 35–39.

5 Johnson, B. (1973) The research thread. [How research is taught to degree students in the Faculty of Nursing, Toronto.] Nursing Papers, 5 (1) Jun 1973, 15–20.

6 King, K. Research in a basic baccalaureate program. Canadian Nurse, 68 (5), May 1972, 21–23.

7 Kissinger, J. F. One approach to teaching clinical inquiry. [A short course in research techniques for baccalaureate students.] Journal of Nursing Education, 14, (2), Apr 1975, 5–9.

8 Kovacs, A. R. Research for the undergraduate student in nursing. Journal of Nursing Education, 13 (1), Jan 1974, 31–36.

9 Krueger, J. C. The value of summer research for undergraduate nursing students. Nursing Research, 21 (2), Mar/Apr 1972, 158–160.

10 Martocchio, B. C. and others Developing a research attitude in nursing students. Nursing Outlook, 19 (6), Jun 1971, 386.

11 North West Thames Nursing Research Bulletin Research and nursing – the preparation of tutors. Report of King's Fund Centre Conference. North West Thames Nursing Research Bulletin, no. 3, Spring 1975, 3–4.

12 Price, J. L. Research problems in the assessment of nursing education. Health Education Journal, 34 (1), 1975, 22–26.

13 Verhonick, P. J. Research awareness at the undergraduate level. Nursing Research, 20 (3), May/Jun 1971, 261–265.

14 Werley, H. H. Research in nursing as input to educational programs. Journal of Nursing Education, 11 (4), Nov 1972, 29–38.

15 Yeaworth, R. C. Alternative to the thesis. [For meeting the research objectives of the masters program.] Hospital Outlook, 21 (5), May 1973, 335–338.

f RESEARCH AND PRACTICE

1 Altschul, A. Beginning and end: the sympathetic assistance of nurse administrators is important to the success of clinical nursing research projects. Nursing Times, 70, 9 May 1974, 718–719.

2 Chow, R. K. Identifying professional nursing practice through research: cardiosurgical patient care. International Journal of Nursing Studies, 9 (3), Aug 1972, 125–134.

3 Diers, D. Finding clinical problems for study. Journal of Nursing Administration, 1 (6), Nov/Dec, 1971, 15–18.

4 Gilchrist, J. M. Practical vision and research. [How research could be implemented in practice.] Nursing Papers, 3 (2), Dec 1971, 6–14.

5 Gortner, S. R. Research for a practice profession. Nursing Research, 24 (3), May/Jun 1975, 193–197.

6 Hanson, R. L. Research: a necessity in nursing service. Journal of Nursing Administration, 3 (3), May/Jun 1973, 14–15, 61–62.

7 Hanson, R. L. Research in nursing service. Nursing Outlook, 19 (8), Aug 1971, 520–523, Nursing Journal of India 63 (2), Feb 1972, 43–44, 59–60.

8 Jacox, A. Nursing research and the clinician. Nursing Outlook, 22 (6), Jun 1974, 382–385.

9 Ketefian, S. Application of selected nursing research findings into nursing practice: a pilot study. [Application of oral mode of temperature determination based on research findings by Nichols and colleagues.] Nursing Research, 24 (2), Mar/Apr 1975, 89–92.

10 Lindeman, C. A. Delphi survey of priorities in clinical nursing research. [Research technique using a series of questionnaires to obtain a consensus of opinion from a group of experts.] Nursing Research, 24 (6), Nov/Dec 1975, 432–441.

11 Lindeman, C. A. Nursing practice research: what's it all about? [Emphasises the role of the nursing administrator in initiating research.] Journal of Nursing Administration, 5 (3), Mar/Apr 1975, 5–7.

12 Lindeman, C.A. Nursing research: a visible, viable component of nursing practice. Journal of Nursing Administration, 3 (2), Mar/Apr 1973, 18–21.

13 Lindeman, C. A. Priorities in clinical nursing research. [Results of a survey.] Nursing Outlook, 23 (11), Nov 1975, 693–698.

14 Lindeman, C. A. Research for nursing: nursing research priorities. [Survey conducted by the Regional Program for Nursing Research Development, Western Interstate Commission for Higher Education.] Journal of Nursing Administration 5 (6), Jul/Aug 1975, 20–21.

15 McKinnon-Mullett, E. L. Circulation research: exploring its potential in clinical nursing research. Nursing Research, 21 (6), Nov/Dec 1972, 494–498.

16 Notter, L. E. The vital significance of clinical nursing research. Cardiovascular Nursing, 8 (5), Sep/Oct 1972, 19–22.

17 Nursing Research Toward more clinical research in nursing. [For the purpose of improving the quality of the practice of nursing.] [Editorial comment on the nursing research sessions at the ANA convention.] Nursing Research, 23 (5), Sep/Oct 1974, 371.

18 Stinson, S. M. Staff nurse involvement in research – myth or reality? Canadian Nurse, 69 (6), Jun 1973, 28–32.

19 Tierney, A. J. Research at ward level. Nursing Times, 70, 9 May 1974, 717–718.

20 Verhonick, P. J. Clinical investigations in nursing. Nursing Forum, 10 (1), 1971, 80–88.

21 Voda, A. M., and others On the process of involving nurses in research. Nursing Research, 20 (3), May/Jun 1971, 261–265.

22 Vredevoe, D. L. Nursing research involving physiological mechanism: definition of the variables. [Through analysis of one physiological adaptive mechanism, the host-antigen relationship and the immune response, a pattern is given for designing a nursing research problem.] Nursing Research, 21 (1), Jan/Feb 1972, 68–72.

23 Werley, H. H. This I believe . . . about clinical nursing research. Nursing Outlook, 20 (11), Nov 1972, 718–720.

24 Western Council on Higher Education for Nursing Regional program for Nursing Research Development. Delphi Survey of clinical nursing research priorities. Boulder, Colorado: Western Interstate Commission for Higher Education, 1974.

25 Western Interstate Commission for Higher Education Communicating nursing research: methodological issues, edited by Marjorie V. Batey. Boulder, Colorado: The Commission, 1970.

26 Western Interstate Commission for Higher Education Communicating nursing research: is the gap being bridged? Edited by Marjorie V. Boulder, Colorado: The Commission, 1971.

27 Williams, C.A. Nurse practitioner research: some neglected issues. [Nurse practitioners should develop clinical trials in primary care rather than concentrate on the quality of care.] Nursing Outlook, 23 (3), Mar 1975, 172–177.

HEALTH SERVICES AND HOSPITALS

28 NURSING AND HEALTH OVERSEAS

a WORLD HEALTH

1 Ammundsen, E. and Newell, K. W. Health service development in the Third World. WHO Chronicle, 29 (1), Jan 1975, 10–11.

2 Babson, J. H. Health care delivery systems: a multinational survey. Pitman Medical, 1972.

3 Berfenstam, R. Cross-national comparative studies on hospital use. [Comparison of health services in Great Britain, Sweden and the USA.] World Hospitals, 9 (4), Oct 1973, 143–149.

4 Bosanquet, N. Talking point – A growing nightmare. [Chances for improvement in world health services.] Nursing Times, 71, 2 Oct 1975, 1562–1563.

5 CIBA Foundation Teamwork for world health. A Ciba Foundation Symposium, 1971.

6 Douglas-Wilson, I. and McLachlan, G., editors Health service prospects: an international survey. Lancet/Nuffield Provincial Hospitals Trust, 1973.

7 Evang, K. Human rights. Health for everyone. World Health, Nov 1973, 3–11.

8 Fry, J. and Farndale, W. A. J., editors International medical care: a comparison and evaluation of medical care services throughout the world. Oxford: Medical and Technical Publishing, 1972.

9 Gale, G. W. Health service problems in developing countries. Royal Society of Health Journal, 93 (1), Feb 1973, 17–19.

10 Godber, G. Basic needs for a healthy life. World Health, 1974, 12–17.

11 Hellberg, J. H. Some thoughts on health planning in developing countries. World Hospitals, 9 (3), Jul 1973, 98–100.

12 Hurst, T. International medical care. [A King's Fund seminar.] Health and Social Service Journal, 85, 1 Mar 1975, 483–484.

13 Mahler, H. Health for all by the year 2000. WHO Chronicle, 29 (12), Dec 1975, 457–461.

14 Morley, D. C. Is the prestigious teaching hospital in the third world a disaster? Nursing Times, 71, 23 Jan 1975, Supplement, 10–11.

15 Murray, D. S. Blueprint for health. [The development of medical care in various countries.] Allen & Unwin, 1973.

16 Newell, K. W., editor Health by the people. Geneva: WHO, 1975.

17 Newell, K. W. Helping the people help themselves. [Problems of rural health in underdeveloped countries.] World Health, Apr 1975, 3–7.

18 Newell, K. W. and others The health care package. [An outline of policies which could be adopted by developing countries.] WHO Chronicle, 29 (1), Jan 1975, 12–18.

19 Office of Health Economics Medical care in developing countries. (Study in current health problems, no. 44.) The Office, 1972.

20 Rudoe, W. Health planning in national development. WHO Chronicle, 27 (1), Jan 1973, 6–7.

21 Thapalyal, L. Manpower for health. [The shortage of trained staff in health services throughout the world.] World Health, May 1974, 4–9.

22 Wade, L. Europe and the British health service. Bedford Square Press/National Council of Social Service, 1974.

23 WHO Chronicle Methods of promoting the development of basic health services. WHO Chronicle, 27 (7/8), Jul/Aug 1973, 333–335.

24 WHO Chronicle Trends in medical manpower. WHO Chronicle, 29 (2), Feb 1975, 46–48.

25 World Health Organization Approaches to national health planning. WHO, 1972. (Public health papers, no. 46.)

26 World Health Organization Modern management methods and the organization of health services. Geneva: WHO, 1974. (Public health papers, no. 55.)

27 World Health Organization. WHO Scientific Group The development of studies in health manpower. Geneva: WHO, 1971, (Technical Report Series no. 481.)

28 World Health Organization and UNICEF Alternative approaches to meeting basic health needs in developing countries. Geneva: WHO, 1975.

29 Yun, S. W. Preventive medicine in developing countries. Nigerian Nurse, 6 (1), Jan/Mar 1974, 18–20.

b ENVIRONMENT AND POLLUTION

1 Ashby, Lord Prospect for pollution. Community Health, 5 (2), Sep/Oct 1973, 92–100.

2 Beattie, A. D. Environmental lead poisoning. Nursing Times, 69, 31 May 1973, 696–697.

3 Croft, H. and Frenkel, S. Children and lead poisoning. [Screening and treatment programs.] American Journal of Nursing, 75 (1), Jan 1975, 102–104.

4 Helmer, R. Controlling water pollution. WHO Chronicle, 29 (11), Nov 1975, 428–434.

5 Hillman, H. The optimum human environment. Nursing Times, 69, 31 May 1973, 692–695.

6 James, C. D. T. Tracing the source of pollution. [An historical account of water supply pollution.] Nursing Times, 70, 4 Jul 1974, 1010–1022.

7 Kazantzis, G. Environmental pollution by cadmium and some other heavy metals. Nursing Mirror, 136, 9 Feb 1973, 12–16.

8 Lamond, N. K. and Muller, O. H. The nurses' role in safeguarding the environment. SA Nursing Journal, 40 (8), Aug 1973, 8–10.

9 Leathem, M. P. Food poisoning from take away foods. Nursing Mirror, 141, 11 Dec 1975, 70.

10 Reed, A. J. Lead poisoning: silent epidemic and social crime. Lamp, 30 (8), Aug 1973, 41–44.

11 Scannell, R. M. Disposal of toxic waste. Occupational Health, 26 (7), Jul 1974, 254–258.

12 Saward, A.C. Pollution of the environment. District Nursing. 15 (9), Dec 1972, 192–193.

13 Waldron, H. A. The Midlands. Health hazards of lead. Nursing Times, 70, 12 Sep 1974, 1406–1409.

14 WHO Chronicle The effect on man of deterioration of the environment. WHO Chronicle, 28 (12), Dec 1974, 549–553.

c WORLD HEALTH ORGANIZATION

1 Brookes, P. Careers extraordinary. WHO's top nurse. Nursing Times, 68, 4 May 1972, 531–532.

2 Burton, J. The WHO fellowships and training programme. WHO Chronicle, 29 (9), Sep 1975, 350–353.

3 Candau, M. G. International public health: some reflections after 25 years. WHO Chronicle, 27 (6), Jun 1973, 225–235.

4 Dorolle, P. Half a century of international health. Royal Society of Health Journal, 95 (1), Feb 1975, 18–19.

5 Mahler, H. Further thoughts on WHO's mission. WHO Chronicle, 29 (7), Jul 1975, 253–256.

6 Mahler, H. Health strategies in a changing world. [A reappraisal of WHO's activities.] WHO Chronicle, 29 (6), Jun 1975, 209–218.

7 Mahler, H. New possibilities for WHO. [Some thoughts on activities at country and regional levels.] WHO Chronicle, 29 (2), Feb 1975, 43–45.

8 Martin, J. The first 25 years of WHO: a full record. International Journal of Health Education, 16 (1), 1973, 2–4.

9 Queen's Nursing Journal Twenty-five years of WHO. Queen's Nursing Journal, 16 (3), Jun 1973, 76, 79.

10 WHO Chronicle WHO celebrates its twenty-fifth anniversary. WHO Chronicle, 27 (7–8), Jul/Aug 1973, 282–285.

11 World Health 25 years, facts and trends. [Issue marking the twenty-fifth anniversary of WHO.] World Health, Apr 1973.

d NURSING: INTERNATIONAL

1 Bauman, M. B. Baccalaureate nursing in a selected number of English speaking countries. [Canada, England, South Africa, India, Philippines.] International Nursing Review, 19 (1), 1972, 12–34.

2 Brink, P. J. Nursing in other cultures: an experimental course. [A course for American nurses preparing for work in undeveloped countries.] International Nursing Review, 19 (3), 1972, 261–265.

3 Commonwealth Nurses Federation Report on activities. Nursing Times, 71, 23 Jan 1975, Supplement 9–16.

4 Commonwealth Nurses Federation Supplements, Nos. 1–4. Nursing Times, 70, 1 Aug 1974, Suppl. 1–8; 71, 23 Jan 1975; 8 May 1975, 17–20; 27 Nov 1975, 25–32.

5 King's Fund Centre Transatlantic nursing seminar. Nursing Times, 68, 14 Sep 1972, Occ. papers, 145–148; 21 Sep 1972; Occ. papers, 149–152.

6 Lavin, M. A. Cross-cultural identification and utilization of nursing approaches applicable to the delivery of health care. [Bolivia, Ecuador and the United States.] International Nursing Review, 20 (3), May/Jun 1973, 73, 77, 84.

7 Moffett, M. B. The third approach. [Nursing in US, UK and Northern Europe.] Australian Nurses' Journal, 1 (4), Oct 1971, 24–26; (5), Nov 1971, 29–31.

8 Lamp Nursing abroad. [Australian Volunteers Abroad.] Lamp, 31 (6), Jun 1974, 25–27.

9 Price, V. Registered nurse training in developing countries. [Zambia, Jordan and Bangladesh.] Nursing Mirror, 141, 28 Aug 1975, 67–70.

10 Trans-Pacific Conference Report of the 1974 Trans-Pacific Nursing Conference – the inaugural conference between the American Nurses' Association and the Royal Australian Nursing Federation. Australian Nurses Journal, 4 (5), Nov 1974, 7–27 (15 pages).

1111 Tulloch, E. E. Some considerations for nursing education with particular reference to developing countries. International Nursing Review, 20, May/Jun 1973, 80–81.

12 Voluntary service nursing overseas. . .with VSO. Nursing Times, 68, 11 May 1972, 588–589.

INTERNATIONAL COUNCIL OF NURSES

13 Cornelius, D. Report of the ICN President, 1973–1975. International Nursing Review, 22 (6), Nov/Dec 1975, 168–176.

14 International Council of Nurses National reports of member associations, 1973: an international statistical survey of nursing. Geneva: ICN, 1973.

15 International Council of Nurses Nurses and nursing: proceedings of the 15th Quadrennial ICN Congress, Mexico City, May 13–18, 1973. Geneva: ICN, 1974. Also reported in American Journal of Nursing, 73 (8), Aug 1973, 1344–1350, 1352–1359; Nursing Times, 69, 10 May 1973, 619; 31 May 1973, 690.

16 International Council of Nurses. Professional Services Committee Prepares proposals on current nursing issues. [Report of meeting, September 1974.] International Nursing Review, 22 (1), Jan/Feb 1975, 4–6.

18 International Nursing Review ICN, 75th anniversary issues, 1899–1974. Basel: Karger, 1974.

19 Kruse, M. ICN at the crossroads: responsible involvement. International Nursing Review, 20 (2), Mar/Apr 1973, 42–46.

20 Magu, J. G. The foundation of the International Council of Nurses. Kenya Nursing Journal, 4 (2), Dec 1975, 35–37.

21 Patten, M. Report of the Council of National Representatives of the International Council of Nurses, Singapore, August, 1975. Australian Nurses' Journal, 5(3), Sep 1975, 14–19.

22 Scott Wright, M. ICN takes some forward looking decisions. [Council of National Representatives, 1975.] Nursing Mirror, 141, 28 Aug 1975, 35; Nursing Times, 71, 28 Aug 1975, 1353.

23 Starr, D. S. ICN meets in Mexico. Canadian Nurse, 69 (8), Aug 1973, 17–28.

24 White, A. ICN: past, present and future. [A student's view.] Irish Nurses' Journal, 4 (8), Aug/Sep 1971, 7–9.

e EUROPE AND EEC

GENERAL

1 Backhouse, N. Towards a Euronurse. Nursing Times, 71, 11 Dec 1975, 1970–1972.

2 Barrowclough, F. European nursing: a personal view. Nursing Times, 67, 24 Jun 1971, 776–777.

3 Bosanquet, N. Talking point. Nurses and the EEC. Nursing Times, 71, 29 May 1975, 835.

4 Council of Europe. European Public Health Committee The situation of doctors and nurses in public health administrations in Council of Europe member states and Finland. Report prepared by Dr. A. de Weyer and others. Strasbourg: The Council, 1974.

5 Cowen, E. Health insurance in the Common Market. Nursing Mirror, 136, 5 Jan 1973, 19–20.

6 Crawford, L. Health care in Sweden, Denmark, and Holland. [Study tour to examine planning objectives in primary health care.] Nursing Mirror, 141, 2 Oct 1975, 65–67.

7 EEC draft directives Further discussions in January meeting. Midwives Chronicle, 88, Mar 1975, 86–87.

8 Ferguson, A. C. British nurses and the Common Market. American Journal of Nursing, 73, (3), Mar 1973, 476–479.

9 Ferguson, A. C. Common Market and nurses, Nursing Times, 67, 11 Nov 1971, Occ. papers 177–179; 18 Nov 1971, Occ. papers, 181–183.

10 Fisek, N. H. Immigrants in Europe: an impact on health. World Health, Oct 1973, 18–25.

11 Florin, M. P. The nursing profession and the European Economic Community. International Nursing Review, 21 (6), Nov/Dec 1974, 183, 184–186.

12 General Nursing Council Nursing in the EEC. A statement. Nursing Times, 68, 23 March 1972, 351–353; Nursing Mirror, 134, 17 Mar 1972, 13–14.

13 Health Professions' Forum E.E.C. Health Professions' Second Conference on E.E.C. British Medical Journal, 3, 15 Jul 1972, Supplement 42–43; Nursing Times, 68, 15 Jun 1972, 728.

14 International Council of Nurses Common Market – threat to nursing standards? Nursing Times, 67, 17 Jun 1971, 738.

15 King's Fund Centre NHS and EEC transcripts of talks given at seminars held at the Centre between June 1973 and June 1974, edited by L. H. W. Paine. The Centre, 1974.

16 Maynard, A. Health care in the European community. Croom Helm, 1975.

17 Maynard, A. Medical care in the European community. New Society, 33, 28 Aug 1975, 466–467.

18 Nursing Mirror The NHS and the EEC: professions in the new Europe. (Conference report.] Nursing Mirror, 141, 20 Nov 1975, 34.

19 Nursing Mirror Nurses represented in Common Market talks. [Parliamentary report.] Nursing Mirror, 133, 5 Nov 1971, 13–14.

20 O'Leary, G. M. Nursing in Iceland. International Journal of Nursing Studies, 9, Mar 1972, 27–30.

21 Orriss, H. D. Health in the Common Market. Nursing Times, 69, 15 Nov 1973, 1530.

22 Permanent Committee of Nurses in liaison with the EEC An examination of the working conditions for first level nurses in the public sector in the EEC countries and the four Nordic countries outside the EEC. The Committee, 1975.

23 Quinn, S. EEC directives on nursing – the final phase. Nursing Mirror, 140, 19 Jun 1975, 40–42.

24 Quinn, S. The EEC – the effect on nursing to date and future trends. NATNews, 11 (9), Dec 1974, 14, 16–17, 20.

25 Royal College of General Practitioners North London Faculty Medicine and the Common Market. [Report of symposium.] Journal of the Royal College of General Practitioners, 23, May 1973, 371–375.

26 Royal College of Nursing Congress report. Second session – The nurse in Europe. Nursing Mirror, 134, 31 Mar 1972, 10; Nursing Times, 68, 30 Mar 1972, 365–366.

27 Royal Society of Medicine Medicine in the Common Market. [Report of a Conference.] British Medical Journal, 4, 17 Nov 1973, 396–411.

28 Smith, G. T. Society at work. Health and the Six. New Society, 17, 18 Feb 1971, 272–273.

29 Turner, A. C. Medical costs in the EEC. [Administrative procedures and medical facilities for UK nationals.] Nursing Mirror, 140, 13 Mar 1975, 63–65.

30 World Health Organization, Regional Office for Europe Directory of schools of nursing in the European region. Copenhagen: WHO, 1971.

31 World Health Organization, Regional Office for Europe Liaison meeting with nursing/midwifery associations on WHOs European nursing midwifery programme: Copenhagen 26–28 June 1974. Copenhagen: WHO, 1975.

32 World Health Organization. Regional office for Europe Trends in European nursing services: report of a working group. Copenhagen: WHO, 1972.

33 World of Irish Nursing The EEC. [Leading article.] World of Irish Nursing, 1 (5), May 1972, 95.

BELGIUM

34 Cowen, E. The six: Social Services. 2. Belgium. Social provisions in the European Economic Community. Nursing Mirror, 134, 14 Apr 1972, 14–15.

35 Nursing Times A meeting with the Belgian nurses. Nursing Times, 69, 22 Feb 1973, 258–259.

36 Paine, L. H. W. NHS and EEC. Health services in Belgium. Health and Social Service Journal, 83, 15 Dec 1973, 2943–2944.

37 Rokeghem, S. Van The nurses are fed up with living outside the law. [Translation of an article from 'Le Soir' on the state and status of nursing in Belgium.] Nursing Mirror, 136, 20 Apr 1973, 30–31.

DENMARK

38 Anderson, B. R. Into Europe. Denmark: the social reform development. Social Work Today, 4, 21 Feb 1974, 728–730.

39 Cannell, S. A. and Dahl, M. A Danish teaching

scheme. [Using three teaching books – a basic text-book, tutor's guide, and student's case book.] Mid-wives Chronicle, 88, Dec 1975, 405.

40 Cowen, E. The Six: Social Services. 8. Denmark. Nursing Mirror, 134, 26 May 1972, 42–43.

41 Davies, R. Voluntary social services in Europe. 5. Denmark. Social Service Quarterly, 49 (3), Oct-Dec 1975, 44–46.

42 McCarrick, H. Into Europe. 6. Denmark. Nursing Times, 69, 8 Nov 1973, 1502–1503.

43 Paine, L. H. W. NHS and EEC. Health Services in Denmark. Health and Social Services Journal, 84, 3 Aug 1974, 1742–1744.

44 Wall, M. and Munns, B. Nursing in Denmark. Report of a scholarship tour. Nursing Times, 70, 18 Jul 1974, 1127–1128.

EIRE

45 Chavasse, J. M. An Irish college of nursing. World of Irish Nursing, 1, Jan 1972, 16–19; 1 Feb 1972, 34–38.

46 Chavasse, J. Nursing in the Emerald Isle. International Nursing Review, 15, Apr 1968, 183–188.

47 Clancy, H. Whither nursing: nurse training and/or nurse education. World of Irish Nursing, 3 (12), Dec 1974, 223, 225.

48 Cowen, E. The Six: Social Services. 9. Eire. Nursing Mirror, 134, 2 Jun 1972, 32–33.

49 Early, B. Management and the Irish health services. Hospital and Health Services Review, 69 (10), Oct 1973, 366–371.

50 Elms, R. R. and others Irish nursing at the cross-roads. International Journal of Nursing Studies, 11 (3), Sep 1974, 163–170.

51 Hensey, B. The health service in Ireland. 2nd ed. Dublin: Institute of Public Administration, 1972.

52 Irish Nurses' Organization Deputation to the Minister for Health. [Editorial.] World of Irish Nursing, 2 (8), Aug 1973, 141–142.

53 Irish Nurses Organization Nursing staff structures. [Committee set up by the Irish Nurses' Organization to study this matter.] World of Irish Nursing, 1 (9), Sep 1972, 178.

54 Keane, K. Summary Report: symposium on higher education in nursing. World of Irish Nursing, 2 (7), Jul 1973, 123, 125.

55 Leydon, I. Development of nurse education in Ireland – training to meet the challenges of the future. International Journal of Nursing Studies, 10 (2), May 1973, 95–100.

56 Nursing Times Nurse education in Eire. Nursing Times, 71, 4 Dec 1975, 1951.

57 O'Carroll, M. F. Restructuring the health care system – an Irish solution. World Hospitals, 7 (2), Apr 1971, 45–49.

58 Paine, L. NHS and EEC. Health services in Ireland. Health and Social Service Journal, 84, 7 Sep 1974, 2034–2036.

59 Taaffe, T. C. Manpower planning and employment opportunities. World of Irish Nursing, 3 (11), Nov 1974, 17; (12), Dec 1974, 221–222.

60 Tierney, B. Nurse education [in the context of the new health services]. World of Irish Nursing, 3 (8), Aug 1974, 137–139.

61 Tierney, B. Nursing in Ireland. International Journal of Nursing Studies, 11 (2), Jul 1974, 111–116.

FRANCE

62 Barrowclough, F. The French connexion – and nursing. Nursing Times, 68, 15 Jun 1972, 735–736.

63 Clarke, F. Hospital at home. [Scheme in Paris for patients who prefer to be cared for at home.] Health and Social Service Journal, 83, 9 Jun 1973, 1311–1312.

64 Clarke, F. Into Europe. Hospital at home. [Statutory centralized service of home care in Paris for patients normally treated in hospital.] Social Work Today, 5 (13), 3 Oct 1974, 387–389.

65 Cowen, E. The Six: social services. 3. France. Nursing Mirror, 134, 21 Apr 1972, 12–13.

66 Fautrel, F. Into Europe. 1. France – apathy and responsibility. Nursing Times, 69, 4 Oct 1973, 1303–1305.

67 Fautrel, F. Into Europe. 2. France – luxury and militancy. [Educational opportunities.] Nursing Times, 69, 11 Oct 1973, 1345–1346.

68 Hinchcliffe, E. Inside a French hospital. [The Institut Calot.] Nursing Mirror, 139, 23 Aug 1974, 76.

69 Hurst, T. W. IHF study tour of France, 1974. [International Hospital Federation.] Hospital and Health Services Review, 71 (2), Feb 1975, 55–61.

70 Maynard, A. Hospital care in Britain and France. Hospital and Health Service Review, 71 (2), Feb 1975, 50–53.

71 New Society French nurses. [Report of a study published in 'Revue Française de Sociologie' to examine the contrast between the nurse's image and the reality of the job.] New Society, 32, 3 Apr 1975, 23.

72 Nursing Times European nurses compare notes. [Conference on nursing roles and medical progress in France.] Nursing Times, 70, 7 Feb 1974, 170.

73 Paine, L. H. W. NHS and EEC. Health services in France. Health and Social Service Journal, 84, 12 Jan 1974, 67–68.

74 Wright, A. F. Primary medical care in France. Journal of the Royal College of General Practitioners, 25, Sep 1975, 664–669.

ITALY

75 Cioni, V. Into Europe. 3. Italy. Hot tempers and cold baths. Nursing Times, 69, 18 Oct 1973, 1382–1383.

76 Cowen, E. The Six: social services. 6. Italy. Nursing Mirror, 134, 12 May 1972, 41–43.

77 Ernandes, J. S. That other Italy. [Nursing in Italy.] Nursing Times, 70, 4 Apr 1974, 516–517.

78 Gubert, S. Nurses in Italy. Nursing Mirror, 140, 23 Jan 1975, 63–66.

79 Paine, L. H. W. NHS and EEC. Health services in Italy. Health and Social Service Journal, 84, 8 Jun 1974, 1274–1275.

NETHERLANDS

80 Cowen, E. The Six: social services. 1. The Netherlands. Nursing Mirror, 134, 7 Apr 1972, 24–26.

81 Lugt, M. Public health in the Netherlands. District Nursing, 15 (4), Jul 1972, 76, 81.

82 McCarrick, H. Into Europe. 4. Holland. Sense and sensibility. Nursing Times, 69, 25 Oct 1973, 1424.

83 Paine, L. H. W. NHS and EEC. Health Services in the Netherlands. Health and Social Service Journal, 83, 6 Oct 1973, 2308–2309, 2311.

84 Vorster, W. P. Personal impressions gained while working in a country hospital in Holland. SA Nursing Journal, 39 (2), Feb 1972, 33, 35–36.

SWEDEN

85 Hazel, N. Into Europe – Sweden – problems of plenty. Social Work Today, 4 (16), 15 Nov 1973, 493–495.

86 Paine, L. H. W. Health services in Sweden. [King's Fund seminar.] Health and Social Service Journal, 85, 26 Jul 1975, 1604–1605.

87 Pendreigh, D. M. Health services organization – Sweden. Health Bulletin, 31 (4), Jul 1973, 204–210.

88 Rabo, M. Nursing in Sweden. International Nursing Review, 18 (4), 1971, 334–346.

WEST GERMANY

89 Cowen, E. The Six: Social Services. 4. The Federal Republic of Germany. Nursing Mirror, 134, 28 Apr 1972, 26–27.

90 McCarrick, H. Into Europe. 5. West Germany. Small wards and paying patients. Nursing Times, 69, 1 Nov 1973, 1460–1461.

91 Paine, L. H. W. NHS and EEC. Health services in West Germany. Health and Social Service Journal, 84, 30 Mar 1974, 721–723.

92 Roebuck, J. P. Working in Germany. Nursing Times, 71, 20 Nov 1975, 1877.

USSR

93 Abdellah, F. Nursing and health care in the U.S.S.R. American Journal of Nursing, 73 (12), Dec 1973, 2096–2099.

94 Bourienkov, S. Multinational health services in the USSR. World Health, Jun 1973, 22–25.

95 Ferguson, M. Nurse or feldsher? A crisis of identity [USSR]. Nursing Times, 69, 25 Oct 1973, 1410–1412.

96 Ryan, T. M. Health services in the Ukraine. [Report of a study tour of doctors, GPs paramedical workers and students to Kiev and Kharkov.] Health and Social Service Journal, 84, 7 Dec 1974, 2826–2827.

97 Stansfield, P. In a Russian hospital. Nursing Times, 67, 17 Jun 1971, 723–725.

98 Tarassova, G. An honoured profession. Union of Soviet Socialist Republics. World Health, Dec 1972, 22–27; Nursing Times, 69, 26 Apr 1973, 527–530.

99 Ussov, I. N. Nurses in the USSR. Nursing Journal of India, 63 (7), Jul 1972, 229.

100 World Health Organization Report on the travelling seminar on nursing in the USSR, 23 March – 14 April 1970. Geneva: WHO, 1971.

OTHER COUNTRIES

101 Cowen, E. The Six: social services. 5. Luxembourg. Nursing Mirror, 134, 5 May 1972, 36–37.

102 Das, M. Much to learn from other Associations. [Nursing in Sweden and Finland.] Nursing Journal of India, 61 (11), Nov 1970, 362–363, 386.

103 Deuchar, E. A. Norwegian nursing experience. New Zealand Nursing Journal, 67 (3), Mar 1974, 4–6.

104 Dittrich, F. Perspectives for nursing in Austria. [Account of a WHO tour to collect impressions of nursing in eight European countries.] International Nursing Review, 20 (6), Nov/Dec 1973, 171–173, 180.

105 Ezban, A. A leap forward. [Health services in Bulgaria.] World Health, Jun 1975, 16–21.

106 Greene, B. Three Yugoslav hospitals. Nursing Times, 69, 14 Jun 1973, 780–781.

107 Kelly, E. M. Nurses of the George Cross island. [Malta.] Nursing Times, 70, 1 Aug 1974, 1210–1211.

108 Kum, E. Nursing in Turkey. International Journal of Nursing Studies, 9 (1), Mar 1972, 51–57.

109 Lamp Health services in Bulgaria – facts and figures. Lamp, 31 (11), Nov 1974, 17–18.

110 Lloyd, J. Decentralization – the Yugoslav way. Health and Social Service Journal, 85, 4 Oct 1975, 2224.

111 Tyrrell, S. M. Social medicine in Poland: a personal view. Community Health, 5 (6), May/Jun 1974, 317–320.

f AFRICA

GENERAL

1 Beck, F. S. Background of nursing. South of the Sahara. International Nursing Review, 18 (3), 1971, 263–270.

2 Bienfait, C. Insight into Africa. Work in a Salvation Army clinic in the African Congo. Nursing Mirror, 133, 16 Jul 1971, 37–40.

3 Bull, D. E. All in a night's work. [Tanzania.] Nursing Mirror, 134, 11 Feb 1972, 46–47.

4 Burgess, D. Nursing in Ethiopia. Nursing Times, 69, 8 Mar 1973, 324–325.

5 Commonwealth Nurses Federation Report of the first All-African Seminar to discuss health problems. Nursing Times, 71, 23 Jan 1975, Supplement 11–12.

6 Cooper-Poole, J. H. A new teaching and referral hospital for Tanzania. World Hospitals, 10 (4), Autumn 1974, 199–201.

7 Cowen E. Algeria – public health in an emergent state. Nursing Mirror, 136, 16 Mar 1973, 33–35.

8 Daintrey, G. Turkana. [The author's work for Voluntary Service Overseas in Kenya.] Nursing Mirror, 136, 20 Apr 1972, 28–29.

9 Davis, A. J. Health problems and nursing practice in sub-Saharan Africa. [Ghana, Nigeria and Kenya.] International Journal of Nursing Studies, 12 (2), Jul 1975, 61–64.

10 Davis, A. J. Preventive intervention healing in West Africa. Journal of Psychiatric Nursing and Mental Health Services, 12 (5), Sep/Oct 1974, 7–9.

11 Dieng, I. Evolution of the nursing profession in Senegal. International Nursing Review, 21 (6), Nov/Dec 1974, 172–173.

12 Gish, C. The way forward. [Health services in Tanzania.] World Health, Apr 1975, 8–13.

13 Guichard, M. T. Nursing in a mission hospital. [Yobondu, Zaire.] Nursing Mirror, 140, 17 Apr 1975, 56.

14 Hewitt, S. Focus on Malawi. 2. Nursing with the church in Malawi. Nursing Mirror, 132, 29 Jan 1971, 24.

15 Hyde, K. J. Missionary nurse in Ovamboland. [South West Africa.] Nursing Mirror, 135, 8 Dec 1972, 30–31.

16 Jegede, S. A. Cultural approach to nursing in Africa. Nigerian Nurse, 7 (3), Jul–Sep 1975, 6–8.

17 McCarthy, N. Nursing in Uganda. In the shadow of the fabled 'Mountains of the Moon'. World of Irish Nursing, 2 (11), Nov 1973, 209–211.

18 Rennie, H. Personal view. [Health and medicine in Malawi.] British Medical Journal, 3, 21 Jul 1973, 168.

19 Swaffield, L. Blending the best of both worlds – nursing in Ghana. Nursing Times, 70, 11 Jul 1974, 1056.

20 Twumasi, P. A. Scientific medicine – the Ghanaian experience. [Impact of scientific medicine on the Ghanaian cultural scene.] International Journal of Nursing Studies, 9 (2), Jun 1972, 63–73.

21 Watts, T. Health centre in Uganda. Health and Social Service Journal, 84, 31 Aug 1974, 1979–1980.

22 WHO Chronicle The place of public health in the economy of Africa. WHO Chronicle, 29 (8), Aug 1975, 317–322.

KENYA

23 Hartwig, M. S. Role and identity: an important distinction. [Education of professional and technical nurses with particular reference to Kenya.] Nursing Outlook, 20 (10), Oct 1972, 665–669.

24 Khachina, J. Some aspects of Kenyatta National Hospital School of Nursing – Medical Training Centre – Nairobi. Kenya Nursing Journal, 1 (1), Jun 1972, 18–21.

25 Kiereini, M. Opening remarks to the National Nurses' Association of Kenya Seminar. 'Effective Nursing Care.' Nairobi, 14 April 1972. Kenya Nursing Journal, 1 (1), Jun 1972, 8–9.

26 Kilty, E. M. In need of our help. [Nursing in Kenya.] Nursing Mirror, 135, 22 Dec 1972, 29–31.

27 Munyua, E. N. Nurse and non-nursing duties in Kenya. Kenya Nursing Journal, 2 (1), Jun 1973, 22–27.

28 What role do our nurses play in the health services of Kenya today? Kenya Nursing Journal, 4 (2), Dec 1975, 5, 47.

NIGERIA

29 Ayo Vaughan-Richards Education and preparation of the nurse to meet the health needs of the nation. Nigerian Nurse, 4 (1), Jan/Mar 1972, 21–22, 24–27.

30 Babayode, D. A. The Nigerian nurse of the future. Nigerian Nurse, 6 (4), Oct/Dec 1974, 51–53.

31 Bailey, A. The Nursing Council and you. [Nursing Council of Nigeria.] Nigerian Nurse, 4 (2), Apr/Jun 1972, 14–18.

32 Barber, R. Health planning in Nigeria. Health and Social Service Journal, 85, 16 Aug 1975, 1790–1791.

33 Chokrich, A. C. Change in nursing in Nigeria. International Nursing Review, 22 (3), May/Jun 1975, 71–79.

34 Davitz, L. J. Becoming a nurse in Nigeria. American Journal of Nursing, 72 (11), Nov 1972, 2026–2028.

35 Davitz, L. J. Identification of stressful situations in a Nigerian school of nursing. Nursing Research, 21 (4), Jul–Aug 1972, 352–357.

36 Jegede, S. A. Nursing in developing countries. [With particular reference to Nigeria.] Nursing Mirror, 136, 9 Mar 1973, 28, 34.

37 Nworolo, F. I. Work and future plans of the Training School, General Hospital. Benin City, Midwest-State, Nigeria. International Journal of Nursing Studies, 8 (4), Dec 1971, 269–273.

38 Oghedegbe, G. U. Towards better nursing in Nigeria. Nigerian Nurse, 5 (4), Oct/Dec 1973, 23, 26.

39 Ogundeyin, W. M. The nurse and the contemporary society [of Nigeria.] Nigerian Nurse, 6 (4), Oct–Dec 1974, 6–9.

40 Okunade, B. The nurse within the health team. [With particular reference to the situation in Nigeria.] International Nursing Review, 22 (2), Mar/Apr 1975, 46–49.

41 Oguntolu, O. A. Identifying the health needs of the nation in the context of the 'role of the nurse in the four year development plan'. Nigerian Nurse, 4 (1), Jan/Mar 1972, 32–33, 35.

42 Schram, R. A history of the Nigerian health services. Ibadan: University Press, 1971.

RHODESIA (ZIMBABWE)

43 Cronje, R. International Nurses Day speech on developments in nursing in Rhodesia. Rhodesian Nurse, 8 (3), Sep 1975, 10–12.

44 Dunaway, M. The community outreach of the Sanyati Baptist hospital. Rhodesian Nurse, 8, Dec 1975, 12–15.

45 Rhodesian Nurse The needs of Rhodesia in the field of progressive nursing education. Rhodesian Nurse, 5 (1), Mar 1972, 13–15, 17–19, 21–24.

46 SA Nursing Journal A school to be proud of. [Salisbury Nurses' Training School, Rhodesia.] SA Nursing Journal, 40 (5), May 1973, 10, 12, 16.

SOUTH AFRICA

47 Boyce, A. N. Changes in education. SA Nursing Journal, 39 (1), Jan 1972, 9–11.

48 The Day Hospital Organization. The first four years. [Cape Peninsula.] [Reprint from S. African Medical Journal, 25 May 1974.] SA Nursing Journal, 12 (12), Dec 1974, 9–10, 12–14.

49 Donn, M. C. South Africa 1975. [Study tour of South African Hospitals.] NATNews, 12 (9), Dec 1975, 11–13.

50 Harrison, P. H. Withdrawal of the South African Nursing Association from the International Council of Nurses. SA Nursing Journal, 40 (9), Sep 1973, 7–8. Reprinted in Nursing Mirror, 137, 2 Nov 1973, 20.

51 Lekhela, E. P. Some aspects of the challenges awaiting Bantu nurses in the Homelands. SA Nursing Journal, 38 (9), Sep 1971, 16–19.

52 Searle, C. The second class doctor and the medical assistant in South Africa. [Further training for nurses to enable them to act as health assistants in the absence of doctors.] SA Nursing Journal, 40 (7), Jul 1973, 12–13, 15, 17.

g MIDDLE EAST

GENERAL

1 Bell, J. Leadership and responsibility. [Nursing in Egypt.] World Health, Dec 1972, 18–21.

2 Church, R. Voluntary nursing in the Yemen. Nursing Times, 69, 3 May 1973, 578–580.

3 Conroy, K. Nursing oasis in Saudi Arabia. Nursing Times, 68, 14 Sep 1972, 1148–1153.

4 Kelly, M. A. Beliefs of Iranian nurses and nursing students about nurses and nursing education. International Nursing Review, 20 (4), Jul/Aug 1973, 108–111.

5 Kelly, E. The Jordanian way. [Nursing and nursing education in Jordan.] Nursing Mirror, 139, 17 Oct 1974, 83–84.

6 Khoury, J. F. Nursing in Kuwait. International Nursing Review, 20 (1), Jan–Feb 1973, 12–21.

7 Logan, W. W. Nursing services in a Gulf sheikhdom. Nursing Mirror, 139, 16 Aug 1974, 61–65.

8 Moutou, L. A glimpse of the nursing profession in Morocco. International Nursing Review, 22 (1), Jan/Feb 1975, 23–24.

9 Rahnema, H. E. M. The role of frontline health workers [in Iran]. WHO Chronicle, 29 (1), Jan 1975, 6–9.

10 Ronaghy, H. A. and others Migration of Iranian nurses to the U.S: a study of one school of nursing in Iran. International Nursing Review, 22 (3), May/Jun 1975, 87–88.

11 Repond, R. House of health. [Health assistants and village health workers bring primary health care to rural communities in Iran.] World Health, Apr 1975, 20–25.

12 Thomas, G. M. Nursing in Lebanon. International Nursing Review, 22 (5), Sep/Oct 1975, 136, 138–143.

13 Tomalin, C. Egypt's health policy – the next five years. Health and Social Service Journal, 85, 16 Aug 1975, 1796.

14 Tomalin, C. A future for health in the Middle East. Health and Social Service Journal, 85, 16 Aug 1975, 1786–1787.

15 Tomalin, C. Medicine in an Arab setting. Health and Social Service Journal, 85, 16 Aug 1975, 1792–1793.

16 Tomiche, F. J. Democratic Yemen. Health builders. World Health, Jul 1975, 24–27.

ISRAEL

17 Affara, F. Nazareth – a nursing experience with a small team from several countries assisting at the establishment and development of new services in a hospital serving the Arab community. International Journal of Nursing Studies, 9 (4), Nov 1972, 235–242.

18 Bergman, R. Professional absorption in Israel of nurse-immigrants from the USSR. International Journal of Nursing Studies, 12 (2), Jul 1975, 73–80.

19 Bergman, R. The Soviet nurse emigre in Israel. [Experiences of three nurses.] Nursing Outlook, 23 (4), Apr 1975, 236–239.

20 Bergman, R. and others Work-life of the Israeli registered nurse. [A survey to facilitate planning for nursing manpower.] International Journal of Nursing Studies, 12 (3), 1975, 133–168.

21 Fisher, D. Health and social services in Israel. Health and Social Service Journal, 84, 6 Apr 1974, 774–775.

22 Golub, S. Nursing in Israel. Nursing Mirror, 136, 15 Jun 1973, 22–25.

23 Margolis, E. Health care in a changing society: the health services of Israel. Medical Care, 13 (11), Nov 1975, 943–955.

24 Nurse in Israel Absorption of immigrant nurses from the USSR. Nurse in Israel, 91 (22), Oct 1974, 2–4.

25 Tel Aviv University. Faculty of Continuing Medical Education. Department of Nursing Research and studies on nursing in Israel, edited by Lea Grief. Tel-Aviv: The University, 1972.

26 Weiss, M. O. Kibbutz nurse. American Journal of Nursing, 71 (9), Sep 1971, 1762–1765.

27 Weiss, O. Nursing in Israel. Australian Nurses' Journal, 2 (4), Oct 1972, 18–19, 25.

h ASIA

GENERAL

1 Chung, H. H. An exploratory study of clinical nursing activities as a preliminary step for planning changes in care delivery system. [Taiwan]. International Nursing Review, 18 (4), 1971, 291–312.

2 Coles, J. A. Nursing in Padang, Indonesia. UNA Nursing Journal, 3, May/Jun 1974, 32–33.

3 Conroy, P. A. Facts about nursing education in Korea. Korean Nurse, 11 (2), 25 Apr 1972, 40–44.

4 Crawford Fourth National Nurses' Convention. [Nursing in Thailand.] New Zealand Nursing Journal, 66 (3), Mar 1973, 7.

5 Dimacall, L. C. The PNA Board at work. [Philippine Nurses Association.] Philippine Journal of Nursing, 44 (1), Jan/Mar 1975, 14–16.

6 Dodds, M. Something new under the sun: an Australian nurse in Indonesia. Australian Nurses' Journal, 1 (9), Mar 1972, 24–26.

7 Donovan, J. My Papua New Guinea experiences: in retrospect. [Work of a volunteer nurse.] Lamp, 32 (7), Jul 1975, 5, 7.

8 Heartfield, M. Nursing at Orokolo [Papua New Guinea]. Tasmanian Nurse, 5 (5), Jun 1971, 8–10.

9 Iu, S. President's address at International Nurses Day celebration. [The development of international nursing with particular reference to the Hong Kong Nurses Association.] Hong Kong Nursing Journal, 17, Nov 1974, 6–9.

10 Koon Guan, H. The status of the nursing service. Nursing Journal of Singapore, 11 (2), Nov 1971, 69–70.

11 Lamp Report on the Asian regional seminar – Asian nurses – problems and challenges. Singapore, 5–15th Dec, 1973. Lamp, 31 (5), May 1974, 15–16.

12 Lo, M. L. L. The education and role of nurses in Taiwan. International Nursing Review, 20 (6), Nov/Dec 1973, 176–177, 180.

13 Palmer, F. New Zealand nurse in Vietnam. [Personal account.] New Zealand Nursing Journal, 69 (7), Jul 1975, 13–14.

14 Valdez, F. M. Trends in nursing. Philippine Journal of Nursing, 44 (1), Jan/Mar 1975, 19–22.

15 Williams, H. W. The nursing profession in South Vietnam. Nursing Times, 67, 25 Feb 1971, 237–240.

16 Yee, L. F. A psychological study of nurses in Singapore. Nursing Journal of Singapore, 13 (1), May 1973, 15–17.

CHINA

17 Branch, M. A black American nurse visits the People's Republic of China. Nursing Forum, 12 (4), 1973, 402–411.

18 Brueton, M. Medical welfare in China. Health and Social Service Journal, 84, 11 May 1974, 1043–1045.

19 Horn, J. S. Community action pays off. [Organization of peasant doctors in China.] World Health, Dec 1975, 22–25.

20 Hsii, F. P. Medicine in China today. Nursing Journal of Singapore, 13 (2), Nov 1973, 126–128.

21 Klintworth, C. General medical care in China. Australian Nurses' Journal, 4 (3), Sep 1974, 33–35.

22 Middlestone, H. J. H. Where health is patriotism. Visit of New Zealand Medical Delegation to China: Aug–Sep 1974. New Zealand Nursing Journal, 68 (4), Apr 1975, 22–23.

23 Philpot, T. Health service advances in China. Health and Social Service Journal, 83, 8 Sep 1973, 2052–2055.

24 Roth, R. B. The health care system in the People's Republic of China. Hospitals, 49 (18), 16 Sep 1975, 57–60.

25 Wen, C. Barefoot doctors in China. Lancet, 1, 18 May 1974, 976–978.

INDIA, PAKISTAN, BANGLADESH

26 Ahad, M. A. Innovations in Indian nursing: a study of foreign returned Indian nurses as innovators. [Research abstract.] Nursing Journal of India, 65 (5), May 1974, 151–152, 158.

27 Anand, D. India, blending old and new. World Health, Feb/Mar 1973, 22–25.

28 Cherian, A. Indian Nursing Council. Nursing Journal of India, 62, 6 Jun 1971, 197.

29 Chioni, R. M. and Schoen, E. Preparing tomorrow's nurse practitioner. Nursing Journal of India, 64 (2), Feb 1973, 49–50, 55–56, 65.

30 Chowdbury, Dr. Health projects in Bangladesh. 2. A community oriented health project. Nursing Times, 71, 8 May 1975, Supplement 19.

31 Ghate, R. Life in Shivangaon: health care in an Indian village. Nursing Mirror, 141 (2), 10 Jul 1975, 69–70.

32 Halim, N. F. Problems of nursing in Pakistan. Pakistan Nursing and Health Review, 1, 1972, 12–18.

33 Kuruvilla, A. Status of nursing in India. Nursing Journal of India, 66 (5) May 1975, 99–100.

34 Malhotra, A. D. Law relating to licensing, registration and practice of nursing. Nursing Journal of India, 66 (1), Jan 1975, 5–6.

35 Powar, J. D. Nursing functions and law in India. Nursing Journal of India, 66 (1), Jan 1975, 4, 21.

36 Price, V. Health projects in Bangladesh. 1. The British Red Cross Society's project. Nursing Times, 71, 8 May 1975, Supplement 18–19.

37 Rao, G. A. J. R. Silver Jubilee of Independence. Nursing in retrospect. Nursing Journal of India, 63 (9), Sep 1972, 298.

38 Sawyer, I. J. Health in rural India. [Two year auxiliary nurse midwife course.] Nursing Times, 69, 25 Oct 1973, 1409.

39 Srivastava, A. L. Nurses in the hospital – a sociological perspective. Nursing Journal of India, 64 (2), Feb 1973, 58.

40 Taylor, E. P. and Cooper, D. K. C. Hospital care in the Indian Punjab. Nursing Times, 68, 20 Jul 1972, 912–914.

41 Tewari, T. R. Nursing survey in India. A CAHP-TNAI undertaking. Nursing Journal of India, 63 (10), Oct 1972, 351.

42 Vichniac, I. Disappearing prejudices. [Nursing in India]. World Health, Dec 1972, 28–33; Nursing Journal of India, 64 (5), May 1973, 157–158, 161.

43 Xaxier, K. G. The 'merit-demerit' system for discipline in nursing schools. Nursing Journal of India, 64 (9), Sep 1973, 314, 321.

i AUSTRALASIA

AUSTRALIA

1 Adams, A. I. Public expectations and the utilization of health services in urban Australia. Medical Care, 10 (4), Jul/Aug 1972, 288–299.

2 Annat, I. M. Economic pressures – and quality nursing. Australian Nurses' Journal, 2 (10), Apr 1973, 36–39.

3 Barnwell, J. The impact of European culture on the health of Australian aborigines. Lamp, 32 (8), Aug 1975, 37–38.

4 Boorer, D. Flying physicians. [Australia's Royal Flying Doctor Service.] Nursing Times, 70, 9 May 1974, 720–721.

5 Boorer, D. 'Hey, Charlie, how long have you had your transplant?' [Impressions of Australian nursing.] Australian Nurses' Journal, 2 (11), May 1973, 30–31.

6 Boorer, D. Nursing in Australia. 1. On the district. Nursing Times, 70, 16 May 1974, 764–765.

7 Boorer, D. Nursing in Australia. 2. Buying time. Victoria's cancer clinic: a nursing ideal. Nursing Times, 70, 23 May 1974, 806–807.

8 Boorer, D. Nursing in Australia. 3. Bush nursing. Nursing Times, 70, 30 May 1974, 844–845.

9 Boorer, D. Nursing in Australia. 4. Impartial efficiency. Nursing Times, 70, 6 Jun 1974, 884–885.

10 Boorer, D. Nursing in Australia. 5. Geography's handicap. Nursing Times, 70, 13 Jun 1974, 926–927.

11 Carroll, P. and Dewdney, J. C. H. Public hospital matrons – a survey. Australian Nurses' Journal, 3 Mar 1974, 26–28; 3 (9), Apr 1974, 20, 22–23.

12 Cowen, E. Health and welfare 'down under'. Nursing Mirror, 136, 22 Jun 1973, 32–34.

13 Dewdney, J. C. H. Australian health services. Wiley, 1973.

14 Donaghue, S. Infusing reality into the health team. Australian Nurses' Journal, 5 (4), Oct 1975, 20–22.

15 Evans, M. Changes in the nursing scene. Australian Nurses Journal, 1 (6), Dec 1971, 19–21.

16 Evans, M. The future role of nurses in the delivery of health care in urban areas. [In Australia.] Australian Nurses' Journal, 3 (6), Dec 1973/Jan 1974, 38–40.

17 Gross, P. F. The future of nursing in Australia: an outsider's realities and strategies. Australian Nurses' Journal, 4 (7), Feb 1975, 33–35.

18 Higham, E. M. A recommended change in the nursing structure: a programme to suit the Australian environment. [The result of a study tour of Britain during 1972.] Lamp, 31 (1), Jan 1974, 32–36.

19 Kalokerinos, A. Poor black health, bad white attitudes. [The health of Australian Aborigines.] Australian Nurses' Journal, 3 (9), Apr 1974, 29–31.

20 Lambert, P. New horizons in nursing. [Implications of the White report on the role of the nurse in Australia and other recent studies of nursing in Australia.] Australian Nurses' Journal, 5 (5), Nov 1975, 31–34, 44.

21 Lamp The role of the nurse in Australia. [Adapted from the National Health and Medical Research Council annual report.] Lamp, 32 (3), Mar 1975, 28–29, (5), May 1975, 27–28.

22 Lickiss, J. N. Community dimensions of health care. Australian Nurses' Journal, 4 (6), Dec 1974/Jan 1975, 29–30, 44.

23 McDonald, G. Diagnosing the problems of the Aborigines. Australian Nurses' Journal, 3 (6), Dec 1973/Jan 1974, 16–18.

24 McDonald, G. Nursing – an organization in the professional mould. [Nursing organizations in Australia]. Australian Nurses' Journal, 1 (2), Aug 1971, 19–21.

25 McPherson, L. A community centre as large as life. [Work of an Australian health centre.] Australian Nurses' Journal, 4 (7), Feb 1975, 39–41.

26 Manock, H. M. How can nursing in Australia grow? Australian Nurses' Journal, 2 (10), Apr 1973, 30–31.

27 Martin, E. M. A white man tries. [Health planning for an Aboriginal settlement.] Lamp, 32 (7), Jul 1975, 27–31.

28 Najman, J. A. Asking the answerable. (Where is nursing going?) [The future of nursing in Australia.] Australian Nurses' Journal, 3 (6), Dec 1973/Jan 1974, 35–37.

29 New South Wales Planning for personal health services. [New South Wales proposals.] Australian Nurses' Journal, 2 (8), Feb 1973, 22–25.

30 Nursing Mirror New courses in field skills prepare Australian nurses for the outback. Nursing Mirror, 137, 19 Oct 1973, 38–40.

31 Nursing Times Flying doctor. [Redevelopment of the Royal Flying Doctor Service.] Nursing Times, 71, 27 Nov 1975, Supplement 26–27.

32 Parkes, M. E. Goals in nursing. [Changes needed in nursing in Australia to meet changing needs of society.] Australian Nurses' Journal, 1 (10), Apr 1972, 35–37.

33 Patten, M.E. Australia, health issues and nursing. Australian Nurses' Journal, 4 (11), Jun 1975, 23–25, 44.

34 Philip, M. Health services and nursing: changing patterns. Australian Nurses' Journal, 2 (3), Sep 1972, 33–34; 2 (4), Oct 1972, 28–30. Feb 1973, 22–25.

35 Routledge, R. H. Past, present and the future of nursing in South Australia. SA Nurses Journal, 5 (15), May/Jun 1971, 14–15.

36 Royal Australian Nurses Federation RANF submission to the Committee on Health Careers (Personnel, Education and Training) established under the auspices of the National Hospital and Health Services Commission. Australian Nurses' Journal, 3 (10), May 1974, 21–23.

37 Schultz, B. Along the way. [Outline history of the Royal Australian Nursing Federation.] Australian Nurses' Journal, 4 (4), Oct 1974, 10–35.

38 Waring, J. E. Focus on change. A comparison of nursing roles – hospital and community. Australian Nurses' Journal, 3 (9), Apr 1974, 39–40.

39 Whittaker, Y. Cultural relativism and outback nursing. Australian Nurses' Journal, 4 (9), Apr 1975, 28–30.

NEW ZEALAND

40 Blazey, M. Work reaches fruition. [New Zealand Nurses' Association.] New Zealand Nursing Journal, 66 (6), Jun 1973, 4–6.

41 Bohm, S. M. A history of our health services. New Zealand Nursing Journal, 67 (12), Dec 1974, 12–13.

42 Chester, T. E. The New Zealand health service: another approach to integration. Hospital and Health Services Review, 71 (9), Sep 1975, 306–311.

43 De Montfort, M. Guidelines for nurses. [Implementation of changes in nursing following the Carpenter Report.] New Zealand Nursing Journal, 66 (3), Mar 1973, 5–6.

44 Fogarty, C. P. From 1900 to the present. [Development of nursing and nursing education.] New Zealand Nursing Journal, 66 (2), Feb 1973, 23–25.

45 Holdgate, E. We have a unique opportunity now. [Nursing in New Zealand.] New Zealand Nursing Journal, 64 (6), Jun 1971, 4–6.

46 Kennedy, D. P. Nursing development. [New Zealand.] New Zealand Nursing Journal, 64 (9), Sep 1971, 17–18.

47 McGuigan, T. Reorganization of the New Zealand health services. Royal Society of Health Journal, 95 (3), Jun 1975, 159–162.

48 Miller, N. R. Manpower planning. [Critical examination of health manpower literature with its relevance for nursing in New Zealand.] New Zealand Nursing Journal, 69 (6), Jun 1975, 25–28.

49 New Zealand. Department of Health A new direction for health. Wellington: The Department, 1975. Summary in New Zealand Nursing Journal, 68 (2), Feb 1975, 17–22.

50 New Zealand Nurses Association Nurses' views on the White Paper. Excerpts from New Zealand Nurses' Association submissions on the Government's White Paper. 'A Health Service for New Zealand'. New Zealand Nursing Journal, 69 (8), Aug 1975, 10–14; 69 (9), Sep 1975, 10–14; 69 (10), Oct 1975, 10–12.

51 New Zealand Nursing Journal Government proposals on restructuring. [New Zealand's health service reorganization and the effects on nursing.] New Zealand Nursing Journal, 69 (6), Jun 1975, 7–9.

52 Thomson, M. Change in nursing education. New Zealand Nursing Journal, 68 (12), Dec 1975, 22–23.

53 Wallis, M. Health services for adulthood [in New Zealand]. New Zealand Nursing Journal, 68 (1), Jan 1975, 10–11.

j CENTRAL AMERICA AND CARIBBEAN

1 Felsted, E. A quarter century of nursing education in Jamaica. Jamaican Nurse, 15 (2), Aug 1975, 15.

2 Galiano, S. Brief history of nursing in Nicaragua. International Journal of Nursing Studies, 12 (4), 1975, 223–229.

3 Glittenberg, J. Adapting health care to a cultural setting. [Guatemala.] American Journal of Nursing, 74 (12), Dec 1974, 2218–2221.

4 Jamaican Nurse Editorial on nursing education in Jamaica. Jamaican Nurse, 14 (2), Aug 1974, 3.

5 Liisberg, E. and Tabizbadeh, I. Revolution in health. [Interview with two WHO observers of health services in Cuba.] World Health, Apr 1975, 14–19.

6 Marshall, S. Regional nursing body [of the Commonwealth Caribbean.] Jamaican Nurse, 13 (1), Apr/May 1973, 18–22.

7 Moreno, G. T. and others Mexican Nurses Association: change for development. International Nursing Review, 19 (4), 1972, 370–376.

8 Mussallem, H. K. A glimpse of nursing in Cuba. Canadian Nurse, 69 (9), Sep 1973, 23–30.

9 Neff, C. and R. Problems and progress in Honduras. International Nursing Review, 22 (2), Mar/Apr 1975, 43–45.

10 Nurses Association of Jamaica Highlights of

NAJ's position paper. 'Blueprint for progress'. Jamaican Nurse, 12 (3), Dec 1972, 31–34.

11 O'Connor, R. 'Volunteering'. [Volunteer nursing in Central America.] World of Irish Nursing, 2 (7), Jul 1973, 129–131.

12 Pincheira, S. Latin America and the Caribbean – the health future. [Report of a meeting called by Pan American Health Office.] International Nursing Review, 20 (6), Nov/Dec 1973, 188–190.

13 Seivwright, M. J. The practice of nursing. [Implications of American theories for Jamaica.] Jamaican Nurse, 15 (2), Aug 1975, 20–21.

14 Tulloch, E. E. Historical perspectives of nursing in Jamaica. International Nursing Review, 18 (1), 1971, 49–57.

15 Vasquez, E. S. and others Nursing resources in Mexico. [Survey being carried out by the Department of Health and Social Welfare, Mexico.] International Nursing Review, 20 (1), Jan/Feb 1973, 22–24.

k NORTH AMERICA

GENERAL

1 Mackie, J. Nursing education in the U.S.A. and Canada. Australian Nurses' Journal, 2 (3), Sep 1972, 30–31.

2 Smith, J. P. Nursing in North America. [Report of a 15 week study tour to examine nursing and nursing education in the USA and Canada.] Nursing Mirror, 139, 28 Nov 1974, 53–56.

CANADA

3 Arcand, L. New health programs in Quebec – a trend for the future. Canadian Nurse, 68 (12), Dec 1972, 27–30.

4 Beswetherick, M. A. What does 'RN' after your name really mean? Canadian Nurse, 68 (10), Oct 1972, 27–28.

5 Clark, J. A. Future health services: British implications for Canadian reform. Canadian Hospital, 50 (7), Jul 1973, 32–37.

6 Germaine, A. Facing the issues. [Nursing education in Canada.] Hospital Administration in Canada, 16 (2), Feb 1974, 19–20.

7 Hill, M. and others Nursing in the sky. [Saskatchewan Air Ambulance Service.] Canadian Nurse, 71 (1), Jan 1975, 23–26.

8 Hospital Administration in Canada Canada's hospitals and health service system. [An overview.] Hospital Administration in Canada, 15 (5), May 1973, S1–S16.

9 Keith, C. W. What is outpost nursing? Canadian Nurse, 67 (9), Sep 1971, 41–44.

10 LaLonde, M. A new perspective on the health of Canadians: a working document. Ottawa: Ministry of National Health and Welfare, 1974.

11 Mustard, J. F. The Mustard report. [Report of the Health Planning Task Force; report commissioned by the Ontario Government.] Hospital Administration in Canada, 16 (11), Nov 1974, 31–34.

12 Pickering, G. L. Education in transition. [Nursing education in Canada.] Hospital Administration in Canada, 16 (2), Feb 1974, 21–22.

13 Rudy, W. A. Planning for comprehensive health care: a planning approach which incorporates all health services, agencies and professionals. Hospital Administration in Canada, 17 (3), Mar 1975, 18–20.

14 Snell, B. Do nurses belong in hospital schools?

[Educational trends in nursing in Canada.] Dimensions in Health Service, 51 (5), May 1974, 41–44.

15 Spruce, J. M. Nursing in Canada. Nursing Times, 69, 22 Nov 1973, 1578–1579.

16 Prichard, M. The education of nurses. Canadian Nurse, 68 (6), Jun 1972, 30–36.

UNITED STATES

17 Allan, A. M. A Britisher looks at American nursing. RN Magazine, 34 (12), Dec 1971, 36–37, 60, 62–64.

18 Altman, S. H. Present and future supply of registered nurses. Washington: US Government Printing Office, 1972.

19 American Journal of Nursing On the health care horizon: nursing issues. [Two articles and a discussion between nursing leaders.] American Journal of Nursing, 75 (10), Oct 1975, 1833–1859.

20 Angelinetta, S. J. Health care in the USA. Health and Social Service Journal, 84, 23 Mar 1974, 668–669.

21 Buttimore, A. A. Aspects of nurse education and service in America. Queen's Nursing Journal, 18 (4), Jul 1975, 110, 115.

22 Cathcart, H. R. Challenge for change. [Health care in the United States.] Hospitals, 49 (1), 1 Jan 1975, 39–43.

23 Coigney, V. Nursing in the U.S.A: a field for dedicated women. World Health, Dec 1972, 12–17.

24 Dunn, A. First things first. [Study tour to report on the health care system in the United States.] Nursing Times, 71, 15 May 1975, 788–789.

25 Dunn, A. Five articles on aspects of nursing in the USA. Nursing Times, 10 Jul 1975, 1082–1091.

26 Dunn, A. The game of the name. [Report of a National League for Nursing convention.] Nursing Times, 71, 19 Jun 1975, 956–957.

27 Frank, R. K. Societal and educational challenges to health care personnel in the United States: an overview of new directions in the education and role of the professional nurse in the United States. International Nursing Review, 19 (2), 1972, 180–185.

28 Freeman, R. H. NLN at twenty: challenge and change. Nursing Outlook, 20, Jun 1972, 376–384.

29 Graves, H. H. Survival in the system. [The role of the professional nurse in the American health system of the future.] Journal of Nursing Administration, 3 (4), Jul/Aug 1973, 26–31.

30 Hodgson, J. Land of contrasts: a surgeon's view of nursing in the USA. Nursing Times, 71, 7 Aug 1975, 1268–1269.

31 Journal of Nursing Administration The changing health scene: impact on and problems for nursing. Journal of Nursing Administration, 4 (2), Mar/Apr 1974, 20–23.

32 Kinsella, C. R. Nursing. [Review of developments in United States 1974 with reference to the literature.] Hospitals, 49 (7), 1 Apr 1975, 101–105.

33 Lord, D. Health services in the USA. Health and Social Service Journal, 83, 18 Aug 1973, 1864.

34 National Commission for the Study of Nursing and Nursing Education. An abstract for action by Jerome P. Lysaught. New York: McGraw-Hill, 1970. Summarised in American Journal of Nursing, 70 (2), Feb 1970, 279–294.

35 National Commission for the Study of Nursing and Nursing Education From abstract into action. New York: McGraw Hill, 1973.

36 National League for Nursing NLN: past, present and future. [Editorial.] Nursing Outlook, 20 (6), Jun 1972, 375.

37 Quin, P. North Carolina Memorial Hospital. Nursing Mirror, 140, 12 Jun 1975, 67–68.

38 Scott, J. M. Federal support for nursing education 1964–1972. [Discussion of its effect on nursing service.] American Journal of Nursing, 72 (10), Oct 1972, 1855–1861.

39 Sharp, B. H. The beginnings of nursing education in the United States: an analysis of the times. Journal of Nursing Education, 12 (2), Apr 1973, 26–32.

40 Simonson, E. Orientation in Alaska. Nursing Times, 68, 7 Dec 1972, 1565.

41 Smith, G. R. From invisibility to blackness. The story of the National Black Nurses' Association. Nursing Outlook, 23 (4), Apr 1975, 225–229.

42 Wilson, J. M. The largest hospital in the world. A visit to Pilgrim State Hospital, New York State. Hospital and Health Services Review, 69 (2), Feb 1973, 55–59.

43 Wilson Barnett, J. Nursing in America. Nursing Times, 70, 27 Jun 1974, 1006–1008.

44 Wright, L. M. Health care services in 1975 – a system or non-system? [A brief review of the United States health service.] AANA Journal, 43 (4), Aug 1975, 394–397.

UNITED STATES: OVERSEAS NURSES

45 Bachu, A. Indian nurses in the United States. International Nursing Review, 20 (4), Jul/Aug 1973, 114–116.

46 Berglas, C. British nurses in New York: some differences between nursing in Great Britain and New York State. Nursing Mirror, 135 (1), 7 Jul 1972, 41.

47 Dudas, S. and Dzik, M. A. Working with the foreign nurse in the United States. Journal of Nursing Education, 10 (1), Apr 1971, 27–31.

48 Dunn, A. USA. 'Wish you were here.' [Recruitment of British nurses and the problems they face.] Nursing Times, 71, 10 Jul 1975, 1087–1088.

49 Jordan, M. Working as a nurse in the USA. Nursing Mirror, 132, 19 Mar 1971, 40–42.

50 Olesen, V. and Davis, A. J. Preliminary findings on factors in the recruitment of foreign students. Nursing Research, 20 (2), Mar/Apr 1971, 159–162.

51 Rayner, R. A. and Jones, B. L. Adaptation. Selected problems of adaptation of the exchange visitor nurse and the seminar approach. [Columbia Presbyterian Medical Centre, New York City.] International Nursing Review, 19 (2), 1972, 140–149.

52 Sweeny, V. K. Working with nurses from overseas. American Journal of Nursing, 73 (10), Oct 1975, 1768–1770.

29 NATIONAL HEALTH SERVICE

a GENERAL

1 Abel-Smith, B. The politics of health. New Society, 18, 29 Jul 1971, 190–192.

2 Abel-Smith, B. Society at work. Managing the health service. New Society, 17, 29 Apr 1971, 721–722.

3 Bosanquet, N. Talking point. Planning the NHS. Nursing Times, 71, 27 Mar 1975, 486.

4 Brown, R. G. S. The changing National Health

Service. Routledge & Kegan Paul, 1973. (Library of Social Policy and Administration).

5 Castle, B. Serious. [The state of the NHS. Address to the conference of the National Association of Health Authorities.] Hospital and Health Services Review, 71 (8), Aug 1975, 257–260.

6 Chisholm, M. K. Maintenance and repair: a Health Visitor's view of the function of the NHS. Nursing Mirror, 140, 23 Jan 1975, 70–71.

7 Forsythe, G. Doctors and state medicine: a study of the British health service. 2nd ed. Pitman, 1973.

8 Godber, G. The health service: past, present and future. Athlone Press, (University of London Heath Clark lectures 1973), 1975.

9 Hardie, M. C. Pointers for the future. Community Medicine, 129, 23 Feb 1973, 379–383.

10 Joseph, Sir K. Sir Keith Joseph surveys the NHS achievements and failures. [Excerpts from Marsden Lecture.] British Medical Journal, 4, 1 Dec 1973, 561–562.

11 Klein, R. An anatomy of the NHS. New Society, 24, 28 Jun 1973, 739–741.

12 McGarrick, H. The first 25 years. . . [Pictorial record of developments in the NHS.] Nursing Times, 69, 23 Aug 1973, 1093–1097.

13 McLachlan, G., editor Challenges for change: essays on the next decade in the National Health Service. Oxford University Press/Nuffield Provincial Hospitals Trust, 1971.

14 McLachlan, G., editor Probes for health: essays from the Health Services Research Centre, University of Birmingham. Oxford University Press/Nuffield Provincial Hospitals Trust, 1975.

15 Mee, B. Crisis in the National Health Service. Midwives Chronicle, 88, Dec 1975, 399–400.

16 Nursing Times Wales. The National Health Service in Wales. Nursing Times, 70, 21 Nov 1974, 1808–1809.

17 Owen, D. Dr. Owen on problems of the NHS. [Extracts from a speech given at the Association of Hospital Secretaries annual conference.] Hospital and Health Services Review, 71 (2), Feb 1975, 62–63.

18 Rayner, C. Centre lunch talk – Priorities in health care. Health and Social Service Journal, 84, 14 Dec 1974, 2875; Hospital and Health Services Review, 70 (12), Dec 1974, 421.

19 Teeling-Smith, G. Health service priorities – hospital or community care? Hospital, 67 (6), Jun 1971, 199–203.

20 Yellowlees, H. The development and future of the National Health Service. District Nursing, 13 (10), Jan 1971, 194–195.

b COMMUNITY HEALTH COUNCILS

1 Dunnell, K. and Owen, J.W. Putting over the patient's view. [Community health councils.] Health and Social Service Journal, 84, 16 Feb 1974, 361–362.

2 Hallas, J. and Fallon, B. Mounting the health guard: a handbook for community health council members. Nuffield Provincial Hospitals Trust, 1974.

3 Health Visitor Community health councils. [Editorial.] Health Visitor, 48 (6), Jun 1975, 197.

4 Hospital and Health Services Review Community health councils. [Review of achievements.] Hospital and Health Services Review, 71 (9), Sep 1975, 320–321. Summary of some annual reports, 71 (12), Dec 1975, 437–438.

5 Johnson, M. CHCs: competing interests. Health and Social Service Journal, 85, 12 Jul 1975, 1467–1468.

6 Klein, R. NHS consumers. [The proposals for a National Council of Community Health Councils.] New Society, 32, 13 Feb 1975, 392.

7 Klein, R. and Lewis, J. Community health councils – the early days. Health and Social Service Journal, 84, 7 Dec 1974, 2824–2825.

8 Klein, R. and Lewis, J. Society at work. NHS brokers or activists? [The work of the community health councils.] New Society, 30, 28 Nov 1974, 547–548.

9 McEwan, P. J. M. Consumer participation in the health service. [The case for elected community health councils.] Community Medicine, 129, 8 Dec 1972, 189–191.

10 Mackeith, J. C. Community participation in health care. Hospital and Health Services Review, 70 (12), Dec 1974, 425–428.

11 Marre, R. M. Community health councils – a personal view. Health Trends, 7 (3), Aug 1975, 45–46.

12 Nash, P. Another body of snoopers? [Community health councils.] Nursing Mirror, 140, 3 Apr 1975, 65–66.

13 Orriss, H. D. Community health councils – watchdogs or lapdogs? Nursing Times, 70, 13 Jun 1974, 928–929.

14 Page, J. A strategy for community health councils. Health and Social Service Journal, 85, 8 Feb 1975, 295–296.

15 Singer, A. W. Membership of a community health council. Queen's Nursing Journal, 18 (1), Apr 1975, 10–11.

16 Taylor, J. E. Community health councils. [In the reorganized NHS] Health and Social Service Journal, 83, 14 Apr 1973, 845–846.

17 Topliss, E. The role of community health councils. Royal Society of Health Journal, 95 (6), Dec 1975, 299–301.

18 Weightman, G. Health councils. [Progress after the first year.] New Society, 32, 5 Jun 1975, 591.

19 Williamson, C. Community health councils and the quality of caring. Hospital and Health Services Review, 71 (8), Aug 1975, 270–271.

c COMPUTERS

1 Abrams, M. E. Health services and the computer. 8. Real-time computing in general practice. Health Trends, 4 (1), Feb 1972, 18–20.

2 Barber, B. and Scholes, M. Health services and the computer. 4. An approach to real-time computing at the London Hospital. Health Trends, 2, Jul 1970, 65–66.

3 Barker, J. Computers in hospitals: two approaches. Hospitals, 67 (8), Aug 1971, 279–282.

4 Bonner, B. B. Medical records and medical care. [Report of King's Fund Centre meeting on the role of the computer.] Health and Social Service Journal, 83, 14 Apr 1973, 857.

5 Grant, D. M. Computer based medical information. Midwife and Health Visitor, 10 (10), Oct 1974, 301–303.

6 Handby, J. G. Health services and the computer. 2. Computers in hospitals. Health Trends, 2 (2), Apr 1970, 41–43.

7 Harbord, W. E. and Knight, J. I. Management information and the computer. Hospital and Health Services Review, 68 (8), Aug 1972, 284–287.

8 Ironside, A. G. and others Use of a computer in an infectious diseases department. [At Monsall Hospital]. Community Medicine, 126 (9), 27 Aug 1971, 136–138.

9 Kenny, D. J. Confidentiality and the growth of computers. Hospital and Health Services Review, 71 (1), Jan 1975, 6–9.

10 Lancet Computers now. [Editorial on the NHS computer research and development programme.] Lancet, 1, 29 Mar 1975, 733–734.

11 The London Hospital computer system. Hospital and Health Services Review, 69 (6), Jun 1973, 220–222.

12 Reekie, D. and others The use of an independent network of semi-intelligent terminals for input to a hospital computer system. [Glasgow Western Infirmary.] Health Bulletin, 33 (5), Sep 1975, 214–219.

13 Rivett, G. C. Health service and the computer 9. Progress in health service computing. Health Trends, 7 (1), Feb 1975, 5–8.

14 Rivett, G. C. Health services and the computer 10. The management of the experimental computer program. Health Trends, 7 (1), Feb 1975, 9–10.

15 Sharratt, M. and Yare, D. Computer monitoring of hospital out-patient clinics: an assessment. Hospital and Health Services Review, 68 (11), Nov 1972, 398–402.

16 Snaith, A. H. Health services and the computer 5. The contribution of the computer to management in the community health services. Health Trends, 3 (1), Feb 1971, 10–11.

17 Spicer, C. C. Health services and the computer. 7. Computers in medical research. Health Trends, 3 (3), Aug 1971, 45–46.

18 Vickers, H. E. and others An inter-hospital comparison of a computerised patient information system which uses a regional computer. [Walton Hospital and Fazakerly Hospital.] Hospital and Health Services Review, 71 (12), Dec 1975, 422–424.

19 WHO Chronicle Hospital computing systems. WHO Chronicle, 26 (7), Jul 1972, 302–307.

20 Yates, J. M. Monitoring in the hospital service. Hospital and Health Services Review, 69 (9), Sep 1973, 322–326.

d FINANCE

1 Bosanquet, N. Talking point. Scrambled budgets. [Pre-31 March spending in the NHS.] Nursing Times, 71, 15 May 1975, 757.

2 British Medical Association and others The financing of the National Health Service [Document sent to the Prime Minister on 31 July 1974 from the British Medical Association, British Dental Association, Royal College of Nursing and the Royal College of Midwives.] British Medical Journal, 4, 2 Nov 1974, 297–300.

3 Castle, B. Cut back in National Health Service financing: Health Authority Chairmen asked to determine priorities. [Letter to health authorities.] Midwives Chronicle, 88, Nov 1975, 376–377.

4 Cooper, M. H. Rationing health. [Use of resources to meet health needs.] New Society, 28, 18 Apr 1974, 131–132.

5 Department of Health and Social Security Resource Allocation Working Party Allocations to regions in 1976/77. First interim report. DHSS, 1975, Chairman J. C. C. Smith.

6 Dunn, A. Hospital land. [Utilization of unused

hospital land as a new revenue source for the NHS.] Nursing Times, 71, 13 Nov 1975, 1804–1806.

7 Gentle, P. H. and Forsythe, J. M.   Revenue allocation in the reorganized Health Service. British Medical Journal, 3, 9 Aug 1975, 382–384.

8 Glass, N. J.   Cost-benefit analysis and health services. Health Trends, 5 (3), Aug 1973, 51–56.

9 Hospital and Health Services Review   Budgetary control in the reorganized health service. Hospital and Health Services Review, 69 (4), Apr 1973, 148–150.

10 Hulse, B. E.   The money game. [Budgetary control in the reorganized NHS.] Health and Social Service Journal, 83, 17 Mar 1973, 596.

11 Jones, D. R. and Bourne, A.   The distribution of resources in the National Health Service. Hospital and Health Services Review, 71 (11), Nov 1975, 382–384.

12 Klein, R.   Health service. [Implications of the First Interim Report of the Resource Allocation Working Party.] New Society, 34, 16 Oct 1975, 150.

13 Klein, R. and Buxton, M.   Health inequities. [Distribution of resources to the Area Health Authorities.] New Society, 30, 7 Nov 1974, 357–359.

14 Royal College of Nursing   Rcn seeks consultation on NHS priorities. 'Savings could be made by rationalising hospital services'. Nursing Times, 71, 25 Dec 1975, 2042.

15 Seabourn, H. W.   Financing the health and personal social services. Health Trends, 4 (3), Aug 1972, 42–46.

16 Tomalin, C.   Efficiency in the NHS. [Symposium on allocation of resources.] Health and Social Service Journal, 85, 12 Apr 1975, 807.

17 Tomalin, C.   Inflation and health expenditure. Health and Social Service Journal, 85, 10 May 1975, 1068.

18 Watkin, B.   Not a special case. [Comment on government expenditure in the health service.] Nursing Mirror, 141, 24 Jul 1975, 39.

19 Whithnell, A. and Barnes, R.   Programme budgeting in a local health authority. Community Medicine, 127 (4), 28 Jan 1972, 41–45.

20 Young, K.   Value for money in the health service. British Medical Journal, 1, 20 Jan 1973, 165–167.

e INFORMATION

1 Alderson, M. R.   Health information systems. WHO Chronicle, 28 (2), Feb 1974, 52–54. Reprinted in Health and Social Service Journal, 84, 2 Mar 1974, 482.

2 Alderson, M. R.   Towards a health information system. [Based on work in the Wessex Medical Information Unit.] Health and Social Service Journal, 83, 7 Jul 1973, 1524–1525.

3 Ashford, J. R. and others   Information requirements for district management in the reorganised NHS. Community Medicine, 129, 26 Jan 1973, 309–317.

4 Barnard, K.   Information services in the NHS. [A King's Fund Centre open day.] Health and Social Service Journal, 84, 14 Dec 1974, 2878–2879.

5 Bryant, D. J. and Mayes, P. E.   Improving information flow in the health service. [Project in Hull.] Hospital and Health Services Review, 69 (8), Aug 1973, 291–293.

6 Cooking, J.   Hospital information services. [As seen by the information officer, West Suffolk HMC.] Hospital and Health Services Review, 70 (2), Feb 1974, 44–45.

7 Elwood, E. J.   Health information systems in the National Health Service. Health and Social Service Journal, 84, 18 Jan 1975, 126–127.

8 Miles, D. P. B.   Information for areas. [Functions of an area information unit.] Health and Social Service Journal, 85, 27 Sep 1975, 2166.

9 Rowe, R. G.   Taking the measure of health service information. Hospital and Health Services Review, 69 (3), Mar 1973, 92–96.

10 Shaw, J. E.   Information rooms – decentralized unit management. [The function of the information room as a co-ordinator in unit organization developed by the Wessex Regional Hospital Board.] Health and Social Service Journal, 84, 7 Dec 1974, 2831.

f MANAGEMENT AND STAFFING

1 Banham, J. M. M.   Managing the reorganised health service. [Followed by discussion.] Hospital and Health Services Review, 69 (6), Jun 1973, 208–213.

2 Barnard, K.   Comprehensive health planning – the state of the art. Community Medicine, 129, 23 Feb 1973, 375–378.

3 Brookes, B.   Background thinking behind the comprehensive health planning seminar. Community Medicine, 129 (16), 2 Feb 1973, 324–325.

4 Brown, R. G. S.   Democracy in the NHS: an open letter to Mrs. Barbara Castle. Health and Social Service Journal, 84, 10 Aug 1974, 1799.

5 Browning, R. H.   The use of statistics in health service planning. [East Dorset field trial.] Health and Social Service Journal, 84, 16 Mar 1974, 598–600.

6 Department of Health and Social Security   Democracy in the NHS. [HSC (1S) 194.] DHSS, 1974. Implementation see Nuring Mirror, 141, 11 Sep 1975, 34.

7 Farham, D. and Burnett, B. J.   Industrial relations training for health service managers. Hospital and Health Services Review, 71 (8), Aug 1975, 265–269.

8 Ferrer, H. P.   Objectives of the NHS. Health and Social Service Journal, 83, 10 Mar 1973, 535–536.

9 Ferrer, H. P., editor   The health services – administration, research and management. Butterworth, 1972.

10 Gatherer, A. and Warren, M. D.   Management and the health services. Oxford: Pergamon, 1971. vice.] Nursing Times, 68, 21 Sep 1972, 1176.

11 Hallas, J.   Two cheers for bureaucracy. [Management arrangement and the health service.] Hospital and Health Services Review, 69 (4), Apr 1973, 123–125.

12 Haywood, S. C.   Managing the health service. Allen and Unwin, 1974.

13 Hunter, T. D.   Planning for health in Scotland. [Functions of the Scottish Health Service Planning Council.] Health and Social Service Journal, 85, 26 Jul 1975, 1600–1601.

14 Jerrome, K.   Industrial relations in the health service – the Southampton way. Nursing Mirror, 136, 5 Jan 1973, 12–13.

15 Jones, A.   Training for personnel in the health service. Personnel Management, 5 (5), May 1973, 35–37.

16 Lemin, B.   Line/staff relationships. [With particular reference to the health service.] Health and Social Service Journal, 83, 11 Aug 1973, 1809.

17 McLachlan, G., editor   Measuring for management: quantitative methods in health service management. Essays by J. R. Ashford and others. Oxford University Press/Nuffield Provincial Hospitals Trust, 1975.

18 March, D. C.   Industrial relations in the health service. Hospital and Health Services Review, 70 (1), Jan 1974, 16–19.

19 Maxwell, R.   Management for health. British Medical Journal, 1, 20 Jan 1973, 160–164.

20 Mowan, A. J.   Management services [in the reorganized NHS.] Health and Social Service Journal, 83, 1973, 1632, 1634.

21 Paine, L. H. W.   An aroma of bureaucracy. [Health service administration.] Health and Social Service Journal, 83, 6 Jan 1973, 27.

22 Picton, G.   Management in the health service – a rejoinder. Hospital and Health Services Review, 71 (3), Mar 1975, 89–90.

23 Piller, G.   Manpower and the National Health Service. Community Health, 3 (1), Jul–Aug 1971, 29–32.

24 Smith, I. G.   Management by objectives and the health service. Health and Social Service Journal, 84, 20 Jul 1974, 1622–1623.

25 Speakman, A. J.   Management in the health service – the myth and the reality. Hospital and Health Services Review, 71, Jan 1975, 19–21.

26 Stubbs, V.   Management/employee relationships in the NHS. Queen's Nursing Journal, 18 (5), Aug 1975, 145–146.

27 Stubbs, V.   Reaching and teaching older staff in the health service. Nursing Mirror, 139, 17 Oct 1974, 78–80.

28 Sugden, J. P.   Personnel – policy and practice in the new NHS. Health and Social Service Journal, 83, 3 Nov 1973, 2554.

29 Sugden, J. P. and Pearce, S. G.   Personnel management – the first year. Achievements, problems, opportunities [after reorganization.] Hospital and Health Services Review, 71 (5), May 1975, 162–165.

30 Tyrell, M.   Using numbers for effective health service management. Heinemann, 1975.

31 Watkin, B.   Management in the reorganised health service. 1. The framework. Nursing Mirror, 140, 16 Jan 1975, 44–46.

32 Watkin, B.   Management in the reorganised Health Service. 2. Talking the language. Nursing Mirror, 140, 23 Jan 1975, 55–56.

33 Watkin, B.   Management in the reorganised Health Service. 3. Awkward relations. Nursing Mirror, 140, 30 Jan 1975, 54–55. Corrected version, 140, 13 Nov 1975, 69–70.

34 Watkin, B.   Management in the reorganised Health Service. 4. A say for the staff. Nursing Mirror, 140, 6 Feb 1975, 60–61.

35 Watkin, B.   Management in the reorganised Health Service. 5. Money matters. Nursing Mirror, 140, 13 Feb 1975, 61–62.

36 Watkin, B.   Management in the reorganised Health Service. 6. Best laid plans. Nursing Mirror, 140, 20 Feb 1975, 51–52.

37 Watkin, B.   Management in the reorganised Health Service. 7. Personnel priorities. Nursing Mirror, 140, 27 Feb 1975, 63–64.

38 Watkin, B.   Management in the reorganised Health Service. 8. Changing times. Nursing Mirror, 140, 6 Mar 1975, 70–71.

39 Wilcox, B.   Questions of monitoring. [A clarification of the management concept of monitoring with particular reference to the health service.] Hospital and Health Services Review, 70 (12), Dec 1974, 428–430.

40 Wiles, B. M. Participative management in the NHS. Health and Social Service Journal, 84, 26 Oct 1974, 2470–2471.

41 Zardin, J. Personnel arrangements in the new service. Hospital and Health Services Review, 69 (12), Dec 1973, 454–456.

g MANAGEMENT PLANNING

1 Draper, P. Value judgements in health planning. Community Medicine, 129 (19), 23 Feb 1973, 372–374.

2 Dummer, J. The planning function. Community Medicine, 129 (17), 9 Feb 1973, 340–343.

3 Eskin, F. The reality of health care planning teams. [Barnsley Area Health Authority.] Health and Social Service Journal, 84, 9 Nov 1974, 2596–2597. Progress report, 85, Nov 1975, 2449.

4 Ferrer, H. P. Data for health planning. Health and Social Service Journal, 83, 25 Aug 1973, 1920.

5 Gooding, D. Planning – strategies, policies and implementation. [In relation to health services.] Community Medicine, 129 (17), 9 Feb 1973, 343–346.

6 Gourlay, J. R. Getting the new team together. [NHS reorganization.] Health and Social Service Journal, 84, 6 Apr 1974, 779–780.

7 Grime, P. Integrated planning in the reorganised NHS. Hospital and Health Services Review, 70 (3), Mar 1974, 90–92.

8 Hallas, J. Team work [in management in the reorganized NHS.] Health and Social Service Journal, 84, 2 Mar 1974, 489.

9 Hardie, M. C. Practical steps towards comprehensive health planning. Community Medicine, 129 (16), 2 Feb 1973, 325–330.

10 Hospital and Health Services Review An NHS planning system. [Circular HRC (73) 8.] Hospital and Health Services Review, 69 (6), Jun 173, 193–194.

11 Howells, W. Importance of teams. [District management teams and health care planning teams in the reorganized NHS.] Health and Social Service Journal, 84, 20 Jul 1974, 1626–1627.

12 Rushworth, V. Manpower planning at district level. Nursing Times, 71, 18 Dec 1975, 2032–2033.

13 Schaefer, M. A management method for planning and implementing health projects. WHO Chronicle, 29 (1), Jan 1975, 18–23.

14 Sharpe, D. Thoughts on team management. [Multi-disciplinary hospital teams]. Hospital and Health Services Review, 70 (8), Aug 1974, 268–270.

15 Sumner, G. The context of comprehensive health planning. Community Medicine, 129 (16), 2 Feb 1973, 331–334.

16 Swaffield, L. 1984 and after. [Development plans outlined by South Glamorgan Area Health Authority.] Nursing Times, 71, 16 Jan 1975, 90–91.

17 Swaffield, L. Teamtalk. [Experiments at West Middlesex Hospital in ward teamwork, involving multi-disciplinary meetings.] Nursing Times, 71, 3 Jul 1975, 1036.

18 Thomas, C. H. Choosing health service teams. [Principles for team organization.] Health and Social Service Journal, 84, 23 Nov 1974, 2708–2709.

19 Watkin, B. Health care planning – comprehensive planning. [Themes to the 'Guide to Planning in the NHS' by B. Watkin.] Health and Social Service Journal, 85, 20 Sep 1975, 2097–2098.

20 Watkin, B. Health care planning – participation and central control. Hospital and Health Service Journal, 85, 27 Sep 1975, 2169–2170.

21 Weddell, J. M. and others Education for health planning [in an integrated health service.] Health and Social Service Journal, 83, 19 May 1973, 1129–1130.

22 Wilcox, B. Teams selected. But what are the rules of the game? A consideration of some aspects of team management. [District management teams in the reorganized NHS.]. Hospital and Health Services Review, 69 (12), Dec 1973, 450–454.

h MANAGEMENT TRAINING

1 Barnwell, M. and others Management courses compared. [Three sets of courses are described and compared.] Health and Social Service Journal, 85, 13 Sep 1975, 2024–2025.

2 Barnwell, M. and others Towards and effective management programme. [Middle management courses at Leicester Polytechnic.] Health and Social Service Journal, 85, 12 Apr 1975, 805–806.

3 Bosanquet, N. NHS organizers. [Report from the Business Graduates Association on inadequate training of senior managers.] New Society, 32, 1 May 1975, 273.

4 Lewin, B. Modular training: an alternative form of management development training. Hospital and Health Services Review, 49 (7), Jul 1973, 248–250.

5 Powell, M. and Maddox, G. R. In the right direction? A viewpoint on training. [An experiment in training supervisors at Nevill Hall Hospital, Abergavenny.] Health and Social Service Journal, 84, 18 Aug 1974, 1858–1859.

6 Watkin, B. Management training for the new NHS. [Six week course in management at the University of Manchester.] Health and Social Service Journal, 83, 16 Jun 1973, 1367–1368.

7 Watkin, B. Teaching methods in management education: [in the heath service]. Nursing Times, 70, 24 Oct 1974, Occ. papers, 89–92.

8 Watkin, B. Training the trainers. [Management education in the health service.] British Hospital Journal and Social Service Review, 82, 30 Sep 1972, 2180.

9 West, C. The role of business schools. [In providing managerial education for health service administrators.] British Hospital Journal and Social Service Review, 82, 30 Sep 1972, 3183–3184.

10 Westbrook, K. Management courses – are they a waste of time? Nursing Times, 71, 30 Jan 1975, 190–191.

11 White, D. Business management for administrators. 1–3. [Assessment of management courses in the NHS.] Health and Social Service Journal, 84, 12 Oct 1974, 2354; 19 Oct 1974, 2414; 26 Oct 1974, 2478.

12 White, D. Management education in health care. Hospital and Health Services Review, 68 (1), Jan 1972, 5–9.

13 Wild, R. Management education and the health service: an opinion. [Role of business management schools and colleges.] Hospital and Health Services Review, 71 (10), Oct 1975, 353–354.

i MEDICAL STAFF

1 Bosanquet, N. Talking point. A very traditional report. [Merrison Committee report.] Nursing Times, 71, 1 May 1975, 679.

2 Carne, S. The Hunter Report. (b) A G.P.'s point of view. Royal Society of Health Journal, 93 (1), Feb 1973, 40–41.

3 Committee of Inquiry into the Regulation of the Medical Profession Report. HMSO, 1975, Cmnd. 6018. Chairman: Dr. A. W. Merrison.

4 Department of Health and Social Security. Working Party on Medical Administrators Report. HMSO, 1972. Chairman: Dr R. B. Hunter.

5 Galloway, T. McL. The Hunter Report. (c) A M.O.H.'s view. Royal Society of Health Journal, 93 (1), Feb 1973, 44–45.

6 Field, I. T. 'Cogwheels.' [The three Cogwheel reports.] Health Trends, 6 (2), May 1974, 25–27.

7 Health Visitors' Association Memorandum to the working party on medical administration. Health Visitor, 44 (5), May 1971, 166.

8 Heath, P. J. The medical administrator in the National Health Service. Community Health, 5 (4), Jan/Feb 1974, 178–182.

9 Howat, H. T. Doctors in management – 1. Cogwheel and multi-disciplinary management in the United Manchester Hospitals. Health and Social Service Journal, 83, 1 Dec 1973, 2816–2818.

10 Hill, S. G. Medical administrators. [Doctors or professional administrators?]. Health and Social Service Journal, 83, 6 Jan 1973, 25–26.

11 Mackenzie, A. S. The region and the regional medical officer. Queen's Nursing Journal, 18 (5), Aug 1975, 136–137.

12 Nuttall, C. S. The doctor as manager: a commentary on the Cogwheel report. Hospital and Health Services Review, 70, Feb 1974, 52–57.

13 Smith, A. The Hunter Report. (a) An academic view. Royal Society of Health Journal, 93 (1), Feb 1973, 42–44.

j PATIENTS' RIGHTS

1 Abel-Smith, B. Society at work. A hospital ombudsman? New Society, 17, 22 Apr 1971, 672–674.

2 Baker, A. Dr. Baker reviews the HAS. [Hospital Advisory Service.] Health and Social Service Journal, 133, 15 Sep 1973, 2114–2115.

3 Barrowclough, F. and Pinel, C. Complaints in geriatric hospitals. Nursing Times, 71, 16 Jan 1975, 118.

4 Bosanquet, N. When things go wrong. [The work of the health ombudsman and Hospital Advisory Service in dealing with complaints from patients.] Nursing Times, 70, 12 Dec 1974, 1920–1921.

5 Brown, R. G. S. Whose hand on the scalpel? [Effect on patient of the NHS new 'unified' structure.] New Society, 25, 6 Sep 1973, 574–576.

6 Bryant, R. J. S. The Health Service Commissioner, his function and how he performs it. Hospital and Health Services Review, 70 (5), May 1974, 149–151.

7 Cooper, P. A glimmer of light: what is reorganization doing for the patient? Nursing Mirror, 141, 13 Nov 1975, 41–42.

8 Cooper, P. What will reorganization do for the patient? Lancet 1, 13 Apr 1974, 670–671.

9 Department of Health and Social Security Committee on Hospital Complaints Procedure. Report. HMSO, 1973. Chairman: Sir Michael Davies.

10 Health and Social Service Journal A patient's right. [Of access to his own medical record. Leading article.] Health and Social Service Journal, 84, 16 Mar 1974, 587–588.

11 Health Service Commissioner Annual report 1973/74 – 1974/75. HMSO, 1974–1975.

12 **Hodgson, H.** Hobson's choice in the NHS. [Patient's rights in the NHS.] Health and Social Service Journal, 85, 6 Sep 1975, 1965.

13 **Hodgson, H.** A service for all. Helen Hodgson [Founder and Chairman of the Patients Association talks to Helen McCarrick.] Nursing Times, 69, 8 Nov 1973, 1500–1501.

14 **Hodgson, H.** Twelve years of patients. [Patients' Association.] Nursing Mirror, 140, 23 Jan 1975, 75–76.

15 **Hospital** Complaints. [Hospital complaints procedures.] Hospital, 67 (8), Aug 1971, 283–284.

16 **Hospital** Ombudsman. [In the hospital and health service.] Hospital, 67 (10), Oct 1971, 340–342.

17 **Hospital Advisory Service** Annual reports 1969/70–1975. HMSO, 1971–1975.

18 **Hospital Advisory Service** HAS finds big gap in communications. [Annual report of Hospital Advisory Service.] Nursing Times, 69, 21 Jun 1973, 785.

19 **Hospital and Health Services Review** Complaints. [Editorial on the Davies Committee.] Hospital and Health Services Review, 70 (2), Feb 1974, 37–39.

20 **Klein, R.** The health commissioner. Lancet, 1, 26 Feb 1972, 482–484.

21 **Klein, R.** Society at work. Hospital grumbles. [Hospital complaints and the work of the Health Commissioner.] New Society, 25, 19 Jul 1973, 143–144.

22 **Klein, R.** Who is the patient's friend? Role of the ombudsman. [Tape recorded discussion.] British Medical Journal, 2, 2 Jun 1973, 528–532.

23 **Marre, A.** The NHS Ombudsman: Sir Alan Marre, the Health Service Commissioner, talks about his work to Pat Young. Nursing Mirror, 140, 23 Jan 1975, 40–41.

24 **Marre, A.** NHS failings highlighted by complaints: the Ombudsman's first annual report. Nursing Mirror, 140, 26 Jun 1975, 36.

25 **Marre, A.** Reflections of the Health Service Commissioner. Queen's Nursing Journal, 18 (9), Dec 1975, 241–242, 244–245.

26 **Metcalfe, D. H. H.** Will the patient care? [Patients' attitudes in the NHS.] Public Health, 87, 5, Jul 1973, 195–198.

27 **Nursing Mirror** Proposals for health service ombudsman. Nursing Mirror, 133, 13 Aug 1971, 7–9.

28 **Robb, B.** Hospital Advisory Service. Nursing Times, 71, 24 Apr 1975, 646–647.

29 **Robb, B.** Sans everything and after. [Events leading to the formation of the Hospital Advisory Service and inquiries into seven longstay hospitals.] Nursing Times, 71, 24 Apr 1975, 644–646.

30 **Royston, R.** Humane laws equal humane hospitals. [MIND conference on the legal position of the patient.] Health and Social Service Journal, 85, 22 Nov 1975, 2610.

31 **Scarlett, J.** Health service commissioner. Nursing Times, 70, 24 Jan 1974, 118–119.

32 **Stacey, M.** Consumer responsibilities and rights in the health service. Queen's Nursing Journal, 18 (2), May 1975, 42, 48.

33 **Stewart, T.** The reorganization of the National Health Service (f) The viewpoint of the patient. Royal Society of Health Journal, 92 (1), Jan/Feb 1972, 32–34.

34 **Swaffield, L.** The first year. [Summary of the Health Service Commissioner's first report.] Nursing Times, 71, 26 Jun 1975, 997.

35 **Townsend, P.** Inequality and the health service. [The right of the sick to free access to health care, irrespective of class or income.] Lancet, 1, 15 Jun 1974, 1179–1190.

36 **University of Sussex Centre for Social Research** The consumer and the Health Service. [Preliminary report criticizing Health Service reorganization proposals.] Health Visitor, 46 (2), Feb 1973, 38–40.

37 **Weaver, N. D. W.** Community participation in the welfare state and hospitals. Hospital, 67 (10), Oct 1971, 347–51.

k PATIENTS' RIGHTS: OVERSEAS COUNTRIES

1 **American Hospital Association** Statement on a patients' bill of rights. Hospitals 47 (4), 16 Feb 1973, 41. Summarized in Nursing Outlook, 21 (2), Feb 1973, 82.

2 **Annas, G. J. and Healey, J.** The patient rights advocate. Journal of Nursing Administration, 4 (3), May/Jun 1974, 25–31.

3 **Bihldorff, J. P.** Personalized care assures patients' rights. [Patient care committee at McMaster University.] Dimensions in Health Service 52 (7), Jul 1975, 36–39.

4 **Goose, M. and Dickinson, A.** Role of the consumer in the USA. [His influence over the development of health care compared to his British counterpart.] Health and Social Service Journal, 84, 13 Apr 1974, 834–835.

5 **International Nursing Review** The patients' rights. Patients' Bill of Rights. International Nursing Review, 20 (5), Sep/Oct 1973, 156.

6 **Morgan, D. M.** At Montreal General: the patient advocate: a new aid for emergency. Canadian Hospital, 50 (8), Aug 1973, 24–25.

7 **Nations, W. C.** Nurse-lawyer is patient-advocate. American Journal of Nursing, 73 (6), Jun 1973, 1039–1041.

8 **New Zealand Nursing Journal** White Paper submissions. [Part of a submission to the Minister of Health on patients' rights.] New Zealand Nursing Journal, 69 (10), Oct 1975, 19–20.

9 **Quinn, N. and Somers, A. R.** The patient's bill of rights: a significant aspect of the consumer revolution. Nursing Outlook, 22 (4), Apr 1974, 240–244.

10 **Rozovsky, L. E.** A Canadian patient's bill of rights. Dimensions in Health Service, 51 (12), Dec 1974, 8–10.

11 **Slavinsky, A. T. and Romoff, V.** Consumer participation, Journal of Nursing Administration, 11 (3), May/Jun 1972, 14–18.

l POLITICS

1 **Bosanquet, N.** The NHS as a vote catcher. [The three major parties' policies towards health.] Nursing Times, 70, 10 Oct 1974, 1565.

2 **Britih Medical Journal** Election manifestos. [Sections on health.] British Medical Journal, 3, 21 Sep 1974, 750–751; 4, 5 Oct 1974, 54.

3 **Howe, Sir G.** The NHS today – the Conservative view. Nursing Mirror's Parliamentary Correspondent talks to Sir Geoffrey Howe, Conservative Shadow Minister for Social Services, about the future of the caring professions. Nursing Mirror, 139, 19 Sep 1974, 33–34.

4 **Owen, D.** Spanning the services. Caroline Tomalin interviews Dr. David Owen, Under-Secretary of State for Health. Health and Social Service Journal, 84, 24 Aug 1974, 1924.

5 **Winstanley, M.** The NHS today – the Liberal view. Nursing Mirror, 139, 26 Sep 1974, 40–41.

m PRIVATE PRACTICE

1 **Bosanquet, N.** Talking point. Private practice. Nursing Times, 70, 25 Jun 1974, 1143.

2 **Cohen, A.** In sickness and in wealth: going private. Compares private nursing with nursing in the NHS. Nursing Mirror, 141, 7 Aug 1975, 67.

3 **Department of Health and Social Security and others** Private practice in National Health Service hospitals. HMSO, (Cmnd. 5270), 1973.

4 **Department of Health and Social Security and others** The separation of private practice from National Health Hospitals: a consultative document. The Department, 1975.

5 **Dicker, K.** Open forum. Private patients – a point of view. Nursing Mirror, 139, 21 Nov 1974, 39.

6 **Drain, G.** The case against private practice. Health and Social Service Journal, 83, 7 Apr 1973, 788.

7 **Fowler, N.** Pay beds – opposition view. [An interview which gives views on proposed legislation to phase out private practice in the NHS.] Nursing Mirror, 140, 22/29 May 1975, 39.

8 **Jolly, C. R.** Independent hospitals. Health and Social Service Journal, 83, 31 Mar 1973, 724–726; 7 Apr 1973, 786–787; 14 Apr 1973, 848–849, 851.

9 **Klein, R.** Is there a case for private practice? British Medical Journal, 4, 6 Dec 1975, 591–592.

10 **Lee, M.** Opting out of the NHS: a review of the private sector of medical care. PEP, 1971.

11 **Lewin, W.** Private medicine will be a key issue in year ahead. [BMA representative meeting report.] Nursing Mirror, 141, 17 Jul 1975, 35.

12 **Midwife Health Visitor and Community Nurse** Private practice. [Editorial.] Midwife Health Visitor and Community Nurse, 11 (5), May 1975, 133.

13 **Nelson, J.** Open forum. Private patients are still patients. Nursing Mirror, 140, 2 Jan 1975, 49.

14 **Nursing Mirror** Pay bed plans disastrous top nurses tell Minister. Nursing Mirror, 141, 30 Oct 1975, 34.

15 **Nursing Times** Pay beds in the NHS. Nursing Times, 70, 25 Jul 1974, 1143.

16 **Nursing Times** Private practice: doctors join forces to prepare for showdown with government. Nursing Times, 71, 9 Oct 1975, 1603.

17 **Royal College of Nursing** Rcn comments on a consultative document: the separation of private practice from NHS hospitals, phasing out of private practice from NHS hospitals. Rcn, 1975.

18 **Royal College of Nursing** Outpatient ban would mean injustice and hardship for the elderly, says Rcn. [Comments on government's proposals on private patients.] Nursing Times, 71, 9 Oct 1975, 1601.

19 **Stevenson, J.** Private and state medicine – the parting of the ways. Nursing Mirror, 140, 22/29 May 1975, 35.

20 **Weightman, G.** How private medicine works out. [The operation of private practice in NHS hospitals and private hospitals.] New Society 31, 6 Mar 1975, 580–582.

21 **Weightman, G.** NHS pay beds. New Society, 31, 27 Mar 1975, 790–791.

30 NATIONAL HEALTH SERVICE REORGANIZATION 1974

a GENERAL

1 Anderson, J. A. D. Re-orientation for 1974. Royal Society of Health Journal, 92 (6), Dec 1972, 277–281.

2 Biddulph, C. Reorganization of the health service. Nursing Times, 70, 28 Mar 1974, 456–457.

3 Bosanquet, N. Reorganisation fiasco? Nursing Times, 70, 13 Jun 1974, 903–905.

4 Brunel Institute of Organization and Social Studies. Health Services Organization Research Unit Working papers on the reorganization of the National Health Service. Revised ed. Brunel University, 1973.

5 Burbridge, D. H. D. National Health Service: the philosophy of change (England). Health Trends, 5 (2), May 1973, 22–23.

6 Burbridge, D. H. D. National Health Service: the philosophy of change (England) 2. Running the district. Health Trends, 5 (3), Aug 1973, 42–44.

7 Burbridge, D. H. D. and Sichel, G. R. M. National Health Service: the philosophy of change (England). 4. The framework of the new structure. [With diagrams.] Health Trends, 6 (1), Feb 1974, 2–6.

8 Burbridge, D. H. D. and Sichel, G. R. M. National Health Service: the philosophy of change (England). 5. Functions and constitutions of managing and advisory bodies before and after re-organization in 1974. Health Trends, 6 (1), Feb 1974, 7–10.

9 Burns, C. Aspects of the reorganized NHS: the community physician in the reorganized Health Service. Midwife and Health Visitor, 10 (5), May 1974, 109, 111, 113.

10 Cullinan, J. Conviction for commitment. NHS reorganization conference [organized by the Industrial Society]. Nursing Times, 69, 21 Jun 1973, 811–812.

11 Davies, W. Health or health service? Reform of the British National Health Service. Knight, 1972.

12 Dearden, R. W. One man's view of reorganization. Nursing Mirror, 137, 5 Oct 1973, 37.

13 Drain, G. The reorganization of the National Health Service (b) The viewpoint of the local authority. Royal Society of Health Journal, 92 (1), Jan/Feb 1972, 16–19.

14 Draper, P. and Smart, T. The future of our health care: a report on the current proposals for the reorganization of the National Health Service. Department of Community Medicine, Guy's Hospital Medical School, 1972.

15 Edwards, B. and Walker, R. Sis vis pacem . . .preparations for change in the National Health Service. Oxford University Press/Nuffield Provincial Hospitals Trust, 1973.

16 Elliott, A. Planning for mismanagement. [A critical summary of NHS reorganization proposals.] British Hospital Journal and Social Service Review 82, 21 Oct 1972, 2347–2348.

17 Fowler, F. J. The reorganization of the National Health Service (d) The viewpoint of the hospital service. Royal Society of Health Journal, 92 (1), Jan/Feb 1972, 24–28.

18 Griffin, S. and Haywood, S. C. Informing staff about reorganization. Hospital and Health Services Review, 70 (4), Apr 1974, 119–122.

19 Hall, C. 'Elaboration is needed'. [Views on proposals for managing the reorganised health service.] Nursing Times, 68, 21 Sep 1972, 1176.

20 Haywood, S. C. The new health service: a progress report. Hospital and Health Services Review, 69 (9), Sep 1973, 326–329.

21 Health Visitors Association National Health Service reorganization. [Comments on the Consultative Document.] Health Visitor, 44 (11), Nov 1971, 377–378.

22 Hudson, B. E. L. Training for NHS reorganization. Hospital and Health Services Review, 69 (5), May 1973, 171–173.

23 Kaprio, L. A. The future of health and social services. Royal Society of Health Journal, 93 (3), Jun 1973, 164–167, 178.

24 Lindars, M. E. Reorganization. Under new management – 1974. Nursing Times, 70, 28 Mar 1974, 454–456.

25 Lovett, W. C. D. National Health Service reorganization in Wales. Health Trends, 6 (2), May 1974, 28–29.

26 Ludkin, S. Community Health Services 1974 – a new structure. Royal Society of Health Journal, 93 (1), Feb 1973, 46–47.

27 Midwife and Health Visitor April 1974 – the shape of things to come in the Health Serivce – Midwife and Health Visitor, 8 (6), Jun 1972, 199, 201.

28 Millard, G. Before it's too late, some urgent thoughts on the reorganization of the NHS. Hospital and Health Services Review, 68 (8), Aug 1972, 279–284.

29 Neill, G. A. W. Consultation – collaboration – consensus [in the reorganized NHS.] Queen's Nursing Journal, 17 (3), Jun 1974, 50–51.

30 New Society Guide to the new NHS. New Society, 27, 28 Feb 1974, 514–517.

31 Northern Ireland Reorganization in practice. The first thirty days in N.Ireland. Health and Social Service Journal, 83, 8 Dec 1973, 2878–2879

32 Nursing Mirror NHS of the future? Nursing Mirror, 135, 15 Sep 1972, 8–9; 22 Sep 1972, 870.

33 Office of Health Economics The National Health Service reorganization. OHE 1974. (Studies of Current Health Problems, no. 48.)

34 Owen, D. Towards a unified health service. Hospital and Health Services Review, 70 (7), Jul 1974, 242–247.

35 Sampson, G. R. Pitfalls of bureaucracy. [Administrative units in the reorganized NHS map, 2239.] Health and Social Service Journal, 83, 29 Sep 1973, 2238–2240.

36 Savage, G. G. 1948 and 1974. Health and Social Service Journal, 83, 1 Sep 1973, 1994.

37 Shepherd, J. The new service. Health and Social Service Journal, 84, 22 Jun 1974, 1385–1386; Hospital and Health Services Review, 70 (7), Jul 1974, 238–242.

38 Smith, E. P. The reorganization of the National Health Service. (a) Outline and general comments on the proposals. Royal Society of Health Journal, 92 (1), Jan/Feb 1972, 12–15.

39 Stanyer, R. L. NHS reorganization and bureaucracy. Hospital and Health Services Review, 70 (4), Apr 1974, 115–119.

40 Stevenson, J. A conspiracy of silence on the health service crisis. Nursing Mirror, 139, 2 Aug 1974, 39–40.

41 University of Hull Department of Social Administration Preparations for change: being the first progress report from the research team studying the reorganization of the National Health Service on Humberside 1972–1975. Hull: The Department, 1973.

42 University of Hull Department of Social Administration The shadow and the substance: being the third progress report from the research team studying the reorganization of the National Health Service on Humberside 1972–1975. Hull: The University, 1974.

43 University of Hull Department of Social Administration Waiting for guidance: being the second progress report from the research team studying the reorganization of the National Health Service on Humberside, 1972–1975. Hull: The University, 1973.

44 University of Hull Institute for Health Studies New bottles: old wine? [Fourth and final interim report on the reorganization project 1972–1975.] Hull: The University, 1975.

45 University of Leeds Nuffield Centre for Health Service Studies NHS reorganization: issues and prospects. The Centre, 1974.

46 White, P. The changes ahead. [Health service reorganization.] Nursing Mirror, 135, 8 Dec 1972, 18–20.

47 Yule, I. G. Prelude to reorganization: a commentary on the preparatory work of joint liaison committees. Health Trends, 6 (4), Nov 1974, 63–65.

b GOVERNMENT DOCUMENTS AND LEGISLATION

1 Department of Health and Social Security Management arrangements for the reorganized National Health Service. HMSO, 1972. [Grey book].

2 Department of Health and Social Security National Health Service reorganization. England. HMSO 1972. (Cmnd 5055). [White paper. Summarized in Nursing Times, 68, 3 Aug 1972, 952–953.]

3 Department of Health and Social Security National Health Service reorganization: consultative document. The Department, 1971.

4 Department of Health and Social Security National Health Service reorganization in Wales. Cardiff: HMSO, 1972 (Cmnd 5057).

5 Parliament National Health Service Reorganization Act, 1973. HMSO 1973.

6 Parliament National Health Service (Scotland) Act, 1972. HMSO, 1972.

7 Welsh Office National Health Service reorganization in Wales: consultative document. Cardiff: Welsh Office, 1971.

8 Welsh Office Management arrangements for the reorganized National Health Service in Wales. Cardiff: HMSO, 1972.

c ASSESSMENT

1 Bompas, R. M. The new NHS – will it work? Hospital and Health Services Review, 71 (11), Nov 1975, 385–387.

2 British Medical Journal Reorganization: the first year. [Conference at Chichester 30–31 May.] British Medical Journal, 2, 28 Jun 1975, 729–738; 3, 5 Jul 1975, 22–29; 3, 12 Jul 1975, 81–86.

3 Chester, T. E. NHS reorganization after one year. One year later – impressions and reflections. Hospital and Health Services Review, 71 (4), Apr 1975, 117–121.

4 Colin-Russ, E. and Duncan, G. D. Reorganization – towards an evaluation – first impressions. (a) Reorganization – its impact – first impressions. Royal Society of Health Journal, 95 (4), Aug 1975, 206–213.

5 Easton, T. R. Reorganized under-financed 'envy of the world'. [Assessment of reorganization including mention of some discouraging signs.] Health and Social Service Journal, 85, 18 Jan 1975, 128.

6 Evans, A. M. [NHS reorganization after one year.] A single-distict AHA(T). Problems and opportunities. Hospital and Health Services Review, 71 (4), Apr 1975, 121–125.

7 Hudson, P. The reorganized health service: the first six months and the next ten years. NATNews, 12 (3), Apr 1975, 10–13.

8 Mitchell, R. NHS reorganization after one year. The first year of the reorganized Scottish health service: a personal viewpoint. Hospital and Health Services Review, 71 (5), May 1975, 159–162.

9 Nursing Times Reorganization. 'A lack of confidence in the consultative machinery.' Nursing Times, 71, 3 Apr 1975, 531–533.

10 Royal Society of Health Reorganization – towards an evaluation. [Conference report.] Hospital and Health Services Review, 71 (7), Jul 1975, 241–242.

11 Watkin, B. Darkness at noon. [Views on reorganization.] Nursing Mirror, 141, 11 Sep 1975, 39.

d INTEGRATION WITH SOCIAL SERVICES

1 Birch, R. A. Social work support for the health service: a review of the working party's report. Health Trends, 7 (1), Feb 1975, 14–17

2 Brotherson, J. Mutual interest in community health. [Integration within the reorganized Health Service.] Community Health, 6, Jan–Feb 1975, 229–235.

3 Burbridge, D. H. D. National Health Service: the philosophy of change [England]. 3. Collaboration with local government. Health Trends, 5 (4), Nov 1973, 72–75.

4 Causey, H. E. After 1974 – collaboration between health and social services. (a) Health and social services post 1974 – an initial view. Royal Society of Health Journal, 94 (2), Apr 1974, 69–73.

5 Evans, W. A. B. Aspects of the reorganized N.H.S. social services and the new health service. Midwife and Health Visitor, 10 (6), Jun 1974, 151–153.

6 Harding, L. Reorganization – unification – integration. Nursing Mirror, 138, 29 Mar 1974, 34–35.

7 Hey, A. and Rowbottom, R. Collaboration between area health and social services authorities. (2) The organization of social work in hospitals and other health care settings. Health and Social Service Journal, 84, 16 Feb 1974, 352–355.

8 Hilditch, C. A. Links between health and social services. British Hospital Journal and Social Service Review, 81, 11 Dec 1971, 2613–2614.

9 Holland, W. W. and Gilderdale, S. Integrated health care – the aim of reorganization. Nursing Mirror, 140, 20 Mar 1975, 46–50.

10 Keywood, O. Local government and NHS reorganization. Nursing Times, 69, 28 Jun 1973, 841–844.

11 Kuensberg, E. V. Reorganization. Integration or disintegration. Nursing Times, 70, 28 Mar 1974, 458–459.

12 Orriss, H. D. Problems of integration. Nursing Times, 69, 25 Oct 1973, 1416–1417.

13 Oxford Conference on Integration Integration should aid understanding. [Speakers included A. M. Lamb, M. Scott-Wright, K. J. Hayes.] Nursing Times, 69, 16 Aug 1973, 1046.

14 Penney, A. O. After 1974 – collaboration between health and social services. (b). Royal Society of Health Journal, 94 (2), Apr 1974, 73–74, 90.

15 Rowbottom, R. and Hey, A. Collaboration between area health and social services authorities. 1. (Working links.) Health and Social Service Journal, 84, 9 Feb 1974, 294–295.

16 Smart, C. J. The future pattern of relationships [between health and social services]. Health and Social Service Journal, 83, 24 Feb 1973, 425.

17 Stevenson, D. P. The effects of the reorganization of the NHS on local authorities and general practitioner services. Royal Society of Health Journal, 93, Aug 1973, 187–191.

18 Stroud, J. Health and social service – the importance of integration. Health and Social Service Journal, 83, 6 Oct 1973, 2305–2306.

19 Wells, K. Kent social services and the new National Health Service. Queen's Nursing Journal, 17 (3), Jun 1974, 54–55.

e NURSING AND REORGANIZATION

1 Bond, J. Reorganization: knowledge and opinions of nurses. Nursing Times, 70, 28 Mar 1974, 460–462.

2 Blenkinsop, D. Nursing within the reorganized health service. Queen's Nursing Journal, 17 (12), Mar 1975, 261–262.

3 Carr, A. Reorganization 1974 or 1984? Where the nurses will stand. [Interview with Mr. Anthony Carr, CNO, Newcastle University Hospitals.] British Medical Journal, 1, 9 Jun 1973, 603–609.

4 Department of Health and Social Security Management arrangements for the reorganized National Health Service. HMSO 1972. Chapter 8, Nursing. Text and details: Nursing Times, 68, 14 Sep 1972, 1166–1168; Nursing Mirror, 135, 22 Sep 1972, 8–10.

5 Devlin, H. B. and others Reorganization and nurse training. [Letter describing the effects of Salmon and NHS reorganization at North Tees General Hospital.] British Medical Journal, 1, 8 Feb 1975, 330.

6 Elias, B. R. Administrators and reorganization. [The position of the new administrators after reorganization with particular reference to the nurse administrator.] Health and Social Service Journal, 84, 16 Nov 1974, 2656.

7 Fairweather, C. Reorganization and nurse training [in the Cleveland Area Health Authority.] [Letter.] British Medical Journal, 22 Feb 1975, 455.

8 Flindall, J. Reorganization. Working for democracy – an ANO's view. Nursing Times, 71, 3 Apr 1975, 526–528.

9 Friend, P. NHS reorganization. Nursing Mirror, 138, 29 Mar 1974, 33.

10 McCarthy, M. K. E. and others Reorganization training for field workers. [Training programme in Leicester for district nurses, midwives and health visitors for NHS reorganization and the introduction of a Mayston management structure.] Nursing Times, 70, 21 Feb 1974, 286–287.

11 Midwives Chronicle The work of the National Staff Committee for Nurses and Midwives in the NHS. Midwives Chronicle, 88, Oct 1975, 337.

12 Nursing Mirror Nursing and midwifery advisory structure in Scotland. Nursing Mirror, 137, 7 Sep 1973, 12–13.

13 Nursing Mirror Staff committee to develop work on personnel policies for nurses. A survey of the activities of the NNSC. Nursing Mirror, 141, 4 Sep 1975, 36.

14 Nursing Times Appointing the top nurses. [Arrangements for the appointments to the top nursing posts in the reorganized NHS] Nursing Times, 69, 3 May 1973, 556.

15 Nursing Times Programme report. A review of the first year's work of the area nursing and midwifery committees – the professional advisory bodies in each AHA which represent the views of clinical nurses. Nursing Times, 72, 29 Jan 1975, 128.

16 Queen's Nursing Journal Professional advisory machinery – nursing and midwifery. [Conference report.] Queen's Nursing Journal, 18 (4), Jul 1975, 120, 125.

17 Richards, S. Responsibility for care. [Interviewed by Jane Cameron, S. Richards discusses issues facing nursing and the health service.] Nursing Times, 71, 29 May 1975, 836–837.

18 Royal College of Nursing Nurses consider N.H.S. reorganization. [Rcn conference.] District Nursing, 15 (8), Nov 1972, 181–182.

19 Scottish Home and Health Department Nurses in an integrated health service: report of a working group. . . Edinburgh: HMSO, 1972. Summarised in Nursing Times, 68, 12 Oct 1972, 1300–1302.

20 Senior, E. Reorganization. Consensus management – an RNO's view. [Development of communication throughout the whole nursing structure.] Nursing Times, 71, 3 Apr 1975, 524–525.

21 Skeet, M. Co-operation between the Health and Social Services in the '70s. (c) The point of view of the nursing officer. Royal Society of Health Journal, 91 (6) Nov/Dec 1971, 276–278.

22 Voss, P. Voice from the bedside. [Formation of area nursing and midwifery committees.] Nursing Times, 71, 12 Jun 1975, 912.

23 White, A. M. W. Reorganization. A more sensitive service – a DNO's view. Nursing Times, 71, 3 Apr 1975, 529–530.

31 HOSPITALS

a GENERAL

1 Anstey, O. E. The concept of a community centred teaching hospital – the impact on nursing. Australian Nurses' Journal, 2 (4), Oct 1972, 22–25.

2 Bennett, A. E. Community hospitals. [The concept of the community hospital as developed in the Oxford Region.] Health Trends, 7 (4), Nov 1975, 66–68.

3 Bosanquet, N. Community hospitals? Nursing Times, 70, 5 Sep 1974, 1371.

4 Bright, K. The hospital – centre for health care. Australian Nurses' Journal, 2 (11), May 1973, 32–33.

5 Davies, R. H. The community hospital. A symposium at the Welsh National School of Medicine. Journal of the Royal College of General Practitioners, 23, Oct 1975, 713–716.

6 Department of Health and Social Security and Welsh Office Community hospitals: their role and development in the National Health Service. HMSO, 1974. Also Circular HCS (IS) 75.

7 Fairley, J. Hospital services – a philosophical review. Royal Society of Health Journal, 93 (2), Apr 1973, 59–61.

8 Gray, M. Cottage hospitals – a new role. [Halfway house before admission to a geriatric or acute unit.] Nursing Mirror, 136, 2 Mar 1973, 11–12.

9 Hospital and Health Services Review Community

hospitals. [Leading article.] Hospital and Health Services Review, 70 (10), Oct 1974, 341–343.

10 Kirk, C. and Bennett, A. E. Management and advice at the grass roots. [Community hospitals in the Oxford Region help to bridge the gap between multiprofessional clinical teams and district management teams.] Lancet, 1, 24 May 1975, 1180–1182.

11 Klein, R. Intensive care. [Changing pattern of hospital use 1959–1973.] New Society, 32, 22 May 1975, 478.

12 Lee-Jones, M. New hospitals – new medical centre – new records. [Wallingford Community Hospital.] Practice Team, no. 32, Jan 1974, 17–21.

13 Maynard, A. Hospital care in Britain and France. Hospital and Health Services Review, 71 (2), Feb 1975, 50–53.

14 Naylor, K. J. and Allardyce, R. N. Diary of a five-day ward. [Lennard Hospital, Bromley.] Nursing Mirror, 139, 21 Nov 1974, 67–69.

15 Nursing Mirror 'Part of the life of the area' – Wallingford Community Hospital. [Mainly illustrations.] Nursing Mirror, 138, 29 Mar 1974, 52–54.

16 The Oxford community hospital [At Wallingford, Berkshire.] Health and Social Service Journal, 83, 9 Jun 1973, 1302–1303.

17 Robinson, G. A. Community hospitals. [Implications of DHSS circular HCS (15) 75.] Hospital and Health Services Review, 71 (7), Jul 1975, 232–233.

18 Robinson, W. Britain's first community hospital. [Wallingford.] Nursing Times, 70, 28 Mar 1974, 483–485.

19 Sergio, A. Evolution of the hospital: old ideas and new concepts. World Hospitals, 9 (2), Apr 1973, 57–59.

20 Smith, J. C. From cottage to community hospital. [Comment on the DHSS memorandum.] Health and Social Service Journal, 84, 23 Nov 1974, 2718.

21 Smith, J. W. and others Comparative study of district and community hospitals. British Medical Journal, 2, 26 May 1973, 471–474.

22 Weaver, N. D. W. On cottage hospitals. Hospitals and Health Services Review, 69 (3), Mar 1973, 90–91.

23 Wycherley, G. J. Administering the community hospital. [Wallingford Community Hospital.] Health and Social Service Journal, 84, 27 Apr 1974, 926–927.

b BED ALLOCATION AND USE

1 Bates, M. M. and Sharratt, M. The King's Fund Emergency Bed Service, London. [Administration, functions and an analysis of use in London.] Health Trends, 7 (4) Nov 1975, 78–82.

2 Chant, A. D. B. and others Hospital beds: a method for evaluating their use. Hospital and Health Services Review, 71 (8), Aug 1975, 263–265.

3 Clarke, M. and Mulholland, A. The use of general practitioner beds. Journal of the Royal College of General Practitioners, 129, Apr 1973, 273–279.

4 Hospital and Health Services Review Determination of bed allocations within the hospital service. Hospital and Health Services Review, 69 (6), Jun 1973, 235–237.

5 Hughes, A. O. and Miller, D. S. The determinants of demand for pre-convalescent beds. [Survey at Nottingham University Hospital Group.] Hospital and Health Services Review, 71 (10), Oct 1975, 350–353.

6 Marshall, R. D. and Spencer, R. I. A more efficient use of hospital beds? [Closure of some acute

beds in an attempt to reduce nurse wastage – experiment at Northampton General Hospital.] British Medical Journal, 3, 6 Jul 1974, 27–30.

7 Spencer, R. I. Determining waiting list admissions: to improve the use of available beds. Hospital and Health Services Review, 70 (9), Sep 1974, 308–311.

8 Stevens, G. C. and others Factors affecting the result of waiting list calls. Hospital and Health Services Review, 69 (12), Dec 1973, 459–461.

9 Wilkes, J. S. Reviewing the bed usage in a children's hospital – a case study in operational research. [Study at the Royal Aberdeen Children's Hospital.] Health Bulletin, 32 (2), Mar 1974, 70–73.

c DISCHARGE AND CONTINUITY OF CARE

1 Bell, J. R. and Shearer, D. S. Economical use of hospital beds. [Planned discharge and after care at Glasgow Royal Infirmary, using district nurse liaison officer.] Nursing Times, 68, 5 Oct 1972, 1264–1265.

2 Bott, M. Can the community cope with patients discharged early from hospital? British Medical Journal, 4, 16 Nov 1974, 390–391, 394.

3 Coleman, V. Integration – an exercise in self analysis. [Study at Glasgow Ear, Nose and Throat Hospital to identify the weak links and improve continuity of patient care.] Nursing Mirror, 140, 1 May 1975, 50.

4 Davey, M. C. Administration and discharge. [Problems of the correct time to discharge patients.] Health and Social Service Journal, 84, 23 Feb 1974, 424.

5 Dickinson, B. H. Getting together – 2. [Co-operation, liaison & communication between hospital & District Nurse.] District Nursing, 14 (1), April 1971, 6–7.

6 Gatt, R. and others Team venture in the North East: a study in co-operation with Aberdeen Royal Infirmary and the domiciliary services. Nursing Mirror, 137, 7 Sep 1973, 35–36.

7 Hayes, K. The extension of progressive patient care in the community of Blackpool. District Nursing, 14 (1), Apr 1971, 20–21.

8 Hingston, C. W. J. and Adam, J. Hospital aftercare: a report of a pilot scheme of hospital/local authority liaison. Medical Officer, 123, 5 Jun 1970, 319–323.

9 Hird, V. Selection and function of staff for hospital and community liaison. Queen's Nursing Journal, 17 (7), Oct 1974, 147–148.

10 Hunt, G. J. W. A hospital and community liaison visiting scheme. [In Reading.] District Nursing, 15 (10), Jan 1973, 229–230.

11 Jamieson, C. W. and Dudley, H. A. F. Another hospital discharge system. Lancet, 2, 11 Aug 1973, 314–315.

12 Journal of the Royal College of General Practitioners Continuity of care. Journal of the Royal College of General Practitioners, 23, Nov 1973, 749–750.

13 Keeling, C. A. A job for the future – liaison health visiting. Nursing Times, 69, 18 Oct 1973, 1385–1386.

14 King's Fund Centre Good neighbours – or plugging gaps? [Place of the volunteer in the continuity of patient care.] Nursing Times, 68, 25 Oct 1972, 1341.

15 King's Fund Centre Home from hospital. Nursing Mirror, 132, 22 Jan 1971, 13–14.

16 Kitchin, C. H. Hospital and after. Nursing Mirror, 132, 19 Mar 1971, 13–14.

17 Lawton, E. E. Home, care of the district nurse. [Pilot scheme for early discharge from hospital in Bolton.] District Nursing, 15 (11), Feb 1973, 245–246.

18 Leonard, M. No bed for the night. [Problems of the homeless after hospital discharge.] Nursing Times, 71, 2 Oct 1975, 1594–1595.

19 Lockwood, E. and McCallum, F. M. Patients discharged from Hospital: an aspect of communication in the Health Service. Health Bulletin, 28 (2), Apr 1970, 75–80.

20 Mellor, H. W. Home from hospital. [Hospital Centre Conference on improvement of services for patients discharged from hospital.] British Hospital Journal and Social Service Review, 82, 9 Dec 1972, 2756.

21 Moore, J. H. and O'Brien, T. Community teams at Moorhaven hospital. [After care service for discharged patients.] Practice Team, 48, May 1975, 2–4.

22 Paxton, C. M. Co-operation and care. [Investigation into liaison schemes.] Nursing Times, 70, 12 Dec 1974; 19/26 Dec 1974, Occ. papers. 113–119.

23 Randall, D. H. Continuity of care for surgical patients. District Nursing, 15 (1), Apr 1972, 8–10.

24 Roberts, I. Discharged from hospital. Rcn, 1975. (Study of nursing care project report series 2, no. 6.)

25 Royal College of Nursing Practical liaison between hospital and community nurses. Rcn, 1973.

26 Stevens, P. F. Discharge from hospital – the problem of adjustment. Nursing Times, 70, 9 May 1974, 700–702.

27 Tulloch, A. J. and others Hospital discharge reports: content and design. [546 reports were reviewed for availability and accessibility of information.] British Medical Journal, 4, 22 Nov 1975, 443–446.

28 White, A. M. Getting together. 1. [Conference bringing together senior nursing staff from hospital and local authority.] District Nursing, 14 (1), Apr 1971, 4–5.

29 Wilson, E. H. Integration of hospital and local authority services in the discharge of patients from a geriatric unit. Lancet, 2, 16 Oct 1971, 864–866.

30 Wilson, E. H. and Wilson, B. O. From hospital to community. [A scheme for elderly patients in Lancaster.] Nursing Mirror, 135, 18 Aug 1972, 17–19.

d DISCHARGE AND CONTINUITY OF CARE: OVERSEAS COUNTRIES

1 Allen, D. V. and others Agencies' perception of factors affecting home care referral. [The assessment of home care program in Detroit.] Medical Care, 12 (10), Oct 1974, 828–844.

2 Ambrose, A. Discharge plans – the weakest link. Hospital Progress, 54 (3), Mar 1973, 58–60.

3 Belanus, R. The forgotten patient. [Importance of the community nurse after discharge from hospital.] Journal of Practical Nursing, 24 (4), Apr 1974, 30–31.

4 Crane, L. M. Home care programs in B. C. [Changes in community services extending home care facilities to acute hospital patients.] Hospital Administration in Canada, 17 (10), Oct 1975, 28–29, 31.

5 Hecht, N. S. and Barringer, V. The liaison nurse: a link between the hospital and community health care centers to ensure continuity of care. Hospitals, 45 (22), 16 Nov 1971, 82, 84, 88, 90.

6 Hook, N. G. Liaison in Australia. Queen's Nursing Journal, 16 (5), Aug 1973, 106, 120.

7 Isler, C. Helping hospital patients – out. [Discharge planning scheme in Brooklyn.] RN Magazine, 38 (11), Nov 1975, 43–44, 46.

8 Lambert, P. Home and hospital: an analysis of a bridging exercise. Australian Nurses' Journal, 4 (9), Apr 1975, 31–33.

9 LaMontague, M. E. and McKeehan, K. M. Profile of a continuing care program emphasizing discharge planning. Journal of Nursing Administration, 5 (8), Oct 1975, 22–33.

10 Lawton, E. E. A visit to Sweden. [Study tour to examine hospital/community liaison in patient discharge.] Queen's Nursing Journal, 18 (1), Apr 1975, 8–9, 11.

11 Morgan, D. Discharge planning: an asset in the continuum of patient care services. Canadian Hospital, 50 (9), Sep 1973, 28–29, 36, 47.

12 Mountford, F. Continuity of patient care in a dynamic era. SA Nursing Journal, 38 (12), Dec 1971, 26–27.

13 Noel, G. E. Continuity of nursing care in Guyana. Health Visitor, 44 (1), Jan 1971, 12–14.

14 Riley, M. E. Teaching nursing referrals by programed instruction. [Teaching importance of continuity of care.] RN Magazine, 36 (1), Jan 1973, 57–58, 60.

15 Rossman, I. The Monteiore Hospital after-care program. Nursing Outlook, 22 (5), May 1974, 325–328.

16 Thomson, H. Assisting patients with post hospitalization plans. Hospitals, 47 (2), 16 Jan 1973, 43–45, 98.

17 Weinbach, R. W. and Dodge, D. D. Educating for discharge planning. Hospitals, 48 (24), 16 Dec 1974, 72, 74, 76.

e EQUIPMENT AND FURNITURE

1 American Journal of Nursing Portable shower for bed patients. American Journal of Nursing, 74 (11), Nov 1974, 2021.

2 Angel, J. C. Aerosols. [The way they work and their application to hospital use.] Nursing Times, 71, 6 Feb 1975, 234–235.

3 Armstrong, K. N. Nonwovens and the raw materials crisis [in relation to disposables in hospitals.] Health and Social Service Journal, 84, 10 Aug 1974, 1807–1808.

4 Asbury, A. J. Electronic equipment in nursing. Nursing Times, 69, 5 Jul 1973, 861–863.

5 Bradshaw, J. S. Disposables: conscientious objections. Nursing Times, 70, 23 May 1974, 783–784.

6 Bretten, P. Hospital beds. [A survey of the different types of beds available.] Nursing Mirror, 139, 24 Oct 1974, 48–55.

7 Dench, J. and Heath, P. Are you sitting comfortably? [Bags filled with polystyrene beads for use with old people.] Nursing Times, 70, 13 Jun 1974, 922–923.

8 Fleet, C. Resuscitation trolley. [In the paediatric Unit at Falkirk and District Royal Infirmary.] Nursing Mirror, 139, 19 Sep 1974, 67–69.

9 Holmgren, J. H. Disposables vs. reusables: the choice hinges on safety, space, time, labor, and cost factors. Modern Hospital, 120 (5), May 1973, 68.

10 Hospital and Health Services Review Notes for students. Equipping a new hospital. Hospital and Health Services Review, 69 (3), Mar 1973, 114–116.

11 Lane, R. J. Disposables: a time for reappraisal. Nursing Times, 70, 23 May 1974, 787–788.

12 Johnson, A. A matter of disposal. Nursing Times, 69, 29 Nov 1973, 1610.

13 Ledger, A. M. and Adams, J. A. Movable slip wards: transportable buildings are used for temporarily 'decanting' patients while their own wards are being redecorated and improved. Health and Social Service Journal, 83, 13 Jan 1973, 84–85.

14 Marett, D. L. and Riley, O. M. Nursing refuse disposal inquiry. Nursing Times, 67, 22 Jul 1971, Occ. papers, 113–115.

15 Nursing Mirror The Egerton Stoke Mandeville tilting and turning bed. [Symposium at Stoke Mandeville Hospital.] Nursing Mirror, 141, 6 Nov 1975, 56–57.

16 Nursing Mirror Harwick geriatric locker. Nursing Mirror, 136, 6 Apr 1973, 43.

17 Nursing Mirror Hospital equipment review. Nursing Mirror, 136, 19 Jan 1973, 43–50.

18 Nursing Mirror O'Malley's paediatric bed. Nursing Mirror, 136, 22 Jun 1975, 46.

19 Nursing Mirror Ward equipment: a review of equipment for use in hospitals, health centres and nursing homes. Nursing Mirror, 140, 20 Mar 1975, 57–60.

20 Rosenhouse, L. More hospitals using waterbeds. Nursing Care, 7 (4), Apr 1974, 26–28.

21 Sale, J. and Wilshire, R. Hoists. Nursing Mirror, 140, 20 Feb 1975, 45–49.

22 Sangster, J. A. Equipping the 'best buy' hospitals. [Involving a multi-disciplinary team.] Health and Social Service Journal, 84, 26 Oct 1974, 2480–2481.

23 Savage, J. A cot drawing board. [Developed at the Brook Hospital, London.] Nursing Times, 71, 21 Aug 1975, 1349.

24 Savage, J. H. Drawing and painting in bed. [A drawing board for patients working in any position.] Nursing Times, 70, 19 Sep 1974, 1478–1479.

25 Scottish Hospital Centre Era of disposables. [Scottish Hospital Centre meeting.] Health and Social Service Journal, 84, 6 Jul 1974, 1510–1511.

26 Spencer, S. R. The development of a new hospital bed. Australian Nurses' Journal, 5 (1), Jul 1975, 36–38.

27 Treasure, C. R. and others Bedsteads – a report from the Central Wirral Group. (King's Fund beds.) Nursing Mirror, 138, 3 May 1974, 67–70.

28 Wakeling, S. G. Disposables: justifiable uses in nursing. Nursing Times, 70, 23 May 1974, 785–786.

f FINANCE

1 Berry, A. K. Stock control forms. [Effect of VAT on hospital purchasing.] Health and Social Service Journal, 83, 31 Mar 1973, 728–730.

2 Coles, J. and others Control of resources: a management research project at Westminster Hospital investigates the possibility of ward teams controlling their own budgets. Health and Social Service Journal, 84, 16 Nov 1974, 2654–2655.

3 Cullis, J. G. and West, P. A. Comparing hospital costs – a reconsideration. Hospital and Health Services Review, 69, Aug 1973, 282–286.

4 Kennerley, J. Statistical data; a platform for further action – but not the final answer [uses of costing and statistical data in the hospital service.] Hospital and Health Services Review, 70, Jul 1974, 231–232.

5 Kramer, L. G. 25 years of hospital accounting.

Hospital and Health Services Review, 70, Apr 1974, 124–127.

6 Opit, L. J. and Cross, K. W. Comparing hospital costs. Hospital and Health Services Review, 69, Feb 1973, 44–49.

7 Sage, B. W. Budgeting by network analysis. [Westminster Hospital.] Health and Social Service Journal, 83, 5 May 1973, 1020–1021.

8 Stirland, M. Behavioural implications of budgetary control. Hospital and Health Services Review, 169 (1), Jan 1973, 14–18.

9 Tatham, L. Hospital banking system. [Computer accounting at West Park Hospital.] Health and Social Service Journal, 83, 17 Feb 1973, 369.

10 Wallace, R. F. and Donnelly, M. Computing quality assurance costs. [Cost benefit analysis of medical audit, nursing audit and utilization review.] Hospital Progress, 56 (5), May 1975, 53–57.

g FIRE AND ACCIDENTS

1 Barlow, J. A. and others Fire precaution methods in hospital. [A research project carried out to broaden the scope of student nurse training.] Nursing Times, 71, 16 Jan 1975, Occ. papers, 1–4.

2 Bringman, M. Safety action sheet keys program. [To help identify causes of accidents, and initiate corrective measures.] Hospitals, 48, 16 Jan 1974, 85–86, 88.

3 Conole, C. P. Safety council innovates. Hospitals, 48 (2), 16 Jan 1974, 88, 90.

4 Considine, J. and Drake, S. J. Safety in hospitals: are nurses expendable? [Identifies the hazards and describes an accident prevention programme.] Lamp, 31 (1), Jan 1974, 7, 9, 15.

5 Department of the Environment and Fire Offices Committee. Joint Fire Research Organization Fires in hospitals by S. E. Chandler. HMSO, 1971. (Fire research technical paper 27).

6 Department of Health and Social Security Committee of Inquiry into the fire at Coldharbour Hospital, Sherbourne on 5 July 1972. Report. HMSO, 1972. Cmnd. 5170. Chairman: D. H. W. Vowden.

7 Department of Health and Social Security. Committee of Inquiry into the Fire at Fairfield Home, Edwalton, Nottinghamshire on 15 Dec 1974 Report. HMSO, 1975. Cmnd. 6149.

8 Dicker, K. Everybody out! [First-hand account of the evacuation of a maternity unit during a fire.] Nursing Mirror, 140, 17 Apr 1975, 70–71.

9 Fischmann, G. S. and others Medical staff, department heads team up for safety's sake. [Electrical safety.] Hospitals, 49 (9), 1 Oct 1975, 89, 92–93.

10 Fletcher, S. and Eales, J. Patient evacuation in a small unit. [Emergency plan using under mattress slings for evacuation in case of fire.] Dimensions in Health Service, 52 (3), Mar 1975, 38–39.

11 Hampton, R. A. Hospital evacuation procedures [in case of fire]. Nursing Times, 49, 7 Dec, 1542–1543.

12 Health and Social Service Journal Fire precautions: the final responsibility. Health and Social Service Journal, 85, 12 Jul 1975, 1478.

13 Health and Social Service Journal Fire safety in hospitals. Health and Social Service Journal, 83, 11 Aug 1973, 1810.

14 Henley, E. S. Fire protection systems tested. Hospitals, 47 (1), Jan 1973, 69–70, 75.

15 Hospital and Health Services Review Accidents in hospitals. Hospital and Health Services Review, 70 (3), Mar 1974, 105–108.

16 **Hospital and Health Services Review** An introduction to fire precautions in hospitals. Hospital and Health Services Review, 70 (6), Jun 1974, 218–219; (7), Jul 1974, 255–257.

17 **Jackson, R. G.** Bomb threats: experience of a new hazard in hospitals. Hospital and Health Services Review, 70 (9), Sep 1974, 317.

18 **Leese, A.** Fire safety in hospitals. Health and Social Service Journal, 83, 19 May 1973, 1132–1133, 1135.

19 **Leese, A.** Tragedy of fire. Health and Social Service Journal, 85, 18 Jan 1975, 125.

20 **Nunn, C.** There's a fire at DRI. [The efficiency of fire precautions following a fire at Dundee Royal Infirmary.] Hospital and Health Services Review, 70 (6), Jun 1974, 202–207.

21 **Nursing Mirror** Fire safety for a happy Christmas. Nursing Mirror, 139, 19 Dec 1974, 43.

22 **Smith, D. E.** Fire safety in hospitals. S. A. Nursing Journal, 42 (4), Apr 1975, 18–19.

23 **Trought, E. A.** Equipment hazards. American Journal of Nursing, 73 (5), May 1973, 858–862.

24 **Walker, P. H.** Detecting electrical hazards in the hospital. Nursing Care, 6 (3), Mar 1973, 11–14.

25 **White, D. C.** Fire precautions in small hospitals. Health and Social Service Journal, 84, 12 Oct 1974, 2358–2359.

26 **White, D. C.** Monitoring fire standards. Health and Social Service Journal, 85, 28 Jun 1975, 1330–1331.

27 **Wright, W. J.** Fire. Nursing Mirror, 139, 5 Jul 1974, 52–53.

h FOOD AND CATERING

1 **Anderson, R. A.** Planning and equipping a catering department. Health and Social Service Journal, 83, 27 Jan 1973, 196–197, 199.

2 **Balk, T. and Dunne, M.** An evaluation of patients' meals. [A method developed by the South East Thames RHA and the Good Food Guide and a report of two surveys.] Health and Social Service Journal, 85, 22 Feb 1975, 428–429.

3 **Beavan, A. J.** The responsibility of the health service district catering manager. Health and Social Service Journal, 85, 15 Nov 1975, 2560.

4 **Davidson, M. J.** Frozen foods in hospital catering. Health and Social Service Journal, 83, 28 Apr 1973, 960–961.

5 **Dunn, A.** Hospital food – catering for all pockets. [The price of food in hospital canteens.] Nursing Times, 70, 28 Feb 1974, 298–300.

6 **Friesen, G.** Ready foods system. Health and Social Service Journal, 83, 28 Apr 1973, 970–971.

7 **Furbank, M.** Improved meals for geriatric patients. [In long-stay hospitals.] Nursing Times, 70, 26 Sep 1974, 1501–1503.

8 **Hospitals** Issue on shared food services in hospitals. Hospitals, 47 (21), 1 Nov 1973, 39–90.

9 **Kincald, J. W.** Patients evaluate cycle menu entrees. [10 day study at Ohio State University Hospital, Columbus.] Hospitals, 49, 1 Nov 1975, 71–73.

10 **Last, K. A.** Tray meal service. [Grundy-Finessa system at Wythenshawe Hospital.] Health and Social Service Journal, 83, 24 Mar 1973, 665.

11 **Lyon, J. and Porritt, B.** Diet and food service in an extended care facility: study conducted at the Penticton Regional Hospital. Hospital Administration in Canada, 17 (9), Sep 1975, 39–40, 43.

12 **Marshall, J. E.** A visit to Australian hospitals. [Catering departments.] New Zealand Nursing Journal, 66 (10), Oct 1973, 4–6.

13 **Millross, J. and others** Consequences of a switch to cook-freeze. [A survey of consumer reaction, nutritional aspects and costs at the Hospital for Women, Leeds.] Hospitals, 48 (17), 1 Sep 1974, 118, 124–126.

14 **Palmer, J.** Evaluating frozen food service in hospital. Hospital Administration to Canada, 17 (8), Aug 1975, 53–55.

15 **Passmore, S. F.** Freeze production catering. [Newcastle project.] Health and Social Service Journal, 83, 24 Feb 1973, 415–416.

16 **Puckett, R.** Questionnaires aid in analysis of department's effectiveness. [Hospital food service.] Hospitals, 47, 16 Jun 1973, 89–90.

17 **Stanley, C.** Hygiene in hospital catering. Health and Social Service Journal, 84, 31 Aug 1974, 1977–1978.

18 **Wilkie, W. M.** Food waste. Health and Social Service Journal, 85, 19 Apr 1975, 870.

i HISTORY

1 **Heyward, J. M.** Institutions of compassion. [Victorian hospitals.] Nursing Mirror, 139, 17 Oct 1974, 87–88.

2 **Howie, W. B.** Consumer reaction: a patients' view of hospital life in 1809. [Poems by Joseph Wilde.] British Medical Journal, 3, 8 Sep 1973, 534–536.

3 **Middlesex Hospital** One hundred years ago. The Middlesex Hospital. Queen's Nursing Journal, 17 (5), Aug 1974, 114.

4 **Osborn, M. L.** Some early foundling hospitals. Midwife and Health Visitor, 9 (3), Mar 1973, 85–87.

j HOUSEKEEPING

1 **Barratt, B.** Staff for 1980? [Domestic staff.] Health and Social Service Journal, 84, 26 Oct 1974, 2483.

2 **Bridges, T.** Process control in linen services. Health and Social Service Journal, 85, 1 Feb 1975, 237–238.

3 **Giancola, D.** The inhouse laundry and linen service. Hospitals, 49 (4), 16 Feb 1975, 97–99.

4 **Health and Social Service Journal** High speed cleaning. [Manor House Hospital, Aylesbury.] Health and Social Service Journal, 83, 31 Mar 1973, 727.

5 **Johnson, A. G.** Case study of a linen distribution system. Hospitals, 48 (2), 16 Jan 1974, 65–66, 68–69.

6 **McElvoy, A.** Efficiency in laundries – old and new. Health and Social Service Journal, 85, 26 Apr 1975, 940.

7 **Maxwell, R.** Conference views on some essentials of laundry services. [Scottish Hospital Centre conference.] Health and Social Service Journal, 84, 13 Apr 1974, 828–829.

8 **Nunn, D. S.** The uniform problem. [Use of Autovalet laundry machine at Central Middlesex Hospital.] Nursing Mirror, 140, 5 Jun 1975, 71.

9 **Packwood, T.** Management research. Hospital housekeeping. Nursing Times, 69, 11 Oct 1973, 1347–1349.

10 **Peet, J. E. and Hibbert, D.** Answers to a linen problem. [Improvement in the laundry service in Doncaster since the two week strike by laundry staff.] Health and Social Service Journal, 84, 17 Aug 1974, 1861.

11 **Pycock, J. E. and Ashton, R.** Spray cleaning. Health and Social Service Journal, 83, 26 May 1973, 1196, 1198.

12 **Rizzo, D. R.** Nursing and the efficient use of linens. Hospitals, 49 (12), 16 Jun 1975, 92–94.

13 **Sladden, J. M.** Low cost cleaning. [Comparison of different methods of cleaning floors.] Health and Social Service Journal, 83, 28 Apr 1973, 964–965.

14 **Spooner, R. R.** Quality control in laundry services. Health and Social Service Journal, 85, 25 Jan 1975, 176–177.

15 **Thynne, C.** The longest washing line. [Central laundry supply system at Clatterbridge Hospital.] Nursing Times, 70, 21 Mar 1974, 444–445.

16 **Turner, D. S.** Work sampling surveys improve housekeeping standards. Hospital Administration in Canada, 16 (3), Mar 1974, 72–74.

k MANAGEMENT

1 **Bompas, R. M.** The administrator. Hospital and Health Services Review, 69 (6), Jun 1973, 204–208.

2 **Bureau, R.** The administrator: the real, the ideal. [Nurses' perception of the role of the hospital administrator.] Canadian Nurse, 71 (3), Mar 1975, 36–37.

3 **Charnock, J.** Leadership and the search for excellence in hospitals: a research study into management by objectives in the Birmingham RHB. Health and Social Service Journal, 84, 16 Mar 1974, 604–605.

4 **Cuming, M. W.** Hospital staff management. Heinemann, 1971.

5 **Dale, A. C.** Management audit in American hospitals. Health and Social Service Journal, 85, 23 Aug 1975, 1865.

6 **Gorman, M. C.** Management for professionals in the health service. [Improving the effectiveness of hospitals by getting more from existing resources.] World Hospitals, 9 (2), Apr 1973, 45–53.

7 **Grant, C.** Hospital management. Churchill Livingstone, 1973.

8 **Harrison, S. E.** Management services – thoughts for the future. [Conference held by the Institute of Work Study Practitioners.] Health and Social Service Journal, 85, 11 Jan 1975, 73–74.

9 **Hill, P. A.** Records, roles and results. [Management by objectives in the Southampton University Hospitals and medical records department.] Health and Social Service Journal, 84, 2 Nov 1974, 2537.

10 **Houslop, P. L.** Clatterbridge industrial zone: concept of industrial departments within the health service. Health and Social Service Journal, 84, 1 Jun 1974, 1235.

11 **Johnson, B. D.** Learning from experience. [Chairman of Group Medical Advisory Committee examines administrative problems while in hospital.] Nursing Times, 71, 8 May 1975, 718–719.

12 **Kay, W. N.** Towards improved administration. [Suggestions of improvements which could be introduced on re-organization.] Hospital and Health Services Review, 69 (11), Nov 1973, 415.

13 **Longest, B. B. Jr.** Human relations in hospital management. Nursing Care, 6 (5), May 1973, 20–22.

14 **McMahon, J. A.** PSROs. . .implications for hospitals. [Professional standards review organizations.] Hospitals, 48, 1 Jan 1974, 53–55.

15 **Martin, F. B.** Implementing accountability management. [Management by objectives.] Hospitals, 47, 16 Jul 1973, 57–59, 212.

16 Millward, R. C. Functions and administration of hospital management committees. Community Health, 4 (4), Jan/Feb 1973, 207–211.

17 Myers, D. The new disease – 'Administration'? British Medical Journal, 2, 21 Jun 1975, 677–679.

18 Robinson, G. A. Functional management: a hospital secretary's view. Hospital and Health Services Review, 71 (4), Apr 1975, 133–134.

19 Savage, G. G. The role of the unit manager. Hospital and Health Services Review, 69 (10), Oct 1973, 374–375.

20 Sutherland, J. G. and others The hospital innovation project. [At Fulbourn Hospital.] Health and Social Service Journal, 84, 26 Jan 1974, 172.

l NOISE

1 British Medical Journal Noise in hospital. [Leading article.] British Medical Journal, 4, 15 Dec 1973, 625–626.

2 Hinks, M. D. 'The most cruel absence of care': report of a follow-up study of noise control in hospital. King's Fund Centre, 1974.

3 Hinks, M. D. They seem to forget. [Study of noise in hospitals.] Health and Social Service Journal, 85, 18 Jan 1975, 130.

4 McArdle, C. Television in the ward. [Letter describing the fitting of a system of individual listening devices to overcome the noise problem.] Lancet, 2, 21 Dec 1974, 1510.

5 Pollitt, W. E. A decibel diagnosis. [Noise levels in three hospital wards.] Community Medicine, 126, 31 Dec 1971, 373–376.

6 Rosenhouse, L. Noise. Nursing Care, 7 (11), Nov 1974, 26–28.

7 Taylor, R. Noise in hospitals. Health and Social Service Journal, 84, 30 Nov 1974, 2770–2771.

8 Whitfield, S. Noise on the ward at night. [A project at Royal West Sussex Hospital, Chichester, which identified areas of noise by means of a questionnaire and made recommendations for their reduction.] Nursing Times, 71, 13 Mar 1975, 408–412.

9 Woods, N. F. and Falk, S. A. Noise stimuli in the acute care area. [Intensive care unit and recovery room.] Nursing Research, 23, Mar/Apr 1974, 144–150.

m NURSING HOMES

1 Davies, R. L. Nuffield Nursing Homes Trust. [Mainly illustrations of different homes.] Nursing Mirror, 140, 24 Apr 1975, 47–50.

2 Hershey, N. Issues in the care of nursing home patients. Journal of Nursing Administration, 3 (2), Mar/Apr 1973, 43–46.

3 Keywood, O. The registration and inspection of nursing homes. Nursing Times, 69, 26 Apr 1973, 544–546.

4 Orstein, S. A nursing home is not a hospital. Nursing Outlook, 21 (1), Jan 1973, 28–31.

5 Schwab, M. Nursing care in nursing homes. American Journal of Nursing, 75 (10), Oct 1975, 1812–1815.

6 Taylor, B. Monday afternoons. [Patient admission at Crumbley House Convalescent Home.] Nursing Mirror, 140, 5 Jun 1975, 69–70.

n OUTPATIENTS (Includes nursing)

1 Babcock, D. W. Screening nurse – Vancouver General Hospital. The patient flow metre. [Adult outpatient department.] Canadian Hospital, 50 (9), Sep 1973, 23–24.

2 Cocking, J. Out-patient clinic planning. Health and Social Service Journal, 83, 1 Sep 1973, 1991.

3 Downey, G. W. Outpatient center improves care, identifies cost. [Beth Israel Ambulatory Center.] Modern Hospital, 120 (6), Jun 1973, 77–80.

4 Eaton, S. Invaluable outcasts: the importance of outpatient work. Nursing Times, 71, 3 Jul 1975, 1068.

5 Evans, P. C. and Murdock, C. The non-attender in an out-patient department. Hospital and Health Services Review, 69 (9), Sep 1973, 333–337.

6 Evans, P. C. and Murdock, C. Non-attenders in outpatient departments. Nursing Times, 69, 1 Nov 1973, 1462–1465.

7 Granstrom, W. P. Outpatient care. [Organizations of one centre.] Hospitals, 47 (13), Jul 1973, 43–45.

8 Hanson, S. Ambulatory nursing standards. [Compiled by the Outpatient Department, University Hospital, Seattle.] Supervisor Nurse, 6 (12), Dec 1975, 10–15.

9 Hauff, W. R. Centralized outpatient care. [St. Mary's Health Center, St. Louis.] Hospitals, 48, 1 Feb 1974, 87–90.

10 Heath, J. L. Out patient efficiency. Health and Social Service Journal, 83, 24 Mar 1973, 660.

11 Metsch, J. M. Administrative evaluation of ambulatory care program effectiveness. Journal of Nursing Administration, 5 (5), Jun 1975, 39–42.

12 Metsch, J. M. and Tilley, F. N. Ambulatory care. Planning integrated, comprehensive services. Hospitals, 49 (12), 16 Jun 1975, 63–66.

13 Pike, N. In hospital. 2. The outpatient's view. [Compiled while on a middle management course.] Nursing Mirror, 140, 1 May 1975, 51.

14 Sandlow, L. J. Quality for walking patients: evaluation of care in out-patient settings. Hospitals, 49 (5), 1 Mar 1975, 95–99.

15 Schiavone, C. Management of patient care in an outpatient department. Nursing Clinics of North America, 8 (2), Jun 1973, 305–311.

16 Thomstad, B. E. and Kaplan, B. H. Nurse clinician: lone commando under fire. [Scheme to improve ambulatory care in an outpatient department.] American Journal of Nursing, 74 (11), Nov 1974, 1993–1997.

17 Vogel, L. C. and Sjoersdma, A. A brief encounter between patient and staff. [Outpatient departments.] Kenya Nursing Journal, 2 (1), Jun 1973, 43–46.

o PLANNING AND DESIGN

1 Breger, W. N. Nurse participation in nursing unit design for health care facilities. Journal of Nursing Administration, 4 (1), Jan/Feb 1974, 52–57.

2 Brigden, R. J. Best buy hospital. 1. Central treatment facilities. Nursing Times, 71, 28 Aug 1975, 1363–1366.

3 British Hospital Journal and Social Service Review The Charing Cross Project, by F. Hart, H. Clift and M. S. Abbott. British Hospital Journal and Social Service Review, 82, 9 Dec 1972, 2746–2748; 16 Dec 1972, 2802–2803; 23 Dec 1972, 2859–2860.

4 Buchanan, D. Moving a ward. [Guidelines laid down at St. Helier Hospital.] Nursing Times, 68, 21 Dec 1972, 1607–1608.

5 Curry, I. How can research assist the nurse in planning capital building projects? North West Thames Nursing Research Bulletin no. 2, Autumn 1974, 17–21.

6 Dix, C. Inside new hospitals. [Building hospitals for patients and staff.] New Society, 28, 4 Apr 1974, 17–18.

7 Friesen, G. A. and Silvin, R. Concepts of health planning. [Integrated approach to hospital design.] World Hospitals, 11 (1), Winter 1975, 35–42.

8 Fry, W. F. and Lauer, J. The planning team: why include nursing membership. Journal of Nursing Administration, 11 (5), Sep/Oct 1972, 71–74.

9 Hamilton, J. Ward room design. Lamp, 32 (3), Mar 1975, 30–36.

10 Hospital and Health Services Review Notes for students. Preparation and approval of individual building schemes. Hospital and Health Services Review, 69 (7), Jul 1973, 272–274.

11 Hospital and Health Services Review Planning guidance material by the DHSS. [Notes for students.] Hospital and Health Services Review, 69, Dec 1973, 479–480.

12 Hughes, J. R. A large nursing unit. [The first in-patient building of the redeveloped Southampton General Hospital (SH University Hospital)]. Nursing Times, 69, 6 Dec 1973, 1660–1661.

13 Isler, C. Nursing in the round. [Cleveland Metropolitan Hospital.] RN Magazine, 35 (11), Nov 1972, 48–51.

14 Lewis, C. J. The Royal Free Hospital – 1. Commissioning training. [For nurses and other staff.] Nursing Times, 70, 3 Oct 1974, 1530–1531.

15 Michaelsen, G. S. Evaluating the hospital environment. Hospitals, 49 (9), 1 May 1975, 69–72.

16 Mikho, E. Hospital building for developing countries: a system approach. World Hospitals, 10 (3), Summer 1974, 150–162.

17 Modern Healthcare One patient, one room: theory and practice. [Survey in California and Utah to examine relative advantages including the gain in quality of care.] Modern Healthcare, 3 (3), Mar 1975, 65–68.

18 Nursing Times Beyond the 'best buy'. Mrs. Castle announces new concept in hospital planning. Nursing Times, 71, 8 May 1975, 713.

19 Rab, K. S. 'Team patient care' room design. Hospital Administration of Canada, 17 (7), Jul 1975, 25–28.

20 Reid, E. A. and Feeley, E. M. Roommates: to have or have not. [Survey of patients in two-bedded rooms.] American Journal of Nursing, 73, Jan 1973, 104–107.

21 Rogers, P. J. Designing for patient care. [Planning a new hospital system.] International Nursing Review, 19 (3), 1972, 267–282.

22 Ryan, J. L. The nursing administrator's growing role in facilities planning. Journal of Nursing Administration, 5 (9), Nov/Dec 1975, 22–27.

23 Shaw, J. E. Commissioning at Southampton. [The use of multidisciplinary user groups for operational policy preparation and management policy at a new teaching hospital.] Health and Social Service Journal, 84, 30 Nov 1974, 2774–2775.

24 Spencer, S. R. A nurse in commissioning. [A nurse as a member of the commissioning team for a new hospital.] Australian Nurses' Journal, 3 (3), Sep 1973, 26–29, 32.

25 Turner, T. M. Best buy hospital – 2. Use of the

central treatment room. [Bury St. Edmunds.] Nursing Times, 71, 4 Sep 1975, 1414–1416.

26 **Voss, P.** Nurse planners. Nursing Times, 71, 14 Aug 1975, 1278–1279.

27 **Woollings, B.A.** Basildon's first hospital: the planning of a new hospital in all its stages, described by a nurse planning officer. Nursing Times, 135, 4 Aug 1972, 21–23.

28 **World Hospitals** Special issues on planning and building health care facilities under conditions of limited resources. World Hospitals, 11 (2/3), Spring/Summer 1975, 55–224; 11 (4), Autumn 1975, 229–248.

p RECORDS AND INFORMATION

1 **Bashook, P. G. and others** Education plan key to POMR success. [Systematic training of staff in use of problem oriented medical records.] Hospitals, 49 (8), 16 Apr 1975, 54–58.

2 **Bonner, B. B.** Problem oriented medical records. Health and Social Service Journal, 83, 17 Feb 1973, 373–374.

3 **De Vries Robbe, P. F.** Useful elements of P.O.M.R. A report of experience. Medical Record, 16 (1), Winter 1975, 13–17.

4 **Ellis-Martin, K. G.** Modernise your master index. [New SISCO system at the Royal Free Hospital, using microfiche.] Health and Social Service Journal, 85, 6 Sep 1975, 1971.

5 **Hill, P. A.** Medical information and patient care. Nursing Mirror, 139, 26 Sep 1974, 52–53.

6 **Jolley, J. L.** Feature cards in the medical field. Medical Record, 14 (2), May 1973, 51–55.

7 **Jones, F. A.** Trends in medical records. Community Health, 7 (1), Jul/Aug 1975, 32–48.

8 **McIntyre, N.** The problem oriented medical record. British Medical Journal, 1, 9 Jun 1973, 598–600.

9 **McNeilly, R. H. and Moore, F.** The accuracy of some hospital activity analysis data. Hospital and Health Services Review, 71 (3), Mar 1975, 93–95.

10 **Murray, A.** Analysing medical records: a Canadian system. Health and Social Service Journal, 84, 21 Sep 1974, 2160–2161.

11 **Pilling, H. J.** Microfilming and computers. [Use for medical records.] Hospital and Health Services Review, 70 (11), Nov 1974, 387–389.

12 **Rossiter, W. J. C.** Disclosure of medical records. Medical Record, 14 (2), May 1973, 41–42.

13 **Smith, G.** A short history of medical records. Medical Record, 16 (2), 1975, 59–64.

14 **Smith, G.** Standard admission form. [Devised by the Association of Medical Records Officers.] Medical Record, 15 (3/4), Summer/Autumn 1974, 89–93.

15 **White, K. J. C.** The integration of records and indices. [A system for bridging the gap between the present storage of medical records and the computer future.] Health and Social Service Journal, 84, 9 Nov 1974, 2598.

q STAFF AND INDUSTRIAL RELATIONS

1 **Armour, W. and Torrington, D.** Industrial relations in hospitals. Health and Social Service Journal, 85, 28 Jun 1975, 1330–1331.

2 **Bishop, T.** Immigrant labour in Britain's hospitals. Personnel Management, 5 (8), Aug 1973, 25–27.

3 **Bosanquet, N.** Talking point. Too many cooks? [The growth of administrative staff in hospitals as a result of reorganization.] Nursing Times, 71, 27 Feb 1975, 326–327.

4 **Burns, J. B.** NHS salary evolution: survival of the fittest? [Analysis changes in pay of various groups of hospital staff 1955–1973.] Health and Social Service Journal, 85, 8 Mar 1975, 544–546.

5 **Carlson, C. E. and Vernon, D. T. A.** Measurement of informativeness of hospital staff members. Nursing Research, 22 (3), May/Jun 1973, 198–205.

6 **Choy, N. K.** Staff orientation. Nursing Journal of Singapore, 14 (1), May 1974, 29–31.

7 **Cuming, M. W.** Industrial action: a note on administrative practice during the action by hospital ancillary staff, Spring, 1973. Hospital and Health Services Review, 70 (4), Apr 1974, 122–124.

8 **Edwards, P. J.** The register of hospital English. International Nursing Review, 21 (6), Nov/Dec 1974, 174–183.

9 **Ford, A.** A department of staff education developed – with success. [University Hospital, London, Ontario.] Hospital Administration in Canada, 16 (7), Jul 1974, 24–29.

10 **Health and Social Service Journal** Breaking the language barrier. [Experimental English language course at St. Bernard's Hospital, Southall.] Health and Social Service Journal, 83, 10 Feb 1973, 311–312.

11 **McDowall, A. and others** Industrial relations in the hospital service, a checklist. King Edward's Hospital Fund for London, 1974.

12 **Meara, R. and others** Industrial relations in the hospital service. [A survey.] Health and Social Service Journal, 84, 9 Mar 1974, 535.

13 **Millard, G.** Personnel management in hospitals. Institute of Personnel Management, 1972.

14 **Miller, R. L.** Collective bargaining: a new frontier for hospitals. Hospital Progress, 56 (2), Feb 1975, 58–60, 65.

15 **Naylor, W. M.** Health expectations. [Presidential address at the 1975 IHSA conference discusses management in the NHS and Whitley machinery.] Hospital and Health Services Review, 71 (6), Jun 1975, 198–202.

16 **O'Connor, V. and Boorer, D.** Northwick Park's powerhouse people. [Personnel department.] Nursing Times, 69, 27 Sep 1973, 1252–1253.

17 **Royston, R.** Breaking the language barrier. [Report of a King's Fund Centre conference dealing with the language problems of foreign hospital workers.] Health and Social Service Journal, 84, 21/28 Dec 1974, 2929.

18 **Veninga, R.** The management of conflict [In hospital staff relationships]. Journal of Nursing Administration, 3 (4), Jul/Aug 1973, 13–16.

19 **Watkin, B.** Management topics – induction. Nursing Mirror, 138, 3 May 1974, 77.

20 **Watkin, B.** Reflections on the hospitals strike. Health and Social Service Journal, 83, 14 Jul 1973, 1575–1576, 1578.

21 **Willey, R.** Hospital relations. [Industrial relations in hospitals.] Nursing Mirror, 140, 20 Mar 1975, 67–69.

r VOLUNTEERS

1 **Boorer, D.** Staff and volunteers. [The relationship between paid and unpaid workers in hospitals.] Health and Social Service Journal, 84, 29 Jun 1974, 1452–1453.

2 **McCarrick, H.** Cheap labour – or a new dimension? [Volunteers]. Nursing Times, 69, 9 Aug 1973, 1030–1032.

3 **McCarrick, H.** The Hospital Saturday Fund – a hundred years on. Nursing Times, 69, 29 Nov 1973, 1618–1619.

4 **McLeod, E.** Hospital volunteers. [A new scheme at Wellington Hospital.] New Zealand Nursing Journal, 67 (12), Dec 1974, 25.

5 **Martin, M.** Patients and volunteers. Health and Social Service Journal, 83, 11 Aug 1973, 1807–1808.

6 **Pinel, C.** Recruitment of volunteers in geriatric hospitals. Nursing Mirror, 137, 5 Oct 1973, 31–32.

7 **Porter, R.** The polka dot girls. [Schoolgirl volunteers in East Cheshire's general and psychiatric hospitals.] Health and Social Service Journal, 84, 24 Aug 1974, 1927.

8 **Stevenson, D.** Objectives of voluntary organizations. Health and Social Service Journal, 83, 8 Sep 1973, 2057.

9 **Twisleton-Wykeham-Fiennes, O.** Voluntary work – a vocation? [Part played by voluntary workers in linking hospital with community and the attitudes of the churches.] Health and Social Service Journal, 83, 21 Apr 1973, 905–906.

COMMUNITY SERVICES

32 COMMUNITY HEALTH

a GENERAL

1 Byrne, P. S. Integrated medicine. [Interdisciplinary work in the community.] Practice Team, 49, Jun 1975, 8–10.

2 Carr, M. Island practice. [Medical services in the Scilly Isles.] Nursing Times, 71, 25 Dec 1975, 2077–2078.

3 Cockcroft, F. Screening tests. Nursing Times, 20 Jun 1974, 955–957

4 Corkill, B. Towards a neighbourhood service [in the London Borough of Tower Hamlets]. Nursing Times, 70, 3 Oct 1974, 1552–1554

5 Davies, J. B. M. Community health and social services. 2nd ed. English Universities Press, 1972

6 Davies, J. B. M. Preventive medicine, community health and social services. 2nd ed. Bailliere, 1971.

7 Donaldson, R. J. Research in community care. [In Teesside.] Public Health, 88 (2), Jan, 1974, 63–70.

8 Dunn, A. The Midlands. Milton Keynes – planning for the year 2001. Nursing Times, 70, 12 Sep 1974, 1410–1413.

9 Evans, E. M. and others Community care: the patient at home, British Broadcasting Corporation, 1972.

10 Farmer, R. Community care – a model system. [The care needs of a modern community.] International Journal of Nursing Studies, 11 (1), Jun 1974, 21–31.

11 Ferrer, H. P. The case for prevention. Health and Social Service Journal, 84, 21/28 Dec 1974, 2935–2936.

12 Grundy, P. F. A rational approach to the 'at risk' concept. Lancet, 2, 29 Dec 1973, 1489.

13 Hall, T. Health screening. Community Health, 6 (1) Jul/Aug 1974, 41–45.

14 Hawthorne, V. M. New dimensions in the discovery of disease. [Screening in preventive medicine.] Nursing Mirror, 136, 22 Jun 1973, 42–44.

15 Jackson, S. M. and Lane, S. Personal and community health. Baillière Tindall, 1975. (Nurses' aids series.)

16 Jones, R. K. and Jones, P. A. Sociology in medicine. English Universities Press, 1975. (Modern nursing series.)

17 Knox, E. G. Screening for disease. Multiphasic screening. Lancet, 2, 14 Dec 1974, 1434–1436.

18 McKeown, T. and Lowe, C. R. An introduction to social medicine. 2nd ed. Oxford: Blackwell, 1974.

19 Maclean, U. Social and community medicine for students. Heinemann Medical, 1971.

20 Markham, J. and Smith, J. P. Community care.

Heinemann, 1975. (For student and pupil nurses.)

21 Oelbaum, C. H. Hallmarks of adult wellness. [Nursing's responsibility to promote wellness and what constitutes this state.] American Journal of Nursing, 74 (9), Sep 1974, 1623–1625.

22 Pesznecker, B. L. and McNeil, J. Relationship among health habits, social assets, psychological well-being, life change, and alterations in health status. [A study by questionnaire of 1,145 residents of Renton, Washington, to examine why some people remain healthy.] Nursing Research, 24 (6), Nov/Dec 1975, 442–447.

23 Stickle, E. A. The objectives of team work. [In community health work.] Nursing Mirror, 134, 16 Jun 1972, 37–39.

24 Taggart, J. McA. Community health services under stress. [Belfast.] Community Health, 5 (4), Jan/Feb 1974, 201–207.

25 Tomalin, C. Rural health care. [Community care in Northumberland.] Health and Social Service Journal 85, 22 Nov 1975, 2606–2607.

26 World Health Organization Mass health examinations. Geneva: WHO, 1971 (Public health papers 45.)

b PRIMARY HEALTH CARE

1 Bloomfield, R. and Follis, P. The health team in action: 18 essays about the general practice health team. BBC Publications, 1974.

2 Bodenstein, J. W. Primary health care: its principles and some of its implications in our South African Development Context. SA Nursing Journal, 42 (11), Nov 1975, 20–24.

3 British Medical Association Board of Science and Education Report of the Panel on Primary Health Care Teams. BMA, 1974.

4 Council for the Education and Training of Health Visitors More team work needed in primary health care. [Report of an enquiry carried out by Edinburgh University's Department of Nursing Studies which examined three health care teams.] Nursing Times, 70, 5 Dec 1974, 1876.

5 Lamberts, H. and Riphagen, F. E. Working together in a team for primary health care – a guide to dangerous country. [Evolution of a multidisciplinary team in Rotterdam.] Journal of the Royal College of General Practitioners, 25, Oct 1975, 745–752.

6 Lloyd, G. and others An interdisciplinary workshop. [Meeting of doctors, district nurses, health visitors and social workers.] Journal of the Royal College of General Practitioners, 23, Jul 1973, 463–473.

7 Malcolm, A. Caring for one another. [A new look at the internal strength of a primary care team.] Queen's Nursing Journal, 17 (10), Jan 1975, 223–224; (11), Feb 1975, 245–246.

8 Pang, H. An approach to primary care. Australian Nurses' Journal 2 (8), Feb 1973, 18, 20, 21.

9 Pritchard, P. M. M. Community participation in primary health care. [The value of obtaining views on general practice from all organizations.] British Medical Journal, 3, 6 Sep 1975, 583–584.

10 Sibbald, R. J. I. Primary medical care in Canada. Journal of the Royal College of General Practitioners, 24, Oct 1974, 727–732.

11 Stickle, E. A. The objectives of team work. [In community health work.] Nursing Mirror, 134, 16 Jun 1972, 37–39.

12 World Health Organization. Regional Office for Europe The definition of parameters of efficiency in primary care and the role of nursing in primary health care: report on two working groups, Reykjavik, 14–18 July 1975. Copenhagen: WHO, 1975.

c GENERAL PRACTICE

1 Brooks, M. B. Management of the team in general practice. Journal of the Royal College of General Practitioners 129, Apr 1973, 239–252.

2 Cooper, B. Social work in general practice: the Derby scheme. Lancet, 1, 13 Mar 1971, 539–542.

3 Gang, S. G. The family doctor and the social worker. [Experiment in social worker attachment.] Practitioner, 214, May 1975, 673–678.

4 Hall, M. S. The diagnosis and treatment of patients in general practice. District Nursing, 3, 18 May 1972, 33–35.

5 Honywood, H. Portrait of a practice – Measham [Leicestershire]. Practice Team, no 42/43, Nov/Dec 1974, 2, 4–7.

6 Hood, J. E. and Farmer, R. D. T. A comparative study of frequent and infrequent attenders at a general practice. International Journal of Nursing Studies, 11 (3), Sep 1974, 147–152.

7 Izzard, R. C. F. The GP and the family health team. 1. Clinical efficiency and job satisfaction. 2. Observations on interprofessional relationships. Nursing Times, 68, 11 May 1972, 572–574.

8 Kuensberg, E. V. Tampoline on cottonwool. [Impact of reorganization on the health team in general practice.] Nursing Times 71, 3 Apr 1975, 533–534.

9 Lloyd-James, A. and Lambert, P. M. An attachment scheme with a difference. [Attachment of a local authority doctor to a group of GPs.] First published in British Medical Journal, 19 Sep 1970. Nursing Times, 67, 7 Jan 1971, 16–17.

10 Marks, J. Aspects of the reorganized NHS. The GP and the new health service. Midwife and Health Visitor, 10 (7), Jul 1974, 183, 185–186.

11 Orriss, H. D. Medical certificates – suggestions for their improvement. Nursing Times, 70, 4 Jul 1974, 1044–1045.

12 Owen, H. The role of the medical secretary. Queen's Nursing Journal, 1975, 170–171.

13 Ratoff, L. More social work for general practice? Journal of The Royal College of General Practitioners, 23, Oct 1973, 736–742.

14 Smallridge, P. W. Social work and medicine. [Relationships between social workers and doctors, with particular reference to group practice.] Health and Social Service Journal, 83, 28 Jul 1973, 1695–1696.

d HEALTH CENTRES

1 Bain, D. J. G. Health centre practice in Livingston New Town. Health Bulletin, 31 (6), Nov 1973, 290–296.

2 Bain, D. J. G. and Haines, A. J. A treatment room survey in a health centre in a new town. Health Bulletin, 32 (3), May 1974, 111–119.

3 Bourns, H. K. Aspects of nursing services in health centres. [Treatment of casualties.] Nursing Times, 70, 18 Apr 1974, 601–602.

4 Duncan, U. C. M. Glasgow's bid for better health. [Woodside health centre.] Nursing Times, 70, 14 Feb 1974, 220–222.

5 Duncan, U. C. M. Nursing services [in Woodside Health Centre]. Health Bulletin, 31 (3), May, 130–132.

6 Follis, P. and Rodgers, A. Wellingborough Health Centre: a study. [Planning study.] Practice Team, no. 44, Jan 1975, 12–16.

7 Health and Social Service Journal Health centre advances. [DHSS conference on planning and design.] Health and Social Service Journal, 83, 21 Apr 1973, 908–909, 911.

8 Health Bulletin The Woodside story. [Special health centre number.] Health Bulletin, 31 (3) May 1973, 106–175.

9 Honywood, H. Prognosis and performance. [The Cleveland Health Centre, Middlesbrough.] Practice Team, no. 38, Jul 1974, 5–9.

10 Jarvis, D. The health centre: a team approach to health care delivery. [Organization of two model health centres in Australia.] Lamp 32 (4) Apr 1975, 15, 17, 19.

11 Laing, S. A. Family health care from health centres. Queen's Nursing Journal, 15 (3), Jun 1973, 63–64, 75

12 MacDonald, M. D. and others Patients' attitudes to the provision of medical care from a health centre. Journal of the Royal College of General Practitioners, 24, Jan 1974, 29–36.

13 McGuire, B. S. Health centre practice and area study. Queen's Nursing Journal, 16 (3), Jun 1973, 58–69, 61.

14 Mills, N. H. N. Health centre satisfaction survey. [Blaenavon Health Centre, Monmouthshire.] Health and Social Service Journal, 83, 29 Sep 1973, 2246–2248, 2251.

15 Morris, J. Mufakose Clinic. [Primary care clinic in Rhodesia.] Rhodesian Nurse, 8 (4), Dec 1975, 6–8.

16 Morton, B. F. Nursing service and education in a comprehensive health care center. Journal of Nursing Administration, 3 (3), May/Jun 1973, 24–26.

17 Munier, S. K. and Richardson, A. A nursing service and education project: development of new nursing roles in a comprehensive health center. Journal of Nursing Administration, 4 (4), Jul/Aug 1974, 44–49.

18 New Zealand Nursing Journal Mosgiel Health Centre. [Seminar paper presented as part of a panel entitled 'Experimentation in Nursing'.] New Zealand Nursing Journal, 69 (10), Oct 1975, 4–5.

19 Nursing Mirror Kent cares for its own. [Dover Health Centre – mainly illustrations.] Nursing Mirror, 136, 4 May 1973, 25–27.

20 Nursing Times Largest health centre for Middlesbrough. [Cleveland Square Health Centre.] Nursing Times, 69, 22 Nov 1973, 1549.

21 Patterson, J. S. Patients' attitudes to health centres. [Review of nine surveys carried out between 1970 and 1973.] Health Bulletin 33 (2), Mar 1975, 52–57.

22 Pattison, F. Community health centre, Roddickton. [Labrador.] Queen's Nursing Journal, 17 (1), Apr 1974, 10, 14.

23 Practice Team Health Centre comments. [Comments and architect's reply to previously published plan of projected health centre.] Practice Team, no. 45, Feb 1975, 10–13.

24 Rae, J. I. and others The treatment rooms in a health centre: report of a pilot study. [Functions of treatment rooms at Woodside Health Centre, Glasgow.] Health Bulletin 33 (4), Jul 1975, 143–152.

25 Stewart, T. I. Reflections on the place of the health centre in the community health team. Practice Team, no 41, Oct 1974, 7, 10–11.

26 Turner, R. M. The Thamesmead project. International Journal of Nursing Studies, 10 (1), Jan 1973, 33–39.

27 University of Kent. Health Services Research Unit Administrative aspects of health centre management. [Conference.] Journal of the Royal College of General Practitioners, 23, Jul 1973, 504–509.

28 Varley, A. The nurse's role in health centre planning. Nursing Times, 69, 12 Jul 1973, 904–907.

29 Walker, J. H. Equipping the Health Centre. Health and Social Service Journal, 83, 23 Jun 1973, 1420–1421.

30 Weston, J. A. B. Getting your communications right. [Communications systems at Chertsey Health Centre.] Practice Team, no. 45, Feb 1975, 2, 4, 6.

31 Woods, J. O. and others Health centres assessed by patients. Journal of the Royal College of General Practitioners, 24, Jan 1974, 23–27.

e HEALTH EDUCATION

1 Ademuwagun, Z. A. The challenge of health education methods and techniques in developing countries. Health Education Journal, 33 (1), 1974, 13–21.

2 British Medical Journal Health education in the reorganized NHS. [Leading article.] British Medical Journal, 1, 1 Feb 1975, 233.

3 Calhoun, J. N. The nurses and health education. Kenya Nursing Journal, 2 (1), Jun 1973, 19–21.

4 Dalzell-Ward, A. J. The health centre as a focal point for health education. Health Education Journal, 34 (2), 1975, 48–50.

5 Dalzell-Ward, A. J. Health education in the 1970s. Community Health, 4 (5), Mar/Apr 1973, 230–238.

6 Dowling, M. A. C. Audiovisual media in health teaching. WHO Chronicle, 26 (1), Jan 1972, 3–6.

7 Eardley, A. and others Health education by chance: the unmet needs of patients in hospital and after. International Journal of Health Education, 18 (1), 1975, 19–25.

8 Elliott, D. S. The health visitor and health education. Community Health, 5 (1), Jul/Aug 1973.

9 Evans, M. W. An introduction to health education in hospital. Nursing Mirror, 139, 10 Oct 1974, 49–50.

10 Ferguson, J. The role of the pharmacist in health education. Mother and Child, 46 (1), Feb 1974, 9–10, 22.

11 Galli, E. Change of attitude – a function of a health educator. SA Nursing Journal, 60 (6), Jun 1973, 23–24.

12 Leininger, M. This I believe . . . about interdisciplinary health education for the future. Nursing Outlook, 19 (12), Dec 1971, 787–791.

13 Milbank, D. J. Aspects of health education. Midwife and Health Visitor, 5 (11), Nov 1969, 449–452.

14 Modern Hospital Making the patient a part of patient care. [Health education for patients in hospital.] Modern Hospital, 121 (4), Oct 1973, 105–110.

15 Pender, N. J. Patient identification of health information received during hospitalization. Nursing Research, 23 (3), May/Jun 1974, 262–267.

16 Pike, L. A. Health education in general practice. Community Health, 4 (4), Jan/Feb 1973, 179–184.

17 Pitcairn-Jones, P. Meeting the needs. [In health education.] Mother and Child, 43 (1), Jan/Feb 1971, 10–13.

18 Rehrmann, D. Health education in industry through audiovisual techniques. Occupational Health Nursing, 20 (1), Jan 1972, 7–8.

19 Ruddick-Bracken, H. The district nurse as health educator. Nursing Times, 69, 13 Sept 1973, 1187–1189.

20 Slovak, S. M. Health education in women's magazines. Nursing Times, 68, 11 May 1972, Occ papers, 73–75.

21 Stewart, R. F. Education for health maintenance. Occupational Health Nursing, 22 (6), Jun 1974, 14–17.

22 Tinch, J. For sickness or for health? The role of the nurse in health education. Nursing Mirror, 140, 24 Apr 1978, 71–72.

23 Waller, P. J. Health education is concerned with the changing of attitudes. Health Visitor, 47 (11), Nov 1974, 310–311.

24 Who Chronicle Health education: a review of the WHO programme. WHO Chronicle, 28 (9), Sep 1974, 401–409.

25 Yarrow, A. Health education in the reorganized health service. Health Trends, 6 (1), Feb 1974, 11–14.

33 COMMUNITY HEALTH NURSING

a GENERAL

1 Barnard, J. M. The links with community nursing. [Similar health goals of occupational health nurses, health visitors and district nurses.] Nursing Mirror, 141, 11 Sep 1975, 65–67.

2 Borlick, M. M. and others Community health nursing 1600 multiple choice questions and reference answers. 2nd ed. Flushing: Medical Examination Publishing Co., 1974. (Nursing examination review book 9.)

3 Bosanquet, N. Community cares. [Problems of conditions of work and allowances for community staff.] Nursing Times, 70, 19 Dec 1974, 1961.

4 Brown, D. E. Regeneration of nursing – and training for a new role. [Community health nurses in a reorganized NHS.] British Hospital Journal and Social Service Review 82, 22 Apr 1972, 887.

5 Buckoke, Y. E. Nursing in the community: a time for reform? [Primary medical care team.] Nursing Times, 67, 26 Aug 1971, Occ. papers, 133–136.

6 Butterworth, J. The community nursing service – the need for change. [Reprinted from journal of the Bradford Royal Infirmary Nurses League.] Health Visitor, 45 (11), Nov 1972, 353–354.

7 Carre, J. Health care in the community [and the role of the community nurse]. Nursing Mirror, 138, 24 May 1974, 54–58.

8 Carson, H. E. A. Nursing services in Wandsworth. District Nursing, 14 (12), Mar 1972, 258–260.

9 Chisholm, M. K. The community – fortress or focal point? Midwife and Health Visitor, 10 (8), Aug 1974, 230–232.

10 Chisholm, M. K. Design, drift and directive. [Changes in the NHS and the recommendations of the Briggs Report as they will affect nurses.] Nursing Mirror, 137, 3 Aug 1973, 33–34.

11 Clark, J. The nurse and primary contact. [Report of conference.] Nursing Times, 67, 9 Dec 1971, 1546–1547.

12 Colliere, M. F. Thoughts on a new approach to public health nursing. International Nursing Review, 22 (3), May/Jun 1975, 80–86.

13 Haigh, E. Team work in Kent. [Community nursing services after reorganisation.] Queen's Nursing Journal, 17 (3), Jun 1974, 52–53.

14 Hasler, J. C. The community nurse in the 70s. Nursing Times, 67, 4 Feb 1971, 146–147.

15 Hockey, L. Use or abuse? A study of the state enrolled nurse in the local authority nursing services. Queen's Institute of District Nursing, 1972.

16 Lamb, A. M. Local authority nursing staff within the future integrated health service. Queen's Nursing Journal, 17 (2), May 1974, 28–30.

17 Lamb, A. M. The public health or community nurse – her duties and responsibilities in the new health service. Royal Society of Health Journal, 93 (6), Dec 1973, 305–308.

18 MacQueen, I. The curious term 'community nurse'. [Lists the different types of nurses who work in the community.] Nursing Mirror, 132, 11 Jun 1971, 10.

19 Stickle, E. A. The triple duty district nursing sister. [Health visitor, district nurse and midwife who functions in some rural areas of Scotland.] Nursing Times, 71, 5 Jun 1975, 900–901.

20 Wilkes, E. 'Increased responsibilities' for the nurse in the community. [Lecture at the annual open meeting of the Queen's Nursing Institute.] Nursing Mirror, 139, 12 Dec 1974, 35.

21 Wilkes, E. The new responsibilities of the nurse in the community. Queen's Nursing Journal, 17 (10), Jan 1975, 214, 216.

22 World Health Organization Expert Committee Community health nursing. Geneva: WHO, 1974. (Technical report series 558.) Summary in Nursing Times 71, 26 Jun 1975, 994; WHO Chronicle, 29 (3) Nov 1975, 91–96.

b MANAGEMENT AND STAFFING

1 Aradine, C. R. and Guthneck, M. The problem oriented record in a family health service. American Journal of Nursing, 74 (6), Jun 1974, 1108–1112.

2 Byatt, J. Management by objectives. [In the nursing management structure in the London Borough of Hillingdon.] Nursing Times, 69, 20/27 Dec 1973, 1736–1737.

3 Conroy, P. Comparative disease study. [A survey in Portsmouth designed to assess future nursing care needs.] District Nursing, 15 (11), Feb 1973, 242–243.

4 Dalton, E. R. and others Changing trends in the staffing levels of community nurses. Community Medicine, 128, 12 May 1972, 97–101.

5 District Nursing Management structure in the local authority nursing services. District Nursing, 14 (12), Mar 1972, 254, 260.

6 Doncaster Area Health Authority Audit for the community nursing servics. Doncaster: The Health Authority, 1975.

7 Few, E. Mayston managed in Buckinghamshire. District Nursing, 14 (12), Mar 1972, 255–257.

8 Hope, P. K. and Goldsberry, J. E. Supervisor to community health nurse clinician. Journal of Nursing Administration, 3 (5), Sep/Oct 1973, 49–54.

9 Horner, J. S. Management by objectives in a local health authority. Community Medicine, 128, 21 Jul 1972, 327–332.

10 Johnson, K. J. and Zimmerman, M. A. Peer review in a health department. [Assessment of leadership potential and working relationships among community health nurses.] American Journal of Nursing, 75 (4), Apr 1975, 618–619.

11 Kissinger, C. L. Community nursing administration: quantifying nursing utilization. Journal of Nursing Administration, 3 (5), Sep/Oct 1973, 42–48.

12 Lamb, A. M. The Mayston report. Midwives Chronicle, 85, Jan 1972, 14–15.

13 Lemin, B. Management and Mayston. District Nursing, 15 (6), Sep 1972, 116, 119.

14 McCarthy, M. K. E. and others Reorganization training for field workers. [Training programme in Leicester for district nurses, midwives and health visitors for NHS reorganization and the introduction of a Mayston management structure.] Nursing Times, 70, 21 Feb 1974, 286–287.

15 Mayers, M. G. A search for assessment criteria. [Of the effectiveness of community health nursing.] Nursing Outlook, 20 (5), May 1972, 323–326.

16 Midwife and Health Visitor Leader on the Mayston Report. Midwife and Health Visitor, 7 (10), Oct 1971, 379.

17 Midwives Chronicle Implementation of Mayston. Midwives Chronicle, 87, Feb 1974, 48–49.

18 Scottish Home and Health Department Nurse staffing (community) survey: book of tables. Edinburgh: The Department, 1975, (Nursing manpower planning report, 4.)

19 Smiley, O. R. The core committee: a model for decision-making within public health units. Nursing Clinics of North America, 8 (2), Jun 1973, 355–359.

20 Smiley, O. R. A management model for public health units. Dimensions in Health Service, 51 (1), 13 Mar 1974, 62–63.

21 Webb, B. B. Community nurse reserve bank. [Leicestershire.] Queen's Nursing Journal, 17 (3), Jun 1974, 60–61.

22 Young, W. C. A work study of nursing staff in a health department. [Burgh of Motherwell and Wishaw and effect of GP attachment.] Health Bulletin, 29 (3), Jul 1971, 154–161.

c OVERSEAS COUNTRIES

1 Adebo, E. O. The expanding roles of the community health nurse in present Nigeria. Nigerian Nurse, 6 (1), Jan/Mar 1974, 36–38.

2 Ademuwagun, Z. A. Toward improved group planning process in public health. Nigerian Nurse, 6 (3), Jul/Sep 1974, 6–13.

3 Anstey, O. E. Community centred care and its effect on nursing. [New South Wales College of Nursing twentieth annual oration.] Lamp, 29 (10), Oct 1972, 21–26.

4 Archer, S. E. and Fleshman, R. P. Community health nursing: a typology of practice. Nursing Outlook, 23 (6), Jun 1975, 358–364.

5 Bactat, J. L. Health care delivery: the expanding role of the community health nurse. Philippine Journal of Nursing, 44 (3), Jul/Sep 1975, 166–172.

6 Beal, J. R. Nurses at work. Growed like Topsy. [The Blue Nursing Service, a domiciliary nursing service in Brisbane.] Australian Nurses' Journal, 4 (6), Dec 1974/Jan 1975, 14–15.

7 Beaton-Mamak, M. The VON: caring since 1898. [Victorian Order of Nurses operating a home nursing service in Canada.] Dimensions in Health Service, 52 (3), Mar 1975, 22–23.

8 Bergman, R. Evaluation of community health nursing. Australian Nurses' Journal, 4 (8), Mar 1975, 39–41.

9 Blair, L. R. Social nursing – or the action station. Australian Nurses' Journal, 2 (10), Apr 1973, 27–29.

10 Byrne, M. and Bennett, F. J. Community nursing in developing countries: a manual for the auxiliary public health nurse. Oxford University Press, 1973.

11 Carl, M. K. Community planning for nursing and nursing education. Nursing Outlook, 20 (8), Aug 1972, 507–509.

12 Davis, M. Community health nursing and the Western Metropolitan health region. Lamp, 30 (8), Aug 1973, 20–21.

13 Dawson, N. and Stern, M. Perceptions of priorities for home nursing care. Nursing Research, 2 (2), Mar/Apr 1973, 145–153.

14 Dorman, M. A health visitor in the Sudan. Mother and Child, 46 (2), Mar 1974, 7–8.

15 Dunn, A. USA. Home health care. [Work of the Visiting Nurse Associations in New York, Chicago and Washington.] Nursing Times, 71, 10 Jul 1975, 1082–1084.

16 Fagin, C. M. and Goodwin, B. Baccalaureate preparation for primary care. [At Herbert H. Lehman College in New York.] Nursing Outlook, 20 (4), Apr 1972, 240–244.

17 Fitzsimons, M. The public health nursing service. World of Irish Nursing, 3 (2), Mar 1974, 39–40.

18 Gawith, M. The nurse's role in community health care. UNA Nursing Journal, Jan/Feb 1974, 36–39.

19 Gray, L. J. Starting a community nursing service in Hong Kong. Queen's Nursing Journal, 17 (9), Dec 1974, 198–201.

20 Hollingworth, P. S. The private practice visiting nurse. Australian Nurses' Journal, 4 (2), Aug 1974, 28–30.

21 Ireland. Ministry of Health Survey of workload of public health nurses: report of working group. Dublin: Stationery office, 1975. Chairman: Dr. Valentine Barry.

22 Kritzinger, E. R. Hospital nursing on wheels.

[District Nursing at the H.F. Verwoerd Hospital, Pretoria.] SA Nursing Journal, 40 (4), Apr 1973, 7, 9, 11.

23 **Killingo, J. S. M.** A nurse in community. Kenya Nursing Journal, 2 (1), Jun 1973, 41–42.

24 **Kusakari, J.** Facts about public health nursing in Japan – changes during the years 1960–1970. International Journal of Nursing Studies, 11 (1), Jun 1974, 3–17.

25 **Maria, S.** A rural community health experiment [at Sokho, India.] Nursing Journal of India, 65 (11), Nov 1974, 295.

26 **Maroldo, P.** A nursing team of peers. [A team of eight qualified public health nurses.] Nursing Outlook, 22 (8), Aug 1974, 515–518.

27 **Mayers, M.** Home visit – ritual or therapy? Nursing Outlook, 21 (5), May 1973, 328–331.

28 **Nursing Clinics of North America** Symposium on community nursing in Canada. Nursing Clinics of North America, 7 (4), Dec 1975, 687–778.

29 **Nursing Times** New type nurse. [28 week diploma course in public health nursing in Western Australia.] Nursing Times, 70, 31 Jan 1974, 155.

30 **O'Connor, M.** Recent emphasis on an 'old' discipline – community health education needs. [Skills required by community health nurses.] Lamp, 32 (11), Nov 1975, 5, 7.

31 **Public health nurses working party** [Recommendations on the McConville Report presented to the Consultative Council on General Medical Practice.] World of Irish Nursing, 4, (3), Mar 1975, 37–38.

32 **Rao, K. S.** Community health nursing today. Nursing Journal of India, 64 (6), Jun 1973, 198–199, 203.

33 **Rhodes, R.** Impressions of a Health Visitor in Rhodesia. Health Visitor, 46 (6), Jun 1973, 190–193.

34 **Risk, M. M.** The community clinical nurse specialist: a two-year perspective. Nursing Clinics of North America, 7 (4), Dec 1975, 761–769.

35 **Slater, P. V.** A pattern for education. [Mainly concerned with the development of community nursing courses for qualified nurses.] Australian Nurses' Journal, 3 (7), Feb 1974, 31–36.

36 **Slater, P. V.** Role of the professions in community health: implications for education. Will our resources make weight? Australian Nurses' Journal, 4 (5), Nov 1974, 36–38, 40.

37 **Stagpoole, J.** Domiciliary nursing – something of special importance. [Sydney Home Nursing Service.] Australian Nurses' Journal, 1 (2), Aug 1971, 30–32.

38 **Stack, J.** The role of the public health nurse. World of Irish Nursing, 3 (8), Aug 1974, 130–131, 133, 135.

39 **Stoeckler, R. A.** A brief history of community nursing in Israel. Australian Nurses' Journal, 2 (12), Jun 1973, 30–33, 42.

40 **Tasmanian Nurse** Home care service in Tasmania. Tasmanian Nurse, 5 (5), Jun 1971, 16, 17, 19.

41 **Wagner, D.** Nursing in an HMO. [Harvard Community Health Plan, a health maintenance organization, where nurses are part of the primary health team.] American Journal of Nursing, 74 (2), Feb 1974, 236–239.

42 **Westwick, J.** On the road to Alaska. American Journal of Nursing, 74 (9), Sep 1974, 1674–1675.

43 **Winstanley, J.** The practice of nursing. Community and family practice. [Implications of the 'Goals in Nursing Education' report.] Australian Nurses' Journal, 5 (3), Sep 1975, 12–14.

44 **Zachariah, S.** The public health nurse in India at a glance. Nursing Journal of India, 64 (6), Jun 1973, 195–196, 207.

d INTERPROFESSIONAL RELATIONSHIPS

1 **Bennett, P. and others** Inter-professional co-operation. [Report of a residential course for general practitioners, health visitors and social workers.] Journal of the Royal College of General Practitioners, 22, Sep 1972, 603–609.

2 **Community Medicine** health visitors and social workers. Community Medicine, 127, 3 Mar 1972, 111.

3 **Gunton, G. F.** Conflict or co-operation? [Between doctors, social workers and health visitors in general practice.] Practice Team, 53, Oct 1975, 10.

4 **Iduna pseud.** Definitions. [Of a health visitor and social worker.] Health Visitor, 47 (8), Aug 1974, 253.

5 **Jefferys, M.** The social worker and the health visitor. Health Bulletin, 31 (2), Mar 1973, 72–75.

6 **Nursing Mirror** Better communications for HVs. [Liaison scheme between health visitors and midwives in the City and Hackney Health District.] Nursing Mirror, 142, 4 Mar 1976, 36.

7 **Powell, M.** The relationship of the specialist in community health to the health visitor and other preventive nursing services. Health Bulletin, 30 (1), Jan 1972, 63–66.

8 **Redmond, B. M.** Health visiting and interpersonal relationships. [Case study of a student nurse taking a community care option in Berkshire.] Health Visitor, 47 (11), Nov 1974, 315–317.

9 **Willmott, P.** Health visitors and social work. British Hospital Journal and Social Service Review, 81, 11 Sep 1971, 1859. Reprinted in Health Visitor 45 (1), Jan 1972, 7–8.

34 FAMILY CARE AND GENERAL PRACTICE NURSING

a GENERAL PRACTICE NURSING

1 **Bohm, S.** The paramedical nurse. [Practice nurse.] New Zealand Nursing Journal, 64 (11), Nov 1971, 16–18.

2 **Cunningham, D. J. and others** The role of the practice nurse from the patient's point of view. [Reactions in a London group practice.] Community Medicine, 128, 6 Oct 1972, 534–538.

3 **Davidson, Y.** 'A trained sympathetic assessor': role of the practice nurse. Nursing Mirror, 135, Jul 1972, 38–40.

4 **Garraway, W. M.** Sickness certification in general practice. [Including brief mention of certification by a community nurse.] Practitioner, 210, Apr 1973, 529–534.

5 **Gilmore, M. and others** The work of the nursing team in general practice. Council for the Education and Training of Health Visitors, 1974.

6 **Hasler, J. C. and others** Training for the treatment-room sister in general practice. British Medical Journal, 1, 22 Jan 1972, 232–234.

7 **Hawthorn, P. J.** The nurse working with the general practitioner: an evaluation of research and a review of the literature. Department of Health, 1971.

8 **Journal of the Royal College of General Practitioners** Nurses in general practice. [Editorial on legal position.] Journal of the Royal College of General Practitioners, 25, Mar 1975, 157–158.

9 **Leifer, N. K.** A course for practice nurses. [A course at Southampton with results of a questionnaire showing activities of twenty-six practice nurses.] Journal of the Royal College of General Practitioners, 25, Jul 1975, 537–538.

10 **Moore, M. F. and others** First-contact decisions in general practice: a comparison between a nurse and three general practitioners. Lancet, 1, 14 Apr 1973, 817–819. For comment on this article see The decision makers, Nursing Times, 69, 26 Apr 1973, 523.

11 **Nursing Times** The practice nurse observed. [Role of the nurse as a primary contract.] Nursing Times, 67, 8 Apr 1971. 425.

12 **Paddock, F. K.** The office nurse. [The functions of the nurse in general practice.] Nursing Care, 7 (10), Oct 1974, 10–13.

13 **Reed, E. M.** Nurses' training and education for the practice team. Practice Team Compendium, Jul/Aug 1975, 163–164.

14 **Reedy, B. L. E. C.** The two faces of general practice. [Current developments particularly in general practitioner/community nurse relations.] Queen's Nursing Journal, 18 (1), Apr 1975, 6–7.

15 **Royal College of Nursing and Royal College of General Practitioners** Report of the joint working party on nursing in general practice in the reorganized National Health Service. The Colleges, 1974. Summarized in Nursing Times, 71, 19 Jun 1974, 952; Queen's Nursing Journal, Sep 1975, 175–177.

16 **Segall, J. and Lee, E.** Co-operation between doctor and nurse. [Letter outlining the duties of a practice nurse as applied to a London NHS practice.] Lancet, 1, 28 Jun 1975, 1420.

17 **Taylor, J. E.** Office nursing in a problem-oriented practice. American Journal of Nursing, 75 (3), Mar 1975, 442–445.

18 **Winter, S. J. and Last, J. M.** Registered nurses in office practice. [A survey of nurses working in doctors' offices in Ottawa, showed the nurses' skills are under used.] Canadian Nurse, 70 (11), Nov 1974, 18–20.

19 **Wrightson, M.** Practice nurses get together. [The work of a practice nurse, and the formation of the Hull Practice Nurses' Association.] Practice Team, no. 32, Jan 1974, 2–4.

b ATTACHED NURSE

1 **Anderson, J. A. D. and others** Medical views on attachment schemes for community nurses. Community Medicine, 126, 19 Nov 1971, 287–290.

2 **Bridges, A.** SEN in the team. [In a group practice.] District Nursing, 15 (3), Jun 1972, 56.

3 **British Hospital Journal and Social Service Review** Leading opinion . . . Health visiting. [Relationship of the practice nurse to the attached health visitor.] British Hospital Journal and Social Service Review, 82, 1 Jul 1972, 1445.

4 **Davies, B. R.** Partnership in care. [Group practice/health visitor attachment from the point of view of the health visitor.] Health Visitor, 46 (4) Apr, 1973, 114–116.

5 **Down, J. and Snaith, A. H.** The deployment of home nurses. [A study of attached nurses in Derbyshire.] British Journal of Preventive and Social Medicine, 29, Mar 1975, 53–57.

6 Fisher, N. Health visitors on secondment – vicarious liability. [Legal aspects.] Health Visitor, 44 (6), Jun 1971, 191–192.

7 Health and Social Service Journal Home nurses at work. [Survey of the amount and type of work done by home nurses attached to general practice at Teesside.] Health and Social Service Journal, 85, 27 Sep 1975, 2161.

8 Hodes, C. Education of nurses and health visitors in group practice. [Reprinted from Journal of the Royal College of General Practitioners.] Nursing Times, 69, 1 Feb 1973, 149–150.

9 Linday, L. H. Group attachment and the SEN. in Birmingham. [Relationship between SEN and SRN in a group scheme.] District Nursing, 15, (3) Jun 1972, 57–58.

10 MacGregor, S. W. The evaluation of a direct nursing attachment in a north Edinburgh practice. Scottish Home and Health Department, 1971. (Scottish Health Service Studies, 18.)

11 Mahoney, S. P. It makes a change: a district nurse becomes attached. [Author's experience.] Nursing Times, 68, 20 Apr 1972, 477.

12 Medical Officer Combined front on nursing attachments. Medical Officer. 125. 8 Jan 1971. 19–20.

13 Mills, A. R. Enlarging the nurse's role. [Attachments to general practice.] Practice Team, no. 52, Sep 1975, 13.

14 Pickworth, K. H. and others Nursing attachments in general practice. Nursing Times, 67, 8 Jul 1971, 838–839.

15 Playfair, C. R. Practice attachment – how yet another did it. [Dunfermline.] Nursing Times, 68, 30 Nov 1972, 1514–1515.

16 Richardson, I. M. General practitioners and district nurses: a study of referral patterns in the City of Aberdeen. British Journal of Preventive and Social Medicine, 28 (3), Aug 1974, 187–190.

c FAMILY CARE AND NURSE PRACTITIONER

1 Aradine, C. R. The challenge of clinical nursing practice in an interdisciplinary office setting. Nursing Forum, 12 (3), 1973, 290–302.

2 Aradine, C. R. Development of a family health service: experiences of a clinical nurse specialist. Journal of Nursing Administration, 4 (1), Jan/Feb 1974, 45–51.

3 Beatty, A. Symposium on family-centered care in a pediatric setting. Nursing Clinics of North America, 7 (1), Mar 1972, 1–93.

4 Becker, M. H. and Green, L. W. A family approach to compliance with medical treatment: a selective review of the literature. International Journal of Health Education, 18 (3), 1975, 173–182.

5 Burnett, B. The nurse practitioner. [A British nurse participates in a family nurse practitioner programme at Indiana University.] Nursing Mirror 140, 19 Jun 1975, 71.

6 College of Nursing, Australia and Royal Australian College of General Practitioners The family practice nurse. [Statement on the developing role.] Australian Nurses' Journal, 4 (7), Feb 1975, 16–18.

7 Edward, P. I. 'How I became a nurse practitioner'. [In a group practice.] Hospital Administration in Canada, 14 (10), Oct 1972, 39, 42, 44.

8 Edwardson, S. The work of the administrator, family practitioner services. Queen's Nursing Journal, 17 (6), Sep 1974, 126–127.

9 Fawcett, J. The family as a living open system: an emerging conceptual framework for nursing. International Nursing Review, 22 (4), Jul/Aug 1975, 113–116.

10 Freeman, R. Nurse practitioners in the community health agency. [Administrative problems.] Journal of Nursing Administration, 4 (6), Nov/Dec 1974, 21–24.

11 Gibson, R. Family care. Queen's Nursing Journal, 16 (5), Aug 1973, 102–105; Health and Social Service Journal, 83, 4 Aug 1973, 1750–1751.

12 Greenidge, J. and others Community nurse practitioners – a partnership. [Private nursing group practice.] Nursing Outlook, 21 (4), Apr 1973, 228–231.

13 Hoffmann, P. Nursing care study. Health visiting. Developments within a large family. Nursing Mirror, 139, 26 Jul 1974, 80–82.

14 Hull, F. M. New roles for nurses in general practice – a lesson from America. [The use of the family nurse practitioner for diagnosis, counselling and follow-up.] Journal of the Royal College of General Practitioners, 15, Feb 1975, 151–153.

15 Hunter, P. Family and health. Mother and Child, 45 (2), Mar/Apr 1973, 14–16, 21.

16 Jolly, H. Families – a nation's strength. [The role of the health visitor in family health care.] Health Visitor, 47, Jul 1974, 216–222.

17 Kergin, D. J. and Spitzer, W. O. A Canadian educational programme in family practice nursing. [McMaster University, Ontario.] International Nursing Review, 22 (1), Jan/Feb 1975, 19–22.

18 Kergin, D. J. and others Changing nursing practice through education. [With particular reference to family practice nurse education at McMaster University.] Canadian Nurse, 69 (4), Apr 1973, 28–31.

19 Kubala, S. and Clever, L. H. Acceptance of the nurse practitioner [as a primary care source]. American Journal of Nursing, 74 (3), Mar 1974, 451–452.

20 Laird, E. B. Mayston . . . Health visiting and the family unit. Health Visitor, 45 (12), Dec 1972, 388–392.

21 Manciaux, M. A new concept – family care. International Nursing Review, 20 (3), May/Jun 1973, 85–88, 95.

22 Martin, L. L. 'I like being an FNP'. [Experiences of a family nurse practitioner.] American Journal of Nursing, 75 (5), May 1975, 826–828.

23 Merenstein, J. H. and others The use of nurse practitioners in a general practice. [Two year study in Pennsylvania.] Medical Care, 12 (5), May 1974, 445–452.

24 Murray, R. H. and Ross, S. A. Training the family nurse practitioner. Hospitals, 47 (21), 1 Nov 1973, 93–94, 96, 98.

25 Parsons, R. Nurse practitioner as medical assistant. [Development of community nurse practitioners in Canada and the USA. with implications for Australia.] Lamp, 32 (11), Nov 1975, 15, 17, 19, 24.

26 Robinson, A. M. M. Lucille Kinlein, RN Independent nurse-practitioner. [First nurse in private practice.] RN Magazine 35 (1), Jan 1972, 40–41, 64, 67–68, 70.

27 Russell, H. General nursing practitioner. Nursing Times, 71, 20 Nov 1975, 1855–1857.

28 Ruybal, S. E. and others Community assessment: an epidemiological approach [to the study of the family in a community nursing course]. Nursing Outlook, 23 (6), Jun 1975, 365–368.

29 Shaw, B. L. The nurse – PA: one experiment that's working. RN Magazine, 34 (6), Jun 1971, 45–47.

30 Slater, P. V. Nurse practitioner, family practice nurse, or physician's assistant. Australian Nurses' Journal, 3 (6), Dec/Jan, 1973/74, 31–34.

31 Smiley, O. R. The family centred approach – a challenge to public health nurses. International Nursing Review, 20 (2), Mar/Apr 1973, 49–50.

32 Sobol, E. G. and Robischon P. Family nursing: a study guide. 2nd ed. St. Louis: Mosby, 1975.

33 UNA Nursing Journal The family practice nurse: the developing role of the nurse. UNA Nursing Journal, 3, May/Jun 1975, 18.

34 Weinstein, P. and Demers, J. L. Rural nurse practitioner clinic [at Darrington, Washington]. American Journal of Nursing, 74 (11), Nov 1974, 2022–2026.

35 Williams, C. A. Nurse practitioner research: some neglected issues. [Nurse practitioners should develop clinical trials in primary care rather than concentrate on the quality of care.] Nursing Outlook, 23 (3), Mar 1975, 172–177.

36 Wiseman, J. Three generations – a health visitor's study. Nursing Times, 70, 21 Nov 1974, 1826–1827.

37 World Health The health of the family. Issue on WHO's activities in promoting family health. World Health, 3 (41), Aug/Sep 1975.

38 Wright, E. Family nurse clinicians: physicians' perspective. [A survey by questionnaire to physicians to determine factors which would help or hinder primary care nurses trained in an expanded role.] Nursing Outlook, 23 (12), Dec 1975, 771–773.

39 Wyn, M. Services for the family. [Community health, including nursing services.] World of Irish Nursing, 3 (4), Apr 1974, 58–62, (5) May, 1974, 81.

d ETHNIC MINORITIES

1 Alder, M. Problems with immigrant families. Nursing Mirror, 137, 27 Jul 1973, 39, 41.

2 Alexander, B. Help for immigrant families: an abridged version of the study of the health visitor's contribution to the well-being of the immigrant patient and his family. Nursing Times, 70, 25 Apr 1974, 632–636.

3 Barnes, G. G. Seen but not heard. Where is home? The isolated West Indian parent and child in London. Social Work Today, 5, 23 Jan 1975, 646–648.

4 Barnes, G. G. Seen but not heard. Work with West Indian parents in distress. Social Work Today, 5, 9 Jan 1975, 606–609.

5 Burrowes, H. P. Immigrant psychiatric problems. Nursing Mirror, 133, 8 Oct 1971, 28–29.

6 Burrowes, H. P. Psychiatric problems in immigrant groups. Royal Society of Health Journal, 92 (3), Jun 1972, 139–140.

7 Cheetham, C. The health of children born to immigrant mothers. District Nursing, 14 (2), May 1971, 34–35.

8 Gans, B. Clinics for immigrant children. [Evening infant welfare clinics.] Midwife and Health Visitor, 9 (12), Dec 1973, 401–404.

9 Health Visitor The children of West Indian immigrants. Health Visitor, (46), Nov 1973, 389, 391–392.

10 Kitzinger, S. Speaking the same language: working with West Indian patients. Practitioner, 213, Dec 1974, 843–850.

11 Pyke-Lees, C. and Gardiner, S. Elderly ethnic minorities. Mitcham: Age Concern, 1974. (Manifesto series, No. 18 specialist report.)

12 Robinson, W. A healthy future. [Preventive care among immigrants in Southall: the work of a chest clinic health visitor.] Nursing Times, 70, 10 Jan 1974, 51–52.

13 Rutter, M. and others The children of West Indian migrants. New Society, 27, 14 Mar 1974, 630–633.

14 Sanderson, S. Immigrant health care. [Immigrant visiting as an increasingly important aspect of health education.] Nursing Times, 70, 14 Feb 1974, 246–247.

e ONE-PARENT FAMILIES

1 Anstice, E. Helping the motherless family. Nursing Times, 69, 5 Apr 1973, 432–433.

2 Barber, D. editor One parent families. Davis-Poynter, 1975.

3 Bourne, J. Pregnant – and alone: the unmarried mother and her child. Royston, Herts: Priory Press, 1971. (Priory care and welfare library 6.)

4 Bramall, M. The Finer committee report [on one parent families.] Health and Social Service Journal, 84, 13 Jul 1974, 1562.

5 Carter, N. J. The lone father. [Increasing number of mothers who now desert their families.] Midwife and Health Visitor, 9 (12), Dec 1973, 399–400.

6 Crellin, E. and others Born illegitimate: social and educational implications. National Foundation for Educational Research, 1971.

7 Department of Health and Social Security. Committee on One-Parent Families Report. HMSO, 1973. 2 vols. Chairman: Sir Morris Finer. Summary in Nursing Times, 70, 25 Jul 1974, 1168.

8 Gingerbread The Association for One-Parent Families. One-parent families – a Finer future? The Association, 1973.

9 Health and Social Service Journal One parent, no prospects. [Organisations which help one-parent families.] Health and Social Service Journal, 84, 9 Feb 1974, 298.

10 Hilton, M. E. Unsupported mothers: a review of 100 expectant mothers booked as unsupported to one midwife during 1971/72. Midwives Chronicle, 86, Jul 1973, 216–218.

11 Hopkinson, A. Families without fathers. Mothers' Union, 1973.

12 Kaseman, C. M. The single-parent family. Canadian Journal of Psychiatric Nursing, 16 (1), Jan/Feb 1975, 16, Mar/Apr 1975, 12–13.

13 Lomax-Simpson, J. M. Some thoughts on the lone mother and her child in Messenger House. [A therapeutic community.] Health Visitor, 48 (6), Jun 1975, 201–203.

14 Marsden, D. Society at work. What action after Finer? New Society, 30, 26 Dec 1974, 817–818.

15 Mothers in Action Various pamphlets. Mothers in Action, 1972–1973.

16 National Council for One Parent Families We need more help, lone parents tell Mrs. Castle. [Report of the annual conference which suggested an extension of health visitor support for these families.] Nursing Times, 71, 27 Feb 1975, 323.

f PROBLEM FAMILIES AND BATTERED WIVES

1 Dewsbury, A. R. Battered wives. (b) Family violence seen in general practice. [Pilot study investigating 15 women.] Royal Society of Health Journal, 95 (6), Dec 1975, 290–294.

2 Frommer, E. A. Families at risk – help for those from broken homes. [Survey to find if families whose mothers were deprived of one of their parents in childhood would become problems.] Nursing Times, 69, 25 Oct 1973, 1408–1409.

3 Gayford, J. J. Battered wives. (a) Research on battered wives. Royal Society of Health Journal, 95 (6), Dec 1975, 288–289.

4 Gayford, J. J. Wife battering: a preliminary survey of 100 cases. British Medical Journal, 1, 25 Jan 1975, 194–197.

5 Harrison, P. Refuges for wives. [Chiswick Women's Aid.] New Society, 34, 13 Nov 1975, 361–364.

6 Hunt, A. Inadequate parents. Mother and Child, 43 (2), Mar/Apr 1971, 14–18.

7 Jobling, M. Battered wives: a survey. Social Service Quarterly, 47 (4), Apr/Jun 1974, 142–144, 146.

8 Marsden, D. and Owens, D. The Jekyll and Hyde marriages. [Survey of 19 battered wives.] New Society, 32, 8 May 1975, 333–335.

9 Pizzey, E. Battered wives. (d) Chiswick Women's Aid. A refuge from violence. Royal Society of Health Journal, 95 (6), Dec 1975, 297–298.

10 Sethi, G. S. Problem families – and what their problems are. Health, 8 (3/4), Autumn/Winter 1971, 20–21.

11 Wilson, E. Battered wives. (c) A social worker's viewpoint. Royal Society of Health Journal, 95 (6), Dec 1975, 294–297.

12 Winn, D. A haven from cruelty. [Chiswick Women's Aid.] Nursing Times, 69, 14 Jun 1973, 775–777.

g WOMEN'S ROLE

1 Ali, A. A. Status of women in India. Nursing Journal of India, 66 (5), May 1975, 105–106.

2 Bartholomew, A. B. Women in industry. Occupational Health Nursing, 23 (7), Jul 1975, 18–19.

3 Blair, P. Are women's hospitals necessary? Health and Social Service Journal, 85, 20/27 Dec 1975, 2790–2791.

4 Dryden, K. G. The deceased husband and the rights of the widow. Queen's Nursing Journal, 18 (8), Dec 1975, 249–250.

5 Dryden, K. G. The rights of the deserted woman – the married woman. Queen's Nursing Journal, 18 (8), Nov 1975, 229–230.

6 Dryden, K. G. The rights of the deserted woman – the mistress. Continuing the series on the district nurse and the law. Queen's Nursing Journal, 18 (7), Oct 1975, 204–205.

7 Guiver, P. Marriage counselling. 2. How counsellors can help. Midwife and Health Visitor, 10 (11), Nov 1974, 343–345.

8 Kearns, J. Women under pressure. [Extract from 'Stress in Industry'.] Occupational Health, 25 (4), Apr 1973, 135–140.

9 Lancaster, J. Coping mechanisms for the working mother. American Journal of Nursing, 75 (8), Aug 1978, 1322–1323.

10 Luthra, P. N. The role of women. Nursing Journal of India, 66 (5), May 1975, 101–102.

11 Maxwell, E. D. The importance of the special education of women in building a healthy community. Community Health, 7 (1), Jul/Aug 1975, 8–12.

12 Miles, H. S. and Hays, D. R. Widowhood. [A therapeutic discussion group organized by the American Red Cross, New York.] American Journal of Nursing, 75, 2, Feb 1975, 280–282.

13 Occupational Health Nursing Why women work. Occupational Health Nursing, 21 (1), Jan 1973, 36–37.

14 Parliament Sex Discrimination Act. HMSO 1975

15 Reid, E. Women at a standstill: the need for radical change. International Labour Review, 3 (6), Jun 1975, 459–468.

16 Rendel, M. Equal opportunity. [An outline of the Sex Discrimination Bill.] New Society, 31, 20 Mar 1975, 724–725.

17 Thornton, G. International Women's Year in the UK Social Service Quarterly, 46 (1), Jul/Sep 1975, 15–18.

18 Tyndall, N. Marriage counselling. 1. Work of marriage guidance councils. Midwife and Health Visitor, 10 (10), Oct 1974, 298–300.

19 Vogel, E. Some suggestions for the advancement of working men. International Labour Review, 112 (1), Jul 1975, 29–43.

20 Warnock, M. The two-career family: problems and adjustment. Mother and Child, 46 (1), Feb 1974, 11, 18–19.

21 Watkin, B. Working wives. Nursing Mirror, 141, 4 Sep 1975, 39.

22 World Health Special issue to mark International Women's Year. World Health, Jan 1975, 4–35.

35 DISTRICT NURSING

a GENERAL

1 Allen, S. The new district nurse. [Special reference to the varicose ulcer.] District Nursing, 14 (7), Oct 1971, 146.

2 British Medical Journal The home nurse. [Editorial.] British Medical Journal, 4, 27 Nov 1971, 551–52.

3 Brown, D. E. Community nurse tutor's view. [Comment on the new district nurse by S. Allen.] District Nursing, 14 (7), Oct 1971, 147.

4 Damant, M. Role of the district trained SEN. in family centred care. Queen's Nursing Journal, 16 (3), Jun 1973, 62, 75.

5 Greggs, S. M. The district nurse. Queen's Nursing Journal, 17 (10), Jan 1975, 225–226.

6 McCarrick, H. Careers in nursing. The district nurse – a new image. Nursing Times, 67, 23 Sep 1971, 1174–1175.

7 McIntosh, J. B. Communication in teamwork: a lesson from the district. The nature and extent of contact and collaboration between district nursing sisters and some of their colleagues in the community health team. A study carried out in Aberdeen. Nursing Times, 70, 17 Oct 1974, Occ. papers, 85–88.

8 McIntosh, J. B. An observation and time study of the work of domiciliary nurses. PhD thesis, Aberdeen University, 1975.

9 Price, I. The present is the foundation for the future. Further comments on the views, expressed in Opinion, on district nursing, Halsbury and Briggs. Queen's Nursing Journal, 17 (8), Nov 1974, 175, 182.

10 Queen's Institute of District Nursing Nursing in the community. A filmstrip presented by The Queen's Institute of District Nursing. [Illustrations only.] Nursing Mirror, 136, 4 May 1973, 11–13; 11 May 1973, 19–21.

11   Queen's Institute of District Nursing. [Series of articles describing its various services.] District Nursing, 15 (1), Apr 1972, 2–7.

12   Queen's Institute of District Nursing [Survey of work.] District Nursing, 14 (9), Dec 1971, 191, 194; 15 (10), Jan 1973, 221–222; Queen's Nursing Journal, 17 (10), Jan 1975, 220–221; 18 (9), Dec 1975, 238, 240, 245.

14   Scott Wright, M. S. Higher targets for district nurses. [Talk given at the annual meeting of the QIDN.] British Hospital Journal and Social Service Review, 82, 2 Dec 1972, 2678.

15   Venables, M. P. Attitudes towards district nursing. Nursing Times, 67, 13 May 1971, 578.

16   Young, E. J. The role of the district nurse. [With the results of a survey of disabled patients helped by district nurses.] Nursing Mirror, 141, 4 Sep 1975, 58–59.

b EDUCATION AND TRAINING

1   Allen, G. Experiment in teaching. [Course in teaching for district nurses.] Nursing Times, 67, 18 Nov 1971, 1453.

2   Buttimore, A. A. An experimental course: a course in practical clinical procedures for nursing sisters in the domiciliary nursing service. Queen's Nursing Journal, 27 (2), May 1974, 41–42.

3   Hockey, L. Research and district nursing. District Nursing. 14 (1), Apr 1971, 14–15.

4   Kratz, C. Training to meet the future needs [in the community]. Queen's Nursing Journal, 17 (12), Mar 1975, 254–255.

5   Matthews, T. W. The panel of assessors for district nurse training: an account of its history and development and its role in the education and training of district nurses in the United Kingdom. Queen's Nursing Journal, 17 (12), Mar 1975, 256–258.

6   Morris, I. H. Research into action: district nursing in Birmingham. District Nursing. 14(1), Apr 1971, 16, 19.

7   Price, I. Correlating theory with practice [in district nurse training]. District Nursing, 14 (9), Dec. 1971, 187–189.

8   Price, I. Evaluation problems of short courses and a trial method. [Applied to a Queen's Institute course in mental health.] Queen's Nursing Journal, 18 (3), Jun 1975, 72–73.

9   Price, I. A personal refresher course. [A tutor spends a short period in district nursing practice.] Queen's Nursing Journal, 17 (6), Sep 1974, 128–130.

10   Price, I. The present is the foundation for the future. [District nurse training.] Queen's Nursing Journal, 17 (8), Nov 1974, 175, 182.

11   Queen's Nursing Institute QNI evidence to working party on District Nurse Training. Queen's Nursing Journal, 18 (5), Aug 1975, 137.

12   Queen's Nursing Journal Training of practical work instructors. Queen's Nursing Journal, 17 (4), Jul 1974, 86.

c MANAGEMENT AND STAFFING

1   Few, E. and others An inquiry into the use of district rooms. Nursing Times, 69, 23 Aug 1973, Occ. papers, 133–136.

2   Fielder, R. District nursing: has a frontline organization some lessons to teach? Nursing Times, 67, 9 Sep 1971, 1132–1133.

3   Groves, W. J. B. The role of the area administrator. Queen's Nursing Journal, 17 (6), Sep 1974, 122–123.

4   Jupp, V. District nursing: an example of front-line organization. Nursing Times, 67, 19 Aug 1971, Occ. papers, 129–31.

5   Lindars, M. E. and Hunt, I. G. W. District nursing in Reading: towards a guideline for future deployment of staff. Community Medicine, 128 (22), 15 Sep 1972, 479–482.

6   Rickard, J. H. The costs of domiciliary nursing care. [A comparative study of two practices.] Journal of the Royal College of General Practitioners, 24, Dec 1974, 839–846.

7   Williams, A. and Anderson, R. Provision of district nurse services at minimum cost. In: Williams, A. and Anderson, R. Efficiency in the social services. Blackwell, 1975, 2, 9–16.

d NIGHT NURSING SERVICE

1   Byatt, J. Night nursing service. [Reply to the recent article by O. Keywood, Nursing Times, 26 Jul 1973.] Nursing Times, 69, 9 Aug 1973, 1029.

2   Humphreys, D. New to the district. [Night nursing service in Reading.] Nursing Times, 68, 4 May 1972, 527.

3   Hunt, G. J. W. Community night nurse. [Scheme in Reading.] Nursing Times, 69, 9 Aug 1973, 1035–1036.

4   Keywood, O. Night nursing 'on the district'. [A 24 hour district nursing service.] Nursing Times, 69, 26 Jul 1973, 974–975.

5   Queen's Nursing Journal Night nursing in the community. [Experiences of a member of the Richmond night nursing team.] Queen's Nursing Journal, 18 (3), Jun 1975, 77.

6   Rogers, J. W. Development of a night nursing service. Queen's Nursing Journal, 16 (8), Nov 1973, 179–180.

36 HEALTH VISITING

a GENERAL

1   Boorer, D. The role of the health visitor. Health Visitor, 47 (9), Sep 1974, 281.

2   British Hospital Journal and Social Service Review Health Visiting. [Research.] British Hospital Journal and Social Service Review, 82, 22 Apr 1972, 870; And the clinical nurse consultant, 13 May, 1972, 1035–1036.

3   British Medical Journal The health visitor. [Training and field of work.] British Medical Journal, 4, 20 Nov 1971, 479–48040

4   Chisholm, M. K. The health visiting scene. 1. The sighs. Nursing Mirror, 134, Mar 1972, 33–34.

5   Chisholm, M. K. The health visiting scene. 2. The satisfactions. Nursing Mirror, 134, 24 Mar 1972, 42–43.

6   Chisholm, M. K. The health visiting scene. 3. Set fair. Nursing Mirror, 134, 31 Mar 1972, 33–34.

7   Chisholm, M. K. The hours between. [Should health visitors provide a 24 hour service?] Nursing Times, 69, Feb 1973, 147–148.

8   Chisholm, M. K. 'I thought we were following the bear'. [Problem of health visitors in identifying and achieving their objectives.] Nursing Times, 71, 8 May 1975, 740–742.

9   Chisholm, M. K. Job specification equals job satisfaction – fact or fiction? [In health visiting.] Midwife and Health Visitor, 8 (3), Mar 1972, 98–101.

10   Chisholm, M. K. Sympathy plus? [Health visiting.] Nursing Mirror, 132, 28 May 1971, 21–23.

11   Chisholm, M. K. What do the consumers pay us for? Aspects of current health visiting practice.] Midwife and Health Visitor, 7 (8), Aug 1971, 297–300.

12   Clark, J. 1. What do health visitors do? 2. The 'New Breed' health visitor. 3. The effect of attachment on the work of the health visitor. Nursing Times, 68, 27 Jul 1972; 68, 3 Aug 1972, Occ. papers, 117, 121–124.

13   Clark, J. The work of the health visitor. MPhil thesis, Department of Politics, Reading University, 1972.

14   Dack, P. The overall umbrella: report on the United Kingdom Conference of the Health Visitors' Association and Scottish Health Visitors' Association. Nursing Mirror, 139, 24 Oct 1974, 40–41.

15   De Silva, J. N. S. How to make proper use of health visitor skills. Health Visitor, 47 (11), Nov 1974, 318–319.

16   Dingwall, R. The health visitors. [Their role and the Briggs proposals.] New Society, 25, 30 Aug 1973, 517–518.

17   Ensing, E. C. Working together. [The work of the health visitor.] Health Visitor, 47 (4), Apr 1974, 100–103.

18   Fisher, N. S. The health visitor and the courts. Health Visitor, 45 (4), Apr 1972, 100–101.

19   Foulds, J. Your choice. [Health visiting in the light of the Briggs Report.] Health Visitor, 46 (5) May 1973, 161, 163.

20   Grey, I. A personal view. [Lack of recognition of the work of the health visitor.] Health Visitor, 46, (7) Jul 1973, 225–226.

21   Health Visitors Association Health visiting in the Seventies and Staffing of the health visiting and school nursing services. [Policy documents.] HVA, 1975. Reprinted in Health Visitor, 48 (9), Sep 1975, 322–333.

22   Hill, C. The role conflicts of the new breed health visitor. Health Visitor, 44 (4), Apr 1971, 120–122.

23   Hill, J. Prevention versus cure. [The work of the health visitor.] Nursing Times, 69, 25 Jan 1973, 128.

24   Hobbs, P. A study of the factors affecting the amount of group teaching undertaken by health visitors. MSc thesis, Salford University, 1971.

25   Hunt, M. The dilemma of identity in health visiting. Nursing Times, 68 (5), 3 Feb 1972, 10 Feb 1972; Occ. papers, 17–20, 23–24.

26   Jameson, A. A career post in health visiting. [Training and salary.] Health Visitor, 46 (3), Mar 1973, 81–82.

27   Keywood, O. The health visitor. [History and present functions.] Practice Team, no. 34, Mar 1974, 5–6, 8–10.

28   Lester, J. Prevention is better than cure. Health Visitors' Association Annual Conference, Stockport. Nursing Mirror, 141, 6 Nov 1975, 41–42.

29   Loveland, M. K. The work of health visitors in an urban and a county area in relation to health visitor training at the University of Surrey. Nursing Times, 67, 3 Jun 1971, Occ. papers, 85–87.

30   McCarrick, H. Careers in nursing. Key figure of the future – the health visitor. Nursing Times, 67, 7 Oct 1971, 1243–1245.

31 Pinder, J. E. A reply to the role conflicts of the new breed health visitor. Health Visitor, 44 (6), Jun 1971, 188–190.

32 Rehin, G. F. The 'point and purpose' of the health visitor: some sociological reflections. Nursing Times, 69, 16 Mar 1972, 304–307.

33 Thorpe, E. Health visiting objectives and the role of the health visitor: a need for organisational research. Health Visitor, 46 (5), May 1973, 156–159.

34 Thorpe, E. and Thorpe, A. Health visiting in the community context. Health Visitor, 44 (12), Dec 1971, 404–408

35 Willmott, P. Future of the health visitor. British Hospital Journal and Social Service Review, 82, 12 Feb 1972, 354–355.

b EDUCATION AND TRAINING

1 Bosanquet, N. Coming out in the open. [Case of Veronica Pickles whose secondment for health visitor training was revoked because of her part in a campaign for homosexual equality.] Nursing Times, 71, 3 Jul 1975, 1037.

2 British Hospital Journal and Social Service Review Health visiting. How useful are the non-health visiting subjects now taught on course such as sociology, social policy and psychology? British Hospital Journal and Social Service Review, 82, 5 Aug 1972. 1726.

3 Clarke-Crutchfield, R. The student. [Personal experiences of becoming a health visitor student.] Health Visitor, 48 (7), Jul 1975, 238.

4 Dingwall, R. W. J. The social organization of health visitor training. PhD thesis, Aberdeen University, 1974.

5 Hicks, V. Reflections on health visitor training. [Integrated course at St. Thomas' and Southampton University.] Nursing Times, 59, 25 Jan 1973, 105–107.

6 James, D. E. and Loveland, M. K. Health visitor students: assessing practical work in Surrey. Nursing Times, 69, 3 May 1973, 563–564. Reprinted in Health Visitor, 46 (11), Nov 1973, 369–370.

7 Lennon, M. A new breed from the youngest statutory body. [Work of the Council for the Training of Health Visitors.] Nursing Times, 67, 18 Mar 1971, 318–320.

8 Mulholland, R. C. A preliminary investigation into the selection and appraisal of health visitors. MSc thesis in applied psychology, Aston University in Birmingham, 1973.

9 New Society Health and revolution. [A health visitor refresher course.] New Society, 18, 5 Aug 1971, 231.

10 North, M. Why sociology? [In the training of health visitors.] Health Visitor, 48 (4), Apr 1975, 113–114.

11 O'Connell, P. Developments in health visitor education. Community Medicine, 129, 3 Nov 1972, 49–51.

12 Rawlinson, K. Field work instructor in group practice. Nursing Mirror, 132, 19 Feb 1971, 34–38.

13 Rice, D. A contribution to health visitor education. Health Visitor, 45 (10), Oct 1972, 316–318.

14 Royal Society of Health Journal The training of health visitors. [Leading article.] Royal Society of Health Journal, 92 (2), Apr 1972, 56.

15 Thorpe, E. The significance of language in the training and work of the health visitor. Health Visitor, 47 (11), Nov 1974, 312–314.

c MANAGEMENT AND STAFFING

1 British Hospital Journal and Social Service Review Health visiting. At long last the regulations have been changed to allow men into health visiting on equal terms with women. British Hospital Journal and Social Service Review, 7 Oct 1972.

2 Burke, M. Bank health visitors. [Letter describing scheme at Melton Mowbray.] Health Visitor, 48 (12), Dec 1975, 479.

3 Kavalier, F. Who said a health visitor should never be a man? [Male health visitors in Aberdeen.] Nursing Times, 68, 5 Oct 1972, 1259–1260.

4 McIntosh, H. T. and Reid, M. T. A study of wastage in health visiting. Health Bulletin, 32 (2), Mar 1974, 51–62.

5 Public Health How best can we deploy our health visitors? Public Health, 89 (6), Sep 1975, 243–246.

6 Tranter, A. W. Health visiting in Lewisham: management by objectives. Setting the targets. [Study based on analysis of information.] Community Medicine, 126, 10 Sep 1971, 157–159.

37 SCHOOL HEALTH

a GENERAL

1 Anderson, C. L. School health practice. 5th ed. St. Louis: Mosby.

2 Bacon, L. Selective school medical inspection in Hampshire. District Nursing, 13 (10), Jan 1971, 199–201.

3 Bender, A. E. and others Survey of school meals. British Medical Journal, 2, 13 May 1972, 383–385.

4 Briault, E. W. H. The school in the community. [Extension of the school's role outside school hours.] Midwife, Health Visitor and Community Nurse, 11 (8), Aug 1975, 259–262.

5 Cook, J. and others A survey of the nutritional status of schoolchildren: relation between nutrient intake and social economic factors. [Survey in Kent.] British Journal of Preventive and Social Medicine, 27 (2), May 1973, 91–99.

6 Department of Education and Science The health of the school child: report of the chief medical officer of the Department of Education and Science. HMSO Annual to 1974.

7 Department of Education and Science The school health service 1908–1974: report of the Chief Medical Officer. HMSO, 1975.

8 Department of Education and Welsh Office. Working Party on the Nutritional Aspects of School Meals. Nutrition in schools, HMSO, 1975.

9 Essex-Cater, A. and Robert-Sargeant, S. Value of school meals. [Survey of Monmouthshire schools to investigate food consumption and nutritional value.] Health and Social Service Journal, 85, 5 Apr 1975, 758–759.

10 Francis, H. W. S. Education and health: the English tradition. [Problems of the school health service illustrated by historical development.] Public Health, 89 (4), May 1975, 129–135; (5), Jul 1975, 181–190; (6), Sep 1975, 273–277.

11 Hackitt, B. S. Of lice and men: incidence of infestation with head lice. Nursing Times, 70, 5 Sep 1974, 1378–1380.

12 Health Education Council The head louse in England: prevalence amongst schoolchildren. The Council, 1975.

13 Jacoby, A. and others Influence of some social and environmental factors on the nutrient intake and nutritional status of schoolchildren. British Journal of Preventive and Social Medicine, 29 (2), Jun 1975, 116–120.

14 Medical Officers of Schools Association Handbook of school health. 15th ed. Lewis, 1975.

15 Richardson, D. P. and Lawson, M. Nutritional value of midday meals of senior schoolchildren. British Medical Journal, 4, 23 Dec 1972, 697–699.

16 Society of Medical Officers of Health The future of the school health service: observations of the Society of Medical Officers of Health to the collaboration working party sub-committee on the future of the school health service. [With an appendix on the work of the School Health Service. Editorial comment 105–107.] Public Health, 86 (3), Mar 1972, 108–118.

17 Webb, E. The educational welfare officer. Midwife, Health Visitor and Community Nurse, 11(1), Jan 1975, 23–25

b HEALTH AND SEX EDUCATION

1 Ascott, M. P. A look at health education in schools. Health Visitor, 48 (5), May 1975, 156–157.

2 Bensley, L. B. An historical overview of school health education in the United Kingdom. Health Education Journal, 32 (3), 1973, 73–76.

3 Boustead, M. C. Health week in an infants' school. Health Education Journal, 33 (1), 1973, 12–14.

4 Clark, J. Learning for living. [A health visitor teaches health and sex education in schools.] Nursing Times, 65, 6 Feb 1969, 181–182.

5 Dwivedi, K. N. and others India: innovations in health education in rural schools. International Journal of Health Education, 16 (2), 1973, 100–106.

6 Ehrman, M. L. Sex education for the young. Nursing Outlook, 23 (9), Sep 1975, 583–585.

7 Evanson, J. 'Grapevine' – a new project. [Action research project in community sex education for the young in Camden and Islington.] Midwife and Health Visitor, 10 (6), Jun 1974, 159–161.

8 Head, M. J. A survey regarding health education in Staffordshire schools. Health Education Journal, 32 (4), 1973, 129–131.

9 Langmaid, W. O. Health education in North Yorkshire junior schools. [Survey.] Health Education Journal, 34 (4), 1975, 121–127.

10 Lewis, D. F. Health education in schools – or little by little. Community Health, 4 (6), May/Jun 1973, 309–314.

11 Murrell, J. Health visitors and teaching in schools. Health Visitor, 46 (2), Feb 1973, 41–43.

12 Norman, M. Health education in schools: health visitor's plea for integrated health education classes. Nursing Times, 71, 17 Apr 1975, 620–621.

13 Ripley, G. D. Human relationships and social responsibility: health education within a school social studies course. [In an English secondary school.] International Journal of Health Education, 18 (3), 1975, 198–201.

14 Ripley, G. D. Sex education. [Syllabus used in secondary schools in Boreham Wood.] Practitioner, 208, Apr 1972, 525–527.

15 Ripley, G. D. Some thoughts on sex education for school children. Midwife and Health Visitor, 7 (12), Dec 1971, 457, 459–461.

16 Robinson, W. The perils of 'La Dolce Vita'. [Necessity for early health education for school children.] Nursing Times, 69, 11 Jan 1973, 64–65.

17 Thompson, C. Health education in junior schools. Nursing Times, 66, 8 Jan 1970, Occ. papers, 7–8.

18 Williams, C. L. Health education in schools: some changes, problems and prospects. Community Health, 5 (4), Jan/Feb 1974, 209–213.

19 Williams, T. Health education as a curricular subject in schools and colleges. (a) Health education and children learning. Royal Society of Health Journal, 95 (4), Aug 1975, 214–216.

c NURSING

1 Bachu, A. Nurses' role in school health programme. Nursing Journal of India, 61 (5), May 1970, 141–142, 173.

2 Bellaire, J. M. School nurse practitioner program. Amcrican Journal of Nursing, 71 (11), 1971, 2192–2194.

3 Birchfield, M. Headstart offers expanded role for the school nurse. Nursing Forum, 12 (4), 1973, 353–363.

4 Bose, R. The role of the nurse in school health programme. Nursing Journal of India, 65 (10), Oct 1974, 267, 286.

5 Brown, J. and others The school nurse in the school health programme. Jamaican Nurse, 13 (3), Dec 1973/Jan 1974, 16–17.

6 Bryan, D. S School nursing in transition. St. Louis: Mosby,1973.

7 Bryant, N. H. School nurse utilization at International School, Bangkok, Thailand. Nursing Research, 22 (2), Mar/Apr 1973, 164–170.

8 Burtz, G. S. Weekend course for school nurses. Nursing Outlook, 19 (5), May 1971, 342–343.

9 Conrad, J. The high school nurse as a pediatric nurse practitioner. Pediatric Nursing, 1 (6), Nov/Dec 1975, 15–17.

10 Fine, L. L. and Bellaire, J. M. The school nurse: an obsolete profession revisited. Pediatric Nursing, 1 (1), Jan/Feb 1975, 25–26, 29.

11 Gettings, B. A school nursing work study in Berkshire. Health Visitor, 44 (9), Sep 1971, 285–288.

12 Hardin, D. The school age child and the school nurse: nursing observation of a well child in school. American Journal of Nursing, 74 (8), Aug 1974, 1476–1478.

13 Hawkins, N. G. Is there a school nurse role? American Journal of Nursing, 71 (4), Apr 1971, 744–751.

14 Health Visitors' Association The future of the school health service. Health Visitor, 45 (6), Jun 1972, 172–174.

15 Health Visitors' Association Staffing of the health visiting and school nursing services. [Policy document.] Health Visitor, 48 (9), Sep 1975, 331–333.

16 Hop, D. C. Discussion on school problems. [Identification of physical and mental disorders.] New Zealand Nursing Journal, 69 (9), Sep 1975, 4–6.

17 Igoe, J. B. The school nurse practitioner. Nursing Outlook, 23 (6), Jun 1975, 381–384.

18 Lewis, M. A. Child-initiated care: a nurse practitioner describes an experimental system in an elementary school. American Journal of Nursing, 74 (4), Apr 1974, 652–655.

19 Royal College of Nursing Professional Nursing Department. Community Health Section. The role of the school nurse: report of a working party. Rcn, 1974.

20 Salami, M. Y. I. The common diseases of the primary school population in Lagos. Nigerian Nurse, 7 (2), Apr/Jun 1975, 30–34.

21 Scott, M. E. What is a school nurse? Nursing Times, 68 (2), Mar 1972, 270–271.

22 Smiley, O. R. Public health nurses and teachers in school health programs: a problem in communication. [Review of school health in Northern Ontario Community.] International Journal of Nursing Studies, 12 (4), 1975, 211–215.

23 Subhadra, V. Public health nurse in school health programmes: a critical study from Calcutta. International Journal of Nursing Studies, 8 (1), Feb 1971, 29–36.

24 Sundell, W. The school nurse practitioner programme. [University of Colorado's School Nurse Practitioner Programme.] International Nursing Review, 21 (1), Jan/Feb 1974, 21–22.

25 Wilson, A. The need for a training course for school nurses. Health Visitor, 44 (9), Sep 1971, 283–284.

38 SOCIAL PROBLEMS

a GENERAL

1 Anstice, E. Tonight and every night. [Centrepoint helps London's homeless young people.] Nursing Times, 68, 21 Dec 1972, 1605. 1606.

2 Blackler, R. Girls alone in London. [A charity for girls under 21 in difficulty.] Midwife and Health Visitor, 10 (4), Apr 1974, 90–91.

3 Boorer, D. Centrepoint people. [Voluntary assistance for homeless young people at risk.] Nursing Times, 69, 30 Aug 1973, 1128–1129.

4 Campaign for the Homeless and Rootless Primary medicine for the homeless. [3 month experiment with a volunteer nurse.] The Campaign, 1975.

5 Chisholm, M. K. Sharing and caring. [Nurse's role in safeguarding the interests of the underprivileged in the community.] Midwife, Health Visitor and Community Nurse, 11 (11), Nov 1975, 360–363.

6 Freeman, R. B. Practice as protest. [Protest and social action are an essential part of nursing practice.] American Journal of Nursing, 71 (5), May 1971, 918–921.

7 Goodman, M. The enclosed environment. [Health hazards of mid-rise accommodation in a new housing estate, with particular reference to 'Captive Wives' and the elderly.] Royal Society of Health Journal, 94 (4), Aug 1974, 165–168.

8 Hansen, R. E. Planning for the underprivileged. [Health care planning teams.] Nursing Mirror, 140, 12 Jun 1975, 72–73.

9 Hodgson, S. Criteria for rehousing on medical grounds. Public Health, 90 (1), Nov 1975, 15–20.

10 Humphrey, P. Learning about poverty and health. [Course to give students insight into problems.] Nursing Outlook, 22(7), Jul 1974, 441–443.

11 Jones, M. Rich man, poor man, beggar . . . [Health visitor notes some of the problems associated with different social classes.] Nursing Times, 68, 10 Feb 1972, 190–191.

12 Kilby-Kelberg, S. A nurse's lesson in humanity from the ghetto. [A public health nurse's experience.] RN Magazine, 38 (6), Jun 1975, 32–34.

13 Leonard, M. No bed for the night. [Problems of the homeless after hospital discharge.] Nursing Times, 71, 2 Oct 1975, 1594–1595.

14 Moore, J. Crime visitors? [Meeting organized by NACRO to show health visitors the part they may play in crime prevention.] Nursing Times, 71, 22 May 1975, 798.

15 Simpson, K. Crime and the nurse. Nursing Times, 68, 13 Jan 1972, 50–52.

16 Sullivan, C. and others Nursing in a society in crisis. [Social issues confronting nurses.] American Journal of Nursing, 72 (2), Feb 1972, 302–304.

17 Timms, W. R. A professional partnership – police and nurses. [From a policeman's point of view.] Nursing Mirror, 139, 21 Nov 1974, 49–51.

18 Toms, K. M. and Walker, F. M. A free clinic for the working poor. [Nurse-staffed clinic in Lancaster, Pennsylvania.] Nursing Outlook, 21 (12), Dec 1973, 770–772.

19 Volante, R. S. and Jackson, S. M. Nursing intervention in housing for health. [East Harlem Environmental Extension Service.] International Nursing Review, 20 (6), Nov/Dec 1973, 178–180.

20 Wai-On, P. The impact of social changes on nursing. Nursing Journal of Singapore, 13 (1), May 1973, 11–13.

21 Wai-On, P. The medical aspect of high-rise and high-density living. [Review of studies from various countries, including Britain.] Nursing Journal of Singapore, 15 (2), Nov 1975, 69–75.

22 Walshe-Brennan, K. S. Family background and antisocial behaviour. [A study of 492 children and adolescents to investigate family background as a main cause of delinquency.] Health Visitor, 48 (12), Dec 1975, 464–465.

23 Wassner, A. Social and racial effects. [Social isolation in urban societies.] New Zealand Nursing Journal, 68 (11), Nov 1975, 14–16.

24 Whitehourse, D. The problems of violence in society. Midwife and Health Visitor, 9 (9), Sep 1973, 291–295.

25 Wright, L. M. A symbolic tree: loneliness is the root – delusions are the leaves. [The concept of loneliness and a case study showing therapeutic nursing intervention.] Journal of Psychiatric Nursing and Mental Health Services, 13 (3), May/Jun 1975, 30–35.

b PRISON NURSING

1 Archer, C. I. Psychiatric nursing behind an iron fence. [In the penitentiary system.] Canadian Journal of Psychiatric Nursing, 14 (5), Sep/Oct 1973, 6–9.

2 Dunn, A. USA. Nursing behind bars. [New York's prison health service.] Nursing Times, 71, 10 Jul 1975, 1084–1085.

3 Holloway Prison Seconded from Holloway. Nursing Times, 67, 1 Apr 1971, 386.

4 Holly, H. Jail matron, RN American Journal of Nursing, 72]9), Sep 1972, 1621–1623.

5 Kennedy, J. A. Health care in prison: a view from inside [by a nurse ex-inmate]. American Journal of Nursing, 75 (3), Mar 1975, 417–420.

6 McDowell, H. M. Change in one city's system.

Leadership at the cell-block level. [Management course for prison nurses in New York.] American Journal of Nursing, 75 (3), Mar 1975, 423–424.

7 McLaren, P. M. and Tappen, R. M. The community nurse goes to jail. Nursing Outlook, 22 (1), Jan 1974, 35–39.

8 Murtha, R. Health care in prison. Change in one city's system, started with a director of nursing. [New York.] American Journal of Nursing, 75 (3), Mar 1975, 421–422.

9 Norens, G. Nurses in prison. Canadian Nurse, 67 (5), May 1971, 37–39.

10 Padberg, J. Nursing and forensic psychiatry. Perspectives in Psychiatric Care, 10 (4), Oct/Nov 1972, 163–167.

11 Protzel, M. S. Nursing behind bars. American Journal of Nursing, 72 (3), Mar 1972, 505–508.

12 Ptak, A. Health care in prison. Change in one city's system: replacing pill pushing with nursing. [Experience in a male prison in New York.] American Journal of Nursing, 75 (3), Mar 1975, 427–428.

13 Strank, R. A. Prison nursing. Nursing Mirror, 140, 27 Feb 1975, 45–47.

14 Wicks, R. J. Vistas in correctional nursing. Occupational Health Nursing, 22 (4), Apr 1974, 19–20.

15 Winstead-Fry, P. Health care in prison. Change in one city's system. Mental health nursing of inmates. [In prison in New York.] American Journal of Nursing, 75 (3), Mar 1975, 425–426.

c ALCOHOLISM

1 Burns, C. R. Alcoholism. New Zealand Nursing Journal, 69 (6), Jun 1975, 4–6.

2 Carbary, L. J. Alcoholism – cirrhosis link delineated. Journal of Practical Nursing, 24 (9), Sep 1974, 28–30.

3 Cassidy, L. Addiction – its challenge to me. New Zealand Nursing Journal, 65 (5), May 1972, 8, 10.

4 Catherine, C. Alcoholism – a family disease. Australian Nurses' Journal, 4 (8), Mar 1975, 34–35, 42.

5 Cooper, P. Progress in therapeutics. Drugs used in alcoholism. Midwife, Health Visitor and Community Nurse, 11 (3), Mar 1975, 85.

6 Dickinson, C. The alcoholic: an unperson? Nursing Forum, 14 (2), 1975, 194–203.

7 Dickson, M. Involvement of the spouse in the treatment of the alcoholic. [With reference to the work of the Unit for the Treatment of Alcoholism, Royal Edinburgh Hospital.] Nursing Mirror, 139, 26 Jul 1974, 77–79.

8 Edwards, G. Demon drink. [Key steps for a national strategy to combat alcoholism.] World Health, Dec 1975, 10–15.

9 Estes, N. J. and Madden, L. P. Alcoholism in fiction: learning from the literature. Nursing Outlook, 23 (8), Aug 1975, 527–530.

10 Funston, F. D. Detoxification: an alternative in transition. Canadian Nurse, 69 (11), Nov 1973, 27–29.

11 Glatt, M. M. The alcoholisms. 1. A complex interdisciplinary disorder. Nursing Times, 71, 1 May 1975, 680–682.

12 Glatt, M. M. The alcoholism. 2. Why and how people become alcoholics. Nursing Times, 71, 8 May 1975, 723–725.

13 Glatt, M. M. The alcoholisms. 3. The 'loss of control' problem. Nursing Times, 71, 15 May 1975, 777–779.

14 Glatt, M. M. The alcoholisms. 4. The birth of the disease concept. Nursing Times, 71, 22 May 1975, 822–823.

15 Glatt, M. M. The alcoholisms. 5. The disease concept – newer developments. Nursing Times, 71, 29 May 1975, 856–858.

16 Glatt, M. M. The alcoholisms. 6. Delirium tremens. Nursing Times, 71, 5 Jun 1975, 887–889.

17 Glatt, M. M. The alcoholisms. 7. The complications of alcoholism. Nursing Times, 71, 12 Jun 1975, 936–938.

18 Glatt, M. M. The alcoholisms. 8. The treatment of alcoholism. Nursing Times, 71, 19 Jun 1975, 974–976.

19 Glatt, M. M. The alcoholisms. 9. The prevention of alcoholism. Nursing Times, 71, 26 Jun 1975, 1018–1020.

20 Glatt, M. M. The challenge of alcoholism. Midwife and Health Visitor, 9 (8), Aug 1973, 262–264.

21 Hannigan, L. Problem drinking. Occupational Health Nursing, 22 (1), Jan 1974, 19–20.

22 Harrison, P. Young people and drink. New Society, 26, 27 Dec 1973, 773–776.

23 Hecht, M. Children of alcoholics are children at risk. American Journal of Nursing, 73 (10), Oct 1973, 1764–1767.

24 James, W. P. and others Alcohol and drug dependence – treatment and rehabilitation. King Edward's Hospital Fund for London, 1972.

25 Keller, C. Alcoholics and their families. New Zealand Nursing Journal, 69 (8), Aug 1975, 4–5.

26 Kirby, A. Detoxification centres: an expensive form of cosmetic surgery. [Work of the Salvation Army's unit, Whitechapel.] Health and Social Service Journal, 85, 4 Oct 1975, 2223.

27 MacIver, C. Increasing 'self-worth': is it an answer for alcoholism? [Alcoholics Anonymous.] Canadian Journal of Psychiatric Nursing, 16 (4), Jul/Aug, 8–10.

28 Madden, J. S. Alcoholism. Nursing Mirror, 137, 31 Aug 1973, 8–10.

29 Mitchell, M. J. One day at a time. Detoxification and rehabilitation. Journal of Practical Nursing, 23 (5), May 1975, 28–30.

30 O'Neill, T. and Orr, J. Alcoholism – yesterday, today and tomorrow. [Treatment programme at Downshire Hospital, Northern Ireland.] Nursing Times, 71, 1 May 1975, 683–686.

31 Orr, J. Frank – an environmental alcoholic? Nursing Times, 71, 8 May 1975, 726–727.

32 Pepys, J. and Simmonds, S. P. Allergic relactions – to alcoholic beverages. Nursing Mirror, 139, 12 Jul 1974, 81–82.

33 Rabbitte, M. and Peters, T. Alcoholism. [The work of the Alcoholism and Drug Dependence Unit, St. Bernard's Hospital, Southall, Middlesex.] Nursing Mirror, 140, 20 Feb 1975, 58–61.

34 RN Magazine, Alcoholism. [Three articles by various authors.] RN Magazine, 37(7), Jul 1974, 31–37.

35 Wilmot, A. McKinnon. [Work of a 20 bed alcoholic and soft drug withdrawal and motivation unit. Sydney.] Australian Nurses' Journal, 5 (4), Oct 1975, 23–25, 32.

36 World Health Alcoholism as a disease. World Health, Jul/Aug 1973, 24–29.

d ALCOHOLISM: NURSING

1 Boyson, M. A. Experiments in nursing: helping the alcoholic cope with . . . sobriety. [Counselling program for alcoholics and their families.] RN Magazine, 38 (7), Jul 1975, 37.

2 Burkhalter, P.K. Alcoholism, drug abuse and drug addiction. [A study by questionnaire to examine the instruction received and its relevance to nursing practice.] Journal of Nursing Education, 14 (2), Apr 1975, 30–36.

3 Burkhalter, P. K. Nursing care of the alcoholic and drug abuser. New York: McGraw-Hill, 1975.

4 Calhoun, B. Alcoholism. A challenge to nursing. Journal of Practical Nursing, 23 (5), May 1973, 24–27.

5 Caruana, S. and Buttimore, A. Nurse's handbook on alcohol and alcoholism. Medical Council on Alcoholism, 1974.

6 Caruana, S. and Scowen, P. Alcohol and alcoholism: health visitor's handbook. Edsall, 1973.

7 Chalke, H. D. The health visitor and 'a family disease'. [Alcoholism.] Health Visitor, 47 (6), Jun 1974, 182–183.

8 Estes, N. J. Counselling the wife of an alcoholic spouse. American Journal of Nursing, 74 (7), Jul 1974, 1251–1255.

9 Gilmour, V. How do nurses feel about alcoholism. New Zealand Nursing Journal, 66 (9), Sep 1973, 31–32.

10 Gurel, M. Should courses for nurses that deal solely with alcoholism be taught at Universities? A preliminary report. Nursing Research, 23 (2), Mar/Apr 1974, 166–169.

11 Heinemann, M. E. Caring for patients with alcohol problems. Journal of Psychiatric Nursing and Mental Health Services, 12 (6), Nov/Dec 1974, 34–38.

12 Heinemann, M. E. and Estes, N. J. A program in alcoholism nursing [at the University of Washington School of Nursing.] Nursing Outlook, 22 (9), Sep 1974, 575–578.

13 Jackson, K. M. Nursing care study. Chronic alcoholism. Nursing Times, 70, 18 Jul 1974, 1104–1107.

14 Maddon, F. Alcohol, alcoholism and the nurse. New Zealand Nursing Journal, 68 (4), Apr 1975, 24–27.

15 Mayfield, D. Managing alcohol problems in geriatric patients. Nursing Care, 7 (7), Jul 1974, 10–11.

16 Mueller, J. F. Treatment for the alcoholic: cursing or nursing? American Journal of Nursing, 74 (2), Feb 1974, 245–247.

17 Mueller, J. F. and Schwerdtfeger, T. H. The role of the nurse in counselling the alcoholic. Journal of Psychiatric Nursing and Mental Health Services, 12 (2), Mar/Apr 1974, 26–32.

18 Orr, J. Nursing care study. Brian, an alcoholic – does he want to be cured? Nursing Times, 71, 15 May 1975, 780–781.

19 Schmid, N. J. and Schmid, D. T. Nursing students' attitudes toward alcoholics. Nursing Research, 22 (3), May/Jun 1973, 246–248.

20 Slater, A. M. Nursing care study. David – an alcoholic. Nursing Times, 71, 6 Feb 1975, 214–216.

21 Strong, F. Wessex. First of his kind. [The first psychiatric community care nurse in alcoholism, the work of the Hampshire Council on Alcoholism and the development of the clinical nurse specialist in alcoholism.] Nursing Times, 71, 29 May 1975, 838–840.

22 Wilkins, R. H. The community nurse and the alcoholic. Nursing Times 69, 16 Aug 1973, 1071–1072.

23 Wilkins, R. H. The health visitor and the alcoholic. Health Visitor, 46 (11), Nov 1973, 366–368.

e ALCOHOLISM: WORK SETTING

1 Bissell, L. C. and others The alcoholic hospital employee. Nursing Outlook, 21 (11), Nov 1973, 708–711.

2 Craig, A. Addiction as seen in industry. Occupational Health, 23 (11), Nov 1971, 358–360.

3 Hughes, J. P. W. A policy on alcoholism. Occupational Health, 25 (3), Mar 1973, 89.

4 Kenyon, W. H. The alcoholic at work. [Alcoholics in industry.] Personnel Management, 6 (7), Jul 1974, 33–36.

5 Nicholson, R. E. and others A seminar on the problem employee. [Alcoholism and drug addiction.] Occupational Health Nursing, 21 (4), Apr 1973, 9–26.

6 Occupational Health Nursing Alcoholism in industry. [Three articles.] Occupational Health Nursing, 22 (4), May 1974, 7–15.

7 Quigley, J. L. and Papas, A. N. A therapy program for hospital employees. Hospitals, 47 (18), 16 Sep 1973, 60–63.

8 Smoyak, S. A. Therapeutic approaches to alcoholism based on systems theories. Occupational Health Nursing, 21 (4), Apr 1973, 27–30.

f DRUG ADDICTION

1 Beckett, H. D. The twisting crutch. [Drugs which carry a danger of dependence.] Nursing Times, 67, 18 Mar 1971, 311–312.

2 Brink, P. J. Behavioral characteristics of heroin addicts on a short-term detoxification program. Nursing Research, 21 (1), Jan/Feb 1972, 38–45.

3 Brink, P. J. Heroin addicts: patterns of behavior during detoxification. Journal of Psychiatric Nursing, 10 (2), Mar/Apr 1972, 12–18.

4 Brink, P. J. Rehabilitating heroin addicts. Journal of Psychiatric Nursing and Mental Health Services, 12 (6), Nov/Dec 1974, 14–19.

5 Caddow, H. G. Diagnosing narcotic addiction in Hong Kong. Nursing Mirror, 140, 10 Apr 1975, 62–63.

6 Caddow, H. G. Low dosage methadone treatment of narcotic dependents in Hong Kong. Nursing Mirror, 139, 19 Jul 1974, 66–70.

7 Cameron, D. C. and Ling, G. M. Fool's paradise. [Preventive measures for drug addiction.] World Health, Dec 1975, 16–21.

8 Canadian Nurses' Association CNA's response to the Le Dain Commission Report. [Commission of Inquiry into the Nonmedical Use of Drugs.] Canadian Nurse, 70 (11), Nov 1974, 32–35.

9 Carney, M. W. P. Bromism – a clinical chameleon. Nursing Times, 69, 5 Jul 1973, 859–861.

10 Ellison, S. Preventing drug dependence. Nursing Times, 70, 23 May 1974, 808–809.

11 Fink, M. and others Narcotic antagonists: another approach to addiction therapy. American Journal of Nursing, 71 (7), July 1971, 1359–1363.

12 Fortuin, B. Drug abuse – a symptom of family breakdown. SA Nursing Journal, 39 (4), Apr 1972, 35.

13 Galli, E. A. Drug abuse – a current family health problem. SA Nursing Journal, 39 (2), Feb 1972, 16, 18, 20.

14 Glatt, M. M. What makes an addict? Nursing Times, 67, 4 Nov 1971, 1382–1386.

15 Gordon, W. C. Drug abuse and its relationship to industry. Occupational Health Nursing, 20 (3), March 1972, 7–8, 45.

16 Houlette, W. N. and Josephine, Sister Responding to drug abuse. [Programs designed to help individuals cope with drug abuse at Little Company of Mary Hospital, Evergreen Park, Illinois.] Hospital Progress, 56 (2), Feb 1975, 34–36.

17 King Edward's Hospital Fund for London Drug Dependency Discussion Group Drugs – the fuzz and the halo. [Work of the drug squad.] Nursing Times, 67, 4 Feb 1971, 152–153.

18 Kramer, J. F. and Cameron, D. C. joint editors A manual on drug dependence compiled on the basis of reports of WHO expert groups and other WHO publications. Geneva: WHO, 1975.

19 Krepick, D. S. and Long, B. L. Heroin addiction: a treatable disease. Nursing Clinics of North America, 8 (1), Mar 1973, 41–52.

20 Lawless, K. An unrecognized danger. [Interview with Kevin Lawless, of Release, founded to help drug addicts.] Nursing Times, 71, 18 Sep 1975, 1491–1493.

21 Long, B. L. and Krepick, D. S. New perspectives on drug abuse. Nursing Clinics of North America, 8 (1), Mar 1973, 25–40.

22 Mitchell, B. Barbiturates. Barbiturate abuse – a growing problem. An eight-year register of drug users seen at the Middlesex Hospital, Accident and Emergency Department.] Nursing Times, 71, 18 Sep 1975, 1488–1490.

23 Morgan, R. Drugs in society. Nursing Times, 70, 25 Jul 1974, 1158–1162.

24 Morton, J. The community view [on prescription of barbiturates for the elderly and confused]. Nursing Times, 71, 18 Sep 1975, 1496.

25 Nursing Times 'Keep away from them'. [Personal story of a drug addict.] Nursing Times, 71, 18 Sep 1975, 1490–1491.

26 Nursing Times Prescription in hospital. [Of barbiturates.] Nursing Times, 71, 18 Sep 1975, 1495–1496.

27 Odom, C. The enigma of drug abuse. Journal of Practical Nursing, 24 (9), Sep 1974, 19–21.

28 Pillari, G. and Narus, J. Physical effects of heroin addiction. [Data collected at Samaritan Halfway Society, New York.] American Journal of Nursing, 73 (12), Dec 1973, 2105–2108.

28 Plant, M. A. Illegal drugtaking – a medical or social problem? Nursing Times, 71, 28 Aug 1975, 1385–1387.

30 Smith, S. E. How drugs act. 27. Drugs and addiction. Nursing Times, 71, 25 Dec 1975, 2072–2073.

31 Tann, I. 'A habit of living'. The therapeutic drug-free community [for the rehabilitation of drug addicts]. Journal of Practical Nursing, 24 (9), Sep 1974, 22–26.

32 Walker, L. Crises of change: a case study of a heroin-dependent patient. Perspectives in Psychiatric Care, 12 (1), Jan/Mar 1974, 20–25.

33 Walker, L. Nutritional concerns of addicts in treatment. Journal of Psychiatric Nursing and Mental Health Services, 13 (3), May/Jun 1975, 21–26.

34 Wells, F. Pioneer practice. [Interview with Dr. Frank Wells who has restricted barbiturate prescriptions in his Ipswich practice.] Nursing Times, 71, 18 Sep 1975, 1494–1495.

35 Willis, J. H. Drug dependence: a study for nurses and social workers. 2nd ed. Faber, 1975.

g DRUG ADDICTION: NURSING

1 Australian Nurses' Journal The nurse's role in the use and abuse of drugs: papers from the 6th national convention of the Royal Australian Nursing Federation. Melbourne, Australian Nurses' Journal Supplement, Jun 1972.

2 Brink, P. J. Nurses' attitude toward heroin addicts. Journal of Psychiatric Nursing, 11 (2), Mar/Apr 7–12.

3 Cox, M. R. Nursing in a drug dependency 'family' unit. [Veterans Administration Hospital, Bedford, Mass.] RN Magazine, 37 (9), Sep 1974, 52–54.

4 Dambacher, B. and Hellwig, K. Nursing strategies for young drug users. Perspectives in Psychiatric Care, 9 (5), Sep/Oct 1971, 201–205.

5 Diver, W. J. Nurses and the drug problem. Queen's Nursing Journal, 17 (1), Apr 1974, 5–6.

6 Doran, M. O. A nursing approach to the treatment of drug addicts: evaluation of an educational programme. International Journal of Nursing Studies, 10 (4), Dec 1973, 217–227.

7 Drug Addiction Unit, St.Clement's Hospital Drug addiction: role of the nurse and the social worker. [Work of the Drug Addiction Unit, St. Clement's Hospital, Bow.] Occupational Therapy, 35 (4), Apr 1972, 246–249.

8 Dy, A. J. and others The nurse in the methadone maintenance program: expansions and transitions in role. Journal of Psychiatric Nursing and Mental Health Services, 13 (3), May/Jun 1975, 17–20.

9 Foreman, N. J. and Zerwekh, J. V. Drug crisis intervention. American Journal of Nursing, 71 (9), Sep 1971, 1736–1741.

10 Greenblatt, D. J. and Shader, R. I. Treating the drug abuser in the ED. RN Magazine, 38 (5), May 1975, OR 1, 5, 8, 10.

11 Henderson, E. H. Problems of children with drug abusing parents. [Experiences of a health visitor.] Nursing Times, 70, 5 Dec 1974, 1890–1892.

12 Huey, F. L. In a therapeutic community. [Drug addiction.] American Journal of Nursing, 71 (5), May 1971, 926–933.

13 Lee, T. F. Nursing care study. John – a drug addict. Nursing Times, 70, 6 Jun 1974, 859–860.

14 Lewis, P. The role of the nurse in a drug crisis center. Journal of Psychiatric Nursing and Mental Health Services, 11 (6), Nov/Dec 1973, 14–17.

15 Martin, R. M. The role of the nurse in drug abuse treatment, preparation and practice: surveys of drug abuse teaching and nursing experience. Kansas City: American Nurses' Association, 1972.

16 Moore, G. E. A new role for the addiction unit nurse: a pilot study of drug abuse in youth clubs. [Survey by nurse.] Nursing Mirror, 137, 6 Jul 1973, 46–47.

17 Morgan, A. J. and Moreno, J. W. Attitudes toward addiction. American Journal of Nursing, 73 (3), Mar 1973, 497–501.

18 Morris, M. L. and McClellan, A. G. The drug dependent patient and the nurse. Nursing Care, 7 (12), Dec 1974, 29–31.

19 Musser, M. V. Journey to today. [A case study which illustrates the role and function of a Drug Dependency Unit.] Journal of Practical Nursing, 24 (11), Nov 1974, 24–27, 33.

20 Nelson, K. The nurse in a methadone maintenance program. American Journal of Nursing, 73 (5), May 1973, 870–874.

21 Newman, R. G. Methadone maintenance treatment [including the role of the nurse]. Journal of Practical Nursing, 24 (10), Oct 1974, 22–23, 40.

22 Roache, M. O. Humanistic learning. [Experiences of a nurse working with drug addicts.] American Journal of Nursing, 74 (8), Aug 1974, 1453–1456.

23 St. John, D. and Soulary, E. Introduction of goal oriented record keeping on an inpatient drug treatment setting. Journal of Psychiatric Nursing and Mental Health Services, 11 (5), Sep/Oct 1973, 20–27.

24 Smith, E. S. Nursing care study. Withdrawal [from amylobarbitone sodium]. Nursing Times, 70, 17 Oct 1974, 1625–1626.

25 Tagliaferri, M. Nursing care of the patient with a drug dependence. Journal of Practical Nursing, 23 (3), Mar 1973, 36.

26 Walker, L. Methadone maintenance [for the use of long term treatment of heroin addicts]. Journal of Psychiatric Nursing and Mental Health Services, 12 (6), Nov/Dec 1974, 25–28.

h SMOKING

1 Bewley, B. R. and others Smoking by children in Great Britain: a review of the literature, by Beulah R. Bewley, Isabel Day and Lovely Ide. Science Research Council and Medical Research Council, 1973.

2 Bramley, S. P. Ban smoking in hospitals. Nursing Times, 68, 10 Feb 1972, 185.

3 Colley, J. Passive smoking in children. Nursing Times, 71, 20 Nov 1975, 1858–1859.

4 Department of Education and Science Smoking and health in schools. The Department, 1973. (Education information.)

5 Dixon, M. Hospital smoke. Is enough being done about smoking on hospital premises? Midwives Chronicle, 88, Jul 1975, 233.

6 Hamby, R. G. Some interesting results from vital capacity data on smoking and non-smoking. Occupational Health Nursing, 23 (3), Mar 1975, 17–20.

7 Horn, D. Why people smoke. World Health, Dec 1975, 26–31.

8 Howard, L. S. Be an exemplar – help people change their smoking behavior. Occupational Health Nursing, 21 (6), Jun 1973, 19, 50.

9 Kessler, S. Protecting nonsmokers in public places. Canadian Nurse, 70 (1), Jan 1974, 32–35.

10 Laycock, E. No smoking in patient rooms – please. [Policy at a Toronto hospital.] Hospital Administration in Canada, 17 (10), Oct 1975, 45–46.

11 Royal College of Physicians of London Smoking and health now: a new report and summary on smoking and its effects on health. Pitman, 1971.

12 Shearman, E. M. Control of smoking in the ward area. Nursing Times, 68, 10 Feb 1972, 185

13 Spain, D. M. and others Cigarette smoking more lethal for women than for men? RN Magazine, 36 (9), Sep 1973, ICU 1 – 4.

14 Swaffield, L. A dying habit. [Action on Smoking and Health conference.] Nursing Times, 71, 22 May 1975, 799.

15 Wake, F. R. and others Nurses, smoking and schoolchildren. Canadian Nurse, 69 (7), Jul 1973, 19–22.

16 WHO Chronicle Smoking and disease: the evidence reviewed. WHO Chronicle 29 (10), Oct 1975, 402–408.

17 World Health Organization Expert Committee. Smoking and its effects on health. Geneva: WHO, 1975. (Technical report series, 568)

18 Young, P. New Government proposals on smoking. Nursing Mirror, 141, 18 Sep 1975, 42.

MATERNITY SERVICES

39 MIDWIFERY AND MATERNITY SERVICES

a MATERNITY SERVICES

1 Berriman, D. A. The Rhesus unit at Lewisham. Midwives Chronicle, 85, Aug 1971, 282–283; Sep 1971, 304–307; 85, Oct 1971, 336–338.

2 Bishop Auckland A new maternity unit. [Bishop Auckland General Hospital, Durham.] Nursing Mirror, 141, 24 Jul 1975, 62–63.

3 Browne, J. C. M. The birthday team. [Ninth Dame Juliet Rhoys Williams memorial lecture.] Midwives Chronicle, 86, Dec 1973, 391–394; 87, Jan 1974, 16–18.

4 Bullock, A. E. Let the GP in out of the cold. [Possible future developments in obstetric care.] Nursing Mirror, 134, 14 Apr 1972, 38–39.

5 Ferster, G. and Pethybridge, R. J. The costs of a local maternity care system. Hospital and Health Services Review, 69 (7), Jul 1973, 243–247.

6 Freeburne, V. P. Opening a general practitioner midwifery hospital. [Tower Hill Maternity Hospital, Armagh.] Midwives Chronicle, 84, Feb 1971, 58–59.

7 Golding, B. M. Home or hospital? Why not both. Queen's Nursing Journal, 16 (4), Jul 1973, 84, 92.

8 Headington Hospital Maternity unit completes first phase at Headington. [Mainly illustrations.] Nursing Mirror, 137, 7 Sep 1973, 28–32.

9 Hope Hospital Mini-stay maternity unit. [Hope Hospital, Salford – 12 hour scheme.] Nursing Mirror, 133, 24 Dec 1971, 25–27.

10 King's Mill Hospital The Dukeries Centre, King's Mill Hospital, Sutton-in-Ashfield. [A new maternity hospital which opened in 1974.] Nursing Mirror, 140, Feb 1975, 40–41.

11 Kingsley, C. Evolution of an emergency obstetric unit [at University College Hospital.] Midwives Chronicle, 87 Dec 1974, 413–414.

12 Kuck, M. The ideal maternity unit. Nursing Mirror, 132, 12 Feb 1971, 26–32.

13 McKendrick, J. A new concept of general practitioner obstetrics. Midwife and Health Visitor, 8 (1), Jan 1972, 16–19.

14 McLachlan G. and Shegog, R. editors In the beginning: studies of maternity services. Oxford University Press for Nuffield Provincial Trust, 1970.

15 Martin, S. M. and Finan, K. M. 'Elegance and luxury'. Both are provided for expectant mothers in Stockport's new maternity unit at Stepping Hill Hospital. Nursing Mirror, 134, 23 Jun 1972, 37–39.

16 Meadow, R. Problems of visiting in neonatal and maternity units. Nursing Mirror, 138, 3 May 1974, 60–61.

17 Midwives Chronicle Teaching on patients in relation to the maternity service. Midwives Chronicle, 88 Oct 1975,343.

18 Moriarty, T. R. and Ward, S. Unification of midwifery services in Walsall. Midwives Chronicle, 86, Aug 1973, 252–253.

19 Pitcairn, L. The National Association for Maternal and Child Welfare. Mother and Child, 45 (6), Dec 1973, 21–22.

20 Scottish Home and Health Department Maternity services: integration of maternity work. Edinburgh: HMSO, 1973.

21 Shotley Bridge The '100 per cent' maternity unit. [Shotley Bridge General Hospital. Mainly illustrations.] Nursing Mirror, 133, 3 Dec 1971, 19–21.

22 Solihull Hospital A bright beginning. New maternity wing at Solihull Hospital, Warwickshire. [Illustrations only.] Nursing Mirror, 136, 15 Jun 1973, 36–41.

23 Staincliffe General Hospital Five into one will go. [New maternity unit at Staincliffe General Hospital. Mainly illustrations.] Nursing Mirror, 136 (13), 30 Mar 1973, 33–35.p

24 Standon-Batt, M. I. Hospital visiting: a survey at the maternity unit, Royal Berkshire Hospital, Reading. Midwives Chronicle, 86, Sep 1972, 284–206.

25 Whipps Cross Whipps Cross new maternity unit – prototype of a new standard design. [Mainly illustrations.] Nursing Mirror, 138, 22 Mar 1974, 78–82.

26 Williams, C. D. and Jelliffe, D. B. Mother and child health: delivering the services. Oxford University Press, 1972.

27 World Health Organization. Regional Office for Europe New trends in maternal and child health: report of a conference, Moscow, 11–15 November 1975. Copenhagen: WHO, 1975.

b TEXTBOOKS

1 Bailey, R. E. Mayes' midwifery: a textbook for midwives. 8th ed. Baillière Tindall, 1972.

2 Bailey, R. E. Obstetric and gynaecological nursing. 2nd ed. Baillière Tindall, 1975. (Nurses' aids series.)

3 Bender, S. Obstetrics for pupil midwives. 2nd ed. Heinemann Medical, 1972.

4 Bentall, A. P. and Fairs, D. J. Notes for students of midwifery. Churchill Livingstone, 1971.

5 Chalmers, J. A. Essential obstetrics for midwives and obstetric nurses. Lancaster: Medical and Technical Publishing, 1973.

6 Garland, G. W. and Quixley, J. M. E. Obstetrics and gynaecology for nurses. 3rd ed. English Universities Press (Modern Nursing series), 1971.

7 Hallum, J. L. Midwifery. English University Press (Modern nursing series), 1972.

8 Law, R. G. and Friedman, M. Midwifery. Staples, 1972.

9 Lerch, C. Workbook for maternity nursing. 3rd ed. St. Louis: Mosby, 1973.

10 Myles, M. F. A textbook for midwives. 8th ed. Churchill Livingstone, 1975.

11 Towler, J. and Butter-Manuel, R. Modern obstetrics for student midwives. Lloyd-Luke, 1973.

c PROFESSIONAL ASPECTS

1 Brain, M. A. 'Salmon'. Midwives Chronicle, 86, Mar 1972, 80–81.

2 Farrer, M. Midwife supervisor's role causes utter confusion. [Royal College of Midwives Symposium.] Nursing Mirror, 141, 20 Nov 1975, 35.

3 Hawkins, D. M. No strike action by college members. President outlines RCM position in AGM speech. Midwives Chronicle, 87, Jul 1974, 234–236.

4 Humphreys, D. Midwife with a motive. [Research midwife.] Nursing Times, 68, 23 Mar 1972, 346–348.

5 King's Fund Centre Launching the 'new breed' of midwives. [Conference on maternity unit care.] Nursing Times, 71, 18 Sep 1975, 1481.

6 Layton, M. E. A. International Congress of Midwives. [October 1972.] Midwives Chronicle, 86 (1021), Feb 1973, 43–45.

7 Midwives Chronicle Independent pay review for nurses and midwives. Midwives Chronicle, 87, Jul 1974, 238–239.

8 Morris, D. The doctor – patient – midwife relationship. Midwife and Health Visitor, 8 (1), Jan 1972, 23–24.

9 Napier, J. G. Scientific and technological advances in midwifery. Midwives Chronicle, 86, Aug 1972, 244–245.

10 Rowe, K. H. Attitudes of nursing staff in three maternity hospitals. [Research project into the effect of change resulting from the implementation of the Salmon recommendations.] Nursing Times, 69, 22 Feb 1973, Occ. papers, 29–32.

11 Royal College of Midwives Midwives and the Industrial Relations Act 1971. Midwives Chronicle, 86, Apr 1972, 122–123.

12 Royal College of Midwives 91st Annual General Meeting, Plymouth – June 14, 1973. Midwives Chronicle, 86, Aug 1973, 243–248.

13 Royal College of Midwives The RCM and the child health services committee. Midwives Chronicle, 87, Jun 1974, 203–204.

14 Royal College of Midwives The Royal College of

Midwives comment on equality for women. Nursing Mirror, 21 Nov 1974, 40–41.

15 Russell, J. K. The midwife's role in research projects. Midwives Chronicle, 85, Aug 1971, 276–277.

16 Ryan, C. Whither midwifery. World of Irish Nursing, 3 (10), Oct 1974, 177, 179.

17 Sheffield Regional Hospital Board The report of the working party to study the hospital midwife. The Board, 1972.

18 Uprichard, M. The midwife in Northern Ireland. Midwives Chronicle, 88, Feb 1975, 44–46.

19 Walker, J. The changing role of the midwife. International Journal of Nursing Studies, 9 (2), Jun 1972, 85–93.

20 Watson, V. Asa Briggs Report as it affects midwives. Nursing Mirror, 136, 20 Apr 1973, 22–26.

21 White, V. Monitoring opportunities in midwifery. Midwife and Health Visitor, 9 (1), Jan 1973, 6–12.

22 Young, P. 17th International Congress of Midwives. Nursing Mirror, 141, 3 Jul 1975, 40–42.

d EUROPE AND THE EEC

1 Bayes, M. The role of the midwife at international level with special emphasis on the EEC. World of Irish Nursing, 2 (3), Mar 1973, 47, 49; (4), Apr 1973, 67, 69.

2 Beck, L. Obstetrics in West Germany – present and future plans. Midwife and Health Visitor, 9 (9), Sep 1973, 297–298.

3 Byatt, J. Study tour of Scandinavia. [Midwifery in Denmark, Sweden, Finland and Norway.] Midwives Chronicle, 87, Mar 1974, 92–93.

4 Denison, M. The midwifery profession in France. Midwives Chronicle, 88, Mar 1975, 87–89; Apr 1975, 124–125.

5 Edgar, L. Home delivery – Dutch style. [Described by a Canadian nurse living in Holland.] Canadian Nurse, 71 (10), Oct 1975, 36–38.

6 Fenney, R. J. The midwife and the Common Market. Midwives Chronicle, 84, May 1971, 151.

7 Grossenbacher, G. The midwifery profession in Switzerland. Midwives Chronicle, 88, Jun 1975, 188–189.

8 Haspels, A. A. Obstetric care in the Netherlands. Public Health, 88 (4), May 1974, 183–188.

9 Hodge, I. Midwife in the EEC. Nursing Mirror, 137, 2 Nov 1973, 18–20.

10 Klapper, R. J. The midwife in Europe. Nursing Times, 69, 3 May 1973, 586–587.

11 Lapre, R. M. The organization of maternity care in the Netherlands, delivery at home or in the hospital. World Hospitals, 10 (3), Summer 1974, 128–131.

12 Lapre, R. M. and Meijer, W. J. Midwifery in Holland. Nursing Mirror, 140, 26 Jun 1975, 62–64.

13 Organisation Nationale des Syndicats de Sages-Femmes. Midwives Chronicle, 86, Sep 1972, 278.

17 Royal College of Midwives EEC draft directives. Midwives Chronicle, 86, Dec 1973, 385–387; 88, Mar 1975, 86–87.

15 Tholstrup, M. F. Having a baby in Finland. [A nurse's experience of Finland's national health service.] American Journal of Nursing, 75 (8), Aug 1975, 1333–1334.

16 Vellay, P. Focus on the EEC. Obstetrics in France – progress and shortcomings. Midwife and Health Visitor, 9 (7), Jul 1973, 225–228.

e OTHER OVERSEAS COUNTRIES

1 American Journal of Nursing Birthing, parenting and nurturing. [Eight articles on maternity and child care services.] American Journal of Nursing, 75 (10), Oct 1975, 1679–1714.

2 Ampofo, D. A. The changing pattern of midwifery practice in Ghana. [First published in the Ghanaian Nurse, 7 (1), Jul 1971.] International Nursing Review, 20 (4), Jul/Aug 1973, 127.

3 Bagnall, D. Obstetric rituals and taboos. [Practised by primitive races.] Nursing Times, 70, 18 Jul 1974, 1130–1133.

4 Bannerman, R. H. O. Maternity care in the developing countries. Midwives Chronicle, 86, Mar 1973, 70–74.

5 Bean, M. A. The nurse-midwife at work. American Journal of Nursing, 71 (5), May 1971, 949–952.

6 Burosh, P. Physicians' attitudes toward nurse-midwives. Nursing Outlook, 23 (7), Jul 1975, 453–456.

7 Canadian Nurses' Association CNA statement on the nurse-midwife. Canadian Nurse, 70 (4), Apr 1974, 12.

8 Clark, L. W. Maternity nursing – challenge or bore? [Attitudes of students.] Nursing Outlook, 19 (9), Sep 1971, 608–610.

9 Denison, M. Joint study group working party in West Africa. Midwives Chronicle, 88, Jan 1975, 16–18.

10 Evans, A. C. Domiciliary midwifery in rural India. Midwives Chronicle, 84, Jan 1971, 18–19.

11 Glanville, M. V. Midwifery in rural Zambia. Midwives Chronicle, Nov 1971, 380–381.

12 Har, K. K. Childbirth customs in Malaysia. Midwives Chronicle, 86, Aug 1972, 249.

13 Haward, L. R. C. Midwifery in Hong Kong. Midwives Chronicle, 86, Apr 1973, 114–115.

14 Hayes, M. African obstetrics. Nursing Mirror, 132, 2 Apr 1971, 34–37.

15 Hayes, P. Midwives? In Canada? Let's hope so! Canadian Nurse, 67 (7), Jul 1971, 17–19.

16 Isler, C. Bright future for OBG nursing. RN Magazine, 37 (1), Jan 1974, 31–37.

17 Jacobi, E. M. Perinatal care in the United States. [Paper from a combined New Zealand/American Nurses' Association conference.] New Zealand Nursing Journal, 68 (3), Mar 1975, 7–8.

18 King, E. The American College of Nurse-Midwives. Midwives Chronicle and Nursing Notes, 86, Jul 1972, 211–212.

19 Kitzinger, S. Having a baby in South Africa. New Society, 33, 24 Jul 1975, 188–191.

20 Lawson, J. Maternity care in the tropics. Nursing Times, 68, 23 Mar 1972, 358–359.

21 McLeod, F. Midwifery among the aborigines. Nursing Mirror, 132, 12 Mar 1971, 28–31.

22 Moss, C. A midwife in a developing country. [Malawi.] Nursing Mirror, 132, 18 Jun 1971, 32–35.

23 Moss, E. P. Focus on Malawi. 1. Twas on a Sunday morning. [Midwifery case study.] Nursing Mirror, 132, 28 Jan 1971, 21–23.

24 Nielson, I. L. A midwife-physician team in private practice. [Eugene, Oregon.] American Journal of Nursing, 75 (10), Oct 1975, 1693–1695.

25 Nurses Association of the American College of Obstetricians and Gynaecologists Obstetric, gynaecologic and neonatal nursing functions and standards. Chicago: The Association, 1973.

26 Nursing Mirror Some thoughts on midwives from the USA, New Zealand and Canada. Nursing Mirror, 134, 21 Jan 1972, 12–13.

27 Obrig, A. M. A nurse-midwife in practice. American Journal of Nursing, 71 (5), May 1971, 953–957.

28 Paul, P. E. Midwifery in a Zambian bush hospital. Midwives Chronicle, 85, Jun 1971, 194–197.

29 Quartly, J. V. Mother and baby services in Toronto and New York City. Health Visitor, 48 (1), Jan 1975, 4–8.

30 Rosamma, N. V. Nurse-midwife – a helper to women in labour. Nursing Journal of India, 54 (7), Jul 1973, 249.

31 Sosanya, R. O. Midwifery services in Nigeria. Nigerian Nurse, 4 (4), Oct/Dec 1972, 18–21.

32 Timberlake, B. The new Life Center. [An innovative maternity unit focusing on the needs of a family at the Family Hospital, Milwaukee.] American Journal of Nursing, 75 (9), Sep 1975, 1456–1461.

33 Turner, M. Nursing care study. Obstructed labour. [In a remote part of Papua New Guinea.] Nursing Mirror, 138, 31 May 1974, 74–75.

34 Verderese, M. and Turnbull, L. M. The traditional birth attendant in maternal and child health and family planning: a guide to her training and utilization. Geneva: World Health Organization, 1975. (WHO offset publication, 18.)

35 Zachariah, S. Midwifery service in rural West Bengal. Nursing Journal of India, 52 (8), Aug 1971, 251–252.

f DOMICILIARY MIDWIFERY (Includes nurse practitioner)

1 Clunes, E. J. Take over in the community: a look towards midwifery in 1974. Nursing Times, 69, 9 Aug 1973, 1033–1034.

2 Freeman, M. Maternity nurse practitioner: need for new specialist nursing roles in the community. Nursing Times, 71, 20 Nov 1975, 1853–1855.

3 Lindars, M. E. and Odell, E. J. Domiciliary midwifery in Reading. Nursing Times, 69, 30 Aug 1973, 1118–1121.

4 Malcolm, M. M. The changing pattern of community care [due to early transfer of babies from hospital.] Midwives Chronicle, 88, May 1978, 152–155.

5 Out of the 'rut' – the domiciliary midwife. Nursing Times, 67, 18 Nov 1973, 1450–1452.

6 Royal College of Midwives Community care programmes and projects: a report by the Midwife Teachers Groups of the RCM. Midwives Chronicle, 86, Nov 1973, 350–352.

7 Royal College of Midwives Domiciliary midwifery and maternity bed needs. [Comment on the Peel Report.] Midwives Chronicle, 84, Feb 1971, 56–57.

8 Savage, E. P. The domiciliary midwife. [Symposium on childbirth.] Nursing Mirror, 141, 3 Jul 1975, 51.

9 Shreeve, J. and Kimmance, K. J. Midwives on the 'bleep'. [The use of pocket radio receivers by domiciliary midwives in Buckinghamshire.] Midwives Chronicle, 87, Dec 1974, 422–423.

10 Wilson, R. Safely delivered. [Advantages of home deliveries and their implications for hospital practice.] Nursing Mirror, 141, 21 Aug 1975, 63.

g EDUCATION AND TRAINING

1 Battle, P. J. Midwifery training at the Frauenklinik, Zurich. Midwives Chronicle, 86, Jun 1973, 190–191.

2 Bender, S. Examinations and the pupil midwife. Nursing Mirror, 134, 11 Feb 1972, 38–39.

3 Bending, B. J. Teachers' page. 3. Some thoughts on the single period training. Midwives Chronicle, 87, Feb 1974, 54–55.

4 Bent, E. A. Midwife teacher training in a Polytechnic. [Newcastle-upon-Tyne.] Midwives Chronicle, 86, May 1972, 148–149.

5 Brigden, V. G. Teachers' page. 4. Objective testing – a time for change? [Objective testing of pupil midwives.] Midwives Chronicle, 87, Apr 1974, 136–137.

6 Chivers, M. I. Educational course for holders of Midwife Teachers Diploma. Midwives Chronicle, 84, Feb 1971, 48–51.

7 Cowell, B. The midwife teachers diploma: marriage of a profession and a university. [Courses based at the Midwife Teachers Training College, Kingston and Surrey University.] Midwives Chronicle, Jan 1975, 7–8.

8 Cowper-Smith, F. Educating the midwife today and tomorrow. Royal College of Midwives Annual Conference, Hull. Nursing Mirror, 141, 24 Jul 1975, 35.

9 Educating more nurse-midwives. [Reprinted from Nursing Outlook, Sep 1970.] Midwives Chronicle, 84, Jan 1971, 16–17.

10 Franklin, M. H. Recent advances in teaching methods. [Midwifery education course at the University of Surrey, July 2 – 4, 1975.] Midwives Chronicle, 88, Oct 1975, 349.

11 Grove, G. J. Practical instructors' course for teaching midwives. Midwives Chronicle, 88, Jan 1975, 9–10.

12 Gurhy, E. New horizons in nursing. [Education in midwifery.] World of Irish Nursing, 4 (2), Feb 1975, 24–25.

13 Harper, H. E. and McCall, N. Community care experience for pupil midwives [in Lancashire]. Midwives Chronicle, 87, Nov 1974, 384–385.

14 James, D. E. Teachers' page. 9. University involvement in midwifery education. Midwives Chronicle, 88, Mar 1975, 80–81.

15 James, D. E. Teachers' page. 10. Midwife tutor courses in Surrey University. Midwives Chronicle, 88, May 1975, 157–158.

16 James, D. E. Teachers' page. 11. Inservice education for senior midwives. Midwives Chronicle, 88, Jul 1975, 229–230.

17 Kilty, J. M. Objective testing and item banking at the RCM. Midwives Chronicle, 87, Sep 1974, 318–320.

18 Kilty, J. M. and Potter, F. W. The midwife teacher's diploma research project: report to the Royal College of Midwives. Royal College of Midwives, 1975.

19 Kitson, L. M. Teachers' page. 2. Obstetric nursing secondment in Scotland, Midwives Chronicle, 86, Dec 1973, 388–389.

20 Kruger, L. A. Midwifery training at North Tees – where the student midwife stays on. Nursing Mirror, 133, 10 Dec 1971, 16.

21 Malcolm, M. Evaluation of a midwifery training programme. [Mothers' Hospital, Salvation Army.] Nursing Mirror, 137, 6 Jul 1973, 22–26.

22 Midwives Chronicle Midwife teachers' representative advisory council. Midwives Chronicle, 86, Aug 1973, 250.

23 Midwives Chronicle Teachers' page. 5. The assessment of pupil midwives. Midwives Chronicle, 87, Jun 1974, 202.

24 Midwives Chronicle The work of the joint study group on the training and practice of midwives and maternity nurses. [Including the definition of a midwife.] Midwives Chronicle, 87, Feb 1974, 59–60.

25 Muscroft, V. P. Teachers' page. 12. Programmed instruction. Midwives Chronicle, 88, Sep 1975, 310–312.

26 Roberts, L. and Large, A. Midwifery refresher courses reviewed. Nursing Mirror, 133, 8 Oct 1971, 13–16.

27 Wessex Midwifery training. [Integrated training in the Wessex region.] Nursing Times, 71, 29 May 1975, 846–848.

h HISTORY

1 Arthure, H. Early English midwifery. Midwife, Health Visitor and Community Nurse, 11 (6), Jun 1975, 187–190.

2 Arthure, H. Midwifery practice in the first half of the 20th century. Midwife, Health Visitor and Community Nurse, 11 (10), Oct 1975, 333–334; (11), Nov 1975, 357–358.

3 Arthure, H. Midwifery today – 400 years of progress. Nursing Times, 70, 21 Feb 1974, 285.

4 Arthure, H. 19th century midwifery and the formation of the CMB. Midwife, Health Visitor and Community Nurse, 11 (8), Aug 1975, 254–256.

5 Biggar, J. When midwives were witches . . . white ones of course. A look at maternity care in the Middle Ages. Nursing Mirror, 134, 26 May 1972, 36–39.

6 Brian, V. A. The intriguing history of obstetrical forceps. Nursing Mirror, 141, 31 Jul 1975, 62–63.

7 Copcutt, D. I. Midwifery in the 17th century. [Reprinted from SA Nursing Journal 1960–1961.] SA Nursing Journal, 42 (4), Apr 1975, 9–10.

8 Copcutt, D. I. Midwifery in the 18th century. [Scotland, Ireland, Germany, England, America and France.] SA Nursing Journal, 42 (10), Oct 1975, 18–22.

9 Donnison, J. E. The development of the profession of midwife in England from 1750–1902. PhD thesis, London University, 1975.

10 Ehrenreich, B. and English, D. Witches, midwives and nurses: a history of women healers. Compendium, 1974. (Glass mountain pamphlet no. 1.)

11 Forbes, T. R. The regulation of English midwives in the eighteenth and nineteenth centuries. Medical History, 15 (4), Oct 1971, 352–362.

12 Gordon, E. Nurses and nursing in Britain. 15. Care of the lying in woman. Midwife and Health Visitor, 8 (4), Apr 1972, 125–130.

13 Hughes, W. H. Changes in infections in midwifery since the 1930s. Midwives Chronicle, 88, Dec 1975, 402–403.

14 Midwives Chronicle and Nursing Notes Our 1000th issue. Midwives Chronicle, 84, May 1971, 159–162.

15 Osborn, L. Mary Tudor and the empty cradle. [False pregnancy.] Midwife and Health Visitor, 10 (10), Oct 1974, 313–316.

16 The Royal College of Midwives of the United Kingdom of Great Britain and Northern Ireland 1881–1972. Midwives Chronicle, 86, Apr 1972, 109–110.

17 Simms, M. Midwives and abortion in the 1930's. [Midwives Institute memorandum in 1937 to the Bir-

kett Committee on Abortion, based on evidence collected from midwives.] Midwife and Health Visitor, 10 (5), May 1974, 114–116.

18 Thornton, A. The past in midwifery services. [In New South Wales.] Australian Nurses' Journal, 1 (9), Mar 1972, 19–33, 26.

19 Thornton, J. L. The first printed English edition of 'Observations in Midwifery' by Percival Willughby (1596–1685). Practitioner, 208, Feb 1972, 295–297.

i MALE MIDWIVES

1 Banks, P. Intimate duties of the midwife. Midwives Chronicle, 88, Jan 1975, 15.

2 Blenkin, T. Male midwives – a feasible prospect? [Opposition to views expressed by P. Banks in Midwives Chronicle, Jan 1975.] Midwives Chronicle, 88, Jun 1975, 191.

3 Clay, T. Male midwives – a male nurse's point of view. Midwife and Health Visitor, 10 (4), Apr 1974, 79, 81.

4 Clayton, S. Male midwives – RCOG supports Collegeviews. Midwives Chronicle, 88, Jan 1975, 3.

5 Donnison, J. Society at work. The sex of midwives. New Society, 26, 1 Nov 1973, 275–276.

6 Hawkes, P. Accoucheur or accoucheuse? [Attitudes of women to male midwives.] Nursing Times, 70, 24 Jan 1974, 119.

7 Keywood, O. Men midwives? An account of a symposium by the South Worcestershire Branch of the Royal College of Midwives. Midwives Chronicle, 86, Jun 1973, 186–187.

8 McCarrick, H. Men in midwifery. [In Scotland.] Nursing Times, 70, 14 Feb 1974, 243–244.

9 Mee, B. D. Sex of midwives. [Letter.] New Society, 26, 25 Nov 1973, 421.

10 Midwife and Health Visitor Male midwives – a midwife's point of view. Midwife and Health Visitor, 10 (2/3), Feb/Mar 1974, 44–45.

11 Nursing Mirror: Parliamentary Correspondent No barriers for male midwives. Nursing Mirror, 140, 26 Jun 1975, 41.

12 Nursing Times Exemption clause could stop male midwives. Nursing Times, 71, 26 Jun 1975, 991; Lords agree to male midwives amendment. Nursing Times, 71, 7 Aug 1975, 1234.

13 Royal College of Midwives Male midwives – Mrs Castle concedes major points to RCM. [Correspondence between the General Secretary of the RCM and Mrs Castle.] Midwives Chronicle, 88, Apr 1975, 128–129; Nursing Times, 71, 13 Mar 1975, 402.

14 Sweet, B. R. Patients' reactions to male midwives. Nursing Times, 70, 17 Oct 1974, 1619–1620.

15 Wakeley, J. Male midwives in UK? Supervisor Nurse, 6 (1), Jan 1975, 47.

16 Watkin, B. Male midwives. Nursing Mirror, 141, 17 Jul 1975, 39.

40 PREGNANCY

a ANTENATAL PREPARATION

1 Ballesty, B. Antenatal preparation. [Symposium on childbirth.] Nursing Mirror, 141, 3 Jul 1975, 52–54.

2 Chamberlain, G. Antenatal education. [Results of surveys by the Research Committee, Royal College of Midwives, and Queen Charlotte's Hospital for Women,

London.] Midwife, Health Visitor and Community Nurse, 11 (9), Sep 1975, 289, 291–292.

3 Craven, R. O. and others Guidelines for teachers of parentcraft and relaxation. [Series of eight parts.] Midwives Chronicle 88; Jan 1975, 11–12; Feb 1975, 55; Mar 1975, 84–85; Apr 1975, 118; May 1975, 155; Jun 1975, 205; Jul 1975, 236; Aug 1975, 266–267.

4 Laughran, M. A project on antenatal health education in Manchester: results of a health visitor training project. Midwife and Health Visitor, 9 (6), Jul 1973, 195–197.

5 Myerscough, P. Health education in pregnancy. Nursing Mirror, 134, 7 Jan 1972, 11–13.

6 Rathbone, B. Focus on new mothers: a study of antenatal classes. (Research Series.) RCN, 1973.

7 St. Luke's Hospital Maternity Research Project Committee Researchers? Of course. [Study to evaluate the effects of prenatal education by nurses untrained in research methodology.] Journal of Nursing Administration, 5 (9), Nov/Dec 1975, 7–9.

8 Williams, M. and Booth, D. Antenatal education: guidelines for teachers. Edinburgh: Churchill Livingstone, 1974.

9 Wright, P. The health visitor's role in antenatal care. [Symposium on childbirth.] Nursing Mirror, 14, 3 Jul 1975, 67–68.

b PREGNANCY

1 Bancroft, A. V. Pregnancy and the counter-culture. Nursing Clinics of North America, 8 (1), Mar 1973, 67–76.

2 Beazley, J. M. Pregnancy – a time for evaluation. Nursing Mirror, 141, 11 Dec 1975, 60–61.

3 Beazley, J. M. and Underhill, R. A. Confinement date unknown. Nursing Times, 67, 11 Nov 1971, 1414–1417.

4 Bomar, P. J. The nursing process in the care of a hostile pregnant adolescent. Maternal-Child Nursing Journal, 4 (2), Summer 1975, 95–100.

5 Bryan-Logan, B. N. and Dancy, B. L. Unwed pregnant adolescents: their mothers' dilemma. Nursing Clinics of North America, 9 (1),Mar 1974, 5–68.

6 Dumoulin, J. G. Some aspects of multiple pregnancy. Nursing Mirror, 137, 31 Aug 1973, 19–20.

7 Eddy, J. W. Multiple pregnancies – fact and fiction. 1 and 2. Midwife and Health Visitor, 9 (8), Aug 1973, 265–267.

8 Elliott, J. Triplet pregnancy. Midwives Chronicle, 86, Jan 1973, 5–8.

9 Frye, B.A. and Barham, B. Reaching out to pregnant adolescents. American Journal of Nursing, 75 (9), Sep 1975, 1502–1504.

10 Hatcher, J. Pregnancy tests. Nursing Times, 67, 18 Feb 1971, 203.

11 Hibbard, E. D. Folate and vitamin B12 metabolism in pregnancy. Midwife and Health Visitor, 8 (8), Aug 1972, 280–282.

12 Hudson, C. N. Multiple pregnancy. Nursing Times, 69, 22 Nov 1973, 1555–1557.

13 Hurford, A. Twin to twin transfusion syndrome. New Zealand Nursing Journal, 64 (7), Jul 1971, 6–7, 9.

14 Iffrig, M. C. Body image in pregnancy: its relation to nursing functions. Nursing Clinics of North America, 7 (4), Dec 1972, 631–639.

15 Lowe, M. L. Relationship between compliance with medical regimen and outcome of pregnancy. Nursing Research, 22 (2), Mar/Apr 1973, 157–164.

16 Moore, R. E. B. Wellbeing of the pregnant. New Zealand Nursing Journal, 66 (9), Sep 1973, 10–12.

17 Oakes, G. K. and others Diet in pregnancy: meddling with the normal or preventing toxemia? American Journal of Nursing, 75 (7), Jul 1975, 1134–1136.

18 Pridmore, B. R. Carbohydrate metabolism in pregnancy. Midwife and Health Visitor, 9 (11), Nov 1973, 351, 353–354.

19 Ranney, J. M. Superstitions of pregnancy. Nursing Care, 6 (2), Feb 1973, 12–15.

20 Rubin, R. Maternal tasks in pregnancy. Maternal-Child Nursing Journal, 4 (3), Fall 1975, 143–153.

21 Wattis, E. Eating for two: the importance of the right type of food in pregnancy. Nursing Times, 69, 27 Sep 1973, 1248–1249.

22 Young, R. Nursing care study. Quintuplets – a community experience. Nursing Mirror, 138, 3 May 1974, 81–82.

c COMPLICATIONS

1 Aiken, D. A. Infection in association with pregnancy. Nursing Mirror, 135, 1 Sep 1972, 12–13.

2 Aiken, D. A. Spontaneous abortion: the most common complication in pregnancy. Nursing Times, 69, 12 Jul 1973, 898–899.

3 Allen, V. M. Two nursing care studies specially for midwives. 2. Diabetes mellitus and pyelonephritis complicating pregnancy. Nursing Mirror, 135, 17 Nov 1972, 28–30.

4 Barnett, D. Nursing care study. Fulminating pre-eclampsia. Nursing Mirror, 137, 21 Sep 1973, 44–48.

5 Barr, M. S. Intra-uterine exchange transfusion. [For severe haemolytic disease.] Midwife and Health Visitor, 7 (12), Dec 1971, 462–464.

6 Beazley, J. M. Sepsis in an obstetric unit. Nursing Mirror, 134, 30 Jun 1972, 22–25.

7 Brant, H. A. Pregnancy and urinary tract infections. Nursing Times, 69, 19 Jul 1973, 919–921.

8 Chamberlain, G. V. Heart disease in pregnancy. Nursing Mirror, 134, 21 Apr 1972, 15–18.

9 Chard, T. Threatened abortion: placental lactogen levels guide. Nursing Mirror, 138, 29 Mar 1974, 50–51.

10 Clarke, C. A. Practical effects of blood group incompatibility between mother and fetus. Nursing Mirror, 136, 19 Jan 1973, 20–23.

11 Davies, P. A. Infection in the foetus and newborn. Midwife and Health Visitor, 8 (9), Sep 1972, 305–310.

12 DiPalma, J. R. Drug therapy today. The ubiquitous anaerobe: cause for concern in OBG. RN Magazine 38 (12), Dec 1975, 61–62, 64, 65.

13 Divine, D. Toxemias in pregnancy. Nursing Care, 8 (3), Mar 1975, 21–22.

14 Edwards, J. How nurse can aid in finding renal disease in pregnancy. Hospital Topics, 50 (7), Jul 1972, 44–45.

15 Grant, M. and Perkins, A. J. Case study: essential hypertension in pregnancy. Midwives Chronicle, 88, Jun 1975, 193–196.

16 Hudson, C. Intestinal disorders in pregnancy. Midwife and Health Visitor, 10 (12), Dec 1974, 378–381.

17 Law, R. G. Minor abnormalities of pregnancy. Midwife and Health Visitor, 9 (9), Sep 1973, 287–290.

18 Low, A. W. Postnatal treatment of toxaemia. Nursing Times, 71, 16 Oct 1975, 1671–1672.

19 McGarry, J. Pre-eclampsia and eclampsia. Nursing Mirror, 137, 20 Jul 1973, 25–27.

20 MacGillivray, I. Investigation and treatment of pre-eclampsia. Midwife and Health Visitor, 10 (4), Apr 1974, 83–86; (5), May 1974, 121–123.

21 McKenzie, A. W. Skin disorders in pregnancy. Nursing Times, 68, 2 Mar 1972, 268–269.

22 Martin, I. C. A. Confused and confusing – hyperemsis gravidarum. Nursing Times, 70, 28 Mar 1974, 473–474.

23 Mather, G. Medical hazards of childbearing. Nursing Mirror, 136, 23 Feb 1973, 21–23.

24 Midwinter, A. Vomiting in pregnancy. Nursing Times, 68, 13 Jan 1972, 42–45.

25 Nash, T. G. Extra-uterine pregnancy. Nursing Times, 70, 17 Oct 1974, 1623–1624.

26 Nursing Mirror Viral infection during pregnancy. Nursing Mirror, 138, 14 Jun 1974, 52.

27 Nye, E. B. The Rhesus factor in pregnancy. Nursing Times, 67, 7 Oct 1971, 1240–1242.

28 Oakley, C. M. Heart disease in pregnancy. Nursing Mirror, 135, 15 Dec 1972, 22–28.

29 Oo, C. H. Nursing care study. A twin pregnancy. [Case of ectopic gestation.] Nursing Times, 70, 2 May 1974, 670–671.

30 Ormerod, T. P. Medical hazards in pregnancy. Nursing Mirror, 134, 5 May 1972, 25–27.

31 Picton, F. C. R. Ectopic gestation. Nursing Times, 70, 2 May 1974, 672–673.

32 Robinson, P. A. Nursing care study. Pregnancy with complications. Nursing Mirror, 136, 16 Mar 1973, 22–24.

33 Spicher, E. Some variables and their relationship to chloasma gravidarum in postpartum women. An exploratory investigation. [Blotchy yellow-brown pigmentation of the face during pregnancy.] Nursing Research, 22 (2), Mar/Apr 1973, 117–122.

34 Walton, S. M. 'A social mess'. [Hyperemesis gravidarum.] Nursing Times, 69, 5 Apr 1973, 452–453.

35 Wingfield, J. G. Thrombo-embolic phenomena associated with childbirth. Midwives Chronicle, 86, Sep 1972, 280–282.

36 Wiser, W. L. and others Toxemias of pregnancy: nursing essentials. Journal of Practical Nursing, 22 (4), Apr 20–22; (5), May 1972, 20–22, 32.

d DRUGS

1 Farquhar, J. B. Drugs in obstetric practice. Midwives Chronicle, 84, Mar 1971, 97–100; Apr 1971, 118–122.

2 Hutton, P. M. L. Nursing care study. How will she fare? [Psychiatric illness in a pregnant drug addicted woman.] Nursing Times, 70, 28 Feb 1974, 303–305.

3 Illingworth, R. S. Drugs in pregnancy. Their possible effect on the fetus. Midwives Chronicle, 86, Feb 1973, 36–37.

4 Overbach, A. M. Drugs used with neonates and during pregnancy. 2. Drugs other than antibiotics, including oxygen. RN Magazine, 37 (11), Nov 1974, 52–56.

5 Overbach, A. M. Drugs used with neonates and during pregnancy. 3. Drugs that may cause fetal damage or cross into breast milk. RN Magazine, 37 (12), Dec 1974, 39–45.

6 Rodman, M. J. Drug therapy today. The pregnant patient: treating her without harming the baby. RN Magazine, 38 (2), Feb 1975, 61–62, 66–68, 70, 72, 74–75.

7 Smith, S. E. How drugs act. 24. Drugs and pregnancy. Nursing Times, 71, 4 Dec 1975, 1948–1949.

8 Towers, S. H. Drugs and the fetus. [The harmful effects on the fetus of drugs taken in pregnancy.] Nursing Mirror, 138, 14 Jun 1974, 70–72.

9 Tsatsaronis, S. Effects of drugs on the foetus. Australian Nurses' Journal, 4 (5), Nov 1974, 34–35.

e FETUS

1 Abramovich, D. Factors affecting volume and composition of liquor amnii. Midwife and Health Visitor, 7 (1), Jan 1971, 15, 17–18.

2 Beazley, J. M. Assessment of fetal maturity. Nursing Mirror, 133, 30 Jul 1971, 19–22.

3 Beazley, J. M. Hazards to fetal development. Nursing Mirror, 138, 22 Mar 1974, 53–54.

4 Beazley, J. M. and Kurjak, A. Prediction of foetal maturity and birthweight by abdominal palpation. Nursing Times, 69, 14 Jun 1973, 765.

5 Case, L. L. Ultrasound monitoring of mother and fetus. American Journal of Nursing, 72 (4), Apr 1972, 725–727.

6 Costello, E. and Duncan, G. R. Graphic guide to progress. The partogram graphic guide to progress. New Zealand Nursing Journal, 69 (10), Oct 1975, 7–9.

7 Dunstan, M. K. Prenatal factors influencing the foetus up to the end of the second trimester. Midwife and Health Visitor, 9 (10), Oct 1973, 319, 321, 323.

8 Edwards, E. M. Hazards of fetal development. Nursing Mirror, 139, 26 Sep 1974, 48–50.

9 Hatcher, J. Amniotic fluid analysis. Midwives Chronicle, 86, Mar 1972, 76.

10 Hibbard, B. M. The private pond. [Amniotic fluid.] Midwives Chronicle, 86, Jun 1972, 180–184.

11 Jeffcoate, N. The unborn child. Nursing Mirror, 134, 28 Apr 1972, 10–14.

12 Kelly, J. Foetal distress. Nursing Times, 68, 27 Jan 1972, 110–117.

13 Kelly, J. Monitoring for the modern midwife. Nursing Mirror, 136, 18 May 1973, 22–27.

14 Lasater, C. Electronic monitoring of mother and fetus. American Journal of Nursing, 72 (4), Apr 1972, 728–730.

15 Lewin, R. Whether ultrasonics in obstetric diagnosis? A penetrating gaze into the womb. Maternal and Child Care, 7 (73), Oct 1972, 85–88.

16 McClure Browne, J. C. Fetal development and care for the patient at risk. [Symposium on childbirth.] Nursing Mirror, 141, 3 Jul 1975, 48–50.

17 McLean, F. H. Assessing gestational age. Canadian Nurse, 68 (3), Mar 1972, 23–26.

18 MacVicar, J. Antenatal assessment of the fetus. Midwives Chronicle, 86, Sep 1973, 286–289.

19 Micallef, T. The nurse in an ultrasound unit. Nursing Times, 71, 31 Jul 1975, 1205–1206.

20 Rothberg, L. A new sound in obstetrics. RN Magazine, 34 (12), Dec 1971, 38–40;

21 Russell, J. G. B. The uses of ultrasound in obstetrics. Lecture given on October 24, 1974 at the 59th London Nursing Conference. Nursing Mirror, 139, 31 Oct 1974, 66–68.

22 Russin, A. W. and others Electronic monitoring of the fetus. American Journal of Nursing, 74 (7), Jul 1974, 1294–1299.

23 Simmons, S. C. Monitoring the foetus during labour. Nursing Times, 68, 26 Oct 1972, 1349–1351.

24 Snaith, L. Hazards to the fetus. Nursing Times, 69, 29 Nov 1973, 1605–1607.

25 Sutherst, J. R. Fetal circulation. Nursing Times, 71, 13 Mar 1975, 413–414.

26 Underhill, R. A. Ultrasound in obstetrics. Nursing Times, 69, 4 Oct 1973, 1278–1281.

27 Wheeler, T. Reading fetal heart-rate records. Nursing Mirror, 141, 30 Oct 1975, 66–69.

28 Wheeler, T. Safety of the fetus during labour. Nursing Mirror, 137, 10 Aug 1973, 20–23.

f FETAL ABNORMALITIES

1 Butler, L. J. Human chromosome abnormalities. 2. Occurrence in spontaneous abortion and antenatal detection by amniocentesis. Midwife and Health Visitor, 7 (3), Mar 1971, 105–108.

2 Cowie, V. Prenatal diagnosis of abnormalities in babies. Nursing Mirror, 135, 21 Jul 1972, 22–23.

3 Crome, L. Pathology of mental handicap. NM Conference Lecture. Nursing Mirror, 138, 7 Jun 1974, 50–53.

4 Dumoulin, J. G. Management of fetal abnormalities. Nursing Mirror, 132, 11 Jun 1971, 26–30.

5 Dunn, P. M. Congenital postural deformities: perinatal associations. Nursing Mirror, 136, 27 Apr 1973, 26–29.

6 Fielding, M. 'Cri du chat' syndrome: a chromosomal abnormality. Australian Nurses' Journal, 2 (1), Jul 1972, 25–26.

7 Gilford, P. 'Black spot' – an exercise in the prevention of mental retardation. [Retrospective study of the light for dates babies born in the St. Thomas's Group 1965–1970 to examine intra-uterine nutrition and growth.] Midwives Chronicle, 88, Feb 1975, 49–54.

8 Lind, T. The clinical uses of amniocentesis. Mother and Child, 43 (5), Sep/Oct 1971, 6–9.

9 Liu, D. T. Y. and Thwaites, P. M. Induced midtrimester abortion [when fetal abnormality is diagnosed.] Nursing Times, 70, 3 Oct 1974, 1543.

10 Nitowsky, H. M. Prenatal diagnosis of genetic abnormality. American Journal of Nursing, 71 (8), Aug 1971, 1551–1557.

11 Nursing Times A vaccine against mental retardation. [To prevent cytomegalovirus infection in utero.] Nursing Times, 70, 7 Feb 1974, 197.

12 Smithells, R. W. The prevention of congenital abnormalities. Midwives Chronicle, 84, May 1971, 152–155.

g PLACENTA

1 Andrews, M. E. Case study: hydatidiform mole. Midwives Chronicle, 88, Oct 1975, 338–339.

2 Bender, S. Placental insufficiency. Nursing Mirror, 132, 5 Feb 1971, 23–24.

3 Blair, R. G. Abruptio placentae. 1. Incidence, aetiology and clinical features. Midwife and Health Visitor, 10 (6), Jun 1974, 147, 149–150.

4 Blair, R. G. Abruptio placentae. 2. Management. Midwife and Health Visitor, 10 (7), Jul 1974, 195–198.

5 Drechsler, Sr. Nursing care study. Pregnancy complicated by a hydatidiform mole. Nursing Mirror, 139, 30 Aug 1974, 71–72.

6 Elder, M. G. Placental function tests and obstetric practice. Midwife and Health Visitor, 9 (4), Apr 1973, 107, 109, 111–112.

7 Hamilton, W. J. The human placenta. Nursing Mirror, 134, 28 Jan 1972, 25–27.

8 Kilker, R. C. and Wilkerson, B. Nursing care in placenta previa and abruptio placentae. Nursing Clinics of North America, 8 (3), Sep 1973, 479–487.

9 Letchworth, A. T. Placental lactogen and fetal distress. Nursing Mirror, 136, 6 Apr 1973, 32–33.

10 Limming, C. Nursing care study. Placental transfusion syndrome. Nursing Times, 71, 16 Jan 1975, 102–104.

11 McDonnell, B. Abruptio placentae. Midwife and Health Visitor, 7 (5), May 1971, 177, 179–81.

12 Manlik, D. Placenta praevia. Midwife and Health Visitor, 7 (2), Feb 1971, 69–72.

13 Symonds, M. Assessment of placental function. Midwife Health Visitor and Maternity Nurse, 11 (6), Jun 1975, 173, 175, 177.

14 Turner, G. Examination of the placenta. Nursing Mirror, 135, 28 Jul, 19–21; 4 Aug 1972, 15–17.

15 Underhill, R. A. Diagnosis of placenta praevia by ultrasound. [A new and safer method of placental localisation.] Midwife and Health Visitor, 10 (11), Nov 1974, 346–350.

16 Willocks, J. Prenatal assessment of placental insufficiency. Nursing Times, 69, 6 Sep 1973, 1154–1156.

h SMOKING IN PREGNANCY

1 Andres, J. Smoking in pregnancy. Midwife and Health Visitor, 8 (7), Jul 1972, 239, 241–243.

2 Collingwood, J. M. Smoking during pregnancy: effects on perinatal mortality and on subsequent intellectual and physical development. Health Visitor, 47 (3), Mar 1974, 68–69.

3 Goldstein, H. Smoking in pregnancy and the health of the baby. Mother and Child, 44 (2), Mar/Apr 1972, 10–11.

4 Halliday, N. P. The pregnant smoker. [Reprinted from 'Update', Sep 1971.] Midwives Chronicle, 86, Jan 1973, 14–15.

5 Jones, P. Smoking and pregnancy. [Survey to measure the effectiveness of Health Education Council publicity campaign by the Buckinghamshire Health Education Service.] Nursing Times, 71, 18 Dec 1975, 2038–2039.

6 McLaren, A. and Rasor, P. A survey of the attitudes of non-pregnant mothers to cigarette smoking during pregnancy and its effects on the child. Midwife and Health Visitor, 9 (11), Nov 1973, 362–365.

7 Midwives Chronicle Smoking in pregnancy: the Rush Green Hospital Project. [Campaign to warn mothers.] Midwives Chronicle, 87, May 1974, 166–171.

8 Richmond, A. and others Smoking during pregnancy. Nursing Mirror, 141, 18 Sep 1975, 50–51.

9 Wood, A. J. Smoking and pregnancy. Nursing Mirror, 137, 12 Oct 1973, 26–28.

41 CHILDBIRTH

a GENERAL

1 Bell, E. J. A personal experience of labour. Nursing Mirror, 136, 12 Jan, 34–36. [Reprinted in Midwife and Health Visitor, 10, Jan 1974, 10–14.]

2 **Cauble, K.** Call me Miss . . . [Problems of the unmarried mother in the maternity unit.] Supervisor Nurse, 6 (5), May 1975, 46–47.

3 **Clark, A. L.** Labor and birth: expectations and outcomes. [Interview with 24 expectant mothers.] Nursing Forum, 14 (4), 1975, 413–428.

4 **Edwards, M. E.** Unattended home birth. American Journal of Nursing, 73 (8), Aug 1973, 1332–1335.

5 **Huntingford, P.** Call for 'safe but happy' approach to childbirth. [Address to the National Childbirth Trust.] Nursing Times, 71, 15 May 1975, 754.

6 **Moore, D. S. and Cook-Hubbard, K.** Comparison of methods for evaluating patient response to nursing care. [Study of obstetric patients.] Nursing Research, 24 (3), May/Jun 1975, 202–204.

7 **Muir, E.** What the patient saw. [Patient comfort in an obstetric ward.] Australian Nurses' Journal, 4 (5), Nov 1974, 41.

8 **Nunnally, D. M. and Aguiar, M. B.** Patients' evaluation of their prenatal and delivery care. Nursing Research, 23 (6), Nov/Dec 1974, 469–474.

9 **Nursing Mirror** A symposium on childbirth: the daily miracle. Nursing Mirror, 141, 3 Jul 1975, 47–68.

10 **RN Magazine** The nursing challenges of OB. [Four articles on maternity nursing.] RN Magazine, 34 (11), Nov 1971, 35–48 [7p].

11 **Shields, D.** The psychology of child birth. Canadian Nurse, 70 (11), Nov 1974, 24–26.

12 **Webster, D. M.** Childbirth in the technological age – the mother's emotional needs. Nursing Mirror, 140, 27 Mar 1975, 55–58.

b ANAESTHESIA AND ANALGESIA

1 **Appleton, P. J. and Yorston, B.** Hazards of obstetric analgesia and anaesthesia. Nursing Mirror, 132, 15 Jan 1971, 22–27.

2 **Burn, J. M. B.** Analgesia in obstetric practice. Nursing Mirror, 134, 18/25 Feb 1972, 28–31.

3 **Burn, J. M. B.** Diazepam in labour: a word of caution. Midwives Chronicle, 87, Oct 1974, 348–349.

4 **Burn, J. M. B.** Hazards of obstetric analgesia and anaesthesia. Nursing Mirror, 137, 24 Aug 1973, 10–14.

5 **Crawford, J. S.** Some hazards of anaesthesia for obstetrics. Midwives Chronicle, 88, Oct 1975, 344–348.

6 **Dillon, J. B.** Obstetric anesthesia (Analgesia.) Journal of the American Association of Nurse Anesthetists, 40 (2), Apr 1972, 108–110, 117–122.

7 **Field, P. A.** Relief of pain in labor. [Psychological aspects of pain and the use of drugs.] Canadian Nurse, 70 (12), Dec 1974, 17–23.

8 **Greiss, F. C. Jr.** Obstetric anesthesia. American Journal of Nursing, 71 (1), Jan 1971, 67–69.

9 **Hendrie, M. J. M.** Liquid food for obstetric patients. [An analysis of two foods given just before labour bearing in mind the possibility of general anaesthesia.] Nursing Times, 71, 9 Jan 1975, 60–62.

10 **Holdcroft, A.** Analgesia and anaesthesia. [Symposium on childbirth.] Nursing Mirror, 71, 3 Jul 1975, 60–63.

11 **Holdcroft, A.** Obstetric epidural analgesia. Nursing Times, 71, 6 Nov 1975, 1773–1775.

12 **Isler, C.** Gastric acid down, OB patient safety up. [Prevention of acid aspiration during obstetrical anesthesia.] RN Magazine, 38 (9), Sep 1975, 39, 42, 45.

13 **Jones, D. H.** Epidural analgesia in obstetrics. Midwives Chronicle, 88, Nov 1975, 367–369.

14 **Jones, P. L. and Rosen, M.** Methoxyflurane in midwifery practice. Midwives Chronicle and Nursing Notes, 85, June 1971, 202–204.

15 **Long, C. F. and Soo, B.** The relationship of significance of nurse-patient relations to pain reaction in labour. [Study to compare a training area and a normal labour ward.] Nursing Journal of Singapore, 15 (1), May 1975, 13–17.

16 **Mills, C. D.** Drugs and the midwife. Nursing Mirror, 138, 12 Apr 1974, 59–61.

17 **Moir, D. D.** Pain relief in labour: a handbook for midwives. Edinburgh: Churchill Livingstone, 1971. 2nd ed. 1975.

18 **Nicholls, A. N. and Keen, S.** Objectives and rewards of research. [Research in the Obstetric Unit at Pembury Hospital, which includes research into pain relief in labour.] Midwives Chronicle, 87, Jun 1974, 208–210.

19 **Pearson, J. F.** Epidural analgesia in practice. Midwife, Health Visitor and Community Nurse, 11 (11), Nov 1975, 364–366.

20 **Perkins, H.** Sparine – its value in obstetrics. Midwives Chronicle, 87, Jan 1974, 10–11.

21 **Rowbotham, C. J. F.** Obstetric pain [and methods of pain relief.] Physiotherapy, 60 (4), Apr 1974, 103–106.

22 **Rubin, A. P.** Anaesthesia and maternal mortality. Midwife and Health Visitor, 8 (6), Jun 1972, 202–205.

23 **Sasmor, J. L. and others** The childbirth team during labor. [Psychoprophylactic method.] American Journal of Nursing, 73 (3), Mar 1973, 444–447.

24 **Steel, G. C.** Epidural nerve block in obstetrics. Nursing Mirror, 138, 19 Apr 1974, 55–58.

25 **Williamson, J. A.** Alternative medicine. Hypnosis in obstetrics. [A comparative study of 70 patients trained in auto-hypnosis, 70 given physiotherapy and 70 with no antenatal training.] Nursing Times, 71, 27 Nov 1975, 1895–1897.

c LABOUR

1 **Beard, R. W.** Fetal intensive care in labour. Nursing Mirror, 136, 4 May 1973, 23–24.

2 **Beazley, J. M.** Inevitable ante-partum haemorrhage. Nursing Times, 67, 12 Aug 1971, 985–987.

3 **Bender, S.** Deep transverse arrest. Nursing Mirror, 137, 26 Oct 1973, 28–29.

4 **Buxton, R. St. J.** Maternal respiration in labour. Nursing Mirror, 137, 7 Sep 1973, 22–25.

5 **Chou, Y.** Effects of an upright position during labor. American Journal of Nursing, 74 (12), Dec 1974, 2202–2205.

6 **Copson, H. A.** Nursing care study. Spontaneous acute inversion of the uterus. Nursing Mirror, 137, 19 Oct 1973, 42–45.

7 **Cushnie, J.** Nursing care in hospital: labour and post partum. [Symposium on childbirth.] Nursing Mirror, 141, 3 Jul 1975, 64–66.

8 **David, T. Y. and others** Aminophylline used for premature labour. Midwives Chronicle, 88, Jul 1975, 230.

9 **Gray, A.** Can labour even be 'natural'? Midwife and Health Visitor, 9 (12), Dec 1973, 396–398. Reprinted in Nursing Mirror, 138, 28 Jun 1974, 70–71.

10 **Greenhalf, J. O.** Concealed accidental antepartum haemorrhage. Nursing Times, 71, 6 Mar 1975, 382–384.

11 **Hibbard, B. M.** Mothers in labour – nature deserves help. Nursing Times, 69, 25 Oct 1973, 1403–1405.

12 **Keaveny, M. E.** Supporting the Lamaze patient in labor. Nursing Care, 6 (5), May 1973, 15–19.

13 **Kopp, L. M.** Ordeal or ideal – the second stage of labor. American Journal of Nursing, 71 (6), Jun 1971, 1140–1143.

14 **Law, R. G.** Prolonged labour. Nursing Mirror, 133, 5 Nov 1971, 24–26.

15 **Limb, D. G. and Thelwall-Jones, H.** Perineal repair. Midwives Chronicle, 88, 1975, 116.

16 **McManus, C. F.** Nursing care study. Postpartum haemorrhage due to hypofibrinogenaemia. Nursing Mirror, 140, 1 May 1975, 69–72.

17 **Morison, C. R.** Mechanism of labour. 1. Normal labour. Nursing Mirror, 133, 15 Oct 1971, 34–38.

18 **Morison, C. R.** Mechanism of labour. 2. Role of the uterine muscle. Nursing Mirror, 133, 22 Oct 1971, 27–31.

19 **Morison, C. R.** Mechanism of labour. 3. Other abnormal positions of the fetus. Nursing Mirror, 133, 29 Oct 1971, 19–25.

20 **Pilkington, R.** Safe delivery. Nursing Mirror, 132, 28 May 1971, 14–15.

21 **Popins, L. S.** Preparation for premature delivery at home. Nursing Care, 6 (12), Dec 1973, 29–30.

22 **Sayle D.** Midwifery care study. The normal delivery of a baby in hospital. Nursing Times, 72, 13 May 1976, 732–735.

23 **Smith, B. A. and others** The transition phase of labor. [Lamaze techniques.] American Journal of Nursing, 73 (3), Mar 1973, 448–450.

24 **Terry, M. F.** Postpartum haemorrhage. Nursing Mirror, 137, 14 Sep 1973, 28–30.

25 **Wagstaff, T. I.** Prolonged labour as an avoidable condition. Midwives Chronicle, 86, Mar 1972, 74–75.

26 **Walker, P. A.** Separation of the placenta. Nursing Times, 71, 28 Aug 1975, 1377–1378.

27 **Wilday, R. J.** Total patient care in labour. Nursing Mirror, 141, 18 Sep 1975, 58–60.

28 **Williams, B.** Care and repair of the perineum. Nursing Times, 70, 28 Feb 1974, 301–302.

29 **Wright, P. A.** Birth interval and malnutrition. Nursing Times, 67, 16 Dec 1971, 1578–1581.

30 **Yeadon, D.** Nursing care study. Uterine inversion. Nursing Mirror, 139, 12 Jul 1974, 88–89.

d INDUCTION

1 **Arthur, H. R.** Active management of labour. Nursing Times, 69, 6 Dec 1973, 1654–1655.

3 **Beard, R. W.** Active management of labour. Midwives Chronicle, 85, Dec 1972, 374–376.

3 **Brown, I.** Active management of labour – the new obstetrics. Midwife and Health Visitor, 9 (7), Jul 1973, 217, 219–221.

4 **Clayton, K.** Daylight midwifery. [Risks involved in the induction of labour for convenience.] Nursing Times, 70, 18 Apr 1974, 595–596.

5 **Elder, M. G.** The use of prostaglandins in the induction of labour. Midwife, Health Visitor and Community Nurse, 11 (4), Apr 1975, 107–111.

6 **Hamlett, J. D.** Mechanised infusion of oxytocics.

[Intravenous infusion of drugs which stimulate uterine muscular activity.] Nursing Mirror, 136, 2 Feb 1973, 10–12.

7 **Holt, E. M.** Induction of labour. Midwife and Health Visitor, 7 (7), Jul 1971, 262–264. Reprinted in Nursing Mirror 135, 24 Nov 1972, 44–45.

8 **Howie, P. W.** Induction of labour. Nursing Mirror, 141, 21 Aug 1975, 56–59.

9 **Kitzinger, S.** Some mothers' experiences of induced labour: submission to the Department of Health and Social Security from the National Childbirth Trust. The Trust, 1975.

10 **Laros, R. K. and others** Prostaglandins. [Use in inducing labor and in abortion.] American Journal of Nursing, 73 (6), Jun 1973, 1001–1003.

11 **Mantle, J. R.** Scheduled delivery – delivered on schedule. Nursing Times, 68, 20 Jul 1972, 898–899.

12 **Nursing Times** Row over pre-Xmas inductions. [National Childbirth Trust claims births are being induced early to clear units.] Nursing Times, 70, 12 Dec 1974, 1914.

13 **O'Driscoll, K.** Active management of labour. Midwife, Health Visitor and Community Nurse, 11 (5), May 1975, 146–148.

14 **Royal Society of Medicine** 'Terrifying experience'. [Report of a conference on induction of labour held at the Royal Society of Medicine.] Nursing Mirror, 140, 17 Apr 1975, 35.

15 **Saggers, D.** Teachers' page – a new series. 1. Active management of labour. Midwives Chronicle, 86, Oct 1973, 312–313.

16 **Tacchi, D.** Active management of labour. Nursing Mirror, 136, 26 Jan 1973, 21–22.

e SURGICAL PROCEDURES

1 **Beynon, C. L.** Some surgical procedures in obstetrics. Nursing Mirror, 136, 13 Apr 1973, 23–26.

2 **Brant, H.** Caesarean section in modern obstetric practice. Midwife and Health Visitor, 7 (9), Sep 1971, 348–350.

3 **Collins, M.** Nursing care study. A longed-for child. [Breech presentation associated with subseptate uterus.] Nursing Mirror, 136, 29 Jun 1973, 21–23.

4 **Dumoulin, J. G.** Breech delivery. Nursing Times, 67, 8 Jul 1971, 825–827.

5 **Hill, J. G.** Breech management. Incorporating the use of fetal blood sampling. Midwives Chronicle, 86, Apr 1973, 104–106.

6 **Jones, O. V.** Surgical procedures in obstetrics. Nursing Mirror, 134, 24 Mar 1972, 28–30.

7 **Pickles, B.** Breech management. Nursing Mirror, 138, 17 May 1974, 62–63.

8 **Sutherst, J. R.** Caesarean section. Nursing Times, 71, 7 Aug 1975, 1247–1249.

9 **Varten, C. K.** Management of breech presentation. Nursing Mirror, 136, 16 Feb 1973, 29–31.

9 **Wingfield, J.** The place of forceps in the management of labour. Midwife and Health Visitor, 9 (12), Dec 1973, 394–395.

f POSTNATAL DEPRESSION AND PSYCHOLOGICAL ASPECTS AND POSTNATAL DEPRESSION

1 **Balchin, P.** The midwife and puerperal psychosis. Midwife, Health Visitor and Community Nurse, 11 (2), Feb 1975, 41–43.

2 **Bardon, D.** Puerperal depression. Midwife and Health Visitor, 8 (1), Jan 1972, 9–11, 13, 15.

3 **Bardon, D.** Puerperal psychosis. Nursing Times, 68, 18 May 1972, 615–617.

4 **Bhagat, M.** The concept of psychology in midwifery. Midwives Chronicle, 88, Sep 1975, 302–304.

5 **Brian, V. A.** Postnatal depression. Nursing Mirror, 140, 1 May 1975, 68.

6 **Brown, C.** Baby blues. [Post-partum depression.] Nursing Mirror, 141, 18 Sep 1975, 61–62.

7 **Burkett, G.** Psychological aspects of the puerperal woman. Jamaican Nurse, 12 (1), Apr 1972, 8–9, 34.

8 **Daysh, E. S.** Nursing care study. Puerperal psychosis. Nursing Mirror, 137, 17 Aug 1973, 43–44.

9 **de Boer, C. H.** Postnatal complications. Nursing Mirror, 137, 17 Aug 1973, 40–42.

10 **Kitzinger, S.** The fourth trimester? [Emotional problems occurring after birth.] Midwife, Health Visitor and Community Nurse, 11 (4), Apr 1975, 118–121.

11 **Melchior, L.** Is the postpartum period a time of crisis for some mothers? [Study of six mothers.] Canadian Nurse, 71 (7), Jul 1975, 30–32.

12 **Oakley, A.** The trap of medicalised motherhood. [The crisis of identity produced by first childbirth.] New Society, 34, 18 Dec 1975, 639–641.

13 **Palmer, R. L.** Psychological and emotional adjustment during pregnancy. Midwife and Health Visitor, 8 (2), Feb 1972, 49, 51–52.

14 **Pitt, B.** Depression after childbirth. Midwives Chronicle, 86, Jun 1973, 184–185.

15 **Protheroe, C.** Puerperal psychiatric illness. Nursing Mirror, 132, 30 Apr 1971, 34–36.

16 **Trick, K. L. K.** Psychological problems following birth and miscarriage. Nursing Mirror, 142, 10 Jul 1975, 61–62.

17 **Tylden, R.** Psychological problems during pregnancy. Midwife and Health Visitor, 8 (9), Sep 1972, 311–314.

18 **Woollaston, M.** Psychiatric consequences of the puerperium – some case histories. Midwife and Health Visitor, 9 (5), May 1973, 145, 147, 149–150.

19 **Zeal, B.** Psychiatry or people. [Case of a young Pakistani woman who took an overdose after the birth of her baby.] Nursing Times, 69, 19 Apr 1973, 513–514.

g MATERNAL DEATHS

1 **Arthure, H.** Avoidable factors in maternal deaths. Midwife and Health Visitor, 7 (10), Oct 1971, 381, 383, 385, 387.

2 **Chamberlain, G.** Maternal deaths. Nursing Times, 68, 15 Jun 1972, 750–754.

3 **Lawson, J. G.** Avoidable factors in maternal deaths. Nursing Mirror, 139, 12 Sep 1974, 48–50.

42 FAMILY PLANNING

a GENERAL AND SERVICES

1 **Anderson, J. A. D.** Economic and environmental aspects of family planning. Midwife, Health Visitor and Community Nurse, 11 (2), Feb 1974, 44–45.

2 **Bone, M.** Family planning services in England and Wales: an enquiry carried out on behalf of the Department of Health and Social Security. HMSO, 1973.

3 **Brook, C.** Family planning in Britain today. Mother and Child, 44 (3), May/Jun 1972, 6–8.

4 **Burns, C.** Family planning in Islington. Midwife and Health Visitor, 9 (11), Nov 1973, 355–358.

5 **Carpenter, C. B.** Psychological aspects of family planning. Occupational Health Nursing, 20 (7), July 1972, 7–12.

6 **Cassidy, J. T.** Teenagers in a family planning clinic. Nursing Outlook, 18 (11), Nov 1970, 30–31.

7 **Deys, C. M.** A personal view of family planning. Health Visitor, 44 (10), Oct 1971, 333.

8 **Family Planning Association** Birth control [in Runcorn and Coalville. Report of a Family Planning Association campaign.] New Society, 30, 19 Dec 1974, 760–761.

9 **Family Planning Association** Free and good: family planning in the National Health Service. The Association, 1973.

10 **Ferrer, H. P.** Survey of local authority practice on family planning services. Community Medicine, 128, 1 Sep 1972, 439–440.

11 **Gabert, J.** A domiciliary family planning service. Health Visitor, 44 (10), Oct 1971, 328–332.

12 **Giles, A.** Post natal family planning. Health Visitor, 44 (5), May 1971, 158–160.

13 **Giles, A. W.** Postnatal family planning at St. Mary's Hospital and Westminster Welfare Centre, London. Midwives Chronicle, 83, Oct 1970, 346–347.

14 **Harris, J. G. M.** Family Planning Association. Midwives Chronicle, 86, Feb 1972, 52–53.

15 **Hordern, A.** Excessive population growth – the problem of inadequate contraceptive practices. Midwife and Health Visitor, 7 (8), Aug 1971, 301–306.

16 **Huntingford, Prof. P. J.** Abortion or contraception? Royal Society of Health Journal, 91 (6), Nov/Dec 1971, 292–294.

17 **Jordan, J. A.** Family planning in the reorganized NHS (d) Hospital planning services in the future. Royal Society of Health Journal, 94 (3), Jun 1974, 138–140.

18 **Kane, A. H.** Contraception – a positive duty? Nursing Mirror, 133, 17 Dec 1971, 36–39.

19 **Kitzinger, S.** Body fantasies. Why do so many women fail to follow birth control advice? It may be that we know too little about their feelings towards their bodies. New Society, 21, 6 Jul 1972, 12–13.

20 **Lamb, B. and Murthwaite, C.** Family planning services. Queen's Nursing Journal, 16 (4), Jul 1973, 82–83.

21 **Lask, S.** Motivation in family planning. Nursing Mirror, 135, 15 Dec 1972, 44–46.

22 **Law, B.** Woman and her fertility. Nursing Mirror, 134, 7 Apr 1972, 34–37.

23 **Lumb, K. M.** The Bradford Family Planning Service. [Reprinted from the IPPF Bulletin.] Health Visitor, 46 (9), Sep 1973, 306–308.

24 **McQueen, I. A. G.** Effective contraceptive services. Health Visitor, 44 (10), Oct 1971, 345.

25 **McQueen, I. A. G.** Family planning in the reorganized NHS. (e) Community family planning services. Royal Society of Health Journal, 94 (3), Jun 1974, 140–143.

26 **Meleis, A. I.** Self-concept and family planning. Nursing Research, 20 (3), May/Jun 1971, 229–236.

27 **Newton, J.** A youth advisory clinic. Midwife and Health Visitor, 7 (4), Apr 1971, 140–142.

28 **Newton, J. and others** Hospital family planning:

a youth advisory clinic. British Medical Journal, 2, 12 Jun 1971, 642–645.

29 **Newton, P.** The complete family planning service at King's College Hospital. Nursing Times, 66, 29 Oct 1970, 1399–1400.

30 **Nursing Times** The Midlands. Coalville – an experiment in family planning. Nursing Times, 70, 12 Sep 1974, 1428.

31 **Office of Health Economics** Family planning in Britain. OHE, 1972. (Studies on current health problems, 40.)

32 **Philpot, T.** Fifty years ago. [Birth control clinics.] Nursing Mirror, 132, 19 Mar 1971, 19–20.

33 **Pleydell, M. J.** Family planning. District Nursing, 14 (6), Sep 1971, 114–115, 120.

34 **Pollock, M.** The need for family planning and its history. Midwives Chronicle, 86, May 1973, 156–157.

35 **Porter, W.** Family planning for better health. World Health, Feb/Mar 1973, 36–39.

36 **Potts, D. M.** Family planning. Community Health, 4 (4), Jan/Feb 1973, 185–190.

37 **Rankin, E.** The problem of birth control. Royal Society of Health Journal, 92 (2), Apr 1972, 81–84.

38 **Robinson, W.** Family planning in the new NHS. Health and Social Service Journal, 84, 2 Mar 1974, 483.

39 **Robinson, W.** Parent planning. [Domiciliary family planning.] Nursing Times, 69, 25 Oct 1973, 1425–1426.

40 **Shapiro, P. and Bate, J.** Taking family planning into the home. New Society, 19, 3 Feb 1972, 229–231.

41 **Sieve, A.** The International Planned Parenthood federation. Mother and Child, 44 (3), May/Jun 1972, 4–5.

42 **Smith, M.** The working of the Family Planning Act in the local authorities. Mother And Child, 44 (3), May/Jun 1972, 9–11.

43 **Taylor, R.** Non-verbal communication in family planning. Midwife and Health Visitor, 9 (5), May 1973, 160–162.

44 **Vaughan, S. J.** Problems in industry. [Unmarried mothers and family planning.] Occupational Health, 22 (5), May 1970, 151–152.

45 **Waite, M. and Mitton, R.** Birth control to homes. [Survey of birth control services carried out in 1970.] New Society, 25, 19 Jul 1973, 139–141.

46 **White, D.** Family planning. New Society, 23, 22 Mar 1973, 647–648.

47 **Wilson, E.** Domiciliary family planning service in Glasgow. British Medical Journal, 4, 18 Dec 1971, 731–733.

48 **Wiseman, A.** Family planning policies and practice in population control. Royal Society of Health Journal, 91 (3), May/Jun 1971, 134–138.

b OVERSEAS COUNTRIES

1 **Benson, E.** Family planning services in Yugoslavia. International Nursing Review, 20 (5), Sep/Oct 1973, 142–146.

2 **Casazza, L. J. and Williams, C. D.** Family health versus family planning. [Need for comprehensive approach to health care in developing countries.] Lancet, 1, 31 Mar 1973, 712–714.

3 **Eraj, M. A.** Control of population growth and family planning. Kenya Nursing Journal, 4 (2), Dec 1975, 16–18.

4 **Fischman, S. H.** Change strategies and their application to family planning programs. American Journal of Nursing, 73 (10), Oct 1973, 1771–1774.

5 **Francis, S. E.** The role of social work in family planning Jamaica. Jamaican Nurse, 11 (1), Apr 1971, 13, 21.

6 **International Planned Parenthood Federation** Family planning in five continents. The Federation, 1971.

7 **Lambo, T. A.** The right to health. [Family planning and welfare in undeveloped countries.] World Health, Jun 1974, 3–5.

8 **Lorig, K.** International family planning. Nursing Mirror, 140, 26 Jun 1975, 66–69.

9 **Manisoff, M.** Family planning democratized. [Progress of family planning services in the United States.] American Journal of Nursing, 75 (10), Oct 1975, 1660–1665.

10 **Morgan, D.** Family planning in Canada. Dimensions in Health Service, 52(4), Apr 1975, 38–39.

11 **Okediji, F. O.** Family planning in Africa: overcoming social and cultural resistances. International Journal of Health Education, 15 (3), 1972, 199–206.

12 **Peng, J. Y. and others, editors** Role of traditional birth attendants in family planning: proceedings of an international seminar, Bangkok and Kuala Lumpur, 19–26 Jul 1974. Ottawa: International Development Research Centre, 1974.

13 **Prakash, V.** Family planning programme in India – facilities and achievement. Nursing Journal of India, 45 (12), Dec 1974, 323–326.

14 **Rosenfield, A. G.** Auxiliaries and family planning. [The use of nurses and other auxiliary personnel in various countries with particular reference to Thailand.] Lancet, 1, 16 Mar 1974, 443–445.

15 **SA Nursing Journal** Issue on family planning. SA Nursing Journal, 41 (10), Oct 1974, 1–31.

16 **Walia, I.** Research abstracts. Multiple factors and multiparity. [Knowledge of family planning techniques of Indian mothers.] Nursing Journal of India, 65 (10), Oct 1974, 275–276.

17 **Wee, A.** Social aspects of family planning. Nursing Journal of Singapore, 13 (2), Nov 1973, 71–72.

18 **World Health** Issue on family planning. World Health, Jan 1974, 3–35.

19 **World Health Organization, Expert Committee** Evaluation of family planning in health services. Geneva: WHO, 1974. (Technical report series no. 569.)

20 **World Health Organization, Expert Committee** Family planning in health services. Geneva: WHO, 1971. (Technical report series, no. 476.)

c NURSE, MIDWIFE AND HEALTH VISITOR

1 **Addo, C.** The midwife in family planning. 1. In Ghana. Nursing Mirror, 133, 3 Dec 1971, 34–35.

2 **Bachu, A.** Population education in family planning curriculum in nursing education in India. International Nursing Review, 19 (3), 1972, 239–243.

3 **Bentley, N.** Family planning service in Manchester. [Role of midwives in providing the service.] Nursing Mirror, 140, 22/29 May 1975, 62–64.

4 **Central Treaty Organization** Cento workshop on education responsibilities of nurses and midwives in relation to family planning in maternal and child health; held in Tehran, Iran, 29 Apr to 4 May 1972. Ankara: Central Treaty Organization, 1972.

5 **Chandy, A. K.** A study on the opinions of first and third year nursing students on family planning – an abstract. [Research study.] Nursing Journal of India, 66 (4), Apr 1975, 83.

6 **Clark, J.** Family planning nurse. [The implications of extending the nurse's role.] Nursing Times, 70, 28 Nov 1974, 1856–1857.

7 **Clark, J.** Family planning nurse specialists? Call for new methods to expand service. [Report of the Family Planning Association annual conference.] Nursing Times, 70, 14 Nov 1974, 1757.

8 **Clark, J.** Family planning nurses must come in from the cold. [Rcn and Family Planning Association Joint Conference.] Nursing Mirror, 140, 1 May 1975, 35.

9 **Edmands, E. M. and others** International pilot study teaching of population/family planning in schools of nursing. International Journal of Nursing Studies, 11 (3), Sep 1974, 173–182.

10 **Hammersmith Health Department** It's up to the woman. [The work of the family planning nurse in the Hammersmith Health Department.] Practice Team, (32), Jan 1974, 4, 6.

11 **Handley, N.** The health visitor and family planning. Nursing Times, 68, 1 Jun 1972, 677–678.

12 **Kakar, D. N.** Role of indigenous midwife in family planning programme. Nursing Journal of India, 63 (1), Jan 1972, 14, 26.

13 **Kamal, I.** Role of the nurse and the midwife in MCH/family planning programme. Pakistan Nursing and Health Review, 6 (1), 1975, 6–15.

14 **Kleinman, R. L. editor** Family planning for midwives and nurses. International Planned Parenthood Federation, 1971.

15 **Law, B.** Family planning in nursing. Crosby Lockwood Staples, 1973.

16 **Law, B.** The nurse and family planning. Nursing Times, 70, 7 Feb 1974, 203–204.

17 **McPartland, D.** Family planning – the team's responsibility. District Nursing, 15 (3), Jun 1971, 54.

18 **Midwife, Health Visitor and Community Nurse** Midwives and family planning. [Editorial.] Midwife, Health Visitor and Community Nurse, 11 (6), Jun 1975, 169.

19 **Mowla, K.** Role of nurses and midwives in population planning. Pakistan Nursing and Health Review, 5 (1), 1974, 8–11.

20 **Mudie, E. N.** The role of the midwife in family planning. [Paper read at the International Confederation of Midwives, June 1975.] Kenya Nursing Journal, 4 (2), Dec 1975, 27, 29.

21 **Norattejananda, S.** The midwife in family planning. 2. In Thailand. Nursing Mirror, 133, 10 Dec 1971, 40–41.

22 **Nursing Mirror** Nurses expand their role. [Conference report on the nurse's role in family planning.] Nursing Mirror, 141, 3 Jul 1975, 35.

23 **Nursing Times** Who should issue the pill? [Nurses in FPA clinics.] Nursing Times, 70, 3 Oct 1974, 1524.

24 **Pettinger, C. M.** Domiciliary family planning and the nurse. [A local authority service in Bradford.] Nursing Mirror, 137, 14 Sep 1973, 50–52.

25 **Pollock, M.** Family planning training for midwives. Midwives Chronicle, 86, Jul 1973, 224–225.

26 **Pollock, M.** Nurses and midwives in family planning. Midwives Chronicle, 86, Jun 1973, 188–189.

27 Rooke, A. The nurse's role in family planning. Nursing Times, 67, 17 Jun 1971, 727–730.

28 Sanyal, R. K. The role of nurses in family planning. Nursing Journal of India, 45 (12), Dec 1974, 317.

29 Shea, F. P. and others Survey of health professionals regarding family planning: preliminary report on nursing students and faculty. Nursing Research, 22 (1), Jan/Feb 1973, 17–24.

30 Stewart, E. Family planning and the nurse. [Ethical considerations.] UNA Nursing Journal, 71, Mar/ Apr 1973, 14–15, 17; Catholic Nurse, Christmas, 3–5.

31 Turnbull, L. M. and Pizurki, H. editors Family planning in the education of nurses and midwives. Geneva: World Health Organization, 1973.

32 Waite, M. Domiciliary midwives and birth control advice 1970–71. [Report of a survey undertaken by the Institute for Social Studies in Medical Care.] Nursing Times, 68, 7 Dec 1972, Occ. papers, 193–195; 14 Dec 1972, Occ. papers, 197–199.

33 Waite, M. Health visitors and birth control advice 1970–71. Nursing Times, 68, 12 Oct 1972, Occ. papers, 157–159; 19 Oct 1972, Occ. papers, 161–164.

34 World Health Organization The role of nurses and midwives in family planning. [Summary of a WHO Seminar in Manila, 16–23 Sep 1974.] WHO Chronicle, 29 (3), Mar 1975, 109.

d METHODS

1 Bickerstaff, E. R. Neurological complications of the pill. Nursing Mirror, 134, 19 May 1972, 19–26.

2 Connell, E. B. The pill and the problems. American Journal of Nursing, 71 (2), Feb 1971, 326–332.

3 Corona, M. Contraception. World of Irish Nursing, 3 (9), Sep 1974, 157, 159, 161–162.

4 DiPalma, J. R. Drug therapy today: the pill, pro and con. RN Magazine, 34 (1), Jan 1971, 61–70.

5 Garrett, N. Choosing contraceptives according to need. Canadian Nurse, 68 (9), Sep 1972, 37–41.

6 Howard, G. Pill or IUD? Midwife, Health Visitor and Community Nurse, 11 (8), Aug 1975, 249–252.

7 Leydon, I. Contraception and abortion. World of Irish Nursing, 3 (7), Jul 1974, 112–113, 115.

8 Llewellyn-Jones, D. Human reproduction and society. Faber, 1974.

9 Loudon, J. D. O. Advantages and problems associated with the intrauterine device. Midwife and Health Visitor, 6 (3), Mar 1970, 97–99.

10 Manisoff, M. T. Intrauterine devices. American Journal of Nursing, 73 (7), Jul 1973, 1188–1192.

11 Mann, J. I. and Inman, W. H. W. Oral contraceptives and death from myocardial infarction. British Medical Journal, 2, 3 May 1975, 245–248.

12 Mann, J. I. and others Myocardial infarction in young women with special reference to oral contraceptive practice. British Medical Journal, 2, 3 May 1975, 241–245.

13 Mowat, J. and Johnstone, A. B. Experience with intra-uterine contraceptive device at a local health authority clinic. Health Bulletin, 32 (1), Jan 1974, 35–37.

14 Patients Association Oral contraceptives – a memorandum to the DHSS. [A policy statement opposing 'the pill off prescription'.] Nursing Times, 71, 23 Oct 1975, 1690–1693.

15 Robinson, A. M. Birth control through sterilization. 2. Sterilization of women. RN Magazine, 36 (4), Apr 1973, 33–35, 56, 58, 60.

16 Smith, A. J. Contraception today. Family Planning Association, 1971.

17 Smith, M. and Kane, P. The pill off prescription. Birth Control Trust, 1975.

18 Stallworthy, Prof. Sir J. Family planning in the reorganized NHS. (a) Family planning techniques for the future. Royal Society of Health Journal, 94 (3), Jun 1974, 127–130.

19 Swenson, I. Oral contraceptives: a review of the literature. Journal of Nurse-Midwifery, 20 (1) Spring 1975, 7–14.

20 Swyer, G. I. M. The pill. Nursing Mirror, 136, 25 May 1973, 10–11.

21 Vessey, M. P. The hazards of oral contraception. Midwife and Health Visitor, 5 (12), Dec 1969, 481–483.

22 Voke, J. Colour vision and the pill. Nursing Times, 70, 31 Jan 1974, 139.

23 Whitehouse, W. L. Useful methods of contraception. Lecture given at the 59th London Nursing Conference. Nursing Mirror, 139, 31 Oct 1974, 77–78.

24 Wilkinson, P. M. Every child a wanted child. Report of a two-day conference on family planning techniques. Nursing Times, 66, 8 Oct 1970, 1308–1309.

25 Wood, C. Contraception explained. Geneva: World Health Organization, 1975.

e STERILIZATION

1 Blandy, J. P. Male sterilization. Nursing Times, 68, 3 Feb 1972, 142–144.

2 Blandy, J. P. Vasectomy as a method of family limitation. Midwife and Health Visitor, 8 (5), May 1972. 161, 163–165.

3 Craig, G. A. Female sterilization. Nursing Mirror, 136, 22 Jun 1973, 8–11.

4 Davis, J. E. Vasectomy. American Journal of Nursing, 72 (3), Mar 1972, 509–513.

5 Foreman, J. R. Vasectomy clinic. American Journal of Nursing, 73 (5), May 1973, 819–821.

6 Fortier, L. Needed: a change in attitudes toward elective sterilization. Canadian Nurse, 69 (1), Jan 1973, 21–22.

7 McBride, B. A new method of tubal ligation. [Using the laparascope.] Canadian Nurse, 69 (4), Apr 1973, 32–33.

8 Main, T. F. People, problems and sterilization. Mother and Child, 44 (3), May/Jun 1972, 12–15.

9 Margaret Pyke Centre One thousand vasectomies. British Medical Journal, 4, 27 Oct 1973, 216–221.

10 Nash, J. L. Vasectomy. Nursing Mirror, 137, 21 Sep 1973, 39.

11 Pond, D. A. Psychological aspects of sterilization. Nursing Times, 67, 18 Nov 1971, 1435–1437.

12 Pryor, J. P. Vasectomy. Nursing Times, 69, 7 Jun 1973, 736–737.

13 Robinson, A. M. Birth control through sterilization. 1. Vasectomy: advantages and limitations. RN Magazine, 36 (4), Apr 1973, 30–33.

14 Siegler, A. M. Tubal sterilization. [Discusses particularly the new method using the laparascope.] American Journal of Nursing, 72 (9), Sep 1972, 1624–1629.

15 Sim, M. Psychiatric aspects of female sterilization. British Medical Journal, 3, 28 Jul 1973, 220–222.

16 Thomas, B. J. The great debate: elective hyster-ectomy for sterilization. RN Magazine, 36 (4), Apr 1973, OR 3–4.

17 Todd, I. A. D. Vasectomy. Canadian Nurse, 67 (8), Aug 1971, 20–23.

18 Wallace, D. M. Vasectomy. Nursing Mirror, 138, 22 Mar 1974, 58–59.

43 TERMINATION OF PREGNANCY

a GENERAL

1 Buckle, A. E. R. Abortion clinics and operating sessions. Nursing Mirror, 136, 9 Mar 1973, 36–38.

2 Hamil, E. and others Psychiatric and social factors in the abortion decision. British Medical Journal, 1, 1974, 229; Summary in Nursing Times, 70, 11 Apr 1974, 554.

3 Hull, M. G. R. and Boylston, S. A. Outpatient pregnancy termination in an NHS hospital. [The Samaritan Hospital for Women, London.] Nursing Times, 70, 3 Oct 1974, 1540–1542.

4 Knight, B. Termination of pregnancy in Wales. [Summary of a review of terminations from July 1969 to December 1972 by G. Jones and D. A. Jones.] Nursing Mirror, 140, 3 Apr 1975, 69–70.

5 Nursing Mirror An inconvenient fetus. [Experiences of a person who survived attempted abortion.] Nursing Mirror, 141, 17 Jul 1975, 76.

6 Potts, M. Abortion – a personal testimony. [The problems of illegal abortions.] Nursing Times, 70, 28 Feb 1974, 314–316; Journal of Psychiatric Nursing and Mental Health Services, 12 (4), Jul/Aug 1974, 34–38.

7 Stone, M. Therapeutic abortion and its aftermath. Midwife, Health Visitor and Community Nurse, 11 (10), Oct 1975, 335–338.

8 WHO Chronicle Induced abortion as a public health problem in Europe. WHO Chronicle, 27 (12), Dec 1973, 525–530.

b LANE COMMITTEE AND LEGISLATION

1 Committee on the Working of the Abortion Act Report. HMSO, 1974, 3 vols. Cmnd. 5579. Chairman: The Hon. Mrs Justice Lane.

2 Nursing Mirror Abortion – an evil necessity. [Editorial on the move to amend the 1967 Abortion Act.] Nursing Mirror, 140, 13 Feb 1975, 33.

3 Nursing Times New Abortion Bill. Nursing Times, 71, 6 Feb, 13 Feb 1975, 200, 239.

4 Queen's Nursing Journal Report of the committee on the working of the Abortion Act. [With reference to the health visitor.] Queen's Nursing Journal, 17 (3), Jun 1974, 55.

5 Royal College of Midwives The report of the Committee on the Working of the Abortion Act. [Comments on the Lane Report.] Midwives Chronicle, 87, Jun 1974, 198; Sep 1974, 309.

6 Royal College of Nursing The working of the Abortion Act. Rcn, 1972.

7 Simms, M. How do we judge the Abortion Act? Reflections on the Lane Committee and the 1967 Abortion Act. Public Health, 87 (5), Jul 1973, 155–164

8 Swaffield, L. Abortion – the story so far. [James White's Abortion (Amendment) Bill.] Nursing Times, 71, 17 Jul 1975, 1120.

9 Swaffield, L.   Whatever happened to Lane? [In the Abortion (Amendment) Bill.] Nursing Times, 71, 28 Aug 1975, 1358–1359.

10 Turner, J.   Talking point. Whose interests? Personal view of the oral evidence to the Select Committee on Abortion by the nursing organizations. Nursing Times, 71, 6 Nov 1975, 1763.

11 World Health Organization   Abortion laws: a survey of world legislation. Geneva: WHO, 1971.

12 Young, P.   Lane Report on the working of the Abortion Act. Nursing Mirror, 138, 19 Apr 1974, 37–38.

c COUNSELLING

1 Blair, M.   Counselling for abortion. Midwife, Health Visitor and Community Nurse, 11 (11), Nov 1975, 355–356.

2 Gedan, S.   Abortion counseling with adolescents. American Journal of Nursing, 74 (10), Oct 1974, 1856–1858.

3 Gill, T.   Variables in abortion counselling. British Journal of Guidance and Counselling, 3 (1), Jan 1975, 56–65.

4 Haszeldine, V.   Abortion – a medical social worker's point of view. Nursing Mirror, 139, 19 Jul 1974, 39–40.

5 Keller, C. and Copeland, P.   Counseling the abortion patient is more than talk. American Journal of Nursing, 72 (1), Jan 1972, 102–106.

6 Kelly, M.   Birthright – alternative to abortion. [An organization to help pregnant women.] American Journal of Nursing, 74 (1), Jan 1974, 76–77.

7 Melville, J.   Testing the lifeline. [Consumer reaction to lifeline – a counselling service for pregnant women.] New Society, 26, 15 Nov 1973, 390.

8 Simms, M.   Abortion counselling – a new profession. World Medicine, 8 (11), 28 Feb 1973, 35–37.

9 Simms, M.   Who needs abortion counselling? World Medicine, 8 (23), 8 Aug 1973, 49, 51–52.

d NURSING

1 Allen, D. V. and others   Factors to consider in staffing an abortion service facility. Journal of Nursing Administration, 4 (4), Jul/Aug 1974, 22–27.

2 Arora, P.   Abortion by vacuum method. Nursing Journal of India, 64 (6), Jun 1973, 205–207.

3 Bellevue Hospital Center   Nurses' feelings a problem under new Abortion Law. American Journal of Nursing, 71 (2), Feb 1971, 350–352.

4 Bourne, P. J.   Influences on health professionals' attitudes. [Attitudes of physicians and nurses toward legal abortion.] Hospitals, 46 (14), 16 Jul 1972, 80–83.

5 Branson, H.   Nurses talk about abortion: a survey of 50 nurses in Hawaii where for two and a half years there has been a liberal abortion law. American Journal of Nursing, 72 (1), Jan 1972, 106–109.

6 Brown, N. K. and others   How do nurses feel about euthanasia and abortion? American Journal of Nursing, 71 (7) Jul 1971, 1413–1416.

7 Clancy, B.   The nurse and the abortion patient. [Nursing care.] Nursing Clinics of North America, 8 (3), Sep 1973, 469–478.

8 Coulson, M. J.   Nurses' attitudes to therapeutic abortion. Lamp, 30 (4), Apr 1973, 11, 13, 15.

9 Danon, A. H.   Organizing an abortion service. With a nurse involved in the planning. Nursing Outlook, 21 (7), Jul 1973, 460–464.

10 Dickens, B. M.   The 'conscience clause' and the law on abortion. Nursing Times, 70, 20 Jun 1974, 968–969.

11 Gardner, J.   Weekend program for tubal ligation. [Accompanied by pre and post operative visits by VON nurses.] Canadian Nurse, 69 (4), Apr 1973, 37–39.

12 Greenhalf, J. O.   Termination of a mid-trimester pregnancy. Nursing Mirror, 134, 2 Jun 1972, 34–36.

13 Harper, M. W. and others   Abortion: do attitudes of nursing personnel affect the patient's perception of care? Nursing Research, 21 (4), Jul/Aug 1972, 327–331.

14 New Society   Abortion. [Gallup poll of nurses, commissioned by the Society for the Protection of Unborn Children.] New Society, 23, 15 Feb 1973, 359.

15 Rosen, R. A. H. and others   Some organizational correlates of nursing students' attitudes towards abortion. Nursing Research, 23 (3), May/Jun 1974, 253–259.

16 Sclare, A. B. and Geraghty, B. P.   Termination of pregnancy – the nurse's attitude. [Results of a questionnaire sent to 50 experienced gynaecological nurses and 113 student nurses in Glasgow.] Nursing Mirror, 140, 16 Jan 1975, 59–60.

17 Traynor, L.   Nursing care study. Post abortive depression. Nursing Mirror, 138, 14 Jun 1974, 77–78.

18 Vegh, R.   Why should nurses know better? [Nurses who have abortions.] World Medicine, 9 (8), 16 Jan 1974, 48, 51, 55.

19 Zahourek, R. and Tower, M.   Therapeutic abortion: the psychiatric nurse as therapist, liaison and consultant. Perspectives in Psychiatric Care, 9 (2), Mar/Apr 1971, 64–71.

CHILD HEALTH

44 CHILD HEALTH SERVICES

a GENERAL

1 Bamford, F. N. and Davis, J. A. Towards an integrated child health service. British Medical Journal, 1, 20 Jan 1973, Supplement, 20–22.

2 Bussey, A. L. and others A computer based medical information system for child health. [West Sussex.] Health and Social Service Journal, 85, 4 Jan 1975, 18–20.

3 Court, S. D. M. Child health in a changing community. British Medical Journal, 2, 17 Apr 1971, 125–131.

4 Donaldson, R. J. Family practitioner services and management towards an integrated child health service. (b) Child health centres evaluated. Royal Society of Health Journal, 94 (4), Aug 1974, 202–204.

5 Forfar, J. O. Child health services, today and tomorrow. Community Health, 4 (4), Mar/Apr 1973, 261–267.

6 Frenkiel, A. L. Prospects of health care planning. [Proposals for a child health planning team at district level.] Health and Social Service Journal, 85, 22 Mar 1975, 654–655.

7 Health Visitors' Association Memorandum to the committee reviewing health services for children. Health Visitor, 47 (5), May 1974, 144–145.

8 Hugh-Jones, K. and Norman-Taylor, W. Child health service. Health and Social Service Journal, 84, 20 Jul 1974, 1620–1621.

9 Jenkins, G. C. Organization of a developmental care programme in general practice. [Care of the under-fives.] District Nursing, 15 (8), Nov 1972, 167–168.

10 McLachlan, G., editor Bridging in health: reports of studies on health services for children. Oxford University Press for Nuffield Provincial Hospitals Trust, 1975.

11 Mellor, D. Aspects of the reorganized NHS Community and hospital paediatrics – change and integration. Midwife and Health Visitor, 10 (4), Apr 1974, 87–89.

12 Moss, P. and others Families and their needs. [Survey of use made of social and health services by mothers of pre-school children with comment on the health visitor.] New Society, 23, 22 Mar 1973, 638–640.

13 National Association for Maternal and Child Welfare Diamond Jubilee Conference, June 27–29, 1973. Mother And Child, 45 (5), Sep/Oct 1973, 16–19.

14 Paterson, M. T. The health of the pre-school child. Queen's Nursing Journal, 16 (4), Jul 1973, 87, 92.

15 Peterson, P. O. The child in society. International Nursing Review, 21 (1), Jan/Feb 1974, 23–24.

16 Pickup, J. D. Recent advances in paediatrics. Nursing Mirror, 137, 14 Sep 1973, 26–28.

17 Richman, N. and Tupling, H. A computerized register of families with children under five in a London borough. Health Trends, 6 (1), Feb 1974, 19–22.

18 Rogers, M. G. H. Preventive child health and the health visitor. Nursing Times, 70, 21 Feb 1974, 274–276.

19 Royal College of Midwives The RCM and the child health services committee. Midwives Chronicle, 87, Jun 1974, 203–204.

20 Scottish Home and Health Department. Joint Working Party on the Integration of Medical (PIM) Work. Towards an integrated child health service: report of a sub-group on the child health service. Edinburgh: HMSO, 1973. Chairman: Sir John Brotherston.

21 Smith, C. S. Some medical aspects of community child health. Community Health, 6 (3), Nov/Dec 1974, 177–181.

22 Stark, G. D. and others Paediatrics in Livingston new town: evolution of a child health service. British Medical Journal, 4, 15 Nov 1975, 387–390.

23 Stroud, C. E. Environment and health [Children]. Maternal and Child Care, 7, Jul/Aug 1971, 58–60.

24 Twomey, J. and Stansbie, P. S. Child health clinics: an evaluation of consumer reaction. [Study by questionnaire in Rugby Health District.] Public Health, 90 (1), Nov 1975, 9–14.

b OVERSEAS COUNTRIES

1 Ambrosio, A. Community help for the young family. [Child health clinics.] Nursing Care, 8 (5), May 1975, 14–16.

2 American Journal of Nursing Care of the well child. American Journal of Nursing, 74 (8), Aug 1974, 1471–1494.

3 Christensen, J. C. Services for children. [A description of services available in New Zealand.] New Zealand Nursing Journal, 67 (12), Dec 1974, 9, 11.

4 Clark, A. L. and others MCH in American Samoa. [Workshops on maternal and child health.] American Journal of Nursing, 74 (4), Apr 1974, 700–702.

5 Coulter, P. Mother and child health care in the Yemen. Nursing Times, 70, 14 Nov 1974, 1764–1765.

6 Davis, S. E. Caring for children in Cape Town. Nursing Mirror, 136, 19 Jan 1973, 40–41.

7 Fox, D. H. A contemporary organization design for maternal and infant care projects. Journal of Nursing Administration 5 (4) May 1975, 26–33.

8 Galli, P. Nursing in a pediatric multiphasic program. [Screening of healthy children.] American Journal of Nursing, 74 (5), May 1974, 892–894.

9 Harris, B. T. Health care for young children in Holland, Belgium and France. Journal of the Royal College of General Practitioners, 24, Oct 1974, 676, 681–686.

10 Hauser, H. Nursing care for toddlers in Israel. Health Visitor, 47 (6), Jun 1974, 176–179, 181.

11 Holleran, C. Mother and child care [in the United States. Paper from a combined New Zealand/ American Nurses' Association conference.] New Zealand Nursing Journal, 68 (3), Mar 1975, 9–10.

12 Johnson, P. M. Impressions of child care in France. Health Visitor, 47 (9) Sep 1974, 274–278.

13 Kitzman, H. The nature of well child care. American Journal of Nursing, 75 (10), Oct 1975, 1705–1708.

14 Nulty, Y. Protection de la Mère et de L'Enfant. An account of six weeks' course at the International Children's Centre, Paris – a digest of facts, events and impressions. Queen's Nursing Journal, 18 (2), May 1975, 38–39, 41.

15 Oduori, M. L. Paediatric out-patient care. Kenya Nursing Journal, 2 (1), Jun 1973, 51–54.

16 Pasternack, S. B. Annual well-child visits. American Journal of Nursing, 74 (8), Aug 1974, 1472–1475.

17 Roberts, A. Child-care customs in Colombia. Nursing Mirror, 140 (15), 10 Apr 1975, 64–66.

18 Symons, E. Patterns of child management: Holland. Mother and Child, 45 (1), Jan/Feb 1973, 13–16.

19 Vernon, C. Special needs of the young child in Jamaica. Jamaican Nurse, 11 (3), Dec 1971, 12–16.

20 Wadsworth, Y. The 'whole new ball game. . .' [The infant welfare nurse.] Australian Nurses' Journal, 5 (4), Oct 1975, 26–28.

21 Woodley, M. G. Cours d'Obstetrique Sociale. [International Children's Centre, Paris – course in child care.] Midwives Chronicle, 88, Jul 1975, 238–239.

22 World Health Organization Child health in the European region. WHO Chronicle, 25 (7), Jul 1971, 319–324.

23 Wynn, M. and Wynn, A. The right of every child to health care: a study of the protection of the young child in France. Council for Children's Welfare, 1974.(Occasional papers on child welfare, no. 2.)

c CHILD DEVELOPMENT AND PSYCHOLOGY

1 Arthur, L. J. H. Small stature. [The examination of small children for possible diseases connected with stature.] Midwife and Health Visitor, 10 (11), Nov 1974, 337–342.

2 **Barnard, K.** Trends in the care and prevention of developmental disabilities. American Journal of Nursing, 75 (10), Oct 1975, 1700–1704.

3 **Boon, W. H.** Child development and guidance. Nursing Journal of Singapore, 13 (2), Nov 1973, 115–120.

4 **Butler, N.** The shrinking world of childhood [the pre-school period]. Maternal and Child Care, 8, Jun/Jul 1972, 55–59.

5 **Chesham, I. and others** Paediatric screening. [An evaluation of a scheme introduced by Cheshire County Council.] Health and Social Service Journal, 85, 8 Feb 1975, 293–294.

6 **Crewe, H. J.** Fears and anxiety in childhood. Public Health, 87 (5), Jul 1973, 165–171.

7 **Krebs, K.** Children and their pecking order: dominant and subordinate behaviour at nursery school. New Society, 32, 17 Apr 1975, 127–129.

8 **Lawton, D. S. and Cobb, S.** Children's functional assessment. British Journal of Occupational Therapy, 37 (10), Oct 1974, 175–177.

9 **McGrew, W. C.** How children react to newcomers. [Study in a nursery school.] New Society, 20, 13 Apr 1972, 55–57.

10 **Mitchell, R. G.** Habilitation in childhood. [Facilitating development of the normal and handicapped child.] Health Bulletin, 33 (6), Nov 1975, 245–248.

11 **Morley, D.** Charts to help with malnutrition and over-population problems. [Growth charts monitoring child development in underdeveloped countries.] Lancet, 1, 20 Apr 1974, 712–714.

12 **National Child Development Study** Child health and education in the seventies. A national study in England, Scotland and Wales of all children born 5th – 11th April 1970. Health Visitor, 48 (3), Mar 1975, 75–76.

13 **New Scientist** Developmental psychology forum. [By various authors.] New Scientist, Mar/Jun 1974.

14 **Parfit, J.** Environmental effects on development. Health Visitor, 46 (7), Jul 1973, 222–225.

15 **Paterson, M. T.** Developmental screening of pre-school children. Community Medicine, 128 (19), 25 Aug 1972, 423–424.

16 **Pearson, R. C. M. and Peckham, C.** Preliminary findings at the age of 11 years on children in the National Child Development Study (1958 Cohort). Community Medicine, 127 (9), 3 Mar 1972, 113–116.

17 **Porter, C. S.** Grade school children's perceptions of their internal body parts. Nursing Research, 23 (5), Sep/Oct 1974, 384–391.

18 **Porter, L. S.** The impact of physical-physiological activity on infants' growth and development. Nursing Research, 21 (3), May/Jun 1972, 210–219.

19 **Porter, L. S.** On the importance of activity [in a child's development.] Maternal-Child Nursing Journal, 2 (2), Summer 1973, 85–91.

20 **Reif, K.** A heart makes you live: what children believe about their hearts. American Journal of Nursing, 72 (6), Jun 1972, 1085.

21 **Robertson, A.** Education in personal relationships. [Helping children towards emotional maturity.] Midwife and Health Visitor, 8 (12), Dec 1972, 422–423.

22 **Robischom, P.** PICA practice and other hand-mouth behavior and children's developmental level. Nursing Research, 20 (1), Jan/Feb 1971, 4–16.

23 **Ross, E. M.** Learning about school leavers. The special role of the health visitor in the National Child Development Study (1958 Cohort). Health Visitor, 46 (12), Dec 1973, 408–410.

24 **Scott, D. V.** The development of language. Queen's Nursing Journal, 17 (3), Jun 1974, 65–66.

25 **Scott, D. V.** Perceptual learning. Queen's Nursing Journal, 17 (1), Apr 1977, 2–3.

26 **Scott, D. V.** Social learning. Queen's Nursing Journal, 17 (5), Aug 1974, 100, 103.

27 **Solomon, R.** The gifted child – a problem of recognition. Nursing Times, 71, 12 Jun 1975, 940–941.

28 **Wilson, R. G.** The clumsy child. Midwife and Health Visitor, 10 (2/3), Feb/Mar 1974, 53–55.

d CHILD PSYCHIATRY

1 **Anonsen, D. C.** The hyperkinetic child. Canadian Nurse, 71 (5), May 1975, 27–29.

2 **Anstice, E.** You mustn't confuse the child with his illness. [St. Thomas's Children's Psychiatric Day Hospital.] Nursing Times, 67, 30 Dec 1971, 1620–1621.

3 **Barker, P.** Antisocial behaviour in children. Nursing Mirror, 136, 13 Apr 1973, 28–30.

4 **Barker, P. and Ward, P. A.** Milieu therapy in a child psychiatry unit. [Charles Burns Clinic, Birmingham.] Nursing Times, 68, 14 Dec 1972, 1579–1581.

5 **Bastow, G. M.** The non-communicating child. Health Visitor, 44 (9), Sep 1971, 290–292.

6 **Blomquist, K. B.** Nurse, I need help: the school nurse's role in suicidal prevention. Psychiatric Nursing and Mental Health Services, 12 (1), Jan/Feb 1974, 22–26.

7 **British Medical Journal** Emotional problems in childhood and adolescence. British Medical Association, 1973.

8 **British Medical Journal** Suicide in children. [Leading article.] British Medical Journal, 1, 15 Mar 1975, 592.

9 **Buchanan, W. J.** Nursing and child psychiatry: developments is the nurse's function. Nursing Mirror, 136, 9 Feb 1973, 41–42.

10 **Chapman, A. H.** Management of emotional problems of children and adolescents. 2nd ed. Philadelphia: Lippincott, 1974.

11 **Cooper, V. G.** How Peter beat his fear of going to school. Nursing Times, 69, 23 Aug 1973, 1091–1092.

12 **Crowdes, N. E.** Group therapy for preadolescent boys. American Journal of Nursing, 75 (1), Jan 1975, 92–95.

13 **Cundell, R.** Children and behaviour problems. Nursing Times, 68, 29 Jun 1972, 807–808.

14 **Dolan, P. J.** School absence. British Hospital Journal and Social Service Review, 82, 16 Dec 1972, 2815.

15 **Dundas, M.** Early childhood autism. Nursing Mirror, 134, 31 March 1972, 22–25.

16 **Fagin, C. M., editor** Nursing in child psychiatry. St. Louis: Mosby, 1972.

17 **Frommer, E. A.** Childhood depression. Midwife and Health Visitor, 9 (9), Sep 1973, 299–300.

18 **Haldane, J. D. and Lindsay, S. F.** Child and family psychiatry in an integrated child health service. Health Bulletin, 31 (2), Mar 1973, 79–85.

19 **Haldane, J. D. and others** Nursing in child, adolescent and family psychiatry. International Journal of Nursing Studies, 8, May 1971, 91–101.

20 **Haldane, J. D. and others** Training nurses in child, adolescent and family psychiatry. Nursing Times, 67, 11 Mar 1971, Occ. papers, 37–40.

21 **Hersov, L.** Truancy and school refusal. Midwife and Health Visitor, 9 (8), Aug 1973, 258–261.

22 **Jeffrey, L. I. H.** Child psychiatry – the need for occupational therapy. Occupational Therapy, 36 (8), Aug 1973, 429–437.

23 **Kahan, V. L.** Mental illness in childhood: a study of residential treatment. Tavistock, 1971.

24 **Lansdown, R. and Bentovim, A.** Hospital day centres. [Pre-school provision for disturbed children.] New Society, 25, 2 Aug 1973, 281–282.

25 **Nicholas, S. C.** Diagnosis and prognosis of autism. (The Greeks have a word for it.) Nursing Times, 70, 17 Oct 1974, 1614–1615.

26 **Pinkerton, P.** Paediatric psychiatry. Nursing Mirror, 141, 20 Nov 1975, 48–49.

27 **Pinkerton, P.** Paediatric psychiatry. 2. Emotional development and the clinical implications. Nursing Mirror, 141, 18 Dec 1975, 48–50.

28 **Pinkerton, P.** The psychosomatic approach to paediatrics. An exercise in interdisciplinary liaison. [Royal Liverpool Children's Hospital admits children with psychosomatic disorders into the paediatric department.] Nursing Times, 68, 16 Mar 1972, 311, 316.

29 **Pratt, S. J. and Fischer, J.** Behavior modification: changing hyperactive behavior in a children's group. Perspectives in Psychiatric Care, 8 (1), Jan/Mar 1975, 37–42.

30 **Sanger, J.** Society at work. Illness is created. [The need for counselling services in school to prevent mental illness.] New Society, 31, 6 Mar 1975, 586–587.

31 **Scannell, J.** Some problems with autistic children. Australian Nurses Journal, 2 (5), Nov 1972, 25–26.

32 **Schechter, M. D. and Primeaux, M.** The utilization of nursing staff in a psychiatric research project. [Care of an autistic child.] Journal of Psychiatric Nursing, 9 (1), Jan/Feb 1971, 7–10.

33 **Schuyler, D.** When a child dies, accident or suicide? RN Magazine, 38 (9), Sep 1975, 21–23.

34 **Shufer, S.** Pediatric mental health nurse clinician. Nursing Outlook, 19 (8), Aug 1971, 543–545.

35 **Sims, P.** Children and suicide. New Scientist, 56, 9 Nov 1972, 339.

36 **Stroh, G.** Autistic children. Nursing Mirror, 132, 9 Apr 1971, 38–41.

37 **Tweddle, E. G.** Establishing a child psychiatric nursing unit. [Post-registration course in the psychological management of children and adolescents run by the Nuffield Child Psychiatry Unit, Newcastle upon Tyne.] Nursing Times, 70, 13 Jun 1974, Occ. papers, 21–24.

38 **Varley, J. E.** Depression in children. Nursing Times, 70, 10 Oct 1974, 1568–1569.

39 **Whitlock, J. and Learner, S.** Role of the occupational therapist in child psychiatry. [Work at the Park Hospital for Children, Oxford.] British Journal of Occupational Therapy, 38 (10), Oct 1975, 222–225.

40 **WHO Chronicle** Suicide and the young. WHO Chronicle, 29 (5), May 1975, 193–198.

e ADOLESCENT PSYCHIATRY

1 **Association for the Psychiatric Study of Adolescents** Report on post-registration training of nurses in psychiatric units for adolescents. The Association, 1972.

2 Carstairs, G. M. Psychiatric help for adolescents. British Hospital Journal and Social Science Review, 81. 5 Jun 1971, 1113.

3 Chapman, G. E. Treating parents and disturbed adolescents. [Parent/adolescent group meetings in the adolescent unit at Cassel Hospital, Richmond.] Nursing Times, 70, 31 Jan 1974, 154–155.

4 Christmas, L. The story of James. [Care study of a boy, disturbed by family instability, in an adolescent unit.] Nursing Mirror, 138, 5 Apr 1974, 70–72.

5 Hanson, J. and others One interdisciplinary planning team: a case study. [Teamwork in an adolescent psychiatric clinic from the nurse's point of view.] Journal of Psychiatric Nursing and Mental Health Services, 11. Nov/Dec 1973, 29–34.

6 Latham, R. W. A programme for disturbed adolescents. [Administration of nursing staff of Meon House. adolescent unit, Knowle Hospital, Hampshire.] Nursing Times. 71, 26 Jun 1975, 1024–1026.

7 Laufer, M. Adolescent disturbance and breakdown. Harmondsworth: Penguin, 1975.

8 Nursing Times 'I was nineteen and I wanted to die'. A young university student describes events which led up to, and his attitude after, admission to a psychiatric day hospital.Nursing Times, 69, 8 Feb 1973, 178.

9 Pond, D. A. Behaviour disorders of the adolescent. Nursing Mirror, 134, 5 May 1972, 33–35.

10 Pulford, A. Effects of stress on the modern adolescent. Midwife, Health Visitor and Community Nurse, 11 (12). Dec 1975, 388–390.

11 Pyle, P. L. Behaviour modification. [Instruction given to parents enabled them to control their disruptive and disobedient son.] Nursing Times, 71, 24 Apr 1975, 665–667.

12 Simpson, R. The development and nurse staffing of adolescent psychiatric units. International Journal of Nursing Studies, 10 (3), Aug 1973, 161–168.

13 Weeks, P. Abnormal emotional reactions in an adolescent. [Case study of patient suffering from depression who eventually responded to a psychological reward system.] Nursing Times, 69, 8 Nov 1973, 1485–1487.

f MOTHER CHILD BONDING

1 Aikens, R. M. and Heah, J. Metabolic balance in babies. [Method of carrying out balance studies on babies in the Special Care Baby Unit, Northwick Park Hospital, which enables the mother to continue to care for her baby throughout the trial.] Nursing Times, 70, 7 Nov 1974, 1736–1737.

2 Barden, D. The setting of childbirth and its effect on mother-neonate interaction. [The effects of professional attitudes and procedures in obstetrics and midwifery on mother-child relationship.] Midwives Chronicle, 87, Oct 1974, 343–346.

3 Black, D. Pain and parenting. [Effect of pain connected with childbirth on physical emotional and mental crippling of children.] Midwife, Health Visitor and Community Nurse, 11 (8), Aug 1975, 263–266.

4 Brown, M. S. Mother-child relationship has lasting effects. [Study at Case Western Reserve University with a review of similar studies elsewhere.] Canadian Journal of Psychiatric Nursing, 16 (5), Sep/Oct 1975, 10–12.

5 Brown, P. W. The use of a descriptive theory in planning nursing intervention. [A study to evaluate Rubin's theory of maternal role attainment. First published in Nursing Research, 14, Summer 1967, 237–

245; Fall 1967, 342–346.] Maternal-Child Nursing Journal, 4 (3), Fall 1975, 171.

6 Cox, B. S. Rooming in. Nursing Times, 70, 8 Aug 1974, 1246–1247.

7 Crummette, B. D. Transitions in motherhood. Maternal-Child Nursing Journal, 4 (2), Summer 1975, 65–73.

8 Dare, C. The 'mother-infant' relationship. Midwife and Health Visitor, 10 (6), Jun 1974, 162–164.

9 Edwards, B. and others Developing relationships between mother and child, with special reference to babies placed in special care units. [Project undertaken on a first line management course.] Health Visitor, 48 (7), Jul 1975, 234–236.

10 Frommer, E. A. Problems of mothers who were deprived as children: indications for preventive measures. [Based on a survey in the Obstetric Department, St. Thomas's Hospital.] Midwife and Health Visitor, 9 (10), Oct 1973, 325–327.

11 Geller, J. J. Developmental symbiosis. [Between mother and child.] Perspectives in Psychiatric Care, 8 (1), Jan-Mar 1975, 10–12.

12 Gleeson, M. A. Giving mother-love its due: an account of an experiment in the introduction of mothers of low birth weight babies into special care-intensive care neo-natal nurseries. Australian Nurses' Journal, 1 (7), Jan 1972, 22–23.

13 Higgs, S. C. The mother-infant relationship. SA Nursing Journal, 42 (6), Jun 1975, 32.

14 Krige, P. D. Development of affection in children and the effect of separation from the mother. SA Nursing Journal, 42 (6), Jun 1975, 26–27.

15 Lochead, G. S. and others Pregnancy and child care. [Project undertaken by student nurses during their obstetric experience to study mothers who experience minor complications of pregnancy and their subsequent attitude towards the child.] Nursing Mirror, 139, 2 Aug 1974, 69–70.

16 Martin, T. B. Rooming-in. SA Nursing Journal, 42 (6), Jun 1975, 28, 36.

17 Nash, F. W. Maternal education and attitudes: 100 first maternities. [Survey in Brighton on events in pregnancy, childbirth and the neonatal period which might have adverse effects on the child.] Health and Social Service Journal, 83, 13 Oct 1973, 2363–2364.

18 Penfold, K. M. Supporting mother love. [Case study of care by the nurse of a hospitalized newborn, the nurse taking the role of a therapeutic intermediary between separated mother and infant.] American Journal of Nursing, 74 (3), Mar 1974, 464–467.

19 Richards, M. Developmental psychology forum. The one-day-old deprived infant. [Maternal deprivation within hours of birth.] New Scientist, 61, 28 Mar 1974, 820–822.

20 Rutter, M. Maternal deprivation reassessed. Harmondsworth: Penguin, 1972. (Penguin science of behaviour.)

21 Schreier, A. Factors influencing the maternal acceptance of a child. SA Nursing Journal, 42 (11), Nov 1975, 11–13.

g PARENTHOOD AND FATHER'S ROLE

1 American Journal of Nursing Babies have fathers, too. American Journal of Nursing, 71 (10), Oct 1971, 1980–1981.

2 Bird, R. H. Parentcraft. [Project at Queen Elizabeth II Hospital to provide a course for expectant parents and to provide experience in parentcraft teach-

ing for trained and student midwives.] Midwives Chronicle, 87, Feb 1974, 61–63.

3 Boorer, D. R. An educational blindspot. [Parentcraft education.] Nursing Times, 69, 15 Nov 1973, 1540–1541.

4 Boorer, D. R. An educational blindspot revisited. [Education for parenthood.] Health Visitor, 47 (12), Dec 1974, 356–357.

5 Boorer, D. R. Psychological needs of parents and babies. Midwives Chronicle, 87, Dec 1974, 421.

6 Branson, H. K. Fathers and pregnancy. Bedside Nurse, 4 (7), Jul 1971, 13–15.

7 Cronenwett, L. R. and Newmark, L. L. Fathers' responses to childbirth. Nursing Research, 23 (3) May/Jun 1974, 210–217.

8 Department of Health and Social Security Dimensions of parenthood. Report of a seminar held at All Souls College, Oxford, 10–13 Apr 1973. HMSO, 1974.

9 Department of Health and Social Security Preparation for parenthood: account of consultations with professional, voluntary and other organizations. HMSO, 1974.

10 Doyle, E. Does anybody know that man waiting out by the elevators? A consideration for practical nursing in obstetrics. [Help for the expectant father.] Journal of Practical Nursing, 24 (5), May 1974, 24–25, 28.

11 Fleming, G. Delivering a happy father. American Journal of Nursing, 72 (5), May 1972, 949.

12 Forbes, R. A new role for expectant fathers. Midwife and Health Visitor, 8 (5), May 1972, 166–168.

13 Furlong, E. N. A mothers' group in Alperton. Nursing Mirror, 140, 12 Jun 1975, 70–71.

14 Griffey, D. The health visitor and the isolated mother. [Especially the role of the mother's group.] Health Visitor, 48 (4), Apr 1975, 111–112.

15 Health and Social Service Journal No new kind of visitor. [Work of health visitor in parental and child guidance.] Health and Social Service Journal, 83, 11 Aug 1973, 1789–1790.

16 Heinz, L. The nurse's role in a parenting process program. [Teaching parents about child development.] Journal of Psychiatric Nursing and Mental Health Services, 13 (2), Mar/Apr 1975, 27–30.

17 Hoffman, P. Nursing care study. Health visiting. A couple expecting their first child. Nursing Mirror, 138, 12 Apr 1974, 76–78.

18 Howells, J. G. Fallacies of child care – that fathering is unimportant. Maternal and Child Care, 7, Sep 1971, 71–74.

19 Hunnisett, F. W. Seminars for parents. [Helping parents cope with the problems they face in bringing up their children.] Hospital Administration in Canada, 16 (10), Oct 1974, 36, 38, 40.

20 Isbister, C. The importance of fathers. Australian Nurses' Journal, 3 (11), Jun 1974, 24–26.

21 Jones, W. L. The emotional needs of the new family. Nursing Mirror, 141, 23 Oct 1975, 49–52.

22 Lilley, M. J. Emotional needs of parents. [Role of the midwife.] Nursing Mirror, 139, 19 Jul 1974, 61–63.

23 Pitcairn, L. Parentcraft education. [In schools and colleges. Contribution of National Association for Maternal and Child Welfare.] Queen's Nursing Journal, 16 (8), Nov 1973, 174–176.

24 Ratsoy, M. B. Maternity patients make decisions. [Learning to parent newborn babies with the nurse's role to judge the degree of assistance and support needed.] Canadian Nurse, 70 (4), Apr 1974, 42–44.

25 **Richman, J. and others** Fathers in labour. [Survey showing the effect of childbirth on the father.] New Society, 34, 16 Oct 1975, 143–145.

26 **Seymour, R. M.** An experimental group for mothers of young children to discuss everyday problems of child development, psychological needs and difficulties. Midwife and Health Visitor, 10 (6), Jun 1974, 154–158.

27 **Shaw, N. R.** Teaching young mothers their role. [Description of a training programme in Boston.] Nursing Outlook. 22 (11), Nov 1974, 695–698.

28 **Shu, C. Y.** Husband-father in delivery room? Obstetricians hold divergent views. Hospitals, 47)18), 16 Sep 1973, 90, 92–94.

29 **Taylor, A. M.** Mothers' club. [Family club for mothers of young children in need of social support.] Health and Social Service Journal, 83, 10 Mar 1973, 549.

30 **Towler, J.** The midwife as an educator of parents. Midwives Chronicle, 84, May 1971, 156–158.

31 **Whitehouse, J.** Mothers go to college. [A description of mothercraft classes run by the Social Services Department in Warwickshire for mothers having problems with children.] Social Work Service, 5, Dec 1974, 23–26.

45 INFANTS AND NEWBORN

a GENERAL AND NURSING

1 **Barrie, H.** The folklore, and facts of circumcision. Midwife and Health Visitior, 9 (2), Feb 1973, 40–44.

2 **British Medical Journal** Neonatal nurse practitioners. [Editorial on this new specialist nurse first used in Arizona and its application to the UK.] British Medical Journal, 1, 18 Jan 1975, 115–116.

3 **Broadribb, V. and Corliss, C.** Maternal child nursing. Philadelphia: Lippincott, 1973.

4 **Brown, M. S. and others** The maternal-child nurse practitoner. Pilot program at the University of Colorado. American Journal of Nursing, 75 (8), Aug 1974, 1298–1299.

5 **Browning, M. H. and Lewis, E., compilers** Maternal and newborn care: nursing interventions. New York: American Journal of Nursing Company, 1973. (Contemporary nursing series.)

6 **Campbell, A. G. M.** Electrolyte imbalance in infants: implications for nursing care. Journal of Practical Nursing, 21 (12), Dec 1971, 20–22; 22 (1), Jan 1972, 22–25, 29.

7 **Chao, Yu-Mei Yu** A comparative study of regain of body weight of newborns during the first ten days of life. International Nursing Review, 18 (1), 1971, 15–21.

8 **Crawford, J. S.** Immediate care of the healthy neonate. Nursing Times, 71, 30 Jan 1975, 178–179.

9 **Davis, J. G. and Gatherer, A.** Microbiological environment of babies. [Survey confirming the importance of mothercraft instruction.] Health and Social Service Journal, 85, 4 Jan 1975, 24–25.

10 **Eoff, M. J. F. and others** Temperature measurement in infants: to determine relationships between infant axillary and rectal temperatures taken with a glass thermometer and telethermometer. Nursing Research, 23 (6), Nov/Dec 1974, 457–460.

11 **Gleason, D. E.** Improved methods of newborn identification. Canadian Hospital, 50 (5), May 1973, 24–26, 28.

12 **Hanid, T. K.** Ethical dilemmas in obstetric and newborn care. Midwife, Health Visitor and Community Nurse, 11 (1), Jan 1975, 9–11.

13 **Health Visitors' Association** New baby. The Association, 1972.

14 **Illingworth, R. S. and Illingworth, C. M.** Babies and young children: feeding and management and care. 5th ed. Churchill Livingstone, 1972.

15 **Johnson, R. W.** The case of the nearly mixed-up babies. [Footprinting as a means of identifying newborn babies.] RN Magazine, 37 (10), Oct 1974, 31.

16 **Jones, K.** Babycare hygiene. Nursing Mirror, 132, 16 Apr 1971, 12–13.

17 **Kidd, D. E.** Neonatal bathing technique. [Infa-Care Hygenic Baby Bath used at King's College Hospital.] Midwives Chronicle, 88(1048), May 1975, 164–165.

18 **Lillington, A. W. and others** The umbilical cord – band, clamps and infection? [A survey to investigate the risks of infection.] Midwives Chronicle, 87, Dec 1974, 417.

19 **McFadden, E. and Kopf, R.** Integrated staffing for a special care unit. [Rotation of nurses between a maternity and special care baby unit provides continuity of care.] Supervisor Nurse 6 (5), May 1975, 26–32, 35.

20 **Malan, A. F.** The priorities of perinatal care. SA Nursing Journal, 42 (6), Jun 1975, 7.

21 **Moore, M. L.** The newborn and the nurse. Philadelphia, Saunders, 1972. (Saunders monographs in clinical nursing, no 3.)

22 **Nursing Clinics of North America** Symposium on care of the newborn. Nursing Clinics of North America, 6 (1), Mar 1971, 1–112.

23 **Nursing Times** Identification of babies. Nursing Times, 67, 1 Apr 1971, 376–377.

24 **Oppe, T. E.** The first 28 days: the vulnerable baby. Midwives Chronicle, 87, Sep 1974, 310–312.

25 **Partridge, J. W.** The baby's first days. Priory Press, 1973. (Care and welfare library.)

26 **Patrick, M. J.** The first 28 days. 2. Management of common minor abnormalities. Midwives Chronicle, 87, Aug 1974, 276–281.

27 **Ramsbottom, E.** [Nursing care study.] Jane – an abandoned baby. Nursing Times, 70, 14 Feb 1974, 224–225.

28 **Richards, M. P. M. and Bernal, J. F.** Feeding, crying and sleeping in infancy. [A follow-up study of 80 home delivered babies.] Midwife and Health Visitor, 10 (12), Dec 1974, 375–377.

29 **Richards, M. P. M. and Bernal, J. F.** Why some babies don't sleep. New Society, 27, 28 Feb 1974, 509–511.

30 **Roberts, J. E.** Suctioning the newborn. American Journal of Nursing, 73 (1), Jan 1973, 63–65.

31 **Robinson, W.** A special baby visitor. Nursing Times. 70, 2 May 1974, 685.

32 **Van Leeuwen, G.** The nurse in prevention and intervention in the neonatal period. Nursing Clinics of North America, 8 (3), Sep 1973, 509–520.

33 **Weitzman, S.** Daily care of the newborn infant with reference to early warning signs of complications. SA Nursing Journal, 42 (2), Feb 1975, 7–8, 10, 14.

34 **Woodley, M. G.** New venture in neonatal care.

[Nottingham City Hospital's Department of Neonatal Medicine and Surgery.] Nursing Mirror, 138, 5 Apr 1974, 55–57.

b ABNORMALITIES AND AT RISK

1 **Agrafiotis, P. C.** Teaching parents about Pierre Robin syndrome. American Journal of Nursing, 72, Nov 1972, 2040–2042.

2 **Befus, M. A. and Martin, E. J.** Nursing care study. A baby with Pierre Robin syndrome. Nursing Times, 71, 16 Oct 1975, 1646–1648.

3 **Breslin, S. J.** Case study: a baby with Pierre Robin syndrome. Midwives Chronicle, 87, Dec 1974, 424–426.

4 **Burland, Y. M.** Nursing care study. Congenital morphinism. Nursing Mirror, 138, 28 Jun 1974, 78–79.

5 **Cowie, V.** Prevention and early detection of abnormalities in babies. Midwives Chronicle, 85, Dec 1971, 402–405.

6 **Cowie, V.** Prevention and early recognition of abnormalities in babies. Nursing Times, 69, 10 May 1973, 593–595.

7 **Cranley, M. S.** When a high-risk infant is born. [Services in the USA with multidisciplinary teams using clinical nurse specialists.] American Journal of Nursing, 75 (10), Oct 1975, 1696–1699.

8 **Daker, M.** Chromosome disorders in babies. Nursing Times, 69, 26 Jul 1973, 952–954.

9 **Eckstein, H. B. and others** Severely malformed children: the problem of selection. [Three papers followed by discussion, including mention of the nurse's attitude.] British Medical Journal, 2, 5 May 1973, 284–289.

10 **Ellis, A.** Nursing care study. Pemphigus neonatorum. Nursing Mirror, 136, 6 Apr 1973, 38–40.

11 **Flatley, A.** Victims of circumstances. 1. [Congenital abnormalities.] Nursing Times, 70, 30 May 1974, 830–833.

12 **Flatley, A.** Victims of circumstance. 2. [Postnatal factors resulting in mental handicap.] Nursing Times, 70, 6 Jun 1974, 869–870.

13 **Fogerty, S.** The nurse and the high risk infant. Nursing Clinics of North America, 8 (3), Sep 1973, 533–547.

14 **Freeman, N. V.** Pyloric stenosis. [Congenital abnormality.] Nursing Times, 72, 7 Oct 1976, 1553–1555.

15 **Friedlander, F. C.** Children at risk. SA Nursing Journal, 42 (6), Jun 1975, 29, 31.

16 **Hecht, M.** Children of alcoholics are children at risk. American Journal of Nursing, 73 (10), Oct 1973, 1764–1767.

17 **Hooper, M. H.** Nursing care study. Louise. [Newborn baby with cystic intramural duplication of the ileum.] Nursing Mirror, 136, Jun 1973, 40–42.

18 **Howat, J. M.** Congenital abnormalities of the small intestine. [In neonates.] Nursing Mirror, 136, 8 Jun 1973, 42–44.

19 **Howat, J. M. and Wilkinson, A. W.** Functional intestinal obstruction in the neonate. Maternal and Child Care, 7, Mar/Apr 1971, 21–25.

20 **Hudson, E. P.** Screening for inborn errors of metabolism in infancy. Nursing Mirror, 141, 28 Aug 1975, 64–66.

21 **Laurence, K. M.** Abnormal babies. 1. Causes. Nursing Mirror, 136, 15 Jun 1973, 11–13.

22 **Laurence, K. M.** Abnormal babies. 2. Prevention. Nursing Mirror, 136, 22 Jun 1973, 39–41.

23 **McElroy, C.** Caring for the untreated infant. [After the decision to withhold active treatment has been made.] Canadian Nurse, 71 (12), Dec 1975, 26–27, 30.

24 **Morgan, D. M.** 'High risk' infants and mothers require special care. Canadian Hospital, 48 (11), Nov 1971, 23–25, 28, 31.

25 **Nursing Clinics of North America** Symposium on maternal and infant care in high risk-families. Nursing Clinics of North America, 8 (3), Sep 1973, 467–565.

26 **Roberts, C. J. and Khosla, T.** An evaluation of developmental examination as a method of detecting neurological, visual, and auditory handicaps in infancy. British Journal of Preventive and Social Medicine, 26 (2), May 1972, 94–100.

27 **Sills, J. A. and others** Social factors and feeding practices in hypernatraemia. [A survey at the Royal Liverpool Children's Hospital shows artificially fed children are 'at risk' from hypernatraemia.] Midwife, Health Visitor and Community Nurse, 11 (9), Sep 1975, 302–305.

28 **Vehrs, S. and Baum, D.** A test of visual responses in the newborn. Maternal and Child Care, 7, Feb 1971, 8–11.

29 **Waechter, E. H.** Developmental consequences of congenital abnormalities. Nursing Forum, 14 (2), 1975, 108–129.

c DISEASES AND DISORDERS

1 **Auld, P. A.** Resuscitation of the newborn infant. American Journal of Nursing, 74 (1), Jan 1974, 68–70.

2 **Brown, J. K. and others** Convulsions in the newborn. Nursing Mirror, 135, 25 Aug 1972, 20–25.

3 **Carroll, M. H.** Preventing newborn deaths from drug withdrawal. RN Magazine, 34 (12), Dec 1971, 34–35.

4 **Chadd, D. M. A.** Haemorrhagic diseases of the newborn. Midwives Chronicle, 86, Jun 1972, 190–191.

5 **Danon, A.** How to resuscitate the depressed newborn. RN Magazine, 38 (6), Jun 1975, 29–31.

6 **Davies, C. C.** Nursing care study. An unusual cause of septicaemia in the neonate. Nursing Mirror, 140, 12 Jun 1975, 79.

7 **Davies, P. A.** Infection in the foetus and newborn. Midwife and Health Visitor, 8 (9), Sep 1972, 305–310.

8 **Davies, P. A.** Intra-uterine and neonatal infection. Nursing Mirror, 139, 28 Nov 1974, 57–58.

9 **Ellis, M. I.** Haemolytic disease of the newborn. Nursing Times, 71, 25 Dec 1975, 2050–2052.

10 **Fielding, M.** A hazard for the newborn. [Hyaline membrane disease.] Australian Nurses' Journal, 5 (1), Jul 1975, 32–33.

11 **Finnegan, L. P. and Macnew, B. A.** Care of the addicted infant. American Journal of Nursing, 74 (4), Apr 1974, 685–693.

12 **Franklin, A. J.** Convulsions in the newborn. Nursing Times, 69, 16 Aug 1973, 1056–1059.

13 **Gamble, S. E.** Nursing care study. Necrotising enterocilitis. Nursing Mirror, 139, 21 Nov 1974, 75–80.

14 **Garvey, J.** Infant respiratory distress syndrome. American Journal of Nursing, 75 (4), Apr 1975, 614–617.

15 **Gillon, J. E.** Behavior of newborns with cardiac distress. American Journal of Nursing, 73 (2), Feb 1973, 254–257.

16 **Gould, E. S.** Nursing care study. A baby with an abdominal wound healing problem. Nursing Times, 71, 2 Jan 1975, 24–26.

17 **Griffith, G.** Respiratory difficulties in low birth-weight infants. Nursing Mirror, 135, 29 Sep 1972, 17–18.

18 **Gudermuth, S.** Mothers' reports of early experiences of infants with congenital heart disease. [Interviews with eight mothers.] Maternal-Child Nursing Journal, 4 (3), Fall 1975, 155–164.

19 **Hibbard, B. M.** The changing face of haemolytic disease of the newborn. Midwife and Health Visitor, 8 (10), Oct 1972, 360–363.

20 **Hodson, C.** Nursing care study. A baby with respiratory distress. Nursing Times, 71, 10 Apr 1975, 565–567.

21 **Isler, C.** Infection: constant threat to perinatal life. RN Magazine, 38 (8), Aug 1975, 23–29.

22 **Jones, P. M.** Nursing care study. Bilateral pneumothoraces in a neonate. Nursing Mirror, 136, 18 May 1973, 31–33.

23 **Kent, M. L.** Necrotizing enterocolitis. SA Nursing Journal, 13 (1), Jan 1975, 12.

24 **Kilman, J. W. and others** Respiratory distress: surgery in the newborn. RN Magazine, 38 (6), Jun 1975, OR 1–2.

25 **Lewis, P.** Infant development distress. [On-going research into psychological infant stress.] New Zealand Nursing Journal, 69 (6), Jun 1975, 18–21.

26 **Marzluf, M. J.** A positive approach to being negative. [RH disease in the newborn.] Nursing Care, 7 (1), Jan 1974, 12–15.

27 **Milner, A. D.** Medical emergencies in the neonatal period. Nursing Mirror, 139, 17 Oct 1974, 64–67.

28 **Minns, H.** A Rhesus incompatible baby. Nursing Times, 69, 24 May 1973, 668–670.

29 **Nalepka, C. D.** The oxygen hood for newborns in respiratory distress. American Journal of Nursing, 75 (12), Dec 1975, 2185–2187.

30 **Raffensperger, J. G.** Respiratory distress in the newborn. RN Magazine, 37 (8), Aug 1974, ICU1-ICU2, ICU4.

31 **Wear, M.** Neonatal hypoglycaemia. Midwives Chronicle, 85, Nov 1972, 344–347.

32 **Williams, G. F.** Resuscitation of the newborn by hyperbaric oxygen. Nursing Mirror, 133, 6 Aug 1971, 30–31.

33 **Williams, S. L.** Phototherapy in hyperbilirubinemia. American Journal of Nursing, 71 (7), Jul 1971, 1397–1399.

34 **Wolf, R. I.** Hypoglycaemia – an important neonatal problem. SA Nursing Journal, 42 (6), Jun 1975, 17, 19.

35 **Wood, B. S.** Developments in jaundice and anaemia in the newborn. Nursing Mirror, 136, 9 Feb 1973, 22–23.

36 **Zaslow, S. S.** Nursing care of the addicted newborn. RN Magazine, 37 (5), May 1974, 50–51.

d INTENSIVE CARE

1 **Babson, S. C. and Benson, R. C.** Management of high-risk pregnancy and intensive care of the neonate. 2nd ed. St. Louis: Mosby, 1971.

2 **Baizley, L.** Whose baby is this? [The rights of parents whose babies are being nursed in a neonatal intensive care unit.] Canadian Nurse, 69 (3), Mar 1973, 27–29.

3 **Barnes, C. M.** Levels of consciousness indicated by responses of children to phenomena in the intensive care unit. Maternal-Child Nursing Journal, 4 (4), Winter 1975, 215–285.

4 **Blair, A. W.** Technology in the nursery. [Machines used in special care baby units.] Nursing Mirror, 135, 18 Aug 1972, 31–33.

5 **Blake, A. M. and others** Transport of newborn infants for intensive care. [Survey at University College Hospital of 222 infants transported from other hospitals in a 50 mile radius.] British Medical Journal, 4, 4 Oct 1975, 13–17.

6 **Burson, I.** In neo-natal ICU nursing. [Mainly illustrations.] Pediatric Nursing, 1 (1), Jan/Feb 1975, 20–23.

7 **Campbell, A. G. M.** The newborn ICU for infants with heart disease. RN Magazine, 35 (11), Nov 1972, ICU 1–2, 4, 6.

8 **Coffey, H. and Koch, C. R.** Psycho-social care of the paralyzed child: a technique in intensive care nursing. Pediatric Nursing, 1 (5), Sep/Oct 1975, 21–23.

9 **Colaianni, J. A.** Parents care in intensive care. [Mainly illustrations of the Children's Hospital, Philadelphia.] Pediatric Nursing, 1 (2), Mar/Apr 1975, 16–19.

10 **Harris, C. H.** Some ethical and legal considerations in neonatal intensive care. Nursing Clinics of North America, 8 (3), Sep 1973, 521–531.

11 **Hey, E.** Keeping babies warm. [In incubators.] Nursing Mirror, 139, 5 Jul 1974, 62–64.

12 **Korones, S. B.** High-risk newborn infants: the basis for intensive nursing care. St. Louis: Mosby, 1972.

13 **May, J. G.** Emotional responses in a pediatric ICU: a psychiatrist looks at the feelings of children, parents and nurses and reports on the important role nurses fulfil. RN Magazine, 36 (10), Oct 1973, ICU-1, 5–6.

14 **Petcavage, E.** Guided tour of an intensive care nursery. Journal of Practical Nursing, 24 (12), Dec 1974, 26–28.

15 **Reynolds, E. O. R.** Neonatal intensive care. Nursing Times, 69, 13 Sep 1973, 1178–1181; 20 Sep 1973, 1220–1221.

16 **RN Magazine** Neonatal ICU transport – a life saver. [Bellevue Hospital, New York.] RN Magazine, 38 (12), Dec 1975, ICU 14–15.

17 **Roberts, K. D. and Edwards, J. M.** Paediatric intensive care: a manual for resident medical officers and senior nurses. 2nd ed. Oxford: Blackwell Scientific, 1975.

18 **Scott, J. E. S.** Special care for infants. [The special care unit.] Nursing Times, 70, 17 Jan 1974, 73–77.

19 **Struthers, J. N. M.** Canada – a wealth of experience. [In a neonatal unit.] Nursing Mirror, 133, 24 Sep 1971, 37–39.

20 **Taylor, M. R. H.** Transport of sick newborn babies. Nursing Times, 67, 6 May 1971, 544–546.

21 Whittington Hospital New neonatal intensive care unit at Whittington Hospital, North London. Nursing Mirror, 138, 3 May 1974, 57–58.

22 Wickes, I. G. Special care for neonates. [Review of 'Report of the expert group on special care for babies, 1971'.] Nursing Mirror, 136, 16 Mar 1973, 28–29.

23 Youngblut, A. C. Specially for the newborn – intensive care in the nursery. Canadian Nurse, 67 (8), Aug 1971, 24–27.

e LOW BIRTH WEIGHT AND PREMATURE

1 Chamorro, I. L. and others Development of an instrument to measure premature infant behaviour and caretaker activities: time sampling methodology. Nursing Research, 22 (4), Jul/Aug 1973, 300–309.

2 Cheetham, C. H. Parenteral nutrition in infancy. Midwife and Health Visitor, 9 (11), Nov 1973, 359–361.

3 Chinn, P. L. Infant gavage feeding. American Journal of Nursing, 71 (10), Oct 1971, 1964–1967.

4 Coutts, N. A. The small-for-dates baby. Midwives Chronicle, 87, Apr 1974, 131–134.

5 Crosse, V. M. The preterm baby and other babies with low birth weight. 7th ed. Churchill Livingstone, 1971.

6 Davies, P. A. An improved outlook for the low birth weight baby. Midwives Chronicle, 85, Aug 1971, 272–274.

7 Doust, R. Nursing care study. [Premature baby with severe pre-eclampsia.] Nursing Mirror, 141, 31 Jul 1975, 52–54.

8 Drillien, C. M. Long-term prognosis for the small for date infant. Midwife and Health Visitor, 7 (4), Apr 1971, 133, 135, 137, 139.

9 Drug and Therapeutics Bulletin Oxygen for premature babies. Drug and Therapeutics Bulletin. 12 (12), 7 Jun 1974, 45–47.

10 Dubowitz, L. M. S. and Dubowitz, V. Assessment of gestational age. Nursing Mirror, 133, 13 Aug 1971, 24–28.

11 Haas, L. Respiratory difficulties in low birth-weight babies. Nursing Mirror, 137, 27 Jul 1973, 42–45.

12 Halman, H. B. Feeding infants of low birth weight by continuous intragastric milk-drip. Nursing Mirror, 140, 2 Jan 1975, 28–29.

13 Jones, C. Intravenous feeding of the newborn. Nursing Times, 69, 18 Oct 1973, 1364–1365.

14 Katz, V. Auditory stimulation and developmental behavior of the premature infant. Nursing Research, 20 (3), May/Jun 1971, 196–201.

15 Kramer, M. and others Extra tactile stimulation of the premature infant. Nursing Research, 24 (5), Sept/Oct 1975, 324–334.

16 McKendrick, T. Return to nursing. 14. Premature babies. Nursing Mirror, 133, 27 Aug 1971, 12–13.

17 Myers, M. S. Mature or immature? Assessing gestational age. RN Magazine, 38 (1), Jan 1975, 22–25.

18 Segall, M. E. Cardiac responsibility to auditory stimulation in premature infants. Nursing Research, 21 (1), Jan/Feb 1972, 15–19.

19 Valman, H. B. and others Continuous intra-gastric milk feeds in infants of low birth weight. British Medical Journal, 3, 2 Sep 1972, 547–550.

20 Warrick, L. H. Family centered care in the premature nursery. American Journal of Nursing, 71 (11), Nov 1971, 2134–2138.

21 Wayburne, S. Mini-babies. SA Nursing Journal, 61 (9), Sep 1974, 7–9.

22 Wharton, B. 'Do we know how to feed premature babies?' Nutrition, 26 (5), Oct 1972, 280–289.

23 Wickes, I. G. Light for dates babies. Maternal and Child Care, 7 (70), May-Jun 1971, 36–40.

f INFANT DEATH AND STILLBIRTH

1 Amiel, G. J. South East. Postmaturity. [A study at Beckenham Maternity Hospital of deliveries from 1953–1957 showed postmaturity factor in asphyxia neonatorum leading to perinatal mortality.] Nursing Times, 71, 20 Mar 1975, 462–463.

2 Arthure, H. G. Perinatal mortality. Nursing Mirror, 132, 14 May 1971, 21–26.

3 Bergman, A. B. Sudden infant death. Nursing Outlook, 20 (12), Dec 1972, 775–777.

4 British Medical Journal Cot deaths. British Medical Journal, 4, 30 Oct 1971, 250–251; 4, 6 Nov 1971, 315–316; 1, 2 Mar 1974, 341–342; 3, 20 Sep 1975, 664.

5 Cameron, J. M. Infanticide. Nursing Times, 67, 4 Nov 1971, 1371–1372.

6 Camps, F. E. Sudden deaths in infants. Midwife and Health Visitor, 9 (4), Apr 1973, 113–116.

7 Camps, F. E. When infant death occurs. Nursing Mirror, 133, 12 Nov 1971, 14–15.

8 Camps, F. E. and Carpenter, R. C. editors Sudden and unexpected deaths in infancy. [Cot deaths.] Bristol: Wright, 1972.

9 Chambers, D. R. Sudden and unexpected death in infancy. Health Visitor, 46 (10), Oct 1973, 334–335.

10 Emery, J. L. The unexpected child death. Midwives Chronicle, 86, May 1973, 148–149.

11 Emery, J. L. Unexpected deaths in infants. Nursing Times, 69, 12 Apr 1973, 474–475.

12 Emery, J. L. Welfare of families of children found unexpectedly dead. ['Cot deaths'.] British Medical Journal, 1, 4 Mar 1972, 612–615.

13 Emery, J. L. What parents are being told about 'cot deaths'. Maternal and Child Care, 7 (71), Jul/Aug 1971, 52–54.

14 Evans, A. T. Help for parents after the sudden death of an infant. [Cot deaths.] Mother and Child, 44 (1), Jan/Feb 1972, 9–10.

15 Evans, A. T. Sudden infant death: an interim report on a home visiting project. Mother and Child, 45 (2), Mar/Apr, 10–11.

16 Foundation for the Study of Infant Deaths Cot deaths. 3. Leaflet for parents. [Full text of an information leaflet.] Health Visitor, 48 (10), Oct 1975, 382–383.

17 Foundation for the Study of Infant Deaths Sudden death in infancy. [Papers given at a conference describing a pilot project in Inner North London boroughs.] Public Health, 89 (4), May 1975, 143–163.

18 Greene, J. Killer disease: sudden infant death syndrome. Nursing Care, 8 (4), Apr 1975, 18–20.

19 Gunther, M. The neonate's immunity gap, breast feeding and cot death. Lancet, 1, 22 Feb 1975, 441–442.

20 Gunther, M. H. D. The relation of infant feeding to cot death. Nutrition, 26 (5), Oct 1972, 290–292.

21 Hagan, J. M. Infant deaths: nursing interaction and intervention with grieving families. Nursing Forum, 13 (4), 1974, 371–385.

22 Hardgrove, C. and Warrick, L. H. How shall we tell the children? [Problems in coping with the death of an expected baby.] American Journal of Nursing, 74 (3), Mar 1974, 448–450.

23 Johnson, J. M. Stillbirth – a personal experience. [Reprinted from American Journal of Nursing, Sep 1972.] Nursing Times, 69, 30 Aug 1973, 1116–1117.

24 Knight, B. Perinatal deaths and the law. Nursing Mirror, 140, 6 Feb 1975, 74–75.

25 Knight, B. Stillbirths and the law. Nursing Mirror, 140, 5 Jun 1975, 53–54.

26 Lancet Cot death. [Survey in North London over a two-year period.] Lancet, 2, 22 Nov 1975, 1024–1025.

27 Larsen, J. V. Achieving a low perinatal mortality rate in rural areas. SA Nursing Journal, 42 (6), Jun 1975, 13–14.

28 Limerick, Countess S. Comment on the legal aspect of sudden infant death. Mother and Child, 45 (2), Mar/Apr 1973, 9.

29 Limerick, Countess S. Cot deaths – 1. The relevance of dehydration in some cot deaths. Health Visitor, 48 (10), Oct 1975, 378–379.

30 Norman, M. G. Sudden infant death syndrome. Canadian Nurse, 70 (7), Jul 1974, 22–23.

31 Nursing Mirror Cot deaths. [Your questions answered series.] Nursing Mirror, 141, 18 Sep 1975, 82.

32 Owen, B. and Portess, M. Cot deaths. 2. Prospective investigation into cot deaths. [Sheffield Child Development Survey.] Health Visitor, 48 (10), Oct 1975, 379–381.

33 Richards, I. D. Unexpected deaths of babies. [NM Conference lecture.] Nursing Mirror, 138, 3 May 1974, 53–55.

34 Seitz, P. M. and Warrick, L. H. Perinatal death: the grieving mother. American Journal of Nursing, 74 (11), Nov 1974, 2028–2033.

35 Spector, W. G. Sudden infant death: the current status of the problem. Mother and Child, 45 (2), Mar/Apr 1973, 6–8.

36 Stewart, A. M. Cot deaths. Nursing Mirror, 141, 11 Dec 1975, 57–58.

37 Teare, D. Silent death in infancy. Nursing Mirror, 136, 23 Mar 1973, 18–19.

38 World Health Organization The prevention of perinatal morbidity and mortality: a report on a seminar. Geneva: WHO, 1972. (Public health papers, no. 42.)

39 Wynn, M. and Wynn, A. Must these babies die of cold? Child Poverty Action Group, 1975. (The poor and the crisis.)

40 Wynn, M. and Wynn, A. Rising infant mortality. Child Poverty Action Group, 1975. (The poor and the crisis.)

41 Yates, S. A. Stillbirth – what a staff can do. American Journal of Nursing, 72 (9), Sep 1972, 1592–1594.

42 Young, J. A mother's grief work following the death of her deformed child. Maternal-Child Nursing Journal, 4 (1), Spring 1975, 57–62.

43 Zahourek, R. and Jensen, J. S. Grieving and the loss of the newborn. American Journal of Nursing, 73 (5), May 1973, 836–839.

46 INFANT FEEDING

a GENERAL

1 Allick, H. D. Infant feeding – change and its implications. Nursing Times, 67, 21 Jan 1971, 77–78.

2 Allick, H. D. Infant feeding in the maternity hospital. Nursing Times, 67, 14 Oct 1971, Occ papers, 161–164.

3 American Journal of Nursing Techniques of infant feeding. New York: American Journal of Nursing Company, 1972. (Reprint.)

4 Bacon, N. C. and McL Hayward, J. Warm feeds – baby's choice or mother's preference. [Results of a survey.] Midwife and Health Visitior, 9 (3), Mar 1973, 72–75.

5 Barrie, H. Sugar intolerance in babies. Midwife and Health Visitor, 9 (12), Dec 1973, 387, 389, 391–393.

6 Blackman, J. Baby scales and tin openers: improvements in child health in our recent past. Mother and Child, 45 (6), Dec 1973, 15–17.

7 British Medical Journal Fashions in infant feeding. [Leading article.] British Medical Journal, 2, 30 Jun 1973, 727–728.

8 Clark, D. Rumination in a failure-to-thrive infant. Maternal-Child Nursing Journal, 4 (1), Spring 1975, 9–22.

9 Coutts, J. Current feeding practices at the Royal Manchester Children's Hospital. Nutrition, 26 (5), Oct 1972, 293–296.

10 Cree, J. E. Problems of neonatal nutrition. Nursing Mirror, 139, 19 Sep 1974, 61–63.

11 Creery, R. D. G. Infant nutrition and obesity. Nursing Mirror, 136, 26 Jan 1973, 34–38.

12 Crow, R. M. Why my babies are bottle fed. American Journal of Nursing, 71, Dec 1971, 2367–2368.

13 Davies, P. Current trends in infant feeding. Health Visitor, 46 (1), Jan 1973, 6–8.

14 Davies, P. A. The first 28 days – feeding in the early weeks. Midwives Chronicle, 87, Jul 1974, 242–244.

15 Davies, P. A. Problems of the newborn. Feeding. British Medical Journal, 4, 6 Nov 1971, 351–354.

16 Department of Health and Social Security Committee on Medical Aspects of Food Policy Panel on Child Nutrition. Working Party on Infant Feeding. Present day practice in infant feeding: report. HMSO, 1974. Chairman: T. E. Oppe. (Reports on health and social subjects 9.) Comment in Nursing Times, 71 (4), Sep 1975, 1394.

17 Dobbing, J. Food for the growing brain. [Feeding between mid-pregnancy and the second or third postnatal year.] Midwife and Health Visitor, 10 (7), Jul 1974, 187–190.

18 Francis, D. E. M. and Thompson, M. Children's hospital gets all bottled up. [Sterile prepacked feeds.] Nursing Times, 67, 24 Jun 1971, 763–765.

19 Grosvenor, P. Health education and infant feeding. Nursing Mirror, 135, 7 Jul 1972, 24–25; 14 Jul 1972, 34–37.

20 Hartog, C. D. Nutrition of infants and children. Royal Society of Health Journal, 91 (3), May/Jun, 1971, 111–114.

21 Hatcher, J. Sir Almroth Wright: pioneer of humanized cows' milk. Midwives Chronicle, 85, Nov 1972, 356.

22 Hill, R. J. Ready-to-feed systems for infants. British Hospital Journal and Social Service Review, 81, 2 Oct 1971, 2030–2031.

23 Hunt, M. Pre-packed feeding in a paediatric ward. Nursing Mirror, 135, 22 Sep 1972, 27–28.

24 Illingworth, R. S. Non-puerperal lactation. Midwives Chronicle, 86, Jun 1972, 188–189.

25 Illingworth, R. S. Some thoughts on infant feeding. Midwives Chronicle, 86, Apr 1972, 120–121.

26 Keen, J. H. The milk of human kindness. [A review of infant feeding practices.] Nursing Mirror, 140, 27 Mar 1975, 63–65.

27 Kenna, A. P. Infant feeding and obesity. [Overfeeding in the first few weeks of life.] Nursing Times, 70, 28 Feb 1974, 312–313.

28 Lahiff, M. Infant feeding and the health educator. Midwife, Health Visitor and Community Nurse, 11 (1), Jan 1975, 12–17.

29 Lee, C. A. Infant feeding. Nutrition, 28 (5), 1974, 339–348.

30 Lobo, E. de H. Milk allergy. Nursing Mirror, 133, 9 Jul 1971, 20–22.

31 Morse, E. Vitamin supplements. [An historical survey of the welfare foods scheme with recommendations for the future.] Queen's Nursing Journal, 17 (9), Dec 1974, 190–191, 193.

32 Noble, T. C. Measure out four spoonfuls of milk powder. [Accuracy in measuring spoons.] Nursing Times, 69, 8 Nov 1973, 1488–1489.

33 Nursing Times New policy sought on clinic milk sales. Nursing Times, 71, 27 Feb 1975, 324.

34 Oates, R. K. Infant-feeding practices. British Medical Journal, 2, 30 Jun 1973, 762–764.

35 Ogilvie, L. A. Ready-to-feed concept. Nursing Mirror, 133, 20 Aug 1971, 34–35.

36 O'Grady, R. S. Feeding behavior in infants. American Journal of Nursing, 71 (4), Apr 1971, 736–739.

37 Rallings, J. L. Current thinking by mothers on infant feeding. Midwives Chronicle, 86, Aug 1973, 258–259.

38 Richards, B. Current thinking by mothers on infant feeding. Midwives Chronicle, 86, Apr 1973, 116–118.

39 Robinson, J. Do nurses tell mothers enough about feeding problems? Lamp, 29 (8), Aug 1972, 7, 9, 11, 13, 15.

40 Royal College of Midwives Review of infant foods. RCM recommendations. Midwives Chronicle, 88, Apr 1975, 117–118.

41 Rundels, J. C. Iron deficiency in children. Nursing Care, 6 (9), Sep 1973, 16–18.

42 Salisbury, D. M. Bottle-feeding: influence of teat-hole size on suck volume. Lancet, 1, 22 Mar 1975, 655–656.

43 Scopes, J. W. Dangers of baby feeds that are too concentrated. Midwife Health Visitor and Community Nurse, 11 (5), May 1975, 143–144.

44 Wilkinson, P. W. and others Inaccuracies in measurement of dried milk powders. British Medical Journal, 2, 7 Apr 1973, 15–17.

45 Wright, P. A. Birth interval and malnutrition. Nursing Times, 67, 16 Dec 1971, 1578–1581.

b BREAST FEEDING

1 Brack, D. C. Social focus, feminism and breast feeding. [Study by questionnaire to identify obstacles to breast feeding.] Nursing Outlook 23 (9), Sep 1975, 556–561.

2 Brian, V. A. Is breast feeding being discouraged? Nursing Mirror, 140, 22/29 May 1975, 83.

3 British Medical Journal Free milk from the sacred cow. [Leading article on childhood nutrition.] British Medical Journal, 4, 27 Oct 1973, 183–184.

4 Brown, M. S. and Hurlock, J. T. Preparation of the breast for breast feeding: to evaluate effectiveness of three commonly suggested methods. Nursing Research, 24 (6), Nov/Dec 1975, 448–451.

5 Clark, J. Lip-service only. [Nursing support for breast feeding.] Nursing Mirror, 140, 16 Jan 1975, 39–40.

6 Close, S. The know-how of breast feeding. Bristol: Wright, 1972.

7 Countryman, B. A. Hospital care of the breast fed newborn. American Journal of Nursing, 71 (12), Dec 1971, 2365–2367.

8 Davies, M. The breast feeding promotion group: [of the National Childbirth Trust.] Health Visitor, 48 (7), Jul 1975, 239–240.

9 Davy, S. T. Human milk banks. [Work of the milk bank, Sorrento Maternity Hospital, Birmingham.] Nursing Times, 71, 15 May 1975, 758–761.

10 Daw, E. and McKinley, C. Lactation inhibition. [Report of trial of natural inhibition against oestrogen inhibition.] Nursing Mirror, 136, 29 Jun 1973, 18–19.

11 Department of Health and Social Security Nurses can help stop decline in breast feeding. [DHSS conference.] Nursing Times, 71, 24 Jul 1975, 1156.

12 Duncombe, M. A. A different kind of famine. [Advantages of breast feeding and the work of milk banks.] Nursing Times, 71, 15 May 1975, 762–763.

13 Gray, A. Breast feeding – a trilogy. 1. The physiologist's tale. Midwife, Health Visitor and Community Nurse, 11 (10). Oct 1975, 339–341.

14 Gray, A. Breast feeding – a trilogy. 2. The psychologist's tale. Midwife, Health Visitor and Community Nurse, 11 (11), Nov 1975, 351, 353–354.

15 Gray, A. Breast feeding – a trilogy. 3. The sociologist's tale. Midwife, Health Visitor and Community Nurse, 11 (12), Dec 1975, 391–394.

16 Jelliffe, D. B. and Jelliffe, E. F. The uniqueness of human milk. WHO Chronicle, 25 (12), Dec 1971, 537–540. Reprinted in Nursing Mirror, 135, 8 Dec 1972, 34–35.

17 Jolly, H. Why breast feeding is good for mother and baby. [Reprinted from The Times.] Midwives Chronicle, 88, Nov 1975, 374–375.

18 Knafl, K. Conflicting perspectives on breast feeding. [Attitudes to breast feeding of nurses and mothers and sources of conflict between them.] American Journal of Nursing, 74 (10), Oct 1974, 1848–1851.

19 Kwok, and Soo, B. Breast feeding in the lower socio-economic group. Nursing Journal of Singapore, 15 (1), May 1975, 6–8.

20 Mobbs, E. J. Breast-feeding, rooming-in, demand-feeding and houses of correction. Lamp, 31 (5), May 1974, 13–14.

21 Muller, M. Breast feeding. New Society, 33, 24 Jul 1978, 197–198.

22 Muller, M. Milk, nutrition and the law. [Trends away from breast feeding in the Third World caused by the promotion campaigns of baby food firms.] New Scientist, 66, 8 May 1975, 328–330.

23 Muller, M. Money, milk and marasmus. [Decline of breast feeding in the Third World and the adequacy of substitutes.] New Scientist, 61, 28 Feb 1974, 530–533.

24 Murdaugh, A. and Miller, L. E. Helping the breast-feeding mother. American Journal of Nursing, 72 (8), Aug 1972, 1420–1423.

25 Newton, N. Shall I breast feed my baby? Jamaican Nurse, 12 (1), Apr 1972, 34, 39.

26 Omololu, A. The importance of breast feeding. Nursing Journal of India, 65 (4), Apr 1974, 111–112, 119.

27 Otte, M. J. Correcting inverted nipples – an aid to breast feeding. American Journal of Nursing, 75 (3), Mar 1975, 454–456.

28 Patterson, B. Promotion and management of breast-feeding. [Paper presented at Midwives Congress.] Jamaican Nurse, 12 (3), Dec 1972, 23–24.

29 Rice, R. H. and Seacome, M. Attitudes of a group of mothers to breast feeding. [Survey in Gloucestershire, 1973.] Midwife, Health Visitor and Community Nurse, 11 (5), May 1975, 149–154; (6), Jun 1975, 179–180, 182–186.

30 Rolles, C. Commercial human milk in the United Kingdom. Midwives Chronicle, 86, Nov 1973, 353–354.

31 Russell, T. V. N. and Chalmers, H. J. Suppression of lactation without oestrogens. An assessment of analgesic and diuretic requirements. [Change of policy at Queen Mother's Hospital, Glasgow.] Nursing Mirror, 141, 28 Aug 1975, 60–62.

32 Soffer, R. The basics of breast feeding. Nursing Care, 7 (3), Mar 1974, 12–16.

33 Williams, J. The importance of breast feeding. Queen's Nursing Journal, 17 (5), Aug 1974, 101–103.

34 Winship, W. S. and Bommen, M. Babies, breasts and bottles. SA Nursing Journal, 42 (6), Jun 1975, 25, 26.

47 PAEDIATRIC NURSING

a TEXTBOOKS

1 Alexander, M. M. and Brown, M. S. Paediatric physical diagnosis for nurses. New York: McGraw-Hill, 1974.

2 Anderson, N. J. Workbook for paediatric nurses. 2nd ed. St. Louis: Mosby, 1974.

3 Armstrong, I. L. and Browder, J. J. Nursing care of children, 4th ed., by Joan Bulger Nast and Margaret Dickens. Philadelphia: Davis, 1973.

4 Bates, S. M. Practical paediatric nursing. Oxford, London and Edinburgh: Blackwell, Scientific, 1971.

5 Brown, M. S. and Murphy, M. A. Ambulatory paediatrics for nurses. New York: McGraw-Hill, 1975.

6 Doig, W. B. and Montford, A. Medical paediatrics. Heinemann Medical. 1972. (Modern practical nursing series, 11.) 1972.

7 Duncombe, M. and Weller, B. F. Paediatric nursing. 4th ed. Bailliere Tindall, 1974. (Nurses' aids series.)

8 Essoka, C. C. and others Paediatric nursing continuing education review: 530 essay questions and referenced answers. Flushing: Medical Examination Publishing Co., 1975.

9 Hamilton, P. M. Basic paediatric nursing. 2nd ed. St. Louis: Mosby, 1974.

10 Kessel, I. The essentials of paediatrics for nurses. 4th ed. Churchill Livingstone, 1972.

11 Leifer, G. Principles and techniques of pediatric nursing. Philadelphia; Saunders, 1972.

12 McKaig, C. and others Self assessment of current knowledge in child health nursing: 1,310 multiple choice questions and referenced answers. Flushing: Medical Examination Publishing Co., 1975. (Nursing examination review book 8.)

13 Meering, A. B. and Stacey, G. E. M. Nursery nursing: a handbook of child care. 5th ed. Bailliere Tindall, 1971.

14 O'Connor, A. B. compiler Nursing of children and adolescents. New York: American Journal of Nursing Company, 1975. (Contemporary nursing series.)

15 Porter, L. S. Child health nursing review. New York: Arco, 1975. (Nursing review series.)

16 Roberts, F. B. Review of paediatric nursing. St. Louis: Mosby, 1974. (Comprehensive review series.)

17 Scipien, G. M. and others Comprehensive paediatric nursing. New York: McGraw-Hill, 1975.

18 Speirs, A. L. Basic paediatrics for nurses. Pitman Medical, 1973.

19 Steele, S. editor Nursing care of the child with long-term illness. New York: Appleton-Century-Crofts, 1971.

20 Wallace, M. A. J. Handbook of child nursing care. New York: Wiley, 1971.

b GENERAL

1 Association of British Paediatric Nurses Doing everything possible but. . . [AGM report.] Nursing Times, 71, 10 Apr 1975, 555.

2 Association of British Paediatric Nurses Newsletter, October 1975. Nursing Times, 71, 30 Oct 1975, ABPN Supplement, 1–8.

3 Barltrop, D. Drug dosage in children. Nursing Mirror, 137, 13 Jul 1973, 29–32.

4 Brandt, P. A. and others IM injections in children. American Journal of Nursing, 72 (8), Aug 1972, 1402–1406.

5 Chadney, B. E. Is Salmon good for children? [Survey showing the effect of Salmon on the status and influence of senior paediatric nursing personnel.] Nursing Times, 69, 22 Mar 1973, 383–385.

6 Cleary, J. Nursing attention in a children's ward: an observer's case against task assignment. Medical Sociology Research Centre, University College of Swansea, 1975. (Occ. paper 8.)

7 Cooper, P. Progress in therapeutics. Sedatives and tranquillisers for children. Midwife and Health Visitor, 8 (10), Oct 1972, 364.

8 Crossley, V. Acting out or acting up? Managing the behavior of pediatric patients. Canadian Nurse, 67 (9), Sep 1971, 45–48.

9 Douglas, E. C. Observation of sick children. Nursing Times, 67, 19 Aug 1971, 1011–1014.

10 Freemon, B. L. and others How do nurses expand their roles in well child care? [Paediatric nurses in extended roles include social, emotional and behavioral issues in well child conferences with mothers.] American Journal of Nursing, 72 (10), Oct 1972, 1866–1871.

11 Genn, N. Where can nurses practice as they're taught? [New policy proposals for a paediatric unit meet with administrative opposition.] American Journal of Nursing, 74 (12), Dec 1974, 2212–2215.

12 Hawthorn, P. J. Nurse – I want my mummy! Rcn, 1974. (Study of nursing care project reports, series 1, no. 3.) Based on A study of some aspects of nursing care in nine paediatric units, with particular reference to the emotional needs of children. PhD thesis, Surrey University, 1973.

13 Jones, R. S. and Owen-Thomas, J. B. Care of the critically ill child. Arnold, 1971.

14 McGaffery, M. Children's responses to rectal temperatures: an exploratory study. Nursing Research, 20 (1), Jan/Feb 1971, 32–45.

15 Neufeld, C. G. We care about the shape they're in: an approach to the dilemma of patient needs vs. nursing resources. [The development and initial testing of a paediatric patient classification system called Nursing Attention Requirement Level.] Hospital Administration in Canada, 16 (5), May 1974, 30, 32–34.

16 Nichols, G. A. and others Measuring oral and rectal temperatures of febrile children. Nursing Research, 21 (3), May/June 1972, 261–264.

17 Nursing Journal of India Paediatric nursing issue. Nursing Journal of India, 64 (3), Mar 1973, 77–95.

18 Orr, E. P. Paediatric nursing in Australia. Nursing Mirror, 141, 4 Sep 1975, 71.

19 Riddle, I. Nursing intervention to promote body image integrity in children. Nursing Clinics of North America, 7 (2), Dec 1972, 651–661.

20 Sirota, A. L. Private care in a public clinic. [Work of nurse co-ordinators in a children's medical clinic.] American Journal of Nursing, 74 (9), Sep 1974, 1642–1643.

21 Tan, L. The role of the nurse in child care. Nursing Journal of Singapore, 12 (1), May 1972, 12–13.

22 Tripp, S. Telephone techniques in paediatric practice. American Journal of Nursing, 71 (9), Sep 1971, 1722–1723.

23 Ullathorne, M. M. Collecting urine from small children. Nursing Times, 67, 21 Jan 1971, 72–74.

24 Weller, B. F. A plea for clinical speciality. [Paediatrics.] Nursing Times, 67, 6 May 1971, 552–553.

c EDUCATION AND TRAINING

1 American Nurses' Association and the American Academy of Pediatrics Guidelines on short-term continuing education programs for pediatric nurse associates. American Journal of Nursing, 71 (3), Mar 1971, 509–512.

2 Brinton, D. and Ogden, S. L. Pediatric experience in an ambulatory care setting. [Preparing students for present and future roles in child care.] Nursing Outlook, 20 (6), Jun 1972, 390–393.

3 Chinn, P. L. and Hunt, V. O. Modules in child nursing instruction. [Self-directed learning modules containing learning objectives and evaluation tools for master's program students.] Nursing Outlook, 23 (10), Oct 1975, 650–653.

4 Glanville, C. L. Multiple student assignment as an approach to clinical problem teaching in pediatric nursing. Nursing Research, 20 (3), May/Jun 1971, 237–244.

5 Henderson, J. L. and Wilkinson, A. W. Children's nursing. [Statement on paediatric nurse training in the light of Rcn evidence to the Briggs Committee.] Lancet, 1, 4 Mar 1972, 531.

6 Julias, R. K. Refresher course in paediatric nursing. Nursing Journal of India, 64 (5), May 1973, 153, 156.

7 Spees, E. and others The making of a PNA. [Establishment of a paediatric nurse associate program at Los Angeles County Hospital.] Pediatric Nursing, 1 (2), Mar/Apr 1975, 7–15.

8 Tomita, H. Japan. [Paediatric nurse education.] Nursing Times, 72, 25 Mar 1976, ABPN Supplement, vii–viii.

9 Vuuren, S. G. van Growth in the training for the paediatric diploma at the Transvaal Memorial Hospital for Children. SA Nursing Journal, 40 (10), Oct 1973, 16–17.

d COMMUNITY NURSING

1 American Journal of Nursing The pediatric nurse practitioner in a neighbourhood center. American Journal of Nursing. 71 (3). Mar 1971, 513–515.

2 Ames, I. Strictly for kids. [The provision of a paediatric home nursing scheme in Southampton by district nursing sisters.] Practice Team, no. 35, Apr 1974, 9–11.

3 Andrews, P. M. and Yankauer, A. The pediatric nurse practitioner. American Journal of Nursing, 71 (3), Mar 1971, 504–508.

4 Birenbaum, A. The pediatric nurse practitioner and preventive community mental health. Journal of Psychiatric Nursing and Mental Health Services, 12 (5), Sep/Oct 1974, 14–19.

5 Bonkowsky, M. L. Adapting the POMR to community child health care. Nursing Outlook, 20 (8), Aug 1972, 515–518.

6 British Paediatric Association and British Association of Paediatric Surgeons Day care [for children] in hospitals: report of the Working Party. British Paediatric Association, 1975. Chairman: Dr. W. J. Appleyard.

7 Davenport, D. Keeping your child out of hospital. [Report at the National Association for the Welfare of Children in Hospital: conference on home care schemes for sick children.] Nursery World, 74, 21 Nov 1974, 12–13.

8 Feldman, M. Cluster visits: group visits alternating with individual visits increase mothers' learning and socializing and PNP's satisfaction. [Paediatric nurse practitioner.] American Journal of Nursing, 74 (8), Aug 1974, 1485–1488.

9 Jenkins, S. M. Home care scheme at Paddington. [A unit at St. Mary's Hospital which visits and treats children at home.] Nursing Mirror, 140, 27 Feb 1975, 68–70.

10 Kehoe, K. The paediatric nurse in the community: attitudes forged by searing experience. Australian Nurses' Journal, 5 (4), Oct 1975, 29–32.

11 Martin, F. R. The nurse's role in the Home Care Unit. [The work of district nurses in the St. Mary's Hospital home care team visiting children at home.] Nursing Mirror, 140, 27 Feb 1975, 70–72.

12 Nursing Times Andrea: a study in co-operation. [Hospital Community liaison.] Nursing Times, 67, 4 Feb 1971, 133–137.

13 O'Brien, M. and others Expanding the public health nurse's role in child care. Nursing Outlook, 23 (6), Jun 1975, 369–373.

14 Strozier, V. and Williams, D. Evolution of a role: pediatric nurse clinician. Supervisor Nurse, 6 (2), Feb 1975, 28, 31, 35–37.

15 Thomstad, B. and others Changing the rules of the doctor-nurse game. [Development of more open doors – nurse communications in a child health centre.] Nursing Outlook, 23 (7), Jul 1975, 422–427.

16 Thorp, R. J. The use of the pediatric nurse practitioner in comprehensive health care. Pediatric Nursing, 1 (3), May/Jun 1975, 33–35.

e SURGERY

1 Cox, A. G. Bowel preparation [before surgery]. Nursing Times, 70, 4 Apr 1974, 502–503.

2 Kenna, A. P. Conditions in the newborn requiring surgery. Nursing Mirror, 139, 23 Aug 1974, 64–68.

3 Russell, H. E. and others Controlling body temperatures of infants with an air-fluidized bed. [During surgery.] RN Magazine, 35 (11), Nov 1972, OR17–18.

4 Scott, J. E. S. Nursing the surgical neonate. Nursing Mirror, 134, 17 Mar 1972, 22–25.

5 Scott, J. E. S. Recent advances in neonatal surgery. Midwives Chronicle, 84, Jan 1971, 8–11.

6 Strathdee, E. D. and Young, D. G. Paediatric surgery. Heinemann, 1971. (Modern practical nursing series 3.)

7 Young, D. G. and Weller, B. F. Baby surgery: nursing management and care. Aylesbury, Bucks: Harvey Miller and Medcalf, 1971.

48 CHILD IN HOSPITAL

a GENERAL

1 Ambrosio, A. The child from the poverty area. [Problems of hospitalization.] Nursing Care, 7 (11), Nov 1974, 10–14.

2 Anstice, E. Who'll be mother? [Emotional needs of children in hospital.] Nursing Times, 69, 31 May 1973, 716–717.

3 Brown, L. Children in hospital. [Hospital Centre conference on emotional needs.] Health and Social Service Journal, 83, 17 Mar 1973, 610.

4 Carter, M. D. Identification of behaviours displayed by children experiencing prolonged hospitalization. [Research study.] International Journal of Nursing Studies, 10 (2), May 1973, 125–133.

5 Chaloner, L. Children and hospitals. [Children as visitors to wards as well as patients.] Nursing Mirror, 134, 14 Jan 1972, 11–12.

6 Chang, M. K. A visit to Peking Children's Hospital. American Journal of Nursing, 72 (12), Dec 1972, 2219–2221.

7 Cooper, C. Substitute mothering of young children in hospital. Mother and Child, 46 (2), Mar 1974, 12–15.

8 Crocker, E. Is your hospital any place for a three-year old? [A study of pediatric units.] Dimensions in Health Service, 52 (7), Jul 1975, 32–33.

9 Crossley, V. Child life programs: an essential ingredient to good patient care. [Emotional well-being of the child in hospital.] Hospital Administration in Canada, 17 (2), Feb 1975, 20–24.

10 Department of Health Hospitals facilities for children. HM (71) 22 and Annex. The Department, 1971.

11 Downey, T. J. All my times in the hospital – a child remembers. American Journal of Nursing, 74 (12), Dec 1974, 2196–2198.

12 Duncombe, M. Children in hospital. [Report of a conference held by the Association of British Paediatric Nurses.] Nursing Times, 69, 15 Mar 1973, 354.

13 Dzik, M. A. The use of motility by a preschool boy during hospitalization. Maternal-Child Nursing Journal, 3 (3), Fall 1974, 169–179.

14 Fleming, J. W. Children's drawings aid researcher in understanding health conditions. [Children in hospital.] Nursing Research Report, 8 (2), Jun 1973, 1–2, 5–6.

15 Hospitals Fantasy, colors reassure pediatric patients. Hospitals, 47 (2), 16 Jan 1973, 34, 38.

16 Jolly, J. D. The bib sister programme – a concept of primary nursing care. [Solving separation anxieties due to staff changes at the Children's Medical Centre, Neurosurgical Unit, Montreal.] Nursing Times, 71, 30 Oct 1975, ABPN 2–3.

17 Jolly, J. D. Children in hospital: the ward granny scheme. Nursing Times, 70, 11 Apr 1974, 537–540.

18 King's Fund Centre Caring for children in hospital: some thoughts and suggestions for those living and working in the ward situation. The Centre, 1974. (King's Fund project paper, 4.)

19 Kverndal, R. J. Caring for children in hospital. [Report of conference of National Association for Welfare of Children in Hospital.] Social Work Today, 3, 11 Jan 1973, 18.

20 Lancet Children in hospital – and after. Lancet, 2, 4 Oct 1975, 649.

21 Lewendon, G. and others A survey of children's thoughts in hospital compared with what mothers feel. [Survey by medical students of children aged 4–14.] Midwife, Health Visitor and Community Nurse, 11 (8), Aug 1975, 257–258.

22 Lillystone, D. Emergency clinic for children. [At Queen Charlotte's Maternity Hospital.] Nursing Times, 71, 25 Sep 1975, 1553.

23 Lindheim, R. and others Changing hospital environments for children. Cambridge, Mass: Harvard University Press, 1972.

24 Lowenstein, H. The handling of distress. [Small children in hospital: the nurse-mother-child relationship.] Nursing Times, 68, 26 Oct 1972, 1363–1364.

25 Lubbers, J. M. Emotional aspects of hospitalized children. SA Nursing Journal, 13 (1), Jan 1975, 24–25.

26 McElnea, J. The psychologically disturbed child in hospital. Nursing Times, 71, 6 Feb 1975, 226–227.

27 Markowitz, R. Adventures in a pediatric unit. [An imaginative environment at Brooklyn Hospital helps to reduce the fears of hospitalization.] Hospitals, 48 (21), 1 Nov 1974, 63–65.

28 National Association for the Welfare of Children in Hospital The child out of hospital. [Twelfth annual conference.] Health and Social Service Journal, 84, 26 Oct 1974, 2466.

29 National Association for the Welfare of Children in Hospital Children in hospital. [Ninth annual conference.] Health Visitor, 45 (3), Mar 1972, 83.

30 Needham, A. Talking it over. [In a children's ward.] Nursing Mirror, 132, 15 Jan 1971, 30–32.

31 Nursery Times Ward granny scheme when comfort is important. Nursery Times, 6, Jan 1974, 4.

32 Pike, N. In hospital. 3. The child's view. Nursing Mirror, 140, 8 May 1975. 67–68.

33 Plank, E. N. Children's creativity under stress of hospitalization. Hospital Topics, 49 (2), Feb 1971, 65–66, 68, 77.

34 Riddoch, M. Llongyfarchiadan. Da Tawn-Cymru. [Review of Welsh Hospital Board report on Children in Hospital.] Nursing Times, 69, 1 Mar 1973, 279.

35 Robertson, J. Young children in hospital. 2nd ed. Tavistock, 1970.

36 Robertson, J. and Robertson, J. Substitute mothering. [For children in hospital.] Nursing Times, 69, 29 Nov 1973, 1611–1614.

37 Roskies, E. and others Emergency hospitalization of young children: some neglected psychological considerations. Medical Care, 8 (7), Jul 1975, 570–581.

38 Shah, G. P. and others Patient care classification of children in hospital. Canadian Hospital, 50 (7), Jul 1973, 38–41, 43–44.

39 Spenner, D. A preschool child copes with hospitalization. Maternal-Child Nursing Journal, 3 (1), Spring 1974, 41–48.

40 Suran, B. G. and Hatcher, R. P. The psychological treatment of hospitalized children with failure to thrive. Pediatric Nursing, 1 (5), Sep/Oct 1975, 10–17.

41 Transvaal Memorial Hospital for Children Golden Jubilee 1923–1973. Special Issue. SA Nursing Journal, 40 (10), Oct 1973, 5–33.

42 Wear, E. T. Separation anxiety reconsidered: nursing implications. [In hospitalized children.] Maternal-Child Nursing Journal, 3 (1), Spring 1974, 9–18.

43 Welsh Hospital Board Children in hospital in Wales: final report of a working party. Cardiff: The Board, 1972. Comment in Nursing Times, 69, 1 Mar 1973, 279.

44 Williams, T. K. Responses of a twelve month old girl to physical restraint during hospitalization. Maternal-Child Nursing Journal, 4 (2), Summer 1975, 109–116.

b ADOLESCENTS

1 American Journal of Nursing The pangs and pains of adolescence. [Five articles.] American Journal of Nursing, 75 (10), Oct 1975, 1723–1744.

2 Benson, S. Nursing care study. Brian – a boy of our times. [Patient treated in Adolescent Unit, Hill End Hospital.] Nursing Mirror, 137, 5 Oct 1973, 34–36.

3 Brinton, H. Adolescents at risk. [Counselling and Advice Centre]. Community Health, 5 (2), Sep/Oct, 85–91.

4 Clark, A. Nursing organization in an adolescents' unit. In Association for the Psychiatric Study of Adolescents. Proceedings of the fifth annual conference, Edinburgh, 1970. The Association, 1971.

5 Davis, J. M. Football as therapy. [Adolescent Unit at the Bethlem Royal Hospital, Kent.] Nursing Mirror, 139, 6 Sep 1974, 58–59.

6 Downes, C. E. and Hall, S. M. An exercise in collaboration. [A disabled adolescent.] Social Work Today, 69, 24 Jul 1975, 258–262.

7 Engs, R. C. Setting up a free clinic for transient youth. Canadian Nurse, 68 (1), Jan 1972, 33–36.

8 Gillespie, J. Problems encountered in an adolescent unit. [Edinburgh.] Nursing Times, 68, 5 Oct 1972, 1248–1251.

9 Ibbotson, J. Psychological effects of physical disability: adolescence. Health and Social Service Journal, 85, 27 Sep 1975, 2158–2159.

10 Isler, C. The adolescent unit: tailored for teenage patients. RN Magazine, 38 (9), Sep 1975, 64, 67, 72.

11 Jones, M. and Beavan, M. Wales. Problems in establishing an adolescent unit. Nursing Times, 70, 21 Nov 1974, 1822–1824.

12 Kalafatich, A. J. editor Approaches to the care of adolescents. New York: Appleton-Century-Crofts, 1975.

13 King's Fund Centre Adolescent unit staff discussion group. Report of a meeting held at the Hospital Centre on 29th March, 1971. The Centre, 1971.

14 Lehberger, L. Responses of an adolescent to immobilization during hospitalization. Maternal-Child Nursing Journal, 2 (3), Fall 1973, 189–195.

15 Lore, A. Adolescents: people, not problems. [Nursing care of the hospitalized adolescent.] American Journal of Nursing, 73 (7), Jul 1973, 1232–1234.

16 Nursing Clinics of North America Symposium on the young adult in today's world. Nursing Clinics of North America, 8 (1), Mar 1973, 1–104.

17 Raven, F. Admission and discharge in an adolescent unit; a case study. [Hill End Hospital, St. Albans.] Social Work Today, 4 (4), 17 May 1973, 98–103.

18 Robinson, W. Banstead Place. An experiment in the assessment of physically handicapped adolescents. Nursing Mirror, 141, 31 Jul 1975, 40–42.

19 Tiedt, E. The adolescent in the hospital: an identity resolution approach. Nursing Forum, 11 (2), 1972, 120–140.

20 Wessell, M. L. Use of humor by an immobilized adolescent girl during hospitalization. Maternal-Child Nursing Journal, 4 (1), Spring 1975, 35–48.

21 White, P. Hospital recreation helps adolescent patients. Canadian Nurse, 68 (7), Jul 1972, 34–35.

c FAMILY

1 Abercrombie, M. I. J. Parent-staff communication in a children's unit. Proceedings of the Royal Society of Medicine, 65, Apr 1972, 335–338.

2 Arnold, A. Children in hospital: some reflections on 'substitute'. [Review of Ann Hales-Tooke's book 'Children in hospital: the parents' view'.] Nursing Times, 70, 11 Apr 1974, 555.

3 Aufhauser, T. R. and Lesh, D. Parents need TLC too: a pediatric nurse clinician teaches and counsels the parents of hospitalized children. Hospitals, 47, 16 Apr 1973, 88, 90–91.

4 Beck, M. Attitudes of parents of pediatric heart patients toward patient care units. Nursing Research, 22 (4), Jul/Aug 1973, 334–338.

5 Boon, W. H. Free visiting in children's wards. Nursing Journal of Singapore, 12 (1), May 1972, 15–18.

6 Burrows, J. M. The child and his family. [The Royal Liverpool Children's Hospital.] Nursing Times, 69, 27 Sep 1973, 1266–1267.

7 Burton, L. The family life of sick children: a study of families coping with chronic childhood disease. Routledge and Kegan Paul, 1975.

8 Chong, S. The relationship between the nursing staff and parents of hospitalized children. Nursing Journal of Singapore, 12 (1), May 1972, 25–27.

9 Feely, W. J. Pediatric nurses teach parents. [To participate in the care of a child in hospital.] Bedside Nurse, 5 (6), Jun 1972, 10–13.

10 Fox, S. Stand-in mothers. [Relieving mothers of other family responsibilities so that they are free to stay with a sick child in hospital.] British Hospital Journal and Social Service Review, 82, 11 Mar 1972, 570–571.

11 Freiberg, K. H. How parents react when their child is hospitalized. American Journal of Nursing, 72 (7), Jul 1972, 1270–1272.

12 Hales-Tooke, A. Children in hospital: the parents' view. Priory Press, 1973. (Care and welfare library.)

13 Hardgrove, C. B. and Dawson, R. B. Parents and children in hospital: the family's role in pediatrics. Boston: Little, Brown, 1972.

14 Hardgrove, C. B. and Rutledge, A. Parenting during hospitalization. [A system used at a San Francisco hospital.] American Journal of Nursing, 75 (5), May 1975, 837–839.

15 Holman, D. The heartbreak continues. [Children in hospital and free visiting.] Nursing Mirror, 132, 28 May 1971, 12.

16 Holman, D. Mother's guide to children in hospital. Ilfracombe: Arthur Stockwell, 1973.

17 Howlett, M. R. Accommodation for mothers in a children's hospital. Hospital Management, 34, May/Jun 1971, 162–163.

18 Jefferies, P. M. Free visiting for children. Nursing Times 69, 6 Dec 1973, 1664–1665.

19 Khoo, H. Rapport between parents and nurses in children's wards. Nursing Journal of Singapore, 12 (1), May 1972, 21–23.

20 Lerner, M. J. and others Hospital care-by-parent: an evaluative look. [An experimental pediatric unit at the University of Kentucky Medical Center]. Medical Care, 10 (5), Sep/Oct 1972, 430–436.

21 Lowenstein, H. Filming in a children's ward [to highlight the problems of separation from parents]. Social Service Quarterly, 48 (3), Jan/Mar.1975, 255–257.

22 McElnea, L. Where resident parents are welcome. Nursing Times, 67, 28 Oct 1971, 1331–1333.

23 McNeur, R. Parents in the paediatric ward. New Zealand Nursing Journal, 68 (11), Nov 1975, 20–21.

24 Meadow, R. Children, mothers and hospitals. [Policy of. unrestricted visiting and medical attitudes.] New Society, 27, 7 Feb 1974, 318–320. Letter from James Robertson, New Society, 27, 14 Feb 1974, 402.

25 Meadow, R. Hospital visiting of children. [Problems of unrestricted visiting.] Proceedings of the Royal Society of Medicine, 65, Apr 1972, 341–342.

26 National Association for the Welfare of Children in Hospital. Visiting children in hospital: a survey. The Association, 1972.

27 Orr, E. P. How nurse-parent relationships mean more than meets the eye. Australian Nurses' Journal, 3 (10), May 1974, 37–38, 49.

28 Parfit, J. Parents and relatives. [Emotional needs of parents with sick children.] Nursing Times, 71, 18 Sep 1975, 1512–1513.

29 Stacey, M. editor Hospitals, children and their families. Routledge, 1970. (Medicine, illness and society.)

30 Sulakshini, M. The hospitalized child and the mother. Nursing Journal of India, 65 (5), May 1974, 136, 138.

d PATIENT TEACHING AND ANXIETY

1 Bell, A. N. Psychological preparation of child contributes to success of surgery. Hospital Topics, 49 (6), Jun 1971, 78–79.

2 Bellack, J. P. Helping a child cope with the stress of injury. American Journal of Nursing, 74 (8), Aug 1974, 1491–1494.

3 Blake, Y. The importance of the nurse's attitude towards a child on admission to hospital. SA Nursing Journal, 38 (10), Oct 1971, 7–8.

4 Brown, M. J. Preadmission orientation for children and parents. Canadian Nurse, 67 (2), Feb 1971, 29–31.

5 Claxton, I. Nurses explain hospitals to children. [An orientation program in the community reduces hospitalization fears.] Hospitals, 49 (13), 1 Jul 1975, 41–42.

6 Crawford, C. F. and Palm, M. L. Can I take my teddy bear? Before a child enters Evanston Hospital his 'special nurse' who will give him moral support in the hospital makes a home visit. American Journal of Nursing, 73 (2), Feb 1973, 286–287.

7 Fujita, M. T. The impact of illness or surgery on the body image of the child. Nursing Clinics of North America, 7 (4), Dec 1972, 641–649.

8 Gooden, D. 'Snorky' helps to allay fears of children before surgery. Hospital Topics, 51 (2), Feb 1973, 53–55.

9 Hospitals Fearless of the familiar. [Procedures used to reassure children at the Johns Hopkins Hospital, Baltimore.] Hospitals, 48, 1 Sep 1974, 23, 26.

10 Jackson, Q. and Hope, G. 'Children's Ladies! [Nurses in the children's ward, St. Andrew's Hospital, Billericay, wear mufti as an experiment.] Nursing Times, 67, 21 Jan 1971, 91.

11 Knudsen, K. Play therapy: preparing the young child for surgery. Nursing Clinics of North America, 7 (4), Dec 1975, 679–686.

12 Leese, S. M. Crisis situations – their effect on children. Nursing Mirror, 137, 5 Oct 1973, 38–39.

13 Litchfield, M. The pediatric nurse – and a child in hospital. New Zealand Nursing Journal, 68 (11), Nov 1974, 17–20.

14 Mead, J. The lemonade party. [Preparing children for going into hospital.] Nursing Outlook, 21 (2), Feb 1973, 104–105.

15 Murphy, D. Night in the hospital. [Child's experience in hospital in story-book form.] Nursing Forum, 11 (2), 1972, 165–176.

16 RN Magazine Children's pre-op visits a problem? Try a 'punch bunch'. [A pre-operative teaching session on what to expect in hospital.] RN Magazine, 37 (2), Feb 1974, OR 16.

17 Schultz, N. V. How children perceive pain. Nursing Outlook, 19 (10), Oct 1971, 670–673.

18 Stainton, C. Preschoolers' orientation to hospital. [For well children.] Canadian Nurse, 70 (9), Sep 1974, 38–40.

19 Tisdale, B. 'Not for admission'. [Pre and post operative home visits by a nurse to children undergoing day surgery.] Canadian Nurse, 68 (12), Dec 1972, 35–39.

20 Whitson, B. J. The puppet treatment in pediatrics. [The use of puppets to prepare a child for treatment.] American Journal of Nursing, 72 (9), Sep 1972, 1612–1614.

21 Wolfer, J. A. and Visintainer, M. A. Pediatric surgical patients' and parents' stress responses and adjustment as a function of psychologic preparation and stress-point nursing care. Nursing Research, 24 (4), Jul/Aug 1975, 244–255.

e PLAY

1 Abbas, A. and Rolinson, J. Children in hospital. A library of toys. Nursing Times, 70, 11 Apr 1974, 564–565.

2 Azarnoff, P. Volunteers assist in child activities. Hospitals, 46 (4), 16 Feb 1972, 61–62.

3 Begue, M. T. A. Play: the hospitalized child's best friend. Hospital Topics, 51 (4), Apr 1973, 45–48.

4 Billington, G. F. Play program reduces children's anxiety, speeds recoveries. Modern Hospital, 118 (4), Apr 1972, 90–92.

5 Butler, A. and others Child's play is therapy. [The pre-school child in hospital.] Canadian Nurse, 71 (2), Dec 1975, 35–37.

6 Castle, D. Christmas games on the ward. Nursing Mirror, 141, 25 Dec 1975, 56–57.

7 Conference on play in hospital Health and Social Service Journal, 85, 19 Jul 1975, 1525.

8 Cooper, D. Journey to catharsis? [Psychological effects of fantasy on children.] Nursing Times, 71, 28 Aug 1975, 1360–1362.

9 Cumming, E. E. Children in hospital: do they need a library service? Book Trolley, 3 (3), Sep 1971, 3–9.

10 David, N. Play: a nursing diagnostic tool. Maternal-Child Nursing Journal, 2 (1), Spring 1973, 49–56.

11 Hales-Tooke, A. Nurse, playleader and parent. Nursing Times, 67, 10 Jun 1971, 713–715.

12 Harding, V. and Walker, S. Let's make a game of it! [Play specialists in the Paediatric Unit, Fulham Hospital.] Nursing Mirror, 135, 22 Dec 1972, 14–17.

13 Harvey, S. and Hales-Tooke, A., editors Play in hospitals. Faber, 1972.

14 Hyde, N. D. Play therapy: the troubled child's self-encounter. American Journal of Nursing, 71 (7), Jul 1971, 1366–1370.

15 Murphy, D. C. Therapeutic value of children's play. Nursing Forum, 11 (2), 1972, 141–156.

16 Myrdal, A. Children's play. Opportunities and dangers in an efficiency-minded society. Maternal and Child Care, 8, Dec 1971/Jan 1972, 8–11.

17 Noble, E. Children in hospital. Why play? [The importance of play in child development.] Nursing Times, 70, 11 Apr 1974, 534–536.

18 Poole, A. and Ruck, P. Remedial play groups for the under-fives in a general hospital. [Paediatric Unit, Poole General Hospital.] Physiotherapy, 58 (4), Apr 1972, 132–134.

19 Routledge, L. Technology, toys and therapy. [The work of the Medical Engineering Research Unit at Queen Mary's Hospital for Children, Carshalton, Surrey.] British Journal of Occupational Therapy, 37 (10), Oct 1974, 178–179.

20 Routledge, L. Toy library attached to a district and regional assessment centre. [Newcomen Toy Library, Guy's Hospital.] British Journal of Occupational Therapy, 38 (2), Feb 1975, 30.

21 Savage, J. H. Aids for children's wards. [Cabinet toy and low-level hand propelled couch.] Nursing Times, 137, 21 Sep 1973, 36–39.

22 Savage, J. H. A cot drawing board. [Developed at the Brook Hospital, London.] Nursing Times, 71, 21 Aug 1975, 1349.

23 Savage, J. H. Model kitchen units for a hospital playgroup. Nursing Mirror, 138, 14 Jun 1974, 59.

24 Savage, J. H. Play telephones. [Construction of telephone kiosks for children in hospital.] Nursing Times, 71, 12 Jun 1975, 946–947.

25 Stephenson, A. Toys: pleasure, learning, fun and fantasy. Mother and Child, 45 (6), Dec 1973, 18–20.

26 White, E. G. and others Bloorview's 'Project Satellite'. What was gained? [Pilot project at Bloorview Children's Hospital, Toronto, in the rehabilitation of the young chronic sick.] Hospital Administration in Canada, 15 (3), Mar 1973, 30–31, 34–35.

f TERMINAL CARE AND DEATH

1 Branson, H. K. The dying child and his family. Bedside Nurse, 5 (2), Feb 1972, 11–15.

2 Craig, Y. The care of a dying child: the needs of the nurses, the patient and parents. Nursing Mirror, 137, 28 Sep 1973, 14–16.

3 Elfert, H. The nurse and the grieving parent. [Helping parents cope with the loss of a child.] Canadian Nurse, 71 (2), Feb 1975, 30–31.

4 Fox, S. The death of a child. Nursing Times, 68, 19 Oct 1972, 1322–1323.

5 Freiberg, J. Teaching children to understand about death. New Society, 31, 6 Feb 1975, 318–320.

6 Gyulay, J. E. Care of the dying child. Nursing Clinics of North America, 11 (1), Mar 1976, 95–107.

7 Gyulay, J. E. The forgotten grievers. [People other than mothers affected by a child's death.] American Journal of Nursing, 75 (9), Sep 1975, 1476–1479.

8 Hopkins, L. J. A basis for nursing care of the terminally ill child and his family. Maternal-Child Nursing Journal, 2 (2), Summer 1973, 93–100.

9 Jackson, P. L. The child developing concepts of death: implications for nursing care of the terminally ill child. Nursing Forum, 14 (2), 1975, 204–215.

10 Lacasse, C. M. A dying adolescent. American Journal of Nursing, 75 (3), Mar 1975, 433–434.

11 Lowenberg, J. S. The coping behaviors of fatally ill adolescents and their parents. Nursing Forum, 9 (3), 1971, 269–287.

12 Maxwell, M. B. A terminally ill adolescent and her family. American Journal of Nursing, 72 (5), May 1972, 925–927.

13 Miya, T. M. The child's perception of death. Nursing Forum, 11 (2), 1972, 214–220.

14 Murray, R. Illness as a crisis: the terminally ill child. Journal of Practical Nursing, 23 (3), Mar 1973, 22–25.

15 Newcomer, B. Analysis of behavior in a terminally ill child. Maternal-Child Nursing Journal, 2 (3), Fall 1973, 157–164.

16 Northrup, F. C. The dying child. American Journal of Nursing, 74 (6), Jun 1974, 1066–1068.

17 Oraftik, N. Only time to touch. [The emotional needs of a young dying patient.] Nursing Forum, 11 (2), 1972, 205–213.

18 Waechter, E. H. Children's awareness of fatal illness. American Journal of Nursing, 71 (6), Jun 1971, 1168–1172.

19 Yakulis, I. M. Anxieties of a fatally ill boy. Maternal-Child Nursing Journal, 2 (2), Summer 1973, 121–128.

20 Yakulis, I. M. Changing concepts of death in a child with sickle cell disease. Maternal-Child Nursing Journal, 4 (2), Summer 1975, 117–120.

49 HANDICAPPED CHILDREN

a GENERAL

1 Baker, J. and D. Nigel John. [10 months to 2¾ years. A handicapped child.] Queen's Nursing Journal, 18 (5) Aug 1975, 134–135.

2 Bond, W. T. F. Aids for the disabled. Design for the handicapped child. Nursing Times, 70, 11 Jul 1974, 1066–1068.

3 Fox, M. HV's role not understood by parents of handicapped children – report. [Report on a study of the families of the handicapped, by Mervyn Fox.] Nursing Times, 71, 5 Jun 1975, 867.

4 Ibbotson, J. Psychological effects of physical disability: adolescence. Health and Social Service Journal, 85, 27 Sep 1975, 2158–2159.

5 Jolly, H. Early management of the handicapped child. Midwives Chronicle, 87, Feb 1974, 52–53.

6 Ledney D. What a difference handling can make to the severely handicapped child. Bedside Nurse, 5 (3), Mar 1972, 24–26.

7 Main, J. C. Assessing the handicapped child. Nursing Mirror, 141, 14 Aug 1975, 69–71.

8 Mason, C. Pool activities with the multiply handicapped child. Nursing Mirror, 141, 25 Sep 1975, 50–52.

9 Nursing Clinics of North America Symposium on the child with developmental disabilities. Nursing Clinics of North America, 10 (2), Jun 1970, 307–405.

10 Rosenbaum, P. Delivery of services for young handicapped children: a look at two treatment centres. Community Health, 5 (4), Jan/Feb 1974, 193–199.

11 Ross, T. Medical engineering helps handicapped children. Nursing Mirror, 141, 21 Aug 1975, 41–42.

12 Whitmore, T. K. The handicapped child. Community Health, 4 (6), May/Jun 1973, 330–337.

b EDUCATION AND PLAY

1 Bartle, R. B. Teaching the handicapped child to learn. [Mabel Liddiard Scholarship 1974.] Midwives Chronicle, 88, Aug 1975, 274–276.

2 Brenton, A. G. and Cowan, C. M. Helping a child develop. [A joint study undertaken by health visitors and medical officers in Portsmouth to measure the effect of a three month period of developmental training for handicapped and retarded children.] Nursing Times, 71, 3 Jul 1975, 1052–1055.

3 Browning, H. H. Education at Chailey Heritage. Nursing Mirror, 140, 9 Jan 1975, 65–70.

4 Bull, K. R. Toy library for handicapped children. Nursing Mirror, 137, 24 Aug 1973, 18.

5 Eddington, C. and Lee, T. Sensory-motor stimulation for slow-to-develop children. A home-centered program for parents. American Journal of Nursing, 75 (1), Jan 1975, 59–62.

6 Faulkner, R. E. Opportunity classes and community care. [For handicapped children.] Health and Social Service Journal, 83, 31 Mar 1973, 731–732.

7 Godfrey, A. B. Sensory-motor stimulation for slow-to-develop children. A specialized program for public health nurses. American Journal of Nursing, 75 (1), Jan 1975, 56–59.

8 Holaday, B. J. Achievement behavior in chronically ill children. The Intellectual Achievement Responsibility questionnaire.] Nursing Research, 23 (1), Jan/Feb 1974, 25–30.

9 Knapp, M. E. and others Teaching Suzi to walk by behavior modification of motor skills. [Case study of a child with a neuromuscular disease.] Nursing Forum, 13 (2), 1974, 158–183.

10 Logue, J. E. and Oliver, W. M. F. Everyone falls over sometimes. [Ullenwood Manor, a college of further education for disabled school leavers run by the National Star Centre.] Nursing Mirror, 140, 19 Jun 1975, 60–62.

11 Lovell, L. M. The Yeovil Opportunity Group: a play group for multiply handicapped children. Physiotherapy, 59 (8), 10 Aug 1973, 251–253.

12 McGeorge, H. The children of SPELD. [Specific Learning Difficulties Association.] Australian Nurses' Journal, 2 (11), May 1973, 20–21.

13 Maser, E. Handicapped children learn written communication. Canadian Nurse, 69 (8), Aug 1973, 29–33.

14 Peto, A. Conductive education. [At the Spastics Society's Ingfield Manor School, Sussex, a single teacher/therapist deals with all the child's handicaps.] Nursing Times, 71, 15 May 1975, 756.

15 Tuckwell, P. Schooling the subnormal child. The Massachusetts System. Nursing Mirror, 141, 18 Sep 1975, 73–74.

16 Warr, D. M. SPELD and the nurse. [The role of the nurse in the community in helping children with learning difficulties.] Australian Nurses' Journal, 3 (4), Oct 1973, 19–22, 32.

c FAMILY

1 Barnes, G. G. Working with mothers of brain-damaged children. Midwife and Health Visitor, 9 (2), Feb 1973, 47–50.

2 Bentovim, A. Emotional disturbances of handicapped pre-school children and their families – attitudes to the child. [Reprinted from the British Medical Journal.] Nursery Journal, 63, Feb 1973, 5–8, 10–14.

3 Brimblecombe, F. S. W. Exeter project for handicapped children. [Infant care units, day units and holiday projects help to diminish the strain on the families of the handicapped.] British Medical Journal, 4, 21 Dec 1974, 706–709.

4 Craig, Y. The ward wants to know where her dad is. [The problems of parents with handicapped children.] Nursing Mirror, 141, 23 Oct 1975, 53–54.

5 Dodd, O. V. D. Aycliffe Hospital Parent Association – a year of achievement. Nursing Mirror, 136, 8 Jun 1973, 36–37.

6 Fox, A. M. Families with handicapped children – a challenge to the caring professions. Community Health, 6, Jan/Feb 1975, 217–223.

7 Fox, S. The needs of normal children [in the family of a handicapped child]. Health and Social Service Journal, 83, 10 Nov 1973, 2629–2630.

8 Freeman, L. Society at work. Sharing trouble. [Mothers of handicapped children form a discussion group.] New Society, 24, 7 Jun 1973, 559–560.

9 Gonzalez, M. T. Nursing support of the family with an abnormal infant. Hospital Topics, 49 (3), Mar 1971, 68–69.

10 Gregory, D. Family assessment and intervention plan. [For parents with a handicapped or impaired child.] Pediatric Nursing, 1 (4), Jul/Aug 1975, 23–29.

11 Griffiths, M. I. The congenitally handicapped – the parent and the child. (a) The congenitally handicapped child. Royal Society of Health Journal, 94 (6), Dec 1974, 296–299.

12 Harrison, P. Handicapped. [Family Fund for congenitally disabled children and their families.] New Society, 25, 9 Aug 1973, 339.

13 Hilton, E. A cry for help. [Work of the Invalid Children's Aid Association.] Midwife and Health Visitor, 9 (4), Apr 1973, 117–118.

14 Hitch, D. The congenitally handicapped – the parent and the child. (b) The parent. Royal Society of Health Journal, 94 (6), Dec 1974, 299–304.

15 Jackson, A. and others The needs of handicapped children and their families in an East London Borough. Community Medicine, 129, 19 Jan 1973, 293–297.

16 Jackson, P. L. Chronic grief. [Case study of parents with an abnormal child.] American Journal of Nursing, 74 (7), Jul 1974, 1288–1291.

17 Jones, A. Parents need facts – not just sympathy. [Involvement of parents in helping handicapped children.] New Psychiatry, 2 (8), 10 Apr 1975, 12–13.

18 Kew, S. Handicap and family crisis: a study of the siblings of handicapped children. Pitman, 1975.

19 McLellan, N. L. The congenitally handicapped – the parent and the child. (c) The community. Royal Society of Health Journal, 94 (6), Dec 1974, 304–306.

20 Mercer, R. T. Mothers' responses to their infants with defects. Nursing Research, 23 (2), Mar/Apr 1974, 133–137.

21 Mercer, R. T. Two fathers' early responses to the birth of a daughter with a defect. Maternal-Child Nursing Journal, 3 (2), Summer 1974, 77–86.

22 Mitchell, R. G. Chronic handicap in childhood: its implications for family and community. Practitioner, 211, Dec 1973, 763–768.

23 Mother and Child Parental reactions to the birth of a handicapped child. Mother and Child, 46 (1), Feb 1974, 4–5.

24 Parfit, J. Cardiac disorders, diabetes and haemophilia in children. [Practical and psychological support for parents.] Health and Social Service Journal, 83, 24 Nov 1973, 2751.

25 Stanko, B. Crisis intervention after the birth of a defective child. Canadian Nurse, 69 (7), Jul 1973, 27–28.

26 Voysey, M. A constant burden: the reconstitution of family life. [Care of disabled child.] Routledge and Kegan Paul, 1975.

27 Wertheimer, A. Combating social handicap. [Parents form a group to give social contacts to their handicapped children.] Mind and Mental Health Magazine, Autumn 1972, 36–44.

28 Wickes, I. G. The malformed infant and his parents. Nursing Mirror, 132, 26 Feb 1971, 24–26.

d HOSPITALS AND UNITS
(Includes chronic sick)

1 Cartwright, R. Physical treatment of the handicapped child at Chailey Heritage. Nursing Mirror, 140, 9 Jan 1975, 57–61.

2 Hardwick, R. O. F. Twyford House. A specially designed unit for the care of the younger disabled person. Royal Society of Health Journal, 94 (1), Feb 1974, 30–32.

3 Hill, E. Mabel Liddiard Memorial Lecture. Eye on morbidity. [Study of handicapped children at the Care and Assessment Unit, East Birmingham Hospital, in order to determine the causes of morbidity.] Midwives Chronicle, 86, Oct 1972, 322–325.

4 Hudson, M. Children unwelcome at home. [Children in long-stay hospitals.] General Practitioner, 8 Jan 1971, 22–23.

5 Kelly, J. and Boxall, N. Not so much a unit – more an aid to life. A report on the Coventry Paediatric Assessment Unit by two nursery nurses. Nursery Journal, 62, Sep 1972, 2–5.

6 Maclennan, W. J. The young chronic sick at home and in hospital. Health Bulletin, 30 (2), Apr 1972, 110–119.

7 Miller, E. J. and Gwynne, G. V. A life apart: a pilot study of residential institutions for the physically handicapped and the young chronic sick. Tavistock, 1972.

8 Nursing Mirror A symposium from Chailey Heritage [Craft School and Hospital] Sussex, on the treatment, rehabilitation and education of the handicapped child. Nursing Mirror, 140, 9 Jan 1975, 45–70.

9 Oswin, M. The empty hours: a study of the week-end life of handicapped children in institutions. Allen Lane, 1971.

10 Oswin, M. Society at work. Hospital children. [Chronically handicapped long stay hospital children.] New Society, 22, 7 Dec 1972, 576–577.

11 Oswin, M. When a child is left. [Parental visiting of chronically handicapped children in hospital.] New Society, 28, 9 May 1974, 317–318.

12 Quibell, E. P. Introduction and assessment. [Chailey Heritage Craft School and Hospital.] Nursing Mirror, 140, 9 Jan 1975, 45–48.

13 Quibell, E. P. Reed Cottage – parents' accommodation [at Chailey Heritage hospital for the handicapped]. Nursing Mirror, 140 (2), 9 Jan 1975, 70.

14 Ring, N. Rehabilitation engineering [at Chailey Heritage hospital for handicapped children]. Nursing Mirror, 140, 9 Jan 1975, 61–65.

15 Robertson, J. and Robertson, J. The importance of substitute mothering for the long-stay child. [Abridged version of a paper given at a DHSS day conference for senior staff from long stay hospitals.] Health and Social Service Journal, 84, 20 Apr 1974, 878–879.

16 Smith, K. E. Nursing care at Chailey Heritage. [Hospital for handicapped children.] Nursing Mirror, 140, 9 Jan 1975, 51–53.

17 Steele, D. The younger disabled. Ward development and organization of activities. [Younger Disabled Unit, Poole Hospital, Nunthorpe.] Nursing Mirror, 138, 14 Jun 1974, 68–69.

18 Stobart, I. Nursing care in the admission/assessment unit. [At Chailey Heritage hospital for handicapped children.] Nursing Mirror, 140, 9 Jan 1975, 53–55.

19 Vernon, B. Queen Mary's Hospital School. [The education of long-stay patients in Queen Mary's Hospital for Children, Carshalton.] British Hospital Journal and Social Service Review, 82, 16 Sep 1972, 2075.

20 Williams, B. T. and Lambourne, A. The younger chronic sick: how many beds? British Journal of Preventive and Social Medicine, 27 (2), May 1973, 129–136.

21 Younger chronic sick unit. [Hamlet House, St. Francis House, Dulwich.] Hospital and Health Services Review, 71 (11), Nov 1975, 394–395.

e CYSTIC FIBROSIS

1 Airlie, M. Cystic fibrosis. [Nursing care study.] New Zealand Nursing Journal, 67 (1), Jan 1974, 12–14.

2 Batten, J. Cystic fibrosis in adolescents and adults. Physiotherapy, 61 (8), Aug 1975, 247–248.

3 Brimblecombe, F. S. W. and Chamberlain, J. Screening for cystic fibrosis. Lancet, 2, 22 Dec 1973, 1428–1431.

4 Burnette, B. A. Family adjustment to cystic fibrosis. American Journal of Nursing, 75 (11), Nov 1975, 1986–1989.

5 Burton, L. Caring for children with cystic fibrosis. Practitioner, 210, Feb 1973, 247–254.

6 Burton, L. Cystic fibrosis – a challenge to family strength. Health Visitor, 46 (6), Jun 1973, 186–189.

7 Burton, L. and others The strain of a sick child. [Cystic fibrosis and genetic advice to parents.] New Society, 27, 3 Jan 1974, 13–15.

8 Carter, C. O. Genetics and incidence of cystic fibrosis. Physiotherapy, 61 (8), Aug 1975, 240–242.

9 Gaskell, D. Physiotherapy for adolescents and adults with cystic fibrosis. Physiotherapy, 61 (8), Aug 1975, 250–252.

10 Hodge, G. J. Physiotherapy for children with cystic fibrosis. Physiotherapy, 61 (8), Aug 1975, 248–249.

11 Holzel, A. The quest for the basic defect in cystic fibrosis. Physiotherapy, 61 (8), Aug 1978, 238–239.

12 Lancet Genetic counselling for cystic fibrosis. [Leading article.] Lancet, 2, 21 Jul 1973, 137–138.

13 Lawson, M. Nutrition and the child with cystic fibrosis. Nutrition, 25 (3), Autumn 1971, 141–147.

14 McCrae, W. M. Emotional problems in cystic fibrosis. Physiotherapy, 61 (8), Aug 1975, 252–254.

15 McCrae, W. M. and Cull, A. M. Cystic fibrosis: parents' response to the genetic basis of the disease. Lancet, 2, 21 Jul 1973, 141–143.

16 Marcotte, A. A. Cystic fibrosis. Canadian Nurse, 71 (7), Jul 1975, 33–37.

17 Mearns, M. B. Inhalation therapy of cystic fibrosis. Physiotherapy, 61 (8), Aug 1975, 244–246.

18 Milner, A. D. Physiotherapy in cystic fibrosis. Maternal and Child Care, 9, Feb/Mar 1972, 30–31.

19 Noakes, S. Nursing care study. Sally – a child with cystic fibrosis. Nursing Times, 71, 5 Jun 1975, 876–877.

20 Norman, A. P. Cystic fibrosis. Health Magazine, 11 (2), Summer/Autumn 1974, 5–7.

21 Norman, A. P. Medical management of cystic fibrosis. Physiotherapy, 61 (8), Aug 1975, 242–244.

22 Pugh, R. J. Cystic fibrosis. Nursing Times, 68, 17 Feb 1972, 209–211.

23 Rodgers, B. and others A screening tool to detect psychosocial adjustment of children with cystic fibrosis. [Clinical assessment by a pediatric nurse practitioner.] Nursing Research, 23 (5), Sep/Oct 1974, 420–426.

f SPINA BIFIDA AND HYDROCEPHALUS

1 Allum, N. Spina bifida: the treatment and care of spina bifida in children. Allen and Unwin, 1975.

2 Aylett, M. J. Spina bifida in general practice. Practitioner, 211, Jul 1973, 75–81.

3 Boothman, R. Some observations on the management of the child with spina bifida. British Medical Journal, 1, 18 Jan 1975, 145–146.

4 Bradley, R. A spina bifida baby. Nursing Times, 68, 3 Feb 1972, 145–147.

5 Braney, M. L. The child with hydrocephalus. American Journal of Nursing, 73 (5), May 1973, 828–831.

6 Burman, D. and others The Bristol Spina Bifida Centre. Hospital and Health Services Review, 68 (12), Dec 1972, 443–445.

7 Colliss, V. Myelomeningocele. Nursing care. Nursing Times, 69, 8 Feb 1973, 174–175.

8 Corcoran, R. The enigma of anencephaly and spina bifida. Midwife, Health Visitor and Community Nurse, 11 (7), Jul 1975, 211–213.

9 Cordingly, S. Myelomeningocele: social problems. Nursing Times, 69, 8 Feb 1973, 175–176.

10 Eckstein, H. B. and Colliss, V. Myelomeningocele – the implications for the district nurse. Queen's Nursing Journal, 16 (8), Nov 1973, 177–178.

11 Ellis, H. L. Parental involvement in the decision to treat spina bifida cystica. British Medical Journal, 1, 2 Mar 1974, 369–372.

12 Foster, M. Towards independence in spina bifida children. British Journal of Occupational Therapy, 38 (10), Oct 1975, 220–221.

13 Hunt, G. M. Implications of the treatment of myelomeningocele of the child and his family. Lancet, 2, 8 Dec 1973, 1308–1310.

14 Ineichen, R. Towards co-ordinated care of spina bifida children. Social Work Today, 4, 23 Aug 1973, 321–324.

15 Isler, C. Compression. Promising new treatment for hydrocephalus. RN Magazine, 37 (7), Jul 1974, 45–47.

16 Kapila, L. Myelomeningocele. Surgical aspects. Nursing Times, 69, 8 Feb 1973, 172–174.

17 Kavalier, F. Hidden dangers in a blighted potato. [Investigation by Dr. James Renwick.] Nursing Times, 69, 8 Feb 1973, 177.

18 Lancet Ethics of selective treatment of spina bifida. Report of a working party. Lancet, 1, 11 Jan 1975, 84–88.

19 Lancet Towards the prevention of spina bifida [by amniocentesis]. Lancet, 1, 11 May 1974, 907.

20 Laurence, K. M. Effect of early surgery for spina bifida cystica on survival and quality of life. Lancet, 1, 23 Feb 1974, 301–304.

21 Lorber, J. Management of spina bifida cystica. 1. Clinical types of spina bifida. Nursing Mirror, 137, 12 Oct 1973, 21–23.

22 Lorber, J. Management of spina bifida cystica. 2. Initial management of the treated child. Nursing Mirror, 137, 19 Oct 1973, 33–35, 37.

23 Lorber, J. Management of spina bifida cystica. 3. Follow up care and further treatment. Nursing Mirror, 137, 26 Oct 1973, 35–37.

24 Lorber, J. Myelomeningocele. New approaches to its management. Nursing Times, 70, 21 Feb 1974, 272–273.

25 Lorber, J. Spina bifida cystica. Part 1. Incidence, causes and prevention. Midwife and Health Visitor, 10 (12), Dec 1974, 371–374.

26 Lorber, J. Spina bifida cystica. 2. Policy of management of the newborn with myelocele related to ultimate prognosis. Midwife, Health Visitor and Community Nurse, 11 (1), Jan 1975, 18–19.

27 Nettles, O. Aids to mobility: for children with spina bifida and hydrocephalus. District Nursing, 15 (5), Aug 1972, 92–93.

28 Nursing Times Spina bifida and anencephaly. [Further studies on potato blight in Ireland, disproving Dr. James Renwick's theory.] Nursing Times, 70, 7 Nov 1974, 1745.

29 Parsch, K. and Koch, F. A team approach to spina bifida. Rehabilitation, no. 93, Apr/Jun 1975, 29–32.

30 Passo, S. D. Outcomes of neurosurgical care for the myelomeningocele child and his family. Journal of Neurosurgical Nursing, 6 (2), Dec 1974, 122–126.

31 Passo, S. D. Positioning infants with myelomeningocele. American Journal of Nursing, 74 (9), Sep 1974, 1658–1660.

32 Renwick, J. H. Spina bifida, anencephaly and the potato's home made antibiotics. [Summary of an article which appeared in the British Journal of Social and Preventive Medicine, May 1972.] Nursing Times, 68, 19 Oct 1972, 1323.

33 Rose, G. K. and others Splintage for spina bifida cystica. Nursing Mirror, 133, 20 Aug 1971, 20–23.

34 Rowland, M. Evaluation of play group children with spina bifida. Social Work Today, 4 (11), 23 Aug 1973, 324–325, 327–330.

35 Taylor, M. A. The spina bifida child. New Zealand Nursing Journal, 66 (12), Dec 1973, 11–14.

36 Tew, B. and Laurence, K. M. Some sources of stress found in mothers of spina bifida children. British Journal of Preventive and Social Medicine, 29 (1), Mar 1975, 27–30.

37 Webster, B. M. Spina bifida. District Nursing, 14 (2), May 1971, 31–33.

50 MENTALLY HANDICAPPED CHILDREN

a GENERAL AND NURSING

1 Anstice, E. One of the family. [Family unit for mentally subnormal children at St. Lawrence's Hospital, Caterham.] Nursing Times, 69, 22 Feb 1973, 244–247.

2 Balthazar, E. E. and others Behavior changes in mentally retarded children following the initiation of an experimental nursing program. Nursing Research, 20 (1), Jan/Feb 1971, 69–77.

3 Carr, J. and others Rehabilitation in Camberwell. [Hilda Lewis House, a hospital unit for severely retarded children.] Nursing Mirror, 139, 14 Nov 1974, 49–52.

4 Davis, S. Nursing care study. Daniel, a developing child. [A severely mentally and physically handicapped boy with Apert's syndrome.] Nursing Times, 70, 18 Apr 1974, 588–589.

5 Densein, E. H. Care of the retarded. [Psychopaedic nursing.] New Zealand Nursing Journal, 66 (2), Feb 1973, 4–7.

6 Department of Health and Social Security Study Group Mentally handicapped children in residential homes: report. HMSO, 1974.

7 Dybwad, G. The mentally handicapped child under five. National Society for Mentally Handicapped Children, 1973.

8 Frew, R. and Peckham, C. Mental retardation: a national study. [The work of the National Child Development Study.] British Hospital Journal and Social Service Review, 82, 16 Sep 1972, 2070–2072.

9 Geiger, J. K. and others Head hitting in severely retarded children: nursing strategies based on behavioral modification. American Journal of Nursing, 74 (10), Oct 1974, 1822–1825.

10 Grover, V. M. The meaning of care for young children in institutions for the mentally retarded. SA Nursing Journal, 42 (5), May 1975, 7–9.

11 Hardley, P. Short-term care for mentally handicapped children. [Hill House Hospital, Rye.] Nursing Mirror, 132, 16 Apr 1971, 34–39.

12 Hughes, N. A. S. Help for mentally handicapped babies through developmental physiotherapy. Mother and Child, 44 (1), Jan/Feb 1972, 11–15.

13 Jennings, A. N. Nursing retarded children in Marsden Hospital. Lamp, 30 (3), Mar 1973, 29–32.

14 Kendall, A. and Moss, P. Integration or segregation? The future of education and residential services for mentally handicapped children. Campaign for the Mentally Handicapped, 1972. (CMH discussion paper, no. 1.)

15 Kerkham, G. Nursing care study. A question of care. [A mentally retarded child.] Nursing Mirror, 137, 31 Aug 1973, 38–40.

16 Kirman, B. H. The mentally handicapped child. Nelson, 1972.

17 Locksway House Mentally handicapped children in the southern half of Portsmouth are catered for in this modern residential unit. Nursing Mirror, 133, 17 Dec 1971, 20–23.

18 Maternal and Child Care Residential needs of the mentally handicapped. [Child.] Maternal and Child Care, 8 (75), Dec 1971/Jan 1972, 3–5.

19 Parfit, J. Spotlight on physical and mental assessment. National Children's Bureau, 1971.

20 Peters, C. Nursing care study. Tuberous sclerosis. [In a six year old child.] Nursing Times, 69, 29 Nov 1973, 1603–1604.

21 Pinewood – teaching the handicapped to be self-reliant. [Adventure playground.] Health and Social Service Journal, 85, 30 Aug 1975, 1912–1913.

22 Raeden Centre New assessment centre for children. [The Raeden Centre in Aberdeen for children suspected of delayed development.] Nursing Mirror, 139, 12 Aug 1974, 49.

23 Rose, V. Preparing for a richer, happier life. [Lufton Manor rural training unit for mentally handicapped boys.] Nursing Mirror, 141, 31 Jul 1975, 70–71.

24 Ross, G. Duston ward. [Ward for mentally handicapped children at Princess Marina Hospital, Northampton.] Nursing Times, 69, 6 Dec 1973, 1669.

25 Royds, E. Riding and mental handicap. [Work of the National Society for Mentally Handicapped Children Riding Fund.] Nursing Mirror, 141, 25 Sep 1975, 52–54.

26 Sears, M. and Sylvester, P. E. Home transport for long-stay children. [Scheme at St. Lawrence's Hospital, Caterham, in which subnormal children go home at weekends.] British Hospital Journal and Social Service Review, 82, 29 Apr 1972, 939–940.

27 Solly, K. The different baby. National Society for Mentally Handicapped Children, 1972.

28 Spencer, D. A. Attitudes of relatives of mentally handicapped persons. [Letter.] British Medical Journal, 4, 2 Nov 1974, 287.

29 Taylor, R. An investment for the future: caring for the handicapped child. Nursing Times, 69, 14 Jun 1973, 766–768.

30 Williams, C. and Price, M. Early days: the initial moves in establishing a ward based token system for severely subnormal children. Kidderminster: Institute of Mental Subnormality, 1973.

31 Wood, E. The Wild Boy of Aveyron. ['Itard's syndrome'? Contribution made by Itard to the teaching of mentally handicapped.] Nursing Mirror, 140, 1 May 1975, 61–63.

32 Woolley, E. Nursing care study. Polly – mental deficiency and schizophrenia. Nursing Times, 69, 6 Dec 1973, 1636–1637.

33 Wright, E. C. and others A study of the interactions between nursing staff and profoundly mentally retarded children. [At Queen Mary's Hospital for Children, Carshalton.] British Journal of Mental Subnormality, 20, Part 1, Jun 1974, 14–17. (Letter from J. Coombes and authors' reply 20, Dec 1974, 100–103.)

b FAMILY

1 Brown, L. K. and Smith, J. Group for mothers: a descriptive account of group work with mothers of mentally handicapped children. Social Work Today, 3 (10), Aug 1972, 15–17.

2 Bush, T. E. C. Nobody's child. [Mentally handicapped children rejected by their parents.] Nursing Mirror, 137, 14 Sep 1973, 12–13.

3 Dyer, B. Every Sunday, 2 to 4 p.m. [A mother's experience of a child in a mental handicap hospital.] New Society, 28, 13 Jun 1974, 633–635.

4 Gallop, M. Involving the parents. [Scheme for parents of mentally subnormal children at Little Plumstead Hospital, Norwich.] Nursing Times, 69, 22 Mar 1973, 363–365.

5 Hannam, C. Parents and mentally handicapped children. Harmondsworth: King's Fund Centre Penguin, 1975.

6 Lockett, J. My son John. [A mother's efforts to keep her mentally handicapped child out of hospital.] Nursing Times, 68, 13 Jul 1972, 867–871.

7 Lord, D. Parents and mental handicap. Health and Social Service Journal, 83, 10 Mar 1973, 550.

8 Maxwell, J. E. Home care for a retarded child. Nursing Outlook, 19 (2), Feb 1971, 112–114.

9 National Association for Mental Health The birth of an abnormal child: telling the parents. Report of a working party. Lancet, 2, 13 Nov 1971, 1075–1077.

10 National Society for Mentally Handicapped Children Stress in families with a mentally handicapped child: a report of a working party. New ed. The Society, 1974. (Subnormality in the seventies no. 9.)

11 Price, J. L. and Buchan, L. G. Counselling parents of the mentally retarded: a function of public health nursing. Health Visitor, 47 (12), Dec 1974, 358–359.

12 Ross, J. When support is needed. [National Society for Mentally Handicapped Children service of voluntary welfare visitors to help parents.] Social Service Quarterly, 49 (2), Oct/Dec 1975, 53–55.

13 Smiley, C. W. Feelings and reactions of parents to their retarded child. Occupational Therapy, 38 (2), Feb 1975, 29.

14 Stutz, S. D. Retarded children: they can't say where they hurt. [A mother's view of problems encountered by nurses.] RN Magazine, 38 (7), Jul 1975, 28–29.

c DOWN'S SYNDROME

1 Belton, M. Neither a 'Mongol' nor an 'Idiot'. [Report of a lecture given by Mr. R. Brinkworth on the advances in the treatment of children with Down's syndrome.] Health Visitor, 48 (3), Mar 1975, 87.

2 Brinkworth, R. The unfinished child: early treatment and training for the infant with Down's syndrome. Royal Society of Health Journal, 95 (2), Apr 1975, 73–78.

3 Carr, J. Young children with Down's syndrome: their development and effect on their families. Butterworth, 1975. (IRMMH monograph 4.)

4 Donovan, V. M. Nursing care study. Rosie. [A three-year old child with Down's syndrome.] Nursing Times, 70, 16 May 1974, 738–739.

5 Durand, B. A clinical nursing study. Failure to thrive in a child with Down's syndrome. Nursing Research, 24 (4), Jul/Aug 1975, 272–286.

6 Emanuel, I. and others Accelerated ageing in young mothers of children with Down's syndrome. Lancet, 2, 19 Aug 1972, 361–363.

7 Greet, D. J. Nursing care study. Brian – a young man with Down's syndrome. Nursing Times, 71, 21 Aug 1975, 1325–1327.

8 Griffith, G. W. The 'prevention' of Down's syndrome. Health Trends, 5 (3), Aug 1973, 59–60.

9 Hawks, D. H. The retarded. 'It's a crime not to care.' [A nurse helps an emotionally retarded child.] RN Magazine, 38 (11), Nov 1975, 62–63, 67, 71.

10 Hyde, N. Behavior therapy and therapy in mental retardation. [Case study of a 26 year old girl with Down's syndrome.] American Journal of Nursing, 74 (5), May 1974, 882–886.

11 Ingalls, T. H. Maternal health and mongolism. Lancet, 2, 29 Jul 1972, 213–215.

12 Marais, E. Society at work. John the painter. [A boy with Down's syndrome.] New Society, 31, 30 Jan 1975, 258–259.

13 Mind/National Association for Mental Health Your mongol baby. The Association, 1972.

14 Mori, W. 'My child has Down's syndrome'. American Journal of Nursing, 73 (8), Aug 1973, 1386–1387.

15 Murphy, A. and Pueschel, S. M. Early intervention with families of newborns with Down's syndrome. Maternal-Child Nursing Journal, 4 (1), Spring 1975, 1–7.

16 Musset, A. The untrodden ways: the story of Lucy. Gollancz, 1975.

17 Smith, D. W. and Wilson, A. A. The child with Down's syndrome (mongolism): causes, characteristics and acceptance, for parents, physicians and persons concerned with his education and care. Philadelphia: Saunders, 1973.

18 Smith, W. W. Judith: teaching our mongol baby. National Society for Mentally Handicapped Children, 1975.

19 Stein, Z. and others Screening programme for prevention of Down's syndrome. Lancet, 1, 10 Feb 1973, 305–310.

20 Wilks, J. and Wilks, E. Bernard: bringing up our mongol son. Routledge and Kegan Paul, 1974.

d PHENYLKETONURIA

1 Cox, A. W. and others Children with phenylketonuria: crisis prevention or crisis intervention? [The involvement of nursing in a multidisciplinary treatment program.] Maternal-Child Nursing Journal, 3 (3), Fall 1974, 157–168.

2 Hawcroft, J. and Hudson, F. P. Screening for phenylketonuria in the United Kingdom. Health Trends, 6, Nov 1974, 72–74.

3 Holton, J. and Tyfield, L. The child with phenylketonuria. National Society for Mentally Handicapped Children, 1974.

4 Hudson, F. P. Phenylketonuria. [Development of screening.] Nursing Times, 71, 1 May 1975, 687–689.

5 Hudson, F. P. Phenylketonuria. A filmstrip photographed at Alder Hey Children's Hospital, Liverpool. [Illustrations only.] Nursing Mirror, 137, 5 Oct 1973, 24–27.

6 Justice, P. and Smith, G. F. PKU – Phenylketonuria. American Journal of Nursing, 75 (8), Aug 1975, 1303–1305.

7 Smith, I. and Wolff, O. H. Natural history of phenylketonuria and influence of early treatment. Lancet, 2, 7 Sep 1974, 540–544.

8 Starr, D. J. T. The collection of Guthrie test samples. [Neonatal testing for PKU.] Midwife and Health Visitor, 7 (7), Jul 1971, 271–275.

9 Stevenson, J. S. and Kennedy, R. The Guthrie test for phenylketonuria and allied diseases in Scotland in 1965–1973. Health Bulletin, 32 (6), Nov 1974, 245–249.

51 CHILD WELFARE

a GENERAL AND DEPRIVATION

1 Bowley, A. H. Children at risk: the basic needs of children in the world today. Edinburgh: Churchill Livingstone, 1975.

2 Brearley, P. The deprivation syndrome: an examination of some theoretical approaches to the effects of deprivation on the behaviour of older and younger people. Nursing Times, 71, 27 Nov 1975, 1914–1915.

3 Elliston, L. The formative years. [Cycle of deprivation and adoptive grandparents.] Health and Social Service Journal, 83, 18 Aug 1973, 1859.

4 Hirksyj, P. Nursing care study. Naomi – a case of neglect. [A deprived child.] Nursing Mirror, 139, 14 Nov 1974, 83–84.

5 Joseph, Sir K. The cycle of deprivation. [Speech given at the Annual Conference of the National Association for Maternal and Child Welfare.] Lancet, 2, 7 Jul 1973, 53.

6 Lewin, D. The cycle of deprivation. The author, 1975.

7 Moore, J. G. Yo-yo children. [Children caught between the quarrels of their parents.] Nursing Times, 70, 5 Dec 1974, 1888–1889.

8 Schrock, R. A. For the love of money. [Child welfare legislation as an example of the achievement of social reform.] Nursing Times, 70, 20 Jun 1974, Occ. papers, 25–28.

9 Starte, G. D. The poor communicating two year old and his family. [A survey showing correlation between delayed language development and psychosocial deprivation.] Journal of the Royal College of General Practitioners, 25, Dec 1975, 880–887.

10 Stone, R. All our children. [Home care for children of drug addicts.] Journal of Practical Nursing, 24 (12), Dec 1974, 18–19.

b FOSTERING AND ADOPTION

1 Andrews, C. Whose responsibility? – parent, foster parent or local authority? (c) A child's right to his own family. Royal Society of Health Journal, 95 (5), Oct 1975, 264–269.

2 Association of British Adoption Agencies The adopted person's need for information about his background. The Association, 1972.

3 Donley, K. Adoption for children with special needs: philosophy and methods. Social Work Today, 5, 27 Jun 1974, 194–197.

4 Fletcher, M. Short-stay foster parents. Social Work Today, 4, 7 Feb 1974, 698–700.

5 Hartnell, M. The professional foster parent. [Pilot scheme in Reading.] Health and Social Service Journal, 84, 20 Jul 1974, 1628–1629.

6 Home Office. Research Unit and Social Survey Division of the Office of Population Censuses and Surveys A survey of adoption in Great Britain, by Eleanor Grey and Ronald M. Blunden. HMSO, 1971. (Research studies 10.)

7 Lafferty, M. Operation orphan. [Treating Vietnamese orphans at Fairfield Hospital, Melbourne.] Australian Nurses' Journal, 5 (5), Nov 1975, 24–30.

8 Mattingly, R. Adoption and the Children Bill. Nursing Mirror, 141, 27 Nov 1975, 69–71.

9 Orriss, H. The problems of fostering. Nursing Mirror, 140, 13 Mar 1975, 60–61.

10 Robinson, J. An experience of fostering. Social Work Today, 4, 3 May 1973, 85–86.

11 Robinson, W. The Ockenden venture. [Keffolds House, provides nursing care for Vietnamese orphans.] Nursing Mirror, 140, 5 Jun 1975, 40–42.

12 Seglow, J. and others Growing up adopted: a long-term national study of adopted children and their families, Slough: National Foundation for Education Research in England and Wales. (A report by the National Children's Bureau.)

13 Thorpe, R. Mum and Mrs So and So. The situation of the long term foster child with regard to his natural parents. Social Work Today, 4, 7 Feb 1974, 691–695.

14 Triseliotos, J. In search of origins: the experience of adopted people. Routledge and Kegan Paul, 1973.

c NON-ACCIDENTAL INJURY

1 Baker, H. A question of witness. [Battered child syndrome.] Nursing Times, 67, 10 Jun 1971, 691–694.

2 Ballard, C. Reaching out to the community – unique program prevents child abuse/neglect. [Presbyterian Medical Centre, Pennsylvania.] Pediatric Nursing, 1 (5), Sep/Oct 1975, 31–33.

3 Bassett, L. B. How to help abused children – and their parents. RN Magazine, 37 (10), Oct 1974, 44–46, 48, 50, 52, 54, 57–58, 60.

4 Bird, H. Battered babies – a social and medical problem. Nursing Times, 69, 22 Nov 1973, 1552–1554.

5 Bluglass, R. Parents with emotional problems. [Battered baby syndrome.] Maternal and Child Care, 7, Jul/Aug 1971, 62–64; Nursing Times, 67, 12 Aug 1971, 1000–1001.

6 British Medical Journal Experts and child abuse. [Leading article on the failure of the experts in the Maria Colwell case.] British Medical Journal, 3, 14 Sep 1974, 641–642.

7 British Paediatric Association Non-accidental injury in children. Introductory comment from BPA and

BAPS and a guide on management prepared by a working party in the Department of Child Care, University of Newcastle upon Tyne. British Medical Journal, 4, 15 Dec 1973, 656–660.

8 Cameron, J. M. The battered baby. Nursing Mirror, 134, 9 Jun 1972, 32–38.

9 Carter, B. D. and others Mental health nursing intervention with child abusing and neglecting mothers. [A study to investigate the effectiveness of nursing intervention.] Journal of Psychiatric Nursing and Mental Health Services, 13 (5), Sep/Oct 1975, 11–15.

10 Carter, J. editor The maltreated child. Priory Press, (Care and Welfare Library, 1974.)

11 Castle, B. Maria Colwell. Extracts from a statement by Mrs. Barbara Castle, Secretary of State for Social Services, following publication of the Maria Colwell Report. Queen's Nursing Journal, 17 (7), Oct 1974, 155.

12 Castle, R. L. and Kerr, A. M. A study of suspected child abuse. National Society for the Prevention of Cruelty to Children, Battered Child Research Department, 1972.

13 Corey, E. J. B. and others Factors contributing to child abuse. [A study of hospitalized battered and non-battered children.] Nursing Research, 24 (4), Jul/Aug 1975, 293–295.

14 Court, J. The battered child syndrome. 1. The need for a multi-disciplinary approach. Nursing Times, 67, 3 Jun 1971, 659–661.

15 Court, J. and Kerr, A. The battered child syndrome. 2. A preventable disease? Nursing Times, 67, 10 Jun 1971, 695–698.

16 Davies, J. M. Detection and prevention. [Symposium on the battered child.] Nursing Mirror, 140, 12 Jun 1975, 56–57.

17 Department of Health and Social Security Non-accidental injury to children. Circular LASSL (14) 13. The Department, 1974. Department of Health and Social Security. Non-accidental injury to children: proceedings of a conference . . . 19 June 1974. HMSO, 1975.

18 Department of Health and Social Security Committee of Inquiry into the Care and Supervision Provided in Relation to Maria Colwell. Report. HMSO, 1974. Chairman: T. G. Field-Fisher.

19 Department of Health and Social Security Committee of Inquiry into the provision and Co-ordination of Services to the family of John George Auckland. Report. HMSO, 1975. Chairman: P. J. M. Kennedy.

20 Ealing Battered Baby Conference Proceedings of a one day conference organized by the Health Department of the London Borough of Ealing, November 1973. Edsall, 1973. Chairman: Dr. Ian Seppelt.

21 Fairburn, A. and Jones, S. Society at work. Beta 5 and battering. [Monitoring of children at risk in Bath.] New Society, 33, 31 Jul 1975, 249–250.

22 Follis, P. Recognising non-accidental injury in children. [The work of an accident consultant at the Royal Infirmary, Preston.] Nursing Times, 71, 18 Dec 1975, 2034–2035.

23 Ford, D. The law. [Symposium on the battered child.] Nursing Mirror, 140, 12 Jun 1975, 58.

24 Franklin, A. W. editor Concerning child abuse: papers presented by the Tunbridge Wells Study Group on non-accidental injury to children. Edinburgh: Livingstone, 1975.

25 Franklin, A. W. editor Non-accidental injury to children: report and resolutions [of the] Tunbridge Wells Study Group, 1973.

26 Gray, J. Hospital based battered child team. Hospitals, 47 (4), 16 Feb 1973, 50–52.

27 Howells, J. G. Remember Maria. Butterworth, 1974.

28 Hyman, C. A. and Mitchell, R. A psychological study of child battering. [Summary of investigation by the National Advisory Centre on the Battered Child.] Health Visitor, 48 (8), Aug 1975, 294–296.

29 Jackson, A. Court procedures in child abuse. Midwife, Health Visitor and Community Nurse, 11 (10), Oct 1975, 329, 331–332.

30 Josten, L. The treatment of an abused family. [Nursing intervention.] Maternal-Child Nursing Journal, 4 (1), Spring 1975, 23–33.

31 Kalisch, B. J. Nursing actions on behalf of the battered child. Nursing Forum, 12 (4), 1973, 365–377.

32 Kempe, C. H. and Helfer, R. H. Helping the battered child and his family. Philadelphia: Lippincott, 1972.

33 Kempe, C. H. and Helfer, R. H. editors The battered child. 2nd ed. Chicago: Chicago University Press, 1974.

34 Learoyd, S. and Williamson, A. Nursing care. [Symposium on the battered child.] Nursing Mirror, 140, 12 Jun 1975, 54–55.

35 Lynch, M. A. Ill-health and child abuse. [Survey to compared abused children with non-abused siblings showing abnormal pregnancy and labour, separation and illnesses in parent or child affected parents' attitudes.] Lancet, 2, 16 Aug 1975, 317–319.

36 Mitchell, B. Working with abusive parents: a caseworker's view. American Journal of Nursing, 73 (3), Mar 1973, 480–482.

37 Mowat, A. P. The battered baby syndrome. District Nursing, 14 (2), May 1971, 26–27.

38 Mundle, G. E. and Fontana, V. J. Child abuse: our responsibility. Journal of Practical Nursing, 24 (12), Dec 1974, 14–17.

39 National Society for the Prevention of Cruelty to Children Yo yo children: a study of 23 violent matrimonial cases. The Society, 1974.

40 Norman, M. A lifeline for battering parents. [The role of the health visitor in reducing cases of child abuse.] Nursing Times, 70, 26 Sep 1974, 1506–1507.

41 Nursing Mirror A symposium on battered children. Nursing Mirror, 140, 12 Jun 1975, 47–58.

42 Nursing Times Theory and practice. [Failure of communication between health and social services in child abuse with reference to Lisa Godfrey.] Nursing Times, 71, 1 May 1975, 678.

43 Orriss, H. D. Lessons from a tragedy. [The Maria Colwell case, and lessons to be learnt from it in social service departments.] Nursing Times, 70, 31 Jan 1974, 140–141.

44 Page, G. Nursing care study. Detection of child abuse. Nursing Mirror, 141, 18 Sep 1975, 53–54.

45 Parker, R. Maria Colwell: the lessons. New Society, 29, 12 Sep 1974, 673–674.

46 Renvoize, J. Children in danger: the causes and prevention of baby battering. Routledge and Kegan Paul, 1974.

47 Royal College of Midwives Non-accidental injury to children. [Comments to DHSS.] Midwives Chronicle, 88, Nov 1975, 380.

48 Royal Society of Health After care needs of battering mothers. [Community nursing session of RSH Conference.] Community Medicine, 128 (3), 5 May 1972, 80.

49 Savino, A. B. and Sanders, R. W. Working with abusive parents: group therapy and home visits. American Journal of Nursing, 73 (3), Mar 1973, 482–484.

50 Smith, S. M. The battered child syndrome. Butterworth, 1975.

51 Smith, S. M. The battered child syndrome – some research findings. [Symposium report.] Nursing Mirror, 140, 12 Jun 1975, 48–53.

52 Smith, S. and Noble, S. Battered children and their parents. New Society, 26, 15 Nov 1973, 393–395.

53 Stainton, M. C. Non-accidental trauma in children. Canadian Nurse, 71 (10), Oct 1975, 26–29.

54 Tunbridge Wells Study Group Non-accidental injury to children. [Resolutions passed at a meeting.] British Medical Journal, 4, 13 Oct 1973, 96–97.

55 Wild, D. Baby battering and its prevention. Midwives Chronicle, 85, Jul 1971, 242–244.

d NURSERIES, PLAYGROUPS, CHILD MINDERS

1 Bamford, T. Play material for the first five years. Health Visitor, 48 (9), Sep 1975, 338, 341–342; (10), Oct 1975, 384–386.

2 Barber, R. M. Report on the setting up of a nursery class in the county of Northumberland 1950–1972. Health Visitor, 45 (6), Jun 1972, 164–166.

3 Bessell, R. Playgroups – a unique contribution to family and society. Health and Social Service Journal, 85, 2 Aug 1975, 1668–1669.

4 Carpenter, E. M. An assessment playgroup in an occupational therapy department. Occupational Therapy, 36 (2), Feb 1973, 129–137.

5 Connolly, M. M. Day care for children. (b) A nurse's view. Royal Society of Health Journal, 95 (5), Oct 1975, 233–234.

6 Chaplin, J. B. Day care for children. (a) The social worker's role in day care. Royal Society of Health Journal, 95 (5), Oct 1975, 229–232.

7 Holman, R. You and research. Day care for the under fives. Social Work Today, 6, 11 Dec 1975, 586–587.

8 Hutton, E. The family day care nurseries of Finland and Sweden. Health Visitor, 47 (12), Dec 1974, 354–355.

9 Jackson, B. The childminders. New Society, 26, 29 Nov 1973, 521–524.

10 Jackson, S. The Childminding Research and Development Unit. Health Visitor, 48 (5), May 1975, 158–160.

11 Jackson, S. The illegal child minders: a report on the growth of unregistered child minding and the West Indian community. Cambridge: Priority Area Children, 1971.

12 Jago, L. Play on adventure playgrounds: an exploratory synthesis of theory and children's activities. Social Work Today, 4, 26 Jul 1973, 257–261.

13 Jones, A. F. Day care in America. [Day nursery schemes.] Health and Social Service Journal, 83, 17 Feb 1973, 364–365.

14 Kerr, K. M. Another look at playgroups. Health Visitor, 46 (9), Sep 1973, 304–305.

15 Knight, B. editor Report of the first National Conference on Childminding, Bradford. April 19, 1975. Cambridge: National Education Research and Development Trust, 1975.

16 Mack, J. The pre-school drive. [Provision of nursery education.] New Society, 34, 4 Dec 1975, 535–537.

17 McKenzie, I. The needs of the smaller child. [Pre-school child.] Health Visitor, 48 (5), May 1975, 160–161.

18 Mawby, R. I. Child-minding and social change. [An historical survey.] Social Service Quarterly, 48 (2), Oct/Dec 1974, 208–211.

19 Parry, W. H. New day nurseries for the city of Nottingham. Medical Officer, 125, 23 Apr 1971, 217–219.

20 Rae, R. The baby demos. [Campaign for creche facilities in colleges.] New Society, 32, 12 Jun 1975, 653.

21 Thayer, P. P. The pre school playgroups association and the social services. Social Work Services, (1), Mar 1973, 10–12.

22 Tyne, M. D. The nurse and nursery planning. Pediatric Nursing, 1 (3), May/Jun 1975, 14–17.

23 Whitton, J. R. Children in an old people's home. [An experimental playgroup for local children at Mossley Hall, Congleton.] Health and Social Service Journal, 84, 2 Feb 1974, 234–235.

24 Wilce, H. Infants in industry. [Industrial day nurseries]. New Society, 20, 22 Jun 1972, 613.

25 Willmott, P. Daily childminders after Seebohm. [Project carried out on a fieldwork instructors' course.] Health Visitor, 46 (8), Aug 1973, 253–254.

26 Willmott, P. Health visitors and pre-school playgroups. Health Visitor, 47 (8), Aug 1974, 250–251.

e HOSPITAL DAY NURSERIES

1 Bodger, K. E. Planning a hospital creche. [Hospital for Sick Children, Great Ormond Street.] Nursing Times, 70, 6 Jun 1974, 871–873.

2 Bodger, K. E. Who needs a creche? [Comment from mothers on the Great Ormond Street Creche.] Nursing Times, 70, 13 Jun 1974, 916–917.

3 Droog, P. M. Day nursery project. [Manchester Royal Infirmary.] Health and Social Service Journal, 85, 18 Oct 1975, 2336–2337.

4 Droog, P. Hospital playgroup. [At Musgrove Park Hospital.] Health and Social Service Journal, 83, 13 Apr 1974, 831–833.

5 Kay, J. Hospital day nurseries, a cost-effectiveness study. Nursing Times, 71, 5 Jun 1975, 898–899.

6 Newman, I. A holiday play group. [For hospital staff in the Tunbridge Wells and Leybourne HMC]. Nursing Times, 69, 31 May 1973, 712.

7 Nursing Times News feature. And now the good news. . . [Day nursery at Manchester Royal Infirmary. Mainly illustrations.] Nursing Times, 71, 16 Oct 1975, 1644.

8 Nursing Times Northern nursery. [Creche in the United Manchester Hospital Group. Mainly illustrations.] Nursing Times, 68, 9 Mar 1972, 278–279.

ELDERLY AND DISABLED

52 ELDERLY AND RETIRED

a GENERAL AND GERIATRICS

1 Abrams, M. The new elderly. [Statistics about the elderly shown in the General Household Survey.] New Society, 32, 26 Jun 1975, 777–778.

2 Agate, J. Geriatrics for nurses and social workers. Heinemann Medical, 1972.

3 American Journal of Nursing Options for the aging. [Six articles.] American Journal of Nursing, 75 (10), Oct 1975, 1799–1815.

4 Anderson, W. F. The elderly at the end of life. Nursing Times, 69, 8 Feb 1973, 193–194.

5 Anderson, W. F. Practical management of the elderly. 2nd ed. Oxford: Blackwell, 1971.

6 Bosanquet, N. New deal for the elderly. Fabian Society, 1975. (Fabian, No. 435.)

7 Bosanquet, N. New deal for the elderly. Nursing Times, 71, 17 Jul 1975, 1121.

8 Brantl, V. M. and Brown, M. R., editors Readings in gerontology. St. Louis: Mosby, 1973.

9 British Medical Journal Medicine in old age: articles published in the British Medical Journal 1973–1974. BMJ, 1974.

10 Brocklehurst, J. C. editor Textbook of geriatric medicine and gerontology. Edinburgh: Churchill. Livingstone, 1973.

11 Bromley, D. Psychological adjustment in late life. Nursing Mirror, 132, 18 Jun 1971, 26–27.

12 Caird, F. I. and Judge, T. G. Assessment of the elderly patient. Pitman Medical, 1974.

13 Cooper, P. Hypnotics and tranquillisers for elderly patients. Midwife and Health Visitor, 8 (11), Nov 1972, 397.

14 Davidson, J. R. Trial of self-medication in the elderly. [For patients about to be discharged.] Nursing Times, 70, 14 Mar 1974, 391–392.

15 Department of Health and Social Security Development Group Social Work Services A life style for the elderly: report of a seminar . . . 18–20 July, 1974. HMSO, 1974.

16 Felstein, I. Living to be a hundred: a study of old age. Newton Abbot: David & Charles, 1973.

17 Foster, H. A. Understanding the senior citizen. Nursing Care, 6 (6), Jun 1973, 27–31.

18 Francis, G. Caring for the elderly. Heinemann, 1973.

19 Gerbauckas, D. A nurse's guide to medications for the geriatric patient. [Includes hypnotics and sedatives.] Journal of Practical Nursing, 21 (8), Aug 1971, 22–25, 30, 34.

20 Gore, I. Thoughts on the problems of ageing. Midwife and Health Visitor, 10 (5), May 1974, 124–126.

21 Harrison, P. Living with old age. New Society, 26, 1 Nov 1973, 265–268.

22 Hayter, J. Biologic changes of aging. Nursing Forum, 13 (3), 1974, 289–308.

23 Hawker, M. Geriatrics for physiotherapists and the allied professions. Faber & Faber, 1974.

24 Hazell, K. Social and medical problems of the elderly. 3rd ed. Hutchinson, 1973.

25 Howell, T. H. Old age: some practical points in geriatrics. 3rd ed. Lewis, 1975.

26 Hyams, D. The care of the aged. Priory Press, 1972. (Care and welfare library.)

27 Isaacs, B. Standing old people on their heads: some thoughts on medical care of the elderly. Community Health, 6 (3), Nov/Dec 1974, 142–144.

28 Isaacs, B. and others Survival of the unfittest: a study of geriatric patients in Glasgow. Routledge & Kegan Paul, 1972.

29 Johnson, M. L. A different normality: the needs and potentialities of older people. Nursing Times, 69, 6 Dec 1973, 1662–1663.

30 Jones, E. H. and others editors Old age. Routledge, 1972. (Themes Series.)

31 Kelly, P. A. An experiment in self-medication for older people. Canadian Nurse, 68 (2), Feb 1972, 41–43.

32 Lefroy, R. B. Geriatric medicine – is it an entity? Australian Nurses' Journal, 3 (11), Jun 1974, 27–29.

33 Manley, G. The biology of ageing. Nursing Times 71, 13 Feb 1975, 246–248.

34 Muhlenkamp, A. F. and others Perception of life change events by the elderly. Nursing Research, 24 (2), Mar–Apr 1975, 109–113.

35 Niland, M. Understanding the elderly. Nursing Forum, 11 (3), 1972, 273–289.

36 Nursing Mirror Open forum. Old age – three viewpoints on a growing problem, by M. Corbally, E. M. Cole and C. Slevin. Nursing Mirror, 133, 10 Sep 1971, 14–15.

37 Rodman, M. J. Drug therapy today. Adjusting medications for the needs of the elderly. RN Magazine, 38 (5), May 1975, 65–89. [13 pages.]

38 Rudd, T. N. Grandparents in the 1970s. Nursing Mirror, 16 Aug 1974, 66–67.

39 Rynerson, B. C. Need for self-esteem in the aged: a literature review. Journal of Psychiatric Nursing, 10 (1), Jan/Feb 1972, 22–26.

40 Schwartz, D. Safe self-medication for elderly outpatients. American Journal of Nursing, 75 (10), Oct 1975, 1808–1810.

41 Williamson, J. Problems of old age in contemporary society. Nursing Times, 67, 4 Mar 1971, 255–257.

42 Wilson, M. Caring for an ageing population: the problem for society. Nursing Times, 69, 12 Apr 1973, 486–488.

b MIDDLE AGE AND RETIREMENT

1 Age Concern National conference on the place of the retired and the elderly in modern society. Mitcham: Age Concern, 1974.

2 American Journal of Nursing Life in the middle years. [Ten articles.] American Journal of Nursing, 75 (10), Oct 1975, 1751–1794.

3 Brown, R. A. 1. Pre-retirement education. 1 and 2. Nursing Times, 69, 29 Mar 1973, 397–398; 69, 5 Apr 1973, 434–436.

4 Buttie, B. Preparation for retirement. Mitcham: Age Concern, 1974. (Manifesto series 20.)

5 Freeman, J. T. A prologue to retirement. [Some psychological and physiological problems of retirement.] Occupational Health Nursing, 22 (10), Oct 1974, 14–22.

6 Gunn, A. D. G. Problems of middle age. Physical disorders. Nursing Times, 71, 4 Dec 1975, 1952–1953.

7 Gunn, A. D. G. Problems of middle age. Psychological disorders. Nursing Times, 71, 4 Dec 1975, 1954–1955.

8 Hargreaves, A. G. Making the most of the middle years. American Journal of Nursing, 75 (10), Oct 1975, 1772–1776.

9 Isaacs, B. The silver age. Just how old does one have to be before one is called 'old'? For many, a vigorous 'silver age' separates middle age from old age. New Society, 30, 14 Nov 1974, 417–418.

10 Lambert, G. The sooner the better – preparing for retirement. Queen's Nursing Journal, 17, Oct 1974, 153–154.

11 Lowery, B. J. Problems of middle age. The middle years family. Nursing Times, 51, 11 Dec 1975, 1994–1996.

12 Peplau, H. E. Mid-life crises. American Journal of Nursing, 75 (10), Oct 1975, 1761–1765.

13 Stewart, M. C. Preparation for retirement. Queen's Nursing Journal, 16 (10), Jan 1974, 227–228.

14 Stubbs, V. Preparation for retirement. Nursing Mirror, 141, 25 Sep 1975, 69–70.

15 Webb, M. Retirement planning. Practice Team, (34), Mar 1974, 11–12.

16 Williams, E. Thoughts on retirement. Nursing Mirror, 141, 4 Sep 1975, 73.

c SERVICES

1 Age Concern Age concern on health: comments of 600 old people on the health and welfare service available to them. National Old People's Welfare Council, 1972.

2 Anderson, W. F. Organisation of an area geriatric service. Nursing Mirror, 136, 23 Mar 1973, 38–40.

3 Beith, E. Operation snowball: how a simple idea for weekend care grew to a service which has virtually eliminated geriatric emergencies in Brighton. District Nursing, 14 (3), Jun 1971, 49, 53.

4 Bricknell, J. G. Geriatric services study group. [Subjects discussed at King's Fund Centre meetings 1971–1974. Concerned for the welfare of the elderly.] Nursing Times, 71, 16 Oct 1975, 1676–1679.

5 British Medical Association Primary care for the elderly. Annual Scientific Meeting, 1975. British Medical Journal, 3, 26 Jul 1975, 221–224.

6 Davies, B. and others Variations in services for the aged. Bell, 1971.

7 Fine, W. Arithmetic of geriatrics. [Includes day hospitals, nurse/patient ratios and housing.] Nursing Mirror, 132, 23 Apr 1971, 24–30.

8 Fine, W. Liverpool geriatrics – the first 25 years. Nursing Times, 70, 21 Mar 1974, 429–432.

9 Gruer, R. Needs of the elderly in the Scottish borders. Scottish Home and Health Department, 1975. (Scottish health series studies, no. 33.)

10 Hobman, D. Practical care of geriatric patients. (a) An old person's view of the health services. Royal Society of Health Journal, 95 (1), Feb 1975, 21–25.

11 Howell, T. H. Four levels of geriatrics. [Geriatrics at the levels of personal care, hospital ward, hospital and area.] Hospital and Health Service Review, 70 (9), Sep 1974, 315–317.

12 Jones, R. H. Policy for older people: an age-old problem. Health and Social Service Journal, 84, 14 Dec 1974, 2880–2882.

13 King's Fund Centre Voluntary help in the care of the elderly. The Centre, 1971.

14 Scammells, B. The administration of health and welfare services: a study of the provision of care to elderly people. Manchester: University Press, 1971. (Studies in social administration.)

15 Scottish Hospital Centre Collaboration in care: services for the elderly in Scotland. Edinburgh: The Centre, 1974.

16 Shenfield, B. and Allen, I. The organization of voluntary service: a study of domiciliary visiting of the elderly by volunteers. Political and Economic Planning, 1972. (Broadsheet 533.)

17 Wells, T. Future trends in geriatric care. Nursing Times, 70, 2 May 1974, 677–678.

18 Williams, T. C. P. Problems in geriatrics. [NM conference lecture.] Nursing Mirror, 138, 19 Apr 1974, 46–50.

d SERVICES: OVERSEAS COUNTRIES

1 Dell, S. Nurses in nursing homes. [Care of the elderly in Alberta.] Hospital Administration in Canada, 16 (12), Dec 1974, 26.

2 Dunn, A. USA. Liberating the aged. Nursing Times, 71, 10 Jul 1975, 1086–1087.

3 Fagan, A. E. Nursing homes, facing the crisis in geriatric care [in Canada]. Dimensions in Health Service, 52 (1), Jan 1975, 27–30.

4 Holdgate, E. M. Cultural aspects of ageing. Social and health problems of the aged. New Zealand Nursing Journal, 68 (1), Jan 1975, 17–19.

5 Isler, C. Reducing the risk in relocating the elderly. [Results of research carried out at University of Michigan, Institute of Gerontology.] RN Magazine, 38, (4), Apr 1975, 48–51.

6 Lambertson, E. C. Elderly citizens and long term care. [Combined New Zealand and American Nurses' Associations conference.] New Zealand Nursing Journal, 68 (4), Apr 1975, 4–7.

7 Low, L. A. A new life for the elderly. [Geriatric Assessment and Rehabilitation Unit, Princess Margaret Hospital, Christchurch, NZ.] New Zealand Nursing Journal, 66 (6), Jun 1973, 12–14.

8 McCall, J. Care of the elderly in the EEC. International Journal of Nursing Studies, 11 (1), Jun 1974, 33–34.

9 Major, K. Denmark's geriatric patients. Community care and after care. Nursing Times, 69, 11 Jan 1973, 46–50.

10 Major, K. West Germany's geriatric patients. Community care and after-care. Nursing Times, 69, 4 Jan 1973, 8–11.

11 Managan, D. and others Older adults: a community survey of health needs. [The Nursing Division of the DuPage County, Illinois.] Nursing Research, 23 (5), Sep/Oct 1974, 426–432.

12 Mealey, M. P. Twilight years in the land of the rising sun. [Care of the elderly in Japan.] Modern Healthcare, 3 (6), Jun 1975, 52–58.

13 Morton, S. L. Simeon and Anna House. [Accommodation for the elderly in Rotterdam.] Nursing Mirror, 136, 27 Apr 1973, 12–14.

14 Quinn, J. L. Triage: coordinated home care for the elderly. [In Connecticut.] Nursing Outlook, 23 (9), Sep 1975, 570–573.

15 Van Zonneveld, R. J. Domiciliary care for the elderly. [In the Netherlands.] Royal Society of Health Journal, 95 (2), Apr 1975, 86–88, 92.

16 World Health Organization Expert Committee on Planning and Organization of Geriatric Services. Geneva: WHO, 1974 (Technical report series, 548.)

e HOSPITAL CARE

1 Ali, M. S. Hospital services for the elderly. Nursing Mirror, 141, 27 Nov 1975, 74–75.

2 Baker, A. A. Hospital care for the elderly. Mitcham: Age Concern, 1974. (Manifesto series, no. 8.)

3 Barrowclough, F. and Pinel, C. Complaints in geriatric hospitals. Nursing Times, 71, 16 Jan 1975, 118.

4 Billinge Hospital A first for Manchester . . . and the elderly who live there. [Purpose-built geriatric unit at Billinge Hospital, near Wigan. Mainly illustrations.] Nursing Mirror, 136, 29 Jun 1973, 36–38.

5 Blair, R. The autumn of life. [Geriatric patients at the Royal Infirmary, Edinburgh.] Nursing Times, 68, 5 Oct 1972, 1247.

6 British Geriatrics Society and Royal College of Nursing Improving geriatric care in hospital: a handbook of guidelines (as extracted from the Working Party). Rcn, 1975.

7 British Geriatrics Society and Royal College of Nursing Improving geriatric care in hospital: report of a working party. Rcn, 1975. Chairman: M. D. Green.

8 Brocklehurst, J. Old people in institutions – their

rights. Age Concern, 1974. (Manifesto series, 10 – specialist report.)

9 Dartington, T. C. C. and others Geriatric hospital care. Tavistock Institute of Human Relations, 1974 (2 vols).

10 Department of Health and Social Security Minimum standards in geriatric hospitals and departments. DHSS, 1972. (DS 95/72.)

11 Downie, B. N. The elderly in Scottish hospitals, 1961–1966. Scottish Home and Health Department, 1972. (Scottish Health Service studies, 21.)

12 Golding, A. M. B. and others Priorities in geriatric hospitals. [Common problems encountered during visits to 33 geriatric hospitals in South East London and Kent.] Health and Social Service Journal, 84, 14 Sep 1974, 2103–2104.

13 Greater Glasgow Health Board [Report of the Committee of Inquiry into Ruchill Hospital, Glasgow.] The Board, 1975. Chairman: Simpson, Stevenson.

14 Halliburton, P. M. and Wright, W. B. Towards better geriatric care: a proposal for monitoring standards and teaching good practice in the geriatric unit. Social Work Today, 5 (4), 16 May 1974, 107–108.

15 Halliburton, P. M. and Wright, W. B. Variations in standard of hospital geriatric care. Lancet, 1, 9 Jun 1973, 1300–1302.

16 Hansen, J. Open forum – the elderly in hospital. Nursing Mirror, 135, 8 Dec 1972, 36.

17 Health and Social Service Journal Ward conversion for geriatric patients. Health and Social Service Journal. 84. 8 Jun 1974, 1280–1281.

18 Hospital Advisory Service Geriatric staff levels are at danger point. [The 1973 annual report shows the problems of geriatric care.] Nursing Times, 70, 12 Dec 1974, 1915.

19 Hospital and Health Services Review Ruchill Hospital and geriatric care. Hospital and Health Services Review, 71 (4), Apr 1975, 113–114.

20 Jefferys, P. M. A new geriatric service. [Northwick Park Hospital.] Nursing Times, 69, 29 Mar 1973, 402–404.

21 McLeod, F. The elderly in hospital. Nursing Times, 68, 29 Jun 1972, 801–803.

22 Memorial Hospital Day House for inpatients. [Mainly illustrations.] Nursing Mirror, 141, 20 Nov 1975, 75–76.

23 Milligan, P. K. Progressive patient care. [In a geriatric assessment unit at West Cumberland Hospital.] Nursing Mirror, 137, 14 Sep 1973, 34–38.

24 Northowram Geriatric Hospital Something new for the old. Northowram Geriatric Hospital, Halifax. Nursing Mirror, 133, 31 Dec 1971, 28–31.

25 O'Brien, T. D. and others No apology for geriatrics. [The geriatric department at Oldham and District General Hospital.] British Medical Journal, 4, 3 Nov 1973, 277–280.

24 Pinel, C. and Barrowclough, F. Accidents in geriatric wards. Nursing Mirror, 137, 28 Sep 1973, 10–11.

27 Reid, S. and others The geriatric sub-hospital. [The Forest Assessment Unit at Carlton Hayes Hospital, Narborough.] Health and Social Service Journal, 84, 6 Jul 1974, 1501–1502.

28 Robb, B. Sans everything and after. [Events leading to the formation of the Hospital Advisory Service and inquiries into seven longstay hospitals.] Nursing Times, 71, 24 Apr 1975, 644–646.

29 Rowlands-Price, J. Fashion for the elderly.

[Clothing for long-stay geriatric patients at Leighton District General Hospital.] Nursing Mirror, 138, 28 Jun 1974, 76–77.

30 Rudd, T. N. Improving the quality of life in hospital. [An outline of policies which might be adopted with particular emphasis on long-stay hospitals.] Nursing Mirror, 139, 5 Dec 1974, 53–54.

31 Saunders-Brown, V. E. A dream come true, with the opening of the new nursing unit at Holy Cross Priory, Heatherfield, Sussex. Nursing Mirror, 137, 27 Jul 1973, 24.

32 Scottish Hospital Centre Ward conversion for geriatric patients. Edinburgh, The Centre, 1974.

33 South Western Hospital To invest again with dignity. [South Western Hospital for geriatric and mentally ill patients. Mainly illustrations.] Nursing Mirror, 137, 17 Aug 1973, 34–38.

34 Topliss, E. P. Staffing in a geriatric hospital. [Change of emphasis in patient care results in satisfactory staffing ratio and good patient/staff relations.] Health and Social Service Journal, 83, 27 Jan 1973, 202–204.

35 West Heath Hospital Recovery – then home. [A new ward block for elderly patients at West Heath Hospital, Birmingham.] Nursing Mirror, 135, 22 Sep 1972, 14–16.

36 Whitaker, M. Rowcliffe Hall: an appreciation of a geriatric hospital. Nursing Mirror, 141, 31 Jul 1975, 67–69.

37 World Hospitals Hospitalization of the older patient. [Series of nine articles with a summary of discussion.] World Hospitals, 9 (4), Oct 1973, 192–225.

53 NURSING THE ELDERLY

a GENERAL

1 American Journal of Nursing Caring for the aged. [Eight articles by various authors.] American Journal of Nursing, 73 (12), Dec 1973, 2049–2066.

2 Anderson, H. C. Newton's geriatric nursing. 5th ed. St. Louis: Mosby, 1971.

3 Australian Nurses' Journal Geriatric special issue. Australian Nurses' Journal, 2 (7), Jan 1973, 11–22.

4 Barrowclough, F. Guidance for the geriatric nurse [newly allocated to a geriatric ward.] Nursing Times, 71, 13 Feb 1975, 268–269.

5 Birchenall, J. and Streight, M. E. Care of the older adult. Philadelphia: Lippincott, 1973.

6 Cogliano, J. F. Providing safety for the aged: a complex issue. [Role of the licensed practical nurse.] Nursing Care, 8 (4), Apr 1975, 29–31.

7 Dawson, D. The changing world of geriatrics. [Personal views of developments after sixteen years absence from nursing.] Nursing Mirror, 140, 22/29 May 1975, 73–74.

8 Donaghue, S. Geriatric care: assumptions to throw overboard. Australian Nurses' Journal, 3 (9), Apr 1974, 36–38.

9 Dunning, J. Nursing care study. A geriatric patient. Nursing Times, 71, 25 Sep 1975, 1534–1535.

10 Fox, N. L. Making geriatric nursing creative: practical nursing notes. Journal of Practical Nursing, 23 (9), Sep 1973, 20–21.

11 Gagle, V. Therapeutic interaction with geriatric patients. Nursing Care, 8 (11), Nov 1975, 14–16.

12 Gorton, J. V. Gerontological nursing: where the action is. Journal of Psychiatric Nursing, 11 (1), Jan/Feb 1973, 9–14.

13 Griffiths, G. M. Geriatrics – more than just basic nursing care. Nursing Mirror, 137, 31 Aug 1973, 30.

14 Hammond, H. Geriatric nursing in Australia. Nursing Mirror, 135, 25 Aug 1972, 37–39.

15 Isaacs, B. Nursing old people at home and away. [Summary of a lecture.] Queen's Nursing Journal, 18 (8), Nov 1975, 223.

16 Isaacs, B. and others Geriatric nursing. Heinemann, 1973. (Modern practical nursing series 13.)

17 Jennings, N. S. It's our last chance to do something for geriatrics. Nursing Care, 7 (2), Feb 1974, 28–32.

18 Kinsella, P. Geriatric nursing: it can be rewarding, fulfilling, exciting. Hospital Administration in Canada, 14 (12), Dec 1972, 52–53.

19 Lindsay, F. Nursing care study. A new lease of life for Mrs. H. [Geriatric patient with a fractured lumbar vertebra.] Nursing Mirror, 141, 24 Jul 1975, 72–74.

20 Millard, P. H. Mixed sex nursing in a scattered geriatric unit. Nursing Times, 69, 28 Jun 1973, 826–827.

21 Moe, M. I. For patient's sake: a book for all personnel who care for the aged. Loring Station, Minneapolis: Geriatric Care, 1972.

22 Nursing Clinics of North America Symposium on putting geriatric nursing standards into practice. Nursing Clinics of North America 7 (2), Jun 1972, 201–309.

23 Nursing Digest Focus on care of the elderly. Wakefield, Massachusetts: Contemporary Publishing, 1975.

24 Nursing Times Thoughts on care for the elderly: a life worth living. Nursing Times, 71, 16 Oct 1975, 1661–1664.

25 Nyapadi, T. J. The qualities of nursing. [Sixteen qualities for geriatric nursing placed in order of importance by 103 nurses taking part in a competition.] Nursing Mirror, 140, 17 Apr 1975, 65–67.

26 Rands, V. H. Geriatric nursing services. [The case for radical reform.] Nursing Times, 68, 24 Aug 1972, 1054–1057.

27 Rankine, R. and others Widening horizons: a fresh approach to geriatric nursing. Nursing Times, 68, 17 Oct 1972, 1310–1319.

28 Royal College of Nursing Interest in geriatric care creates new Rcn society. [Conference report.] Nursing Mirror, 141, 11 Dec 1975, 35.

29 Stevens, M. K. Geriatric nursing for practical nurses, 2nd ed. Philadelphia: Saunders, 1975.

30 Tuck, B. R. The geriatric nurse, pioneer of a new specialty. RN Magazine, 35 (8), Aug 1972, 35–38.

31 Unwin, F. T. Coping with geriatrics. [The role of the nurse.] Nursing Times, 69, 13 Dec 1973, 1692–1693.

32 Wells, T. Towards understanding nurses' problems in care of the hospitalized elderly. PhD thesis, Manchester University, 1975.

33 Williams, T. C. P. Problems in geriatrics. [Conference lecture.] Nursing Mirror, 138, 19 Apr 1974, 46–50.

b ATTITUDES

1 Campbell, M. E. Study of the attitudes of nursing personnel towards the geriatric patient. Nursing Research, 20 (2), Mar/Apr 1971, 147–151.

2 Gillis, M. Attitudes of nursing personnel toward the aged. Nursing Research, 22 (6), Nov/Dec 1973, 517–520.

3 Gunter, L. M. Students' attitude toward geriatric nursing. Nursing Outlook, 19 (7), Jul 1971, 466–469.

4 Hardie, M. W. Geriatric patient care: opinions of a sample of nurses. [Research study of female nurses in four hospital groups and seven local authorities in Scotland.] Nursing Times, 71, 26 Jun 1975, Occ. papers, 61–64.

5 Kayser, J. S. and Minnigerode, F. A. Increasing nursing students' interest in working with aged patients. [Results of the Tuckman-Lorge Attitude questionnaire which measures stereotypes and misconceptions.] Nursing Research, 24 (1), Jan/Feb 1975, 23–26.

c EDUCATION AND TRAINING

1 Ashworth, A. M. Caring for the elderly. [Report of an experimental course.] Queen's Nursing Journal, 18 (8), Nov 1975, 227–228.

2 Purcell, R. One person's opinion. Specialist training in geriatric nursing? Nursing Mirror, 141, 4 Dec 1975, 61.

3 Safier, G. Nursing students and their learning experiences in geriatrics [at the University of California, San Francisco.] Journal of Psychiatric Nursing and Mental Health Services, 10 (3), May/Jun 1974, 34–41.

4 Scott, M. L. To learn to work with the elderly. [Nursing Student assigned visits to senior citizens.] American Journal of Nursing, 73 (4), Apr 1973, 662–664.

5 World Health Organization Regional Office for Europe Education and training in long-term and geriatric care: report of working group . . . Florence, 10–13 November 1970. Copenhagen: WHO, 1973.

54 COMMUNITY CARE FOR THE ELDERLY

a GENERAL AND NURSING

1 Age Concern Care is rare: a report on homecoming for the elderly patient, prepared by G. M. Amos, Liverpool: Age Concern, 1973.

2 Age Concern, Liverpool Going home? The care of the elderly patients after discharge from hospital: report on the continuing care project of Age Concern, Liverpool. Liverpool: Age Concern, 1975.

3 Anders, T. Nursing care study: caring for an individual in society. [A retired bachelor under the care of the district nurse.] Nursing Mirror, 137, 26 Oct 1973, 15–16.

4 Anderson, W. F. Community medicine and geriatrics. Public Health, 89 (2), Jan 1975, 53–56.

5 Barnard, C. J. The helping of Mrs. X: medical and social services co-operate to preserve the independence of Mrs. X who is elderly and handicapped. Nursing Times, 70, 14 Nov 1974, 1772–1773.

6 Barrowclough, F. Continuing care for the elderly. [Community support services for the elderly at home.] Nursing Mirror, 139, 30 Aug 1974, 59–61.

7 Carter, M. E. Teamwork in the care of the elderly. [Co-operation between hospital and local authority in the care of the elderly at home in the Teesside area.] Health and Social Service Journal, 84, 26 Jan 1974, 173–174.

8 Charlton, C. Practical care of geriatric patients. (b) 'The home – no substitute for home'. Royal Society of Health Journal, 95 (1), Feb 1975, 25–28.

9 Cheeseman, D. and others Neighbourhood care and old people: a community development project. National Council of Social Service, Bedford Square Press, for the Nottingham Council of Social Service, 1972.

10 Clark, A. N. G. The Diogenes syndrome. [Investigation of old people in Brighton living in squalor due to self neglect.] Nursing Times, 71, 22 May 1975, 800–802.

11 Cox, J. Practical care of geriatric patients. (e) Geriatric care in general practice. Royal Society of Health Journal, 95 (1), Feb 1975, 35–37.

12 Curnow, R. N. and others Visiting the elderly. [An experimental scheme at Reading.] Health and Social Service Journal, 85, 4 Jan 1975, 79–80.

13 Dawar, A. M. Bedfast at home. [Needs of the elderly or disabled at home.] Nursing Mirror, 141, 13 Nov 1975, 73–74.

14 Elliott, A. E. and Stevenson, J. S. K. Geriatric care in general practice. Journal of the Royal College of General Practitioners, 23, Sep 1973, 615–625.

15 Gillet, J. A. Health education of the elderly. Community Health, 4 (5), Mar/Apr 1973, 254–260.

16 Hodes, C. Care of the elderly in general practice. British Medical Journal, 4, 6 Oct 1973, 41–42.

17 How, N. M. A team caring for the elderly at home. Journal of the Royal College of General Practitioners, 23, Sep 1973, 627–637.

18 Jefcoate, R. Cause for alarm. [Alarm systems for the elderly and disabled at home.] Queen's Nursing Journal, 18 (8), Nov 1975, 220–222.

19 Johnson, E. Aspects of geriatric care. Health education and the elderly. [Pilot scheme introduced in Durham.] Midwife, Health Visitor and Community Nurse, 11 (3), Mar 1975, 71–73.

20 Kettle, D. J. Health of the elderly project. An experiment in voluntary visiting of old people [in Newcastle-upon-Tyne]. Health Visitor, 46 (12), Dec 1973, 402–407.

21 McGuire, M. C. Preventive measures to minimize accidents among the elderly. [At home.] Occupational Health Nursing, 19 (4), Apr 1971, 13–18.

22 McHugh, J. G. and Chughtai, M. A. The importance of teamwork in geriatric care. [Primary care team.] Nursing Times, 71, 23 Jan 1975, 140–142.

23 Mullan, G. My elderly lady: the unobtrusive care of the health visitor helps an independent old lady to pass her last years with dignity in her own home. Nursing Times, 71, 17 Jul 1975, 1138–1140.

24 National Corporation for the Care of Old People Service for the elderly at home: a review of current needs and problems. The Corporation, 1972.

25 Orriss, H. D. Concealed crises of communal care. [Care of the elderly in the reorganized health service.] Nursing Times, 70, 14 Feb 1974, 223–224.

26 Osborne, P. On being a district nurse. [Studies of two elderly patients.] Nursing Times, 70, 28 Nov 1974, 1862–1864.

27 Pathy, M. S. and others Role for the specialist health visitor in the geriatric team. [Attached to a hospital geriatric department in Cardiff.] Community Medicine, 127, 4 Apr 1972, 206–208.

28 Pinkerton, F. Nursing care study. What can an auxiliary do? [Nursing care study of a neglected old lady by a nurse on the district.] Nursing Mirror, 141, 25 Sep 1975, 48–49.

29 Practice Team Tackling the care of the elderly. 1. Teamwork in the Wirral. [Includes details of assessment by nurse.] Practice Team, no. 49, Jun 1975, 2, 4.

30 Robinson, W. Caring for the elderly in Camden. [Including scheme of 'geriatric visitors'.] Nursing Times, 69, 5 Apr 1973, 439–441.

31 Royle, G. A. Practical care of geriatric patients. (c) Community care of the elderly – can we get it right? Royal Society of Health Journal 95 (1), Feb 1975, 28–31.

32 Rudd, T. N. Further steps in geriatric management. [Teamwork designed to improve quality of life for old people.] Nursing Mirror, 137, 6 Jul 1973, 40–45.

33 Rudd, T. N. Paying the price of home care. [The inadequacy of home care services for the elderly.] Health and Social Service Journal, 84, 4 May 1974, 983–985.

34 Scott Wright, M. Healthy old age – working together in domiciliary care. [Effective working of the multi-disciplinary primary care team.] Royal Society of Health Journal, 95 (2), Apr 1975, 89–92.

35 Wilson, E. H. and Wilson, B. C. From hospital to community. [A scheme for elderly patients in Lancaster.] Nursing Mirror, 135, 18 Aug 1972, 17–19.

36 Yeardon, J. The elderly dropout. [Case study describing the rehabilitation of a neglected old man by a district nurse.] Nursing Times, 71, 2 Jan 1975, 38–39.

b DAY HOSPITALS AND SHORT STAY (See also Psychogeriatrics)

1 Brocklehurst, J. C. Role of day hospital care. British Medical Journal, 4, 27 Oct 1973, 223–225.

2 Callow, D. L. Towards a happy old age. [St. Pancras Geriatric Day Hospital.] Nursing Mirror, 137, 27 Jul 1973, 14–16.

3 Drug and Therapeutics Bulletin Day hospitals for the elderly. Drug and Therapeutics Bulletin, 11, 27 Apr 1973, 34–36.

4 Feldscher, B. A walking version of ECF. [Day care centre provides medical, social and psychiatric support.] Hospitals, 49, 1 Mar 1975, 75–77, 80.

5 Hospital Centre Day care for the elderly. Nursing Mirror, 132, 15 Jan 1971, 18–19.

6 Lamden, R. S. and Greenstein, L. N. Partnership in outpatient day care [for geriatrics]. Hospitals, 49, 16 Oct 1975, 87–89.

7 Morley, D. Day care and leisure provision for the elderly. Mitcham: Age Concern, 1974.

8 Novick, L. J. Day care meets geriatric needs. Hospital based program provides activities and services for patients who otherwise might have to reside in an institution. Hospitals, 47, 16 Nov 1973, 47–50.

9 Otway, J. Home for the weekend. [Report of a study day.] Health Visitor, 48 (1), Jan 1975, 26.

10 Parnell, J. W. and Naylor, R. Home for the week-end – back on Monday: a study of a five-day ward for the rehabilitation of geriatric patients. Queen's Institute of District Nursing, 1973.

11 Parnell, J. W. and Naylor, R. New developments in five-day care. [Geriatric ward at Lennard Hospital, Bromley.] Nursing Times, 69, 1 Nov 1973, 1454–1455.

12 Scottish Hospital Centre Day hospitals for geriatric patients. Edinburgh: The Centre, 1973.

13 Shell, S. M. and others Home for the week-end – back on Monday: two views of a five-day ward for rehabilitation of geriatric patients. British Journal of Occupational Therapy, 37 (2), Feb 1974, 23.

14 Silcock, J. An experimental hostel ward. [At Park Hospital, Liverpool.] Nursing Mirror, 139, 2 Aug 1974, 56–57.

15 Stone, S. Local authority holidays for the elderly and physically handicapped. HMSO, 1973. (Department of Health and Social Security, Social Science Research Unit, Study no. 2.)

16 Twelve views on geriatric day hospitals. Conclusions reached at a recent geriatric day hospital conference at Hastings. British Journal of Occupational Therapy, 37 (6), Jan 1974, 105.

17 Williams, E. P. Geriatric day centre in North Wales. Nursing Times, 69, 1 Mar 1973, 280–282.

18 Ziman, D. The five-day ward. [For the rehabilitation of geriatric patients at Lennard Hospital, Bromley. Report of Hospital Centre conference.] Health and Social Service Journal, 84, 20 Apr 1974, 874–875.

c FAMILY

1 Gallaghan, J. and Silver, C. R. Relatives' corner. [Scheme at St. Matthew's Hospital, London, to enable relatives and visitors to play a more active part in the care of geriatric patients.] Nursing Mirror, 138, 14 Jun 1974, 76.

2 National Council for the Single Woman and her Dependants The single woman keeping a job and caring for the old. The Council, 1971.

3 Powell, C. Caring for the relatives of the elderly. [During and after hospital admission.] Social Work Today, 6, 10 Jul 1975, 226–229.

4 Sandford, J. R. A. Tolerance of debility in elderly dependants by supporters at home: its significance for hospital practice. [Survey at University College and Whittington Hospitals analyzing the problems which if alleviated would restore a tolerable situation at home.] British Medical Journal, 3, 23 Aug 1975, 471–473.

d SCREENING, SURVEYS AND 'AT RISK'

1 Ascott, M. P. Health checks on the Costa Geriatrica: routine screening of the over 65's in a rural general practice [by nursing staff]. Practice Team, no. 52, Sep 1975, 2–4.

2 Ashley, P. J. Medical assessment of the elderly patient. District Nursing, 15 (8), Nov 1972, 171–173, 175.

3 Bara, E. Supporting the elderly. [Establishment of a register of the elderly needing support by a district nurse.] Nursing Mirror, 141, 21 Aug 1975, 65.

4 Cheraskin, E. and Ringsdorf, W. M. Risk factors in the aging process. Royal Society of Health Journal, 93 (6), Dec 1973, 302–304.

5 Currie, G. and others Medical and social screening of patients aged 70 to 72 by an urban general practice health team. British Medical Journal, 2, 13 Apr 1974, 108–111.

6 Dewar, M. M. Providing for elderly people at risk. [Report from Age Concern, Scotland.] Health and Social Service Journal, 85, 1 Feb 1975, 232.

7 Exe Vale Hospital Health screening service for the elderly? [Exe Vale Hospital's seminar on psychogeriatrics.] Nursing Times, 71, 3 Apr 1975, 520.

8 Heath, P. J. and Fitton, J. M. Survey of over-80 age group in a GP population based on urban health centre. [To ascertain the potential workload.] Nursing Times, 71, 23 Oct 1975, Occ. papers, 109–112.

9 Hiscock, E. and others A screening survey of old people in a general practice. Practitioner, 210, Feb 1973, 271–277.

10 Isaacs, B. and others Studies of illness and death in the elderly in Glasgow. Scottish Home and Health Department, 1971. (Scottish Health Service Studies, no. 17.)

11 Kneer, G. M. Country life: a survey of the needs of old people in a rural area. [A health visitor's interviews in Somerset, highlighted the need for improved social and welfare services.] Nursing Times, 71, 23 Oct 1975, 1714–1716.

12 Livingston, C. The Caversham project. [The work of two health visitors involved in a pilot scheme identifying the needs of the elderly in Reading.] Nursing Times, 70, 10 Oct 1974, 1591–1593.

13 Loveland, M. L. and Hillman, H. A survey of people over 65 years of age living alone in contact with welfare authorities. Health Visitor, 44 (7), Jul 1971, 226–229.

14 MacLeod, R. C. and Morgan, D. C. Survey of the elderly in Sidmouth [to obtain information on general living conditions and availability of welfare services.] Public Health, 89 (3), Mar 1975, 103–108.

15 Madden, G. and Shepherd, F. S. The needs of the elderly. [Research study by questionnaire to 388 general practitioners.] Hospital and Health Services Review, 71 (7), Jul 1975, 226–229.

16 Moore, D. M. A geriatric survey. [In an urban general practice.] Health Visitor, 46 (9), Sep 1973, 302–303.

17 Naylor, H. M. The elderly at risk. [A survey in a rural area.] Health Visitor, 46 (12), Dec 1973, 407.

18 Practice Team Tackling the care of the elderly. 2. An assessment scheme in Glasgow. Practice Team, no. 49, Jun 1975, 4–6.

19 Shaw, S. The role of the nurse in assessing the health of elderly people. In McLachlan, G. editor. Probes for health. Oxford University Press, 1975. Chapter 6, 109–123.

20 Spicer, J. and Gray, J. A. M. Brainwashing in Oxfordshire. [Survey undertaken by district nurses to detect isolation and loneliness in old people.] Queen's Nursing Journal, 18 (6), Sep 1975, 166, 168.

21 Steckler, A. A pilot study: home safety education for the elderly. International Journal of Health Education, 16 (2), 1973, 136–141.

22 Swartz, F. C. and Tobin, S. S. Psychological factors influencing the safety of the elderly. [Includes advice for elderly on accident prevention.] Occupational Health Nursing, 19 (2), Feb 1971, 7–15.

23 Wallace, C. M. Assessment of the elderly by a district nursing sister attached to a group practice. Health Bulletin, 31 (5), Sep 1973, 258–270; Reprinted in Nursing Mirror, 140, 27 Feb 1975, 54–60.

24 Williams, I. A follow-up of geriatric patients after sociomedical assessment. Journal of the Royal College of General Practitioners, 24, May 1974, 341–346.

e HYPOTHERMIA

1 Exton-Smith, A. N. Medicine in old age. Accidental hypothermia. British Medical Journal, 4, 22 Dec 1973, 727–729.

2 Fox, R. H. and others Body temperatures in the elderly: a national study of physiological, social and environmental conditions. British Medical Journal, 1, 27 Jan 1973, 200–206.

3 Fox, R. H. and others Problem of the old and the cold. [Study of elderly people in Portsmouth.] British Medical Journal, 1, 6 Jan 1973, 21–24.

4 Green, M. F. Hypothermia and the elderly. Queen's Nursing Journal, 18 (8), Nov 1975, 23–25.

5 Harrison, P. Old and cold. [Heating needs of the elderly.] New Society, 23, 8 Mar 1973, 535.

6 Illner-Paine, O. Why the old stay cold. New Society, 26, 29 Nov 1973, 531–532.

7 Irvine, R. E. Hypothermia in old age. Practitioner, 213, Dec 1974, 795–800.

8 Knapman, Y. Nursing care study. Out in the cold. [Hypothermia in an elderly woman.] Nursing Times, 70, 10 Jan 1974, 56–57.

9 Nursing Times Hypothermia in the elderly. Nursing Times, 69, 29 Mar 1973, 406.

10 Pinel, C. Accidental hypothermia in the elderly. Nursing Times, 71, 20 Nov 1975, 1848–1849.

11 Roberts, M. Hypothermia: an aid for the elderly. [Experimentation at Hounslow with an electric low-voltage underblanket suitable for the elderly.] Nursing Times, 70, 12 Dec 1974, 1926–1927.

12 Stuart, M. Why winter is a killer. [For old people.] [Reprinted from the Guardian Weekly, 3 Feb 1973.] Nursing Times, 69, 29 Mar 1973, 407.

13 Tolman, K. G. Why is hypothermia overlooked? Canadian Nurse, 67 (9), Sep 1971, 35–37.

14 Williams, M. Accidental hypothermia. Nursing Mirror, 135, 24 Nov 1972, 38.

f NUTRITION AND DIET

1 Bender, A. E. Nutrition of the elderly. Royal Society of Health Journal, 91 (3), May–Jun 1971, 115–121.

2 British Medical Journal Old people's nutrition. British Medical Journal, 1, 9 Feb 1974, 212–213.

3 Brocklehurst, J. C. Nutrition in old age. Nutrition, 26 (3), Jun 1972, 172–178.

4 Davies, L. Nutritional needs of the elderly. Mitcham: Age Concern. (Manifeso series, no. 14.)

5 Department of Health and Social Security A nutrition survey of the elderly: report by the Panel on Nutrition of the Elderly. HMSO, 1972. (Reports on health and social subjects, no. 3.)

6 Eddy, T. P. Nutritional needs of the old. Nursing Times, 70, 26 Sep 1974, 1499–1500.

7 Exton-Smith, A. N. and others Nutrition of housebound old people. King Edward's Hospital Fund for London, 1972.

8 Felstein, I. Nutrition in the over-sixties. Midwife and Health Visitor, 10 (1), Jan 1974, 18–20.

9 Furbank, M. Improved meals for geriatric patients [in long-stay hospitals.] Nursing Times, 70, 26 Sep 1974, 1501–1503.

10 Johnston, H. and Holmen, C. Nutrition for the aged and handicapped. Nursing Care, 6 (9), Sep 1973, 12–15.

11 Judge, T. G. Nutrition of the elderly. Physiotherapy, 62 (6), Jun 1976, 178–179.

12 Latchford, W. Nutritional problems of the elderly. Community Health, 6 (3), Nov/Dec 1974, 145–149.

13 Lonergan, M. E. Nutritional survey of the elderly. Nutrition, 25 (1), Spring 1971, 30–36.

14 Milne, H. Nutrition for the aged. Canadian Hospital, 49 (6), Jun 1972, 40–41.

15 Sharman, I. M. Nutrition for the elderly. Nursing Mirror, 134, 11 Feb 1972, 43–45.

16 Stanton, B. Meals for the elderly: a report on meals on wheels and luncheon clubs in two north London boroughs. King Edward's Hospital Fund for London, 1971.

17 Stephen, J. M. L. Nutrition of the elderly. Health Trends, 4 (4), Nov 1972, 76–77.

18 Young, E. J. Food for geriatrics – a special case in hospitals? Health and Social Service Journal, 85, 15 Nov 1975, 2567.

g REHABILITATION

1 Austin, B. D. Nursing care study. A patient in the geriatric rehabilitation ward. Nursing Times, 71, 29 May 1975, 852–853.

2 Berrington-Jones, N. Activities for the elderly. Royal Society of Health Journal, 95 (2), Apr 1975, 96–98.

3 Clark, M. Advance the advanced – the role and work of nurses in a multidisciplinary geriatric team. [The nurse's role in rehabilitation.] Nursing Times, 69, 1 Nov 1973, 1452–1453.

4 Clark, M. Rehabilitating the elderly patient. [Nurses' involvement in remedial therapy in a medium sized geriatric hospital.] Nursing Mirror, 139, 5 Dec 1974, 51–52.

5 Davies, E. M. Let's get moving: group activation of elderly people. Mitcham: Age Concern, 1975.

6 Davis, W. Rehabilitation by participation [with geriatric patients]. Nursing Times, 67, 25 Nov 1971, 1472–1474.

7 Garden, J. Mobility and the elderly. Mitcham: Age Concern, 1974. (Manifesto series, no. 21.)

8 Harnor, J. Morale in geriatric rehabilitation. Nursing Times, 67, 9 Dec 1971, 1525–1526.

9 Hodkinson, H. M. Medicine in old age. Rehabilitation of the elderly. British Medical Journal, 4, 29 Dec 1973, 777–778.

10 Howard, R. J. Rehabilitation flat. [Part of a pre-discharge geriatric assessment unit in the Tower Hamlets geriatric service.] Health and Social Service Journal, 83, 26 May 1973, 1192–1193.

11 Lennard Hospitals Time to go home. [An intensive rehabilitation unit for geriatric patients at the Lennard Hospitals, Bromley.] Nursing Times, 68, 20 Jul 1972, 896–897.

12 Liell, J. Group variety to flavour a long life. [Group occupational therapy sessions with geriatric patients.] British Journal of Occupational Therapy, 37 (8), Aug 1974, 137–138.

13 Long, J. M. editor Caring for and about elderly people: a guide to the rehabilitation approach. New York: Rochester Regional Medical Program/University of Rochester School of Nursing, 1972.

14 Okotie, P. Patient care study. Determination to regain independence. [Rehabilitation of a patient with a fracture.] Queen's Nursing Journal, 18 (3), Jun 1975, 74.

15 Pathy, M. S. Rehabilitation of the elderly. Queen's Nursing Journal, 16 (10), Jan 1974, 229–231.

16 Phillips, A. E. and others [Case histories of the rehabilitation of four geriatric patients.] Nursing Times, 70, 9 May 1974, 696–699.

17 Rankine, R. and others Widening horizons. [A fresh approach to geriatric nursing based on a team approach to rehabilitation.] Nursing Times, 68, 19 Oct 1972, 1310–1319.

18 Ransome, H. Rehabilitation principles applied to geriatric physiotherapy. Rehabilitation, no. 92, Jan–Mar 1975, 23–33.

19 Traill, L. and McEwan, C. Bonnybridge leisure centre. [Its use in a study of the most successful means of keeping the elderly fit.] Health and Social Service Journal, 84, 12 Oct 1974, 2364.

20 Wall, B. A. Entertaining the elderly. Nursing Mirror, 134, 9 Jun 1972, 44–46.

h RESIDENTIAL CARE AND HOUSING

1 Banks, R. Designing for the elderly. [Living accommodation.] Royal Society of Health Journal, 92 (3), Jun 1972, 151–152, 158.

2 Carstairs, V. and Morrison, M. The elderly in residential care: report of a survey of homes and their residents. Scottish Home and Health Department, 1971. (Scottish Health Service Studies, no. 19.)

3 Crease, A. M. Residential homes of the future. Health and Social Service Journal, 83, 2 Jun 1973, 1260–1261.

4 Elderly Invalids Fund Nursing homes for elderly people and old persons' homes. The Fund, 1975.

5 Liddiard, R. Pioneer home for the elderly in Bath. Health and Social Service Journal, 83, 10 Feb 1973, 317.

6 Moberly, P. Housing for the elderly. Queen's Nursing Journal, 18 (8), Nov 1975, 217–218.

7 Robinson, J. and Fletcher, P. Perception of residents entering old people's homes. [Different criteria used in assessing old people by different types of staff.] Health and Social Service Journal, 83, 20 Oct 1973, 2433–2434.

8 Rudd, T. N. Being human in homes. Public Health, 87, (1/2), Nov 1972/Jan 1973, 5–8.

9 Taylor, E. A. Residential care for the elderly [Improvement of care by amalgamating schemes used at present.] Health and Social Service Journal, 85, 12 Apr 1975, 808–809.

10 Trohear, C. Traffic in souls. [Assessing elderly people for residential care.] Social Work Today, 2, 21 Oct 1971, 25–27.

11 Vogelaar, G. A. M. Housing for elderly people in the Netherlands. Royal Society of Health Journal, 95 (2), Apr 1975, 99–102.

55 PSYCHOGERIATRICS

a GENERAL

1 Age Concern Mental deterioration. The Society, 1974. (Manifesto series, no. 12.)

2 Arie, T. Dementia in the elderly: diagnosis and assessment. British Medical Journal, 4, 1 Dec 1973, 540–543.

3 Arie, T. Dementia in the elderly – management. British Medical Journal, 4, 8 Dec 1973, 602–604.

4 Baker, A. A. Why psychogeriatrics? Lancet, 1, 27 Apr 1974, 795–796.

5 Butler, R. N. and Lewis, M. I. Ageing and mental health: positive psychosocial approaches. St. Louis: Mosby, 1973.

6 Chambers, H. J. Why bother? [The plight of the psychogeriatric.] UNA Nursing Journal, 2, Mar/Apr 1974, 9–10, 12–13.

7 Fine, W. Cerebral sympotomatology in old age. Nursing Mirror, 132, 30 Apr 1971, 37–39.

8 Mitchell, R. Advances in psychiatry – 9. Senile disorders. Nursing Times, 70, 22 Aug 1974, 1305–1307.

9 Neale, S. Society at work. The age of forgetting. [Senile dementia.] New Society, 33, 17 Jul 1975, 137–138.

10 Pitt, B. Psychogeriatrics: an introduction to the psychiatry of old age. Churchill Livingstone, 1974.

11 Szanto, S. Dementia in the elderly. Nursing Mirror, 140, 19 Jun 1975, 64–65.

12 Whitehead, A. and Fannon, D. Dangers in the diagnosis of dementia. Nursing Mirror, 135, 7 Jul 1972, 33–34.

13 Whitehead, J. A. Myths of mental illness in the elderly. Nursing Mirror, 133, 27 Aug 1971, 18–20.

14 Whitehead, J. A. The senile dementia myth. World Medicine, 7 (10), 2 Feb 1972, 47, 49, 52, 55.

15 Wynn-Jones, A. The elderly in subnormality hospitals: a survey into geriatric wards in hospitals for the mentally handicapped in the south-west of England. Health and Social Service Journal, 84, 23 Nov 1974, 2716–2717.

16 Young, J. P. R. Psychiatric morbidity in the elderly. Nursing Mirror, 139, 23 Aug 1974, 60–62.

b NURSING

1 Baker, A. A. How lucky you are on a psychogeriatric ward. Nursing Times, 71, 16 Oct 1975, 1663–1664.

2 Baltes, M. M. and Lascomb, S. L. Creating a healthy institutional environment for the elderly via behavior management: the nurse as a change agent. [A research study.] International Journal of Nursing Studies, 12 (1), Mar 1975, 5–12.

3 Birkett, M. Nursing care study. Secondary dementia. Nursing Mirror, 136, 5 Jan 197 , 34–36.

4 Boore, J. Confusion in the elderly. [A structure which can be used to examine and help confused patients.] Nursing Times, 71, 13 Nov 1975, 1816–1820.

5 Browne, L. J. and Ritter, J. I. Reality therapy for the geriatric psychiatric patient. Perspectives in Psychiatric Nursing. 10 (3), 1972, 135–139.

6 Burnside, I. M. editor Psychosocial nursing care of the aged. New York: McGraw-Hill, 1973.

7 Cooper, C. F. J. The inability to co-operate: the hallmark of the psychogeriatric ward. Nursing Times, 68, 4 May 1972, 549–550.

8 Elphick, D. and others Kardex re-design for nursing reports on patients in the psychogeriatric area of care: progress report. St. Albans: Hill End Hospital.

9 Folsom J. and Folsom, G. Team method of treating senility may contain seed for medical revolution. [Successful treatment of psychogeriatric patients.] Nursing Care, 6 (12), Dec 1973, 17–23.

10 Gersholowitz, N. L. R. and Plant, J. The potential for growth in aged mentally retarded patients. [A developmental model which used group activity to stimulate interest.] SA Nursing Journal, 42 (3), Mar 1975, 17.

11 Gimbel, L. The pathology of boredom and sensory deprivation. [Implications for nursing care particularly with geriatric patients.] Canadian Journal of Psychiatric Nursing, 16 (5), Sep-Oct 1975, 12–13.

12 Gollicker, J. Nursing care study. A new life at 77. [For a psychiatric patient.] Nursing Mirror, 137, 13 Jul 1973, 34–37.

13 Hanley, T. Practical care of geriatric patients.

(d) The organization of psychogeriatric care. Royal Society of Health Journal, 95 (1), Feb 1975, 31–35.

14 Heaney, M. W. and Brooks, M. Never too old to climb. [A nurse administered program designed to help elderly psychiatric patients achieve more independence.] Journal of Psychiatric Nursing and Mental Health Services, 13 (6), Nov/Dec 1975, 37–41.

15 Isler, C. Who says senile geriatric patients are untreatable? [Nursing involvement in intensive rehabilitation by a mental health team.] RN Magazine, 38 (6), Jun 1975, 39–40, 42, 44, 48–50.

16 Lancet Death of Miss A. [Case history of a psychogeriatric patient.] Lancet, 2, 3 Nov 1973, 1017–1018; Editorial comment – The unacceptable patient, 1011–1012.

17 McEvoy, P. Nursing care study. James – a psychogeriatric patient. Nursing Mirror, 139, 12 Sep 1974, 82–83.

18 Mulligan, A. P. and O'Grady, C. P. Reducing night sedation in psychogeriatric wards. Nursing Times, 67, 2 Sep 1971, 1089–1091.

19 Phillips, D. F. Reality orientation: the apparent success of a new therapeutic mode, based on consistent positive reinforcement, attacks some common assumptions about senility. Hospitals, 47 (13), Jul 1973, 46–49, 101.

20 Pitts, J. Y. Psychogeriatric care: a programme for hospital treatment. [Cedar Ward, Bevendean Hospital, Brighton.] Nursing Times, 70, 29 Aug 1974, 1342–1343.

21 Prinsley, D. M. Nursing in a psychogeriatric ward. Nursing Times, 70, 27 Jun 1974, 994–997.

22 Prinsley, D. M. Psychogeriatric ward for mentally disturbed elderly patients. [Guisborough General Hospital.] British Medical Journal, 3, 15 Sep 1973, 574–577.

23 Putman, M. Looking for normality – on a psychogeriatric ward. Nursing Mirror, 139, 19 Sep 1974, 52–53.

24 Roberts, R. E. Nursing care study. Senile dementia and depression, and rehabilitation of the patient. Nursing Times, 71, 4 Dec 1975, 1931–1933.

25 Savage, B. J. Rethinking psychogeriatric nursing care [in Denbigh Ward, Fulbourn Hospital, Cambridge.] Nursing Times, 70, 21 Feb 1974, 282–284.

26 Savage, B. J. Psychogeriatrics. Revising the use of nursing resources. Two studies carried out at Fulbourn Hospital, Cambridge, to determine how staff spend their working times, and to assess patients' capacities and needs, have proved to be of immense value in improving patient care. Nursing Times, 70, 5 Sep 1974, 1372–1374; 12 Sep 1974, 1424–1427.

27 Scott, D. and Crowhurst, J. Reawakening senses in the elderly. [Sensory retraining in a psychiatric setting using activities such as singing, tasting and marching.] Canadian Nurse, 71 (10), Oct 1975, 21–22.

28 Scott, D. and Parker, J. H. On to the pub or is it worth it? [Pub provided for psychogeriatric patients as form of sociotherapy.] Canadian Journal of Psychiatric Nursing, 15 (6), Nov/Dec 1974, 5–7.

29 Whitehead, J. A. Helping old people with mental illness. In an attempt to improve patient care, a leaflet is now issued to all staff. Nursing Mirror, 138, 22 Mar 1974, 76–77.

30 Wilkiemeyer, D. S. Affection: key to care for the elderly. American Journal of Nursing, 72 (12), Dec 1972, 2166–2168.

31 Witts, H. Nursing care study. Who will help him now? [Depression in a geriatric patient.] Nursing Times, 71, 9 Jan 1975, 52–53.

c SERVICES

1 Alderton, Miss Psychogeriatric care. Therapeutic activities. [At Bevendean Hospital, Brighton. Mainly illustrations.] Nursing Times, 70, 29 Aug 1974, 1344.

2 Arie, T. and Dunn, T. A 'do-it-yourself' psychiatric-geriatric joint patient unit. Lancet, 2, 8 Dec 1973, 1313–1316.

3 Fairfield Hospital A psycho-geriatric problem. [Report on the transfer of patients from Fairfield to Rossendale Hospital.] Hospital and Health Services Review, 71 (5), May 1975, 149–150; Nursing Times, 71, 24 Apr 1975, 635.

4 Greenwood House revisited. [A hostel for the elderly mentally infirm.] Nursing Times, 71, 6 Feb 1975, 219–221.

5 Meacher, M. Taken for a ride: special residential homes for the elderly mentally infirm. A study of separatism in social policy. Community Medicine, 128, 21 Apr 1972, 30–32.

6 Meacher, M. Taken for a ride: special residential homes for confused old people: a study of separation in social policy. Longman, 1972.

7 Millar, A. K. 'Port and lemon please.' [A holiday for four psychogeriatric long-stay patients at Dingleton Hospital.] Nursing Times, 70, 17 Oct 1974, 1636–1637.

8 Mind/National Association for Mental Health Now tell us how to solve the psychogeriatric problem of the psychiatric hospitals. The Association, 1972. (Mind report, no. 6.)

9 Mind/National Association for Mental Health Psychogeriatric services – the questions answered? The Association, 1973. (Mind report no. 9.)

10 Mitchell, M. Rehabilitating psychogeriatric patients. [Scheme at Manor Park Hospital, Bristol.] Nursing Times, 70, 18 Jul 1974, 1123–1124.

11 Roberts, L. South East. The care of psychogeriatric patients. [Services in the Thanet area.] Nursing Times, 71, 20 Mar 1975, 458–461.

12 Robinson, R. A. Organising a psychogeriatric service. [An approach based on DHSS recommendations.] Health and Social Service Journal, 84, 11 May 1974, 1050–1052.

13 Tindall, A. and Hubbard, E. Old and confused. [Residential accommodation at Ketts Lodge, Norfolk.] New Society, 27, 7 Mar 1974, 579–580.

14 Whitehead, A. Planning against neglect. [Psychogeriatrics.] Mind and Health Magazine, Spring 1973, 16–20.

15 Whitehead, J. A. Psychogeriatric care: community and hospital services in Brighton. Nursing Times, 70, 29 Aug 1974, 1340–1341.

16 Williams, I. E. I. and Wilson, T. S. A psychogeriatric service in West Cornwall. Nursing Mirror, 138, 26 Apr 1974, 59–63.

d COMMUNITY, DAY AND NURSING HOSPITALS (Including nursing)

1 Arie, T. and Slattery, Z. Psychogeriatrics and the health visitor. Midwife and Health Visitor, 9 (6), Jun 1973, 188–190.

2 Barker, A. and Black, S. An experiment in integrated psychogeriatric care. [Domiciliary service run by St. John's Hospital, Stone, and Buckinghamshire County Council.] Nursing Times, 67, 11 Nov 1971, 1395–1399.

3 Barker, C. Psychogeriatric day patient assessment. 1. Making a visual aid book. [Used at Elgar

House, Powick Hospital, Worcester.] Nursing Times, 71, 14 Aug 1975, 1292–1298.

4 Barker, C. Psychogeriatric day patient assessment. 2. Recording and interpreting the data. Nursing Times, 71, 21 Aug 1975, 1328–1333.

5 Dolan, F. and others Growth of a day hospital. Psychogeriatric Unit at St. Francis Hospital, Sussex.] Nursing Mirror, 135, 22 Sep 1972, 22–24.

6 Griffiths, A. Psychogeriatric liaison health visitor [at Thornhill House, Southampton]. Nursing Times, 70, 31 Jan 1974, 152–153.

7 Leopoldt, H. and others Hospital based community psychiatry nursing in psychogeriatric care. [12 months progress report of a scheme in the Isis Group of Hospitals.] Nursing Mirror, 141, 18 Dec 1975, 54–56.

8 McArthur, R. A day in the life of. . . A psychogeriatric day hospital at Bevendean Hospital, Brighton. Nursing Mirror, 133, 1 Oct 1971, 24–27.

9 Martin, I. Slow motion suicide. [A psychogeriatric patient at risk in the community.] New Society, 30, 31 Oct 1974, 263.

10 Moore, J. H. Planning comprehensive care. [Psychiatric team of nurses and social workers at Noorhaven Hospital, Plymouth, plan a scheme for care within the community.] Practice Team, no. 30/31, Nov/Dec 1973, 2–5.

11 White, D. M. D. Organizing psychogeriatric care in the community. Nursing Times, 69, 18 Jan 1973, 97–98.

12 White, D. M. D. Psychogeriatrics and community care. Lancet, 1, 4 Jan 1975, 27–29.

56 DISABLED PEOPLE
(See also under particular conditions, eg Spinal injuries)

a GENERAL

1 Agerholm, M. Handicaps and the handicapped: a nomenclature and classification of intrinsic handicaps. Royal Society of Health Journal, 95 (1), Feb 1975, 3–8.

2 Alias, R. C. G. Housing and residential accommodation. [For the disabled.] Physiotherapy. 60, 8, Aug 1974, 239–243.

3 Bartha, M. Meeting the needs. [Day care for the handicapped at Fairways, Staines.] Health and Social Service Journal, 85, 20 Sep 1975, 2104–2105.

4 Battye, L. Caring for the disabled. [The problems of residential homes with particular reference to the Cheshire Foundation.] Social Service Quarterly, 48 (4), Apr–Jun 1975, 298–300.

5 Bodington, M. C. Provision of a nursing service [for the disabled at the Royal Hospital and Home for Incurables, Putney]. Nursing Mirror, 141, 25 Sep 1975, 56–58.

6 Central Office of Information Reference Division Care of disabled people in Britain. HMSO, 1975. (Reference pamphlet no. 131.)

7 Chartered Society of Physiotherapy Handling the handicapped: a guide to the lifting and movement of disabled people. Cambridge: Woodhead-Faulkner, 1975.

8 Cheshire Homes for the Disabled The acknowledgement of spiritual needs. [Mainly illustrations.] Nursing Mirror, 138, 14 Jun 1974, 133–136.

9 Cowen, E. Towards independence: the provisions of the Chronically Sick and Disabled Persons Act, 1970. Nursing Mirror, 131, 13 Nov 1970, 18–19.

10 Dale, S. Using the literature: the handicapped person in the community. Milton Keynes: Open University Press, 1975.

11 Doherty, E. Integration in society: a new deal for the disabled. Social Work Today, 4 (7), 28 Jun 1973, 216–218.

12 Firth, B. General practitioners and social help for the handicapped. [A study undertaken to discover 22 general practitioners' knowledge of the Chronically Sick and Disabled Persons Act and how this has been communicated to disabled patients.] Journal of the Royal College of General Practitioners, 25, Jan 1975, 21–26.

13 Goldie, V. and others 'My side of the fence.' [Experiences of three disabled professional workers.] Rehabilitation, no. 95, Oct/Dec 1975, 5–11.

14 Hamilton, Lady A full life for handicapped people. [Conference paper by the Chairman of the Disabled Living Foundation.] Community Health, 6 (6), May–Jun 1975, 345–350.

15 Health and Social Service Journal Handicapped. [Idea of a Ministry for the Handicapped.] Health and Social Service Journal, 83, 17 Feb 1973, 357.

16 Hobbs, M. Hints for disabled people. Nursing Mirror, 136, 29 Jun 1973, 10.

17 Howarth, W. Living with a disability. [The problems of the female quadriplegic, told by an ex-nurse.] Nursing Mirror, 139, 2 Aug 1974, 52–55.

18 Kushlick, A. Some ways of setting, monitoring and attaining objectives for services for disabled people. [Research being undertaken by the Wessex Regional Health Authority.] British Journal of Mental Subnormality, 21, Part 2, Dec 1975, 84–192.

19 Marsham, Baroness Why do they write to me? [Problems of the disabled]. Royal Society of Health Journal, 93 (5), Oct 1973, 268–270.

20 May, C. M. Wheelchair patient for a day: simulating paraplegia to study architectural barriers to wheelchair travel, a student discovered interesting human reactions to her 'condition'. American Journal of Nursing, 73 (4), Apr 1973, 650–651.

21 Morris, A. New horizons for the disabled. Health and Social Service Journal, 83, 28 Apr 1973, 975–976.

22 Orriss, H. D. Failing the disabled. [Chronically Sick and Disabled Persons Act 1970]. Nursing Times, 67, 25 Mar 1971, 338.

23 Orriss, H. D. New benefits for the sick and disabled. Nursing Times, 71, 13 Mar 1975, 436–437.

24 Robinson, W. New unit for Stoke Mandeville. [Sir Ludwig Guttmann Hostel for 40 severely disabled.] Nursing Mirror, 41, 30 Oct 1975, 60–63.

25 Townsend, P. Society at work. Help for the disabled. [Financial problems.] New Society, 33, 24 Jul 1975, 193–194.

b AIDS, EQUIPMENT AND CLOTHING

1 Barlow, A. J. Aids for the disabled. A measure of independence. Nursing Times, 70, 11 Jul 1974, 1072–1073.

2 Bretten, P. Aids for bathing the disabled. Nursing Times, 70, 7 Nov 1974, 1741–1745.

3 British Red Cross Society People in wheelchairs: hints for helpers. British Red Cross Society, 1973.

4 Chaplin, M. Aids for the disabled. Garden tools. Nursing Times, 70, 11 Jul 1974, 1069–1071.

5 Clements, G. Aids for the disabled. Do-it-yourself hospital. [St James's Hospital, King's Lynn.] Nursing Times, 70, 11 Jul 1974, 1076.

6 Clulow, E. E. Clothes for the handicapped. Journal of the Royal College of General Practitioners, 24, May 1974, 362–366.

7 Conacher, G. Electric 'home helps' for the disabled housewife. Mother and Child, 43 (4), Jul/Aug 1971, 15–16.

8 Cornwell, M. Early years. [Aids for the disabled mother.] Disabled Living Foundation, 1975.

9 Design Council Aids for the handicapped. Design Council Awards 1975. [Mainly illustrations.] Nursing Mirror, 140, 22/29 May 1975, 69–70.

10 Drug and Therapeutics Bulletin Clothing for the disabled. Drug and Therapeutics Bulletin, 11 (1), 5 Jan 1973, 1–3.

11 Dunk, C. Research for the handicapped. [Research at St Bartholomew's Hospital into equipment improvement to alleviate stress in nursing staff and families of the handicapped.] Queen's Nursing Journal, 18 (7), Oct 1975, 195–197.

12 Fanshawe, E. Aids to independence. Queen's Nursing Journal, 16 (10), Jan 1974, 232–233, 242.

13 Fanshawe, E. Self-propelling wheelchairs. Health and Social Service Journal, 83, 21 Apr 1973, 916–917.

14 Health and Social Service Journal Comfortable clothes. [Mail order catalogue of clothes for disabled, based on the results of research by the Shirley Institute.] Health and Social Service Journal, 83, 17 Mar 1973, 612.

15 Hyde, D. C. Electronic aids for the disabled. Possum selector unit type 1. Nursing Times, 67, 1 Apr 1971, 371–373.

16 Jefcoate, R. Cause for alarm. [Alarm systems for the elderly and disabled at home.] Queen's Nursing Journal, 18 (8), Nov 1975, 220–222.

17 Jefcoate, R. M. Electronic equipment for the handicapped. Nursing Times, 71, 27 Mar 1975, 510.

18 Jefcoate, R. Independence for the disabled. [The increasing significance of mechanical aids.] Health Visitor, 48 (2), Feb 1975, 47,48.

19 Jefcoate, R. The latest aids for the disabled. Queen's Nursing Journal, 18 (7), Sep 1975, 164–165.

20 Jefcoate, A. G. Possum – the role of the district nurse. [In obtaining Possum equipment for the disabled.] District Nursing, 15 (7), Oct 1972, 142–143.

21 Langston, P. Alarm systems for the elderly and handicapped. Social Work Today, 5, 18 Apr 1974, 44–45.

22 Lyth, M. R. Disabled people's view on their aids. Rehabilitation, (84), Jan/Mar 1973, 48–50.

23 McCarrick, H. Aids for the disabled. Learning to live with it. [Rheumatoid arthritis.] Nursing Times, 70, 11 Jul 1974, 1078–1081.

24 Nursing Mirror Post office aids for the disabled. Nursing Mirror, 140, 6 Feb 1975, 54–57.

25 Nursing Times Reverse gear? [The controversy of the invalid tricycle versus the modified car for the disabled.] Nursing Times, 71, 27 Nov 1975, 1886–1888.

26 Occupational Therapy Lord Snowdon's chairmobile. Occupational Therapy, 35 (6), Jun 1972, 404–405.

27 Occupational Therapy Telephone aids for the disabled. Occupational Therapy, 36 (9), Sep 1973, 465–467.

28 Orriss, H. D. A failure in communications? [The author wonders why the Possum, an electronic aid for the handicapped, is not more widely used.] Nursing Mirror, 130, 8 May 1970, 43–44.

29 Parish, J. G. Possum. [Patient Operated Selector Mechanism.] Health Trends, 4 (1), Feb 1972, 15–16.

30 Parr, E. Small aids for disabled people. Queen's Nursing Journal, 17 (2), Feb 1975, 243–244.

31 Queen's Nursing Journal Organizations which foster independence. Queen's Nursing Journal, 16 (10), Jan 1974, 235.

32 Robinson, W. Disabled Living Foundation. [Work of the Aids Centre, with illustrations.] Nursing Mirror, 141, 23 Oct 1975, 68–71.

33 Sale, J. and Wilshere, E. R. Aids for the disabled. Individual assessment. Nursing Times, 70, 11 Jul 1974, 1058–1060.

34 Sharp, Lady E. Mobility of physically disabled people. HMSO, 1974.

35 Waters, P. D. Simple home environment control for the disabled. [Possum Environmental Control Units.] Queen's Nursing Journal, 17 (9), Dec 1974, 202.

36 Waters, P. D. and Jobson, P. M. The future role of technology and electronic aids in the social services, education and employment. Rehabilitation, (93), Apr–Jun 1975, 21–27.

c COMMUNITY AND HOME CARE

1 Bayley, M. The community can care. [Self-help is achieved by the families of the handicapped and the job of official services.] New Society, 26, 25 Oct 1973, 207–209.

2 Booth Hall Unit, Ladywell Hospital Life at home for the disabled. [Assessment and rehabilitation centre.] Nursing Mirror, 134, 30 Jun 1972, 11.

3 Dawar, A. M. Bedfast at home. [Needs of the elderly or disabled at home.] Nursing Mirror, 141, 13 Nov 1975, 73–74.

4 Evans, D. The severely disabled at home: a picture drawn from statistics of Attendance Allowance in Great Britain, 1973–1974. Health Trends, 6 (4), Nov 1974, 66–69.

5 Grant, W. R. Managing the disabled at home. Practitioner, 208, Jan 1972, 140–145.

6 Howarth, W. Living at home as a totally disabled person. International Nursing Review, 17 (3), 1970, 238–253.

7 Johnson, J. Hope for housebound disabled. Community Health, 5 (3), Nov/Dec 1973, 149–151.

8 MacMillan, C. A. Physiotherapy for the handicapped in the community. Physiotherapy, 60 (8), Aug 1974, 230–231.

9 Osborne, P. Crossroads care attendant scheme. [To train volunteers to help the disabled in their own homes.] Nursing Times, 71, 23 Jan 1975, 149–151.

d PSYCHOLOGICAL AND SEXUAL ASPECTS (Includes sexual problems)

1 Comarr, A. E. and Gunderson, B. B. Sexual function in traumatic paraplegia and quadriplegia. American Journal of Nursing, 75 (2), Feb 1975, 250–255; Midwife, Health Visitor and Community Nurse, 11 (3), Mar 1975, 74–76.

2 Gable, R. Sex counselling for the disabled. [Research Institute for Consumer Affairs meeting.] British Journal of Occupational Therapy, 38 (9), Sep 1975, 206.

3 Greengross, W. Sex problems of the disabled. Rehabilitation, (93), Apr–Jun 1975, 9–13.

4 Ibbotson, J. Psychological effects of physical disability. Health and Social Service Journal, 84, 21 Sep 1974, 2167–2168.

5 Ibbotson, J. The psychological effects of physical disability. [The problems of the congenitally handicapped.] Health and Social Service Journal, 85, 22 Feb 1975, 423–424.

6 Shakespeare, R. The psychology of handicap. Methuen, 1975. (Essential psychology series.)

7 Shearer, A. A right to love? Mind and Mental Health Magazine, Summer 1972, 14–17.

8 Shearer, A. A right to love? A report on public and professional attitudes towards the sexual and emotional needs of handicapped people. Spastics Society, and National Association for Mental Health, 1972.

9 Shearer, A. Sex and handicap. New Society, 20, 11 May 1972, 295–296.

10 Smith, J. and Bullough, B. Sexuality and the severely disabled person. American Journal of Nursing, 75 (12), Dec 1975, 2194–2197.

11 Stewart, W. F. R. Sex and the physically handicapped: the report of a research project. Horsham: National Fund for Research into Crippling Diseases, 1975. (Action research for the crippled child monograph.)

12 Wolff, I. S. Acceptance. [Defining the concept in relation to the physically handicapped.] American Journal of Nursing, 72 (8), Aug 1972, 1412–1415.

e REHABILITATION AND EMPLOYMENT

1 Beidell, L. C. The role of the nurse in hiring the handicapped. Occupational Health Nursing, 23 (7), Jul 1975, 14–17.

2 Birmingham Industrial Rehabilitation Unit Back to work. [The Birmingham Industrial Rehabilitation Unit for the handicapped.] Nursing Mirror, 139, 28 Nov 1974, 66–67.

3 Brooke, G. A. G. Riding for the disabled. District Nursing, 14 (6), Sep 1971, 122–123.

4 Brooke, G. A. G. Riding for the disabled. Social Service Quarterly, 46 (3), Jan/Mar 1973, 98–100.

5 Brooke, G. A. G. Riding for the disabled. A progress report. Health and Social Service Journal, 83, 24 Feb 1973, 418–420.

6 Greaves, M. Centre lunch talk. Dig for victory. [The Disablement Income Group.] Health and Social Service Journal, 83, 8 Dec 1973, 2874.

7 Greaves, M. Employment of disabled people. Physiotherapy, 60 (8), Aug 1974, 232–235.

8 Griffiths, D. Camping for the disabled. Social Service Quarterly, 47 (1), Jul/Sep 1973, 18–19.

9 Guttmann, L. Sport and recreation for the mentally and physically handicapped. Royal Society of Health Journal, 93 (4), Aug 1973, 208–212, 217.

10 Lane, K. Resettlement – helping the disabled back to work. [Work of a disablement resettlement officer at Northwick Park Hospital.] Nursing Mirror, 141, 28 Aug 1975, 55.

11 O'Leary, J. A. Work for the disabled. [Protected Work Centre at Vauxhall Motors.] Occupational Health, 25 (9), Sep 1973, 328–331.

12 **Perring, S.** Personal view. [Disabled nurse who ran a rehabilitation unit for disabled housewives.] British Medical Journal, 1, 31 Mar 1973, 797.

13 **Remploy** Health and Social Service Journal, 83, 7 Apr 1973, 796.

14 **Robinson, W.** Ability in disability. [Rehabilitation of the disabled by a disabled professional worker.] Nursing Mirror, 141, 14 Aug 1975, 40–41.

15 **Robinson, W.** Sport and recreation for the mentally and physically handicapped. Nursing Times, 69, 12 Jul 1973, 895–897.

16 **Spinks, M.** Working in a rehabilitation centre. Nursing Times, 69, 1 Feb 1973, 162–163.

17 **White, A. and Lake, C.** Gardening for the disabled. Nursing Times, 69, 24 May 1973, 678–680.

18 **Whiteman, D. A.** Employment services for the handicapped in Holland. Health and Social Service Journal, 85, 27 Sep 1975, 2162–2163.

MEDICINE AND THERAPEUTICS

57 MEDICINE AND SCIENCE

a ANATOMY AND PHYSIOLOGY

1 Bilger, A. J. and Greene, E. H. editors Winter's protective body mechanics: a manual for nurses. Rev. ed. New York, Springer, 1973.

2 Brooks, S. M. Basic facts of body water and ions. 3rd ed. New York, Springer, 1973.

3 Broome, W. E. and Ogden, E. C. Tables, charts and diagrams for nurses. Butterworth, 1971. (Nursing in depth series.)

4 Del Bueno, D. J. Electrolyte imbalance: how to recognize and respond to it. RN Magazine, 38 (2), Feb 1975, 52–54, 56; (3), Mar 1975, 54–55.

5 Devlin, B. Development of the human intestinal tract. Nursing Mirror, 138, 10 May 1974, 73–75.

6 Dickens, M. L. Fluid and electrolyte balance: a programmed text. 2nd ed. Philadelphia: Davis, 1970.

7 Ellis, H. Hyperhidrosis. [Excessive sweating.] Nursing Mirror, 136, 13 Apr 1973, 31–33.

8 Gotwald, W. H. Anatomy and physiology made relevant. American Journal of Nursing, 72 (12), Dec 1972, 2206–2209.

9 Grant, M. M. and Kubo, W. M. Assessing a patient's hydration status. American Journal of Nursing, 75 (8), Aug 1975, 1306–1311.

10 Hatcher, J. Plasma electrolytes and flame photometry. Nursing Mirror, 136, 16 Feb 1973, 38–39.

11 Hugh, A. Respiratory, alimentary, genitourinary and lymphatic systems. Butterworths, 1971. (Programmed primers of anatomy and physiological functions, 5.)

12 Joannides, S. C. Anatomical drawing. 1. Basic concepts. [A guide for examinations.] Nursing Times, 71, 2 Oct 1975, 1574–1576.

13 Joannides, S. C. Anatomical drawing. 2 and 3. Organs of the digestive system – 1 and 2. Nursing Times, 71, 9 Oct 1975, 1620–1621; 71, 16 Oct 1975, 1659–1660.

14 Joannides, S. C. Anatomical drawing. 4. The gall bladder, the heart and ciruclation. Nursing Times, 71, 23 Oct 1975, 1703–1704.

15 Joannides, S. C. Anatomical drawing. 5. Respiratory organs, (and) the ear. Nursing Times, 71, 30 Oct 1975, 1742–1743.

16 Joannides, S. C. Anatomical drawing. 6. The brain, (and) male genito-urinary system. Nursing Times, 71, 6 Nov 1975, 1778–1779.

17 Joannides, S. C. Anatomical drawing. 7. Female reproductive organs, (and) the kidneys. Nursing Times, 71, 13 Nov 1975, 1821–1822.

18 Keele, K. D. Leonardo on anatomy. Nursing Times, 70, 13 Jun 1974, 899–902.

19 Lee, C. A. and others Extracellular volume imbalance. American Journal of Nursing, 74 (5), May 1974, 888–891.

20 Metheny, N. M. and Snively, W. D. Nurses handbook of fluid balance. 2nd ed. Philadelphia: Lippincott, 1974.

21 Miller, A. Systems of life. Nos 5 and 6. Muscles – 1 and 2. Nursing Times, 71, 1 May 1975, [4 pages]; 5 Jun 1975, [4 pages].

22 Raeburn, J. K. and Raeburn, H. A. Anatomy, physiology and hygiene. 4th ed. Murray, 1975.

23 Rhodes, C. E. Circadian rhythms. [Includes implications for patient care.] Occupational Health, 23 (2), Feb 1971, 45–50.

24 Sharer, J. E. Reviewing acid-base balance. American Journal of Nursing, 75 (6), Jun 1975, 980–983.

25 Sheehan, J. M. Embryology made easy. 5. Development of the intestinal tract and related organs. [Respiratory system.] 6. The central nervous system. Nursing Times, 67, 7 Jan 1971, 10–11; 67, 14 Jan 1971, 43–44.

26 Snively, W. D. and Roberts, K. T. The clinical picture as an aid to understanding body fluid disturbances. Nursing Forum, 12 (2), 1973, 133–159.

27 Uttley, M. Sweat glands and perspiration. Nursing Mirror, 133, 26 Nov 1971, 35–38.

b DIAGNOSTIC TECHNIQUES

1 Blackwell, C. A. PEG and angiography: a patient's sensations. [Reactions to carotid arteriogram and pneumoencephalogram.] American Journal of Nursing, 75 (2), Feb 1975, 264–266.

2 Clarke, C. A. Non disease – the fallibility of tests and procedures. Nursing Times, 70, 4 Apr 1974, 508.

3 Earl, R. Using the laboratory. Queen's Nursing Journal, 16 (6), Sep 1973, 129, 134.

4 Evans, D. M. D. Special tests and their meanings. 8th ed. Faber, 1973.

5 French, R. M. Guide to diagnostic procedures. 4th ed. New York: McGraw Hill, 1975.

6 Hatcher, J. Bacterial serological diagnostic tests. Nursing Mirror, 139, 19 Jul 1974, 56–57.

7 Hatcher, J. Diagnostic aids – a history. Nursing Times, 69, 8 Nov 1973, 1493.

8 Hatcher, J. Electrophoresis in medicine. Nursing Mirror, 135, 7 Jul 1972, 36–37.

9 Hatcher, J. Microscopy of surgical specimens. Nursing Mirror, 139, 2 Dec 1974, 56–57.

10 Hatcher, J. Spectroscopy in medicine. Nursing Mirror, 139, 12 Sep 1974, 59–60.

11 Humphreys, D. What's on the programme today sister? [Sister in charge of the Programmed Investigation Unit, Manchester Royal Infirmary.] Nursing Times, 68, 16 Mar 1972, 308–310.

12 Institute of Medical Laboratory Sciences Information Department The professions supplementary to medicine. Medical laboratory sciences. Nursing Mirror, 141, 20 Nov 1975, 54–55.

13 Litmann, D. Stethethoscopes and auscultation. American Journal of Nursing, 72, Jul 1972, 1239–1241.

14 Longson, D. Programmed investigation unit [at Manchester Royal Infirmary]. Nursing Times, 70, 22 Aug 1974, 1322–1324.

15 Paterson, C. R. Bone biopsy. Nursing Times, 70, 7 Feb 1974, 195–197.

16 Riley, A. and Martin, B. G. We took the strain out of nursing and lab relations. [Nurses and medical technologists work together during a three month period.] RN Magazine, 38 (10), Oct 1975, 45–46.

17 Watson, E. M. Clinical laboratory procedures. Canadian Nurse, 70 (2), Feb 1974, 25–44.

18 Whittingham, T. A. Hand-held ultrasonic scanning arrays. [Use in viewing moving structures.] Nursing Mirror, 141, 18 Sep 1975, 69–70.

c GENETICS AND GENETIC COUNSELLING

1 Beighton, G. The role of the nurse in clinical genetics. SA Nursing Journal, 42 (8), Jul 1975, 17–19.

2 Carter, C. O. Genetic counselling and prenatal diagnosis. Nineteenth Sir William Power Memorial Lecture. Midwives Chronicle, 87, Mar 1974, 88–90.

3 Collingwood, J. M. Genetic disease – early prenatal diagnosis. Nursing Times, 70, 11 Jul 1974, 1061–1063.

4 Crawfurd, M. d'A. Genetic counselling. Nursing Times, 67, 28 Oct 1971, 1351–1352.

5 Emery, A. E. H. Genetic counselling – or what can we tell parents? Practitioner, 213, Nov 1974, 641–646.

6 Emery, A. E. H. and others Social effects of genetic counselling. British Medical Journal, 1, 24 Mar 1973, 724–726.

7 Greenberg, R. C. Genetics and mental disorder. Midwife and Health Visitor, 6 (6), Jun 1970, 219–221.

8 Kirman, B. Genetic counselling for parents of mentally handicapped children. Maternal and Child Care, 8, Dec/Jan 1971, 5–7.

9 Kirman, B. and Angeli, E. Genetic counselling in relation to mental retardation. Nursing Mirror, 132, 1 Jan 1971, 21–24.

10 Maclean, D. Genetics. [An introduction.] Nursing Mirror, 140, 27 Mar 1975, 50–54.

11 Siminovitch, L. Genetic manipulation: now is the time to consider controls. Canadian Nurse, 69 (11), Nov 1973, 30–34.

12 Stevenson, A. C. A changing scene in patterns of genetic advice. Mother and Child, 43 (4), Jul/Aug 1971, 6–9.

13 World Health Organization Facts about human genetics. Information from WHO. International Nursing Review, 21 (6), Nov/Dec 1974, 190–192.

d MATHEMATICS AND METRICATION

1 Arton, M. Teachers page. 13. A brief look at SI Units. Midwives Chronicle, 88, Nov 1975, 370–371.

2 Baron, D. N. Contemporary themes. SI Units. [A revised and extended metric system. 'Systeme International d'Unites' be used in British medicine by Autumn 1975.] British Medical Journal, 4, 30 Nov 1974, 509–512.

3 British Medical Journal SI Units. [Leading article.] British Medical Journal, 4, 30 Nov 1974, 490.

4 Forno, C. You are going SI, nurse! 10. Can you metricate? [Quiz to summarize the previous articles in the series.] Nursing Mirror, 141, 6 Nov 1975, 75–76.

5 Fream, W. C. and Davies, R. P. Arithmetic in nursing. 4th ed. Baillière Tindall, 1972. (Nurses' aids series.)

6 Glister, B. A. Changing to metric. Health and Social Service Journal, 83, 1 Sep 1973, 1992, 1994.

7 Goodsell, D. Coming to terms with SI metric. Nursing Mirror, 141, 27 Nov 1975, 55–59.

8 Greenway, B. You and the metric system. Nursing Times, 69, 13 Sep 1973, 1198–1199.

9 Harris, B. Are you ready for the switch to the metric system? Nursing Care, 8 (3), Mar 1975, 12–14.

10 Kilgour, O. Have you gone SI, nurse? [Metrication.] Nursing Mirror, 136, 5 Jan 1973, 18.

11 Kilgour, O. F. G. Have you gone SI, nurse? 2. Height and fluid balance. Nursing Mirror, 136, 12 Jan 1973, 14.

12 Kilgour, O. Have you gone SI, nurse? 3. Where has specific gravity gone? Nursing Mirror, 136, 19 Jan 1973, 42.

13 Kilgour, O. Have you gone SI, nurse? 4. Calories don't count. Nursing Mirror, 136, 26 Jan 1973, 33.

14 Kilgour, O. Have you gone SI, nurse? 5. Blood pressure – kilopascals. Nursing Mirror, 136, 2 Feb 1973, 29.

15 Kilgour, O. You are going SI, nurse. 1. Counting the change. Nursing Mirror, 141, 4 Sep 1975, 46–47.

16 Kilgour, O. You are going SI, nurse! 2. The lengths we go to with SI. Nursing Mirror, 141, 11 Sep 1975, 69–70.

17 Kilgour, O. You are going SI, nurse! 3. Covering and filling up with SI. Nursing Mirror, 141, 18 Sep 1975, 55–56.

18 Kilgour, O. You are going SI nurse! 4. Weighing up SI. Nursing Mirror, 141, 25 Sep 1975, 59.

19 Kilgour, O. You are going SI, nurse! 5. A mere mole shows the amount in SI. Nursing Mirror, 141, 2 Oct 1975, 55–56.

20 Kilgour, O. You are going SI, nurse! 6. The energetic joule. Nursing Mirror, 141, 9 Oct 1975, 75–76.

21 Kilgour, O. You are going SI, nurse! 7. TPR and BP in SI. Nursing Mirror, 141, 16 Oct 1975, 57–58.

22 Kilgour, O. You are going SI, nurse! 8. Food and SI. Nursing Mirror, 141, 23 Oct 1975, 67.

23 Kilgour, O. You are going SI, nurse! 9. Electricity and SI. Nursing Mirror, 141, 30 Oct 1975, 65.

24 Kotchek, L. D. Numbers in nursing. They aren't as precise as we like to think they are. Nursing Outlook, 19 (10), Oct 1971, 653–655.

25 Lansley, T. S. Going metric in the NHS. Health and Social Service Journal, 85, 26 Jul 1975, 1602–1603.

26 Lansley, T. S. Metrication, scientific services and the hospital. British Hospital Journal and Social Service Review, 81, 16 Jan 1971, 121–124.

27 Martin, J. L. Metrication and decimalization. Nursing Times, 67, 11 Feb 1971, 165–167.

e MEDICINE

1 Barr, R. D. and Laird, E. H. R. Adult medicine. Heinemann Medical, 1971. (Modern practical nursing series 9.)

2 Cable, J. V. Principles of medicine: an integrated textbook for nurses. 5th ed. Christchurch, NZ: N. M. Peryer, 1974.

3 Cooke, R. G. A summary of medicine for nurses and medical auxiliaries. 6th ed. Revised by Ann C. Miller. Faber, 1973.

4 Culclasure, D. F. Medical benefits from space research. American Journal of Nursing, 74 (2), Feb 1974, 275–278.

5 Fricker, R. The Medical Research Council: an explanation for nurses. Nursing Times, 68, 24 Feb 1972, 245–248.

6 Gibson, J. Modern medicine for nurses. 3rd ed. Oxford: Blackwell, 1975.

7 Hatcher, J. Fame is a name. [Medical eponyms.] Nursing Times, 68, 12 Oct 1972, 1298–1299.

8 Hector, W. and Fairley, G. H. Textbook of medicine for nurses. 2nd ed. Heinemann Medical, 1973.

9 Newbold, G. F. 'Things are not always what they seem.' [The practice of 'medicine of the whole person'.] Nursing Mirror, 140, 2 Jan 1975, 43–44.

10 Roberts, A. P. 3. Over-treatment. Nursing Mirror, 137, 28 Sep 1973, 25–27.

11 Toohey, M. Medicine for nurses. 11th ed. Churchill Livingstone, 1975.

f MEDICINE, ALTERNATIVE

1 Armstrong, M. E. Acupuncture. American Journal of Nursing, 72 (9), Sep 1972, 1582–1588.

2 Armstrong, M. E. Acupuncture. Canadian Nurse, 69)2), Feb 1973, 26–31.

3 Barrins, P. C. Nursing care of the hypnotized patient. Nursing Care, 8 (12), Dec 1975, 10–11.

4 Barrins, P. C. What nurses need to know about hypnosis. RN Magazine, 38 (1), Jan 1975, 37, 40, 45–46, 50, 52, 54.

5 Blackie, M. G. Homoeopathy. Nursing Times, 68, 22 Jun 1972, 784–787.

6 Bloomfield, B. Natural therapeutics.When the doctors fail? Health Visitor, 48 (6), Jun 1975, 198–200.

7 Bodman, F. Homoeopathy. Nursing Mirror, 133, 8 Oct 1971, 36–37.

8 Breeden, S. A. and Kondo, C. Using biofeedback to reduce tension. American Journal of Nursing, 75 (11), Nov 1975, 2010–2012.

9 Byram, R. S. My friends the witchdoctors. Nursing Times, 68, 28 Sep 1972, 1220–1221.

10 Capperauld, I. Acupuncture and acupuncture anaesthesia. NATNews, 12 (1), Jan 1975, 11, 12, 14.

11 Capperauld, I. An appraisal of acupuncture in China. Nursing Mirror, 138, 5 Apr 1974, 66–69.

12 Cullinan, J. Anaesthesia by acupuncture. Nursing Times, 68, 17 Aug 1972, 1019–1020.

13 Edwards, H. Alternative medicine: the science of spiritual healing. Nursing Times, 71, 18 Dec 1975, 2008–2010.

14 Hamson, L. An outline of hypnotherapy – a method, not magic. Nursing Times, 67, 29 Jul 1971, 919–920.

15 Harling, M. Alternative medicine. Homoeopathy. Nursing Times, 71, 23 Oct 1975, 1694–1696.

16 Johnson, B. Alternative medicine. Hypnosis in medicine. Nursing Times, 71, 27 Nov 1975, 1898–1899.

17 Rigby, B. Alternative medicine. Transcendental meditation. Nursing Times, 71, 7 Aug 1975, 1240–1242.

18 Rosenhouse, L. Acupuncture in your hospital? Nursing Care, 8 (5), May 1975, 10–12.

19 Ryan, B. J. Biofeedback training: the voluntary control of mind over body and mind. Nursing Forum, 14 (1), 1975, 48–55.

20 Sterman, L. T. Clinical biofeedback. [Appreciation of automation to achieve a modification of physiological functions.] American Journal of Nursing, 75 (11), Nov 1975, 2006–2009.

21 Stuart, M. R. Alternative medicine. Herbalism. Nursing Times, 71, 25 Sep 1975, 1528–1531.

22 Wall, P. Acupuncture – an eye on the needle. [Reprinted from New Scientist, 20 Jul 1972.] Nursing Times, 68, 24 Aug 1972, 1061–1063.

23 Weber, J. P. Nursing students' opinions about acupuncture and Chinese medicine. Nursing Research, 24 (3), May/Jun 1975, 205–206.

24 Wilks, C. G. W. Alternative medicine. Hypnosis in dentistry. Nursing Times, 71, 27 Nov 1975, 1897–1898.

25 Willey, R. Relax with yoga. Nursing Mirror, 134, 3 Mar 1972, 32–34.

g MICROBIOLOGY AND PARASITOLOGY

1 Baker, B. H. Medical bacteriology: infection and resistance. Bedside Nurse, 5 (5), May 1972, 16–20.

2 Baker, B. H. Medical bacteriology: the 'WBC' and 'DIFF'. Nursing Care, 6 (8), Aug 1973, 25–30.

3 Bocock, E. and Parker, M. J. Microbiology for nurses. 4th ed. Baillière Tindall, 1972. (Nurses' aids series.)

4 Caplan, H. Candida infection. Nursing Times, 71, 10 Apr 1975, 568–569.

5 Carter, D. E. Parasitic invasion. Nursing Times, 69, 3 May 1973, 568–570.

6 Cartwright, R. Y. Commensal bacteria of the human gastrointestinal tract. Nursing Times, 70, 9 May 1974, 705–706.

7 Chuan, H. B. Ectoparasites of man in Singapore. Nursing Journal of Singapore, 14 (1), May 1974, 4–7.

8 Hare, R. Bacteriology and immunity for nurses. 3rd ed. Churchill Livingstone, 1971.

9 Hatcher, J. A bug by any other name. . . Nursing Mirror, 136, 11 May 1973, 38–39.

10 Horrobin, D. F. Essential biochemistry, endocrinology and nutrition: a guide to important principles for nurses and allied professions. Aylesbury, Bucks: Medical and Technical Publishing Co, 1971.

11 Ingram, J. T. The magic of dermatology. 3. Animal parasites. Nursing Times, 69, 18 Jan 1973, 86–87.

12 Kaminsky, D. and others, editors Microbiology: 1500 multiple choice questions and referenced answers. 3rd ed. Flushing: Medical Examination Publishing Co., 1974. (Nursing examination review book, vol 7.)

13 Lewis, J. G. Gram-negative bacteraemia. Nursing Mirror, 139, 5 Dec 1974, 47–49.

14 Maisey, M. A. Bacteriology. [In order to understand pathology reports, a nurse spends a week in the bacteriology laboratory.] Nursing Times, 70, 31 Jan 1974, 142–145.

15 Noble, W. C. Commensal bacteria of human skin. Nursing Times, 69, 4 Oct 1973, 1287–1288.

16 Williamson, F. Louis Pasteur. Microbes. 3. Nursing Times, 69, 29 Nov 1973, 1621–1622.

17 Williamson, F. Microbes. 4. Robert Koch: anthrax bacilli isolated. Nursing Times, 69, 6 Dec 1973, 1652–1653.

18 Williamson, F. Microbes. 5. Elie Metchnikoff: advocate for phagocytes. Nursing Times, 69, 13 Dec 1973, 1702–1703.

19 Winner, H. I. Microbiology in modern nursing. Nursing Mirror, 132, 9 Apr 1971, 28–29.

20 Zaman, V. Intestinal nematodes of man. Nursing Journal of Singapore, 13 (2), Nov 1973, 111–113.

h RADIOLOGY

1 Bentley, H. B. The professions supplementary to medicine. Radiography. Nursing Mirror, 141, 23 Oct 1975, 58–61.

2 Best, M. C. and Warrick, C. K. The 10-day rule. [The dangers of X-rays in early pregnancy.] Nursing Times, 70, 19 Sep 1974, 1474.

3 Bliss, A. and others The emergency room nurse orders X-rays of distal limbs in orthopedic trauma. Nursing Research, 20 (5), Sep/Oct 1971, 440–443.

4 Chesney, D. N. and Chesney, M. O. Care of the patient in diagnostic radiotherapy. 4th ed. Oxford: Blackwell, 1973.

5 Goldman, M. A nurse's guide to the X-ray department. 2nd ed. Churchill Livingstone, 1972.

6 Haynes, P. Radiography in the operating theatre. NATNews, 12 (5), Jul 1975, 12–14.

7 Isler, C. Radiation therapy. 2. The nurse and the patient. RN Magazine, 34 (3), Mar 1971, 48–51.

8 Jolles, K. E. The cathetron may revolutionize radiotherapy. Nursing Times, 68, 27 Jul 1972, 937–938.

9 Mould, R. F. Physics and scanning. 1. Radioactive isotopes. Nursing Times, 71, 10 Apr 1975, 562–564.

10 Mould, R. F. Physics and radiotherapy. 1. Introduction. Nursing Times, 70, 7 Mar 1974, 336–338.

11 Mould, R. F. Physics and radiotherapy. 3. Radiation treatment technique. Nursing Times, 70, 21 Mar 1974, 426–428.

12 Mould, R. F. Physics and radiotherapy. 4. Radiation protection. Nursing Times, 70, 28 Mar 1974, 468–470.

13 Mould, R. F. Physics and scanning. 2. Scanning equipment. Nursing Times, 71, 17 Apr 1975, 612–614.

14 Mould, R. F. Physics and scanning. 3. Scan images. [Work with simulated patient organs and actual patients.] Nursing Times, 71, 24 Apr 1975, 657–659.

15 Nebe, D. E. and Gavaghan, M. Lymphography and patients' reactions. American Journal of Nursing, 73 (8), Aug 1973, 1366–1368.

16 Nursing Times Scanning the brain. [The EMI-Scanner.] Nursing Times, 70, 25 Jul 1974, 1170.

17 Padilla, G. V. and Baker, V. E. Variables affecting the preparation of the bowel for radiologic examination. Nursing Research, 21 (4), Jul–Aug 1972.

18 Powell, N. W. Handbook for radiologic technologists and special procedures nurses in radiology. Springfield: Thomas, 1974.

19 Sherwood, T. The intravenous urogram. Nursing Times, 71, 8 May 1975, 730–731.

20 Simpson, J. D. Nuclear medicine. [Radio-isotopic tracer technique.] Nursing Times, 70, 15 Aug 1974, 1260–1263.

21 Skinner, M. X-rays in perspective. Nursing Mirror, 132, 7 May 1971, 24–25.

22 Spencer, R. M. Transvaal Memorial Hospital for Children. Is a Sister necessary in a X-ray department? [Description of her duties.] SA Nursing Journal, 40 (11), Nov 1973, 14.

23 Szur, L. Radiotherapy in benign skin disease. Nursing Times, 69, 25 Oct 1973, 1413–1415.

24 Vaithilingam, K. Preparation of patient for X-ray examinations. Nursing Journal of Singapore, 13 (1), May 1973, 23–31, 35.

25 Watson, J. C. Patient care and special procedures in radiologic technology. 4th ed. St. Louis: Mosby, 1974.

i SCIENCE

1 Durkin, N. Basic science education and the nursing profession. Kenya Nursing Journal, 1 (1), Jun 1972, 39–40.

2 Ellis, R. Values and vicissitudes of the scientist nurse. Nursing Research, 19 (5), Sep/Oct 1970, 440–445.

3 Flitter, H. H. An introduction to physics in nursing. 6th ed. St Louis: Mosby, 1972.

4 Gratz, P. Science for the health professions: a comprehensive, 2-semester course in human ecology to replace the traditional separate science courses in the basic curriculum. Nursing Outlook, 18 (10), Oct 1970, 60–62.

5 Kilgour, O. F. G. An introduction to the chemical aspects of nursing science. Heinemann Medical, 1972.

6 Kilgour, O. F. G. An introduction to the physical aspects of nursing science. 2nd ed. Heinemann, 1972.

7 Mutton, C. J. Blood pH-1. The ABC of acid-base chemistry. Nursing Times, 71, 19 Jun 1975, 968–971.

8 Mutton, C. J. Blood pH-2. Acidosis and alkalosis. Nursing Times, 71, 26 Jun 1975, 1010–1012.

9 Nelson, J. Science matters. Nursing Mirror, 140, 26 Jun 1975, 55.

10 Nolan, R. J. The development of teaching methods in human biology within nurse training schools. MEd thesis, Manchester University, 1973.

11 Wilson, K. J. W. A study of the biological sciences in relation to nursing. Edinburgh: Churchill Livingstone, 1975. Based on PhD thesis Edinburgh University, 1972. Rcn Research Society Summary, Nursing Times 73, 9 Jun 1977, Occ. papers, 84.

j TROPICAL MEDICINE

1 Adams, A. R. D. and Maegraith, B. G. Tropical medicine for nurses. Heinemann, 1975.

2 Chesterman, C. C. Importable tropical disease. Nursing Mirror, 138, 29 Mar 1974, 59–61.

3 Lenczner, M. M. Tropical and parasitic diseases: new challenge to health teams. Canadian Nurse, 69 (9), Sep 1973, 34–36.

4 Rowland, H. A. K. Lassa fever. Nursing Mirror, 140, 26 Jun 1975, 54.

5 Shattock, F. M. Tropical medicine for the health team. [Training nurses at the Liverpool School of Tropical Medicine.] Nursing Times, 71, 23 Jan 1975, 143–145.

6 Tomkins, A. M. and James, W. P. T. Tropical sprue. [Severe malabsorption and secondary malnutrition.] Nursing Times, 71, 16 Oct 1975, 1649–1650.

7 Turner, A. C. Symptomatology of common imported disease. Nursing Times, 70, 22 Aug 1974, 1296–1299.

8 Williamson, F. Man against insect. 2. David Bruce v sleeping sickness. Nursing Times, 70, 25 Jul 1974, 1163–1164.

9 Williamson, F. Man against insect. 3. Walter Reed v yellow fever. Nursing Times, 70, 1 Aug 1974, 1202–1203.

58 PHARMACOLOGY

a GENERAL AND TEXTBOOKS

1 Bailey, R. E. Pharmacology for nurses. 3rd ed. Bailliere Tindall, 1971.

2 Bergersen, B. S. and Sakalys, J. A. Review of pharmacology in nursing. St. Louis: Mosby, 1974. (Comprehensive review series.)

3 Boyle, J. A. Lecture notes in pharmacology and therapeutics for nurses. 2nd ed. Edinburgh: Churchill Livingstone, 1974.

4 Coleman, V. The top drugs. Nursing Times, 69, 26 Apr 1973, 531; 69, 3 May 1973, 571; 69, 10 May 1973, 618.

5 Del Bueno, D. J. Verifying the nurse's knowledge of pharmacology. Nursing Outlook, 20 (7), Jul 1972, 462–463.

6 Del Bueno, D. J. and others Teaching pharmacology – a team approach. Nursing Outlook, 19 (6), Jun 1971, 414–415.

7 DiPalma, J. R. Drug therapy today. What you need to know about bioavailability. [The percentage of the administered drug that reaches the bloodstream.] RN Magazine, 38 (9), Sep 1975, 114, 116, 118.

8 DiPalma, J. R. Drug therapy today. DESI ratings, a revolution in the making. [A system of rating drugs as to their effectiveness for specific indications.] RN Magazine, 36 (6), Jun 1973, 51–54, 56, 60, 62.

9 DiPalma, J. R. Drug therapy today. Postaglandins, the potential wonder drugs. RN Magazine, 35 (10), Oct 1972, 51–52, 55–56, 61.

10 DiPalma, J. Radiopharmaceuticals: nuclear age drugs for diagnosis and treatment. RN Magazine, 38 (3), Mar 1975, 59–62, 64–65.

11 Dison, N. Simplified drugs and solutions for nurses, including arithmetic. 5th ed. St Louis: Mosby, 1972.

12 Geddes, A. M. Antibiotics today. Nursing Mirror, 138, 12 Apr 1974, 55–57.

13 **Gibson, J.** The nurse's materia medica. 3rd ed. Oxford: Blackwell Scientific, 1975.

14 **Heinemann, H. L. and others** Bailliere's pocket book of ward information revised by L. Ann Jee. 12th ed. Baillere, 1971. (Formerly entitled 'Nurses' Pharmocopoeia.)

15 **Hopkins, S. J.** Drugs and pharmacology for nurses. 5th ed. Churchill Livingstone, 1971. 6th ed. 1975.

16 **Hopkins, S. J.** New drugs for old. 2. Antibiotics and others. Nursing Times, 68, 13 Jul 1972, 879–81.

17 **Hopkins, S. J.** Principal drugs: an alphabetical guide. 4th ed. Faber, 1973.

18 **Hull, E. J. and others** The arithmetic of drug dosage: Part 1: Administration by mouth. English Universities Press, 1972. (Modern nursing series – programmed texts for nurses.)

19 **Jones, B. R.** Pharmacology for student and pupil nurses and student pharmacy technicians. Rev. ed. Heinemann Medical.

20 **Kline, N. S. and Davis, J. M.** Psychotropic drugs. American Journal of Nursing, 73 (1), Jan 1973, 54–62.

21 **Lee, R. V.** Antimicrobial therapy. American Journal of Nursing, 73 (12), Dec 1973, 2044–2048.

22 **Lessof, M. H.** Immunosuppressive drugs. Nursing Times, 69, 6 Dec 1973, 1648–1649.

23 **Lewis, J. B.** Therapeutics. 2nd ed. English Universities Press, 1972.

24 **Lowenthal, W.** Factors affecting drug absorption. Programmed instruction. American Journal of Nursing, 73 (8), Aug 1973, 1391–1408.

25 **Morgan, A. J.** Minor tranquilizers, hypnotics and sedatives. American Journal of Nursing, 73 (7), Jul 1973, 1220–1222.

26 **Pitlick, W. H. and Plein, E. M.** Evaluation of clinical pharmacy by nurses. [Survey showing nurses' need of pharmacy information.] Nursing Research, 22 (5), Sep/Oct 1973, 434–437.

27 **Richens, A.** Developments in drug therapy. Nursing Mirror, 137, 28 Sep 1973, 30–32.

28 **Rodman, M. J.** Drug therapy today. Adrenergic drugs and adrenergic blockers. RN Magazine, 37 (4), Apr 1974, 55, (9 pages).

29 **Schultz, W. L. and Muha, K. M.** Penicillins in review. Nursing Care, 8 (11), Nov 1975, 17–19.

30 **Sears, W. G.** Materia medica for nurses: a textbook on drugs and therapeutics. 7th ed. Arnold, 1971.

31 **Skelley, E. G.** Medications and mathematics for the nurse, and instructor's guide. New York: Delmar, 1971.

32 **Smith, S. E.** Drug therapy 1972. 10. Biological drugs and vaccines. Nursing Times, 68, 3 Aug 1972, 965–966.

33 **Smith, S. E.** Drug therapy 1972. 13. The safety of drugs. Nursing Times, 68, 24 Aug 1972, 1067–1068.

34 **Smith, S. E.** How drugs act. 1. How drugs are absorbed. Nursing Times, 71, 26 Jun 1975, 998–999.

35 **Smith, S. E.** How drugs act. 2. How drugs reach their destination. Nursing Times, 71, 3 Jul 1975, 1043–1044.

36 **Smith, S. E.** How drugs act. 3. Elimination and cumulation. Nursing Times, 71, 10 Jul 1975, 1101–1102.

37 **Smith, S. E.** How drugs act. 8. Adrenocortical steroids. Nursing Times, 71, 14 Aug 1975, 1301–1302.

38 **Smith, S. E.** How drugs act. 9. Antibacterial drugs. Nursing Times, 71, 21 Aug 1975, 1339–1340.

39 **Smith, S. E.** How drugs act. 25. Biological drugs and vaccines. Nursing Times, 71, 11 Dec 1975, 1992–1993.

40 **Smith, S. E.** How drugs act. 27. Drugs and addiction. Nursing Times, 71, 25 Dec 1975, 2072–2073.

41 **Trounce, J. R.** Pharmacology for nurses. 6th ed. Churchill Livingstone, 1973.

42 **Williamson, K. C. and White, S. J.** Pharmacology competence ensured. [Assessment techniques are used to test pharmacology knowledge of nursing personnel.] Hospitals, 98, 16 Sep 1974, 95–96, 98.

43 **Worley, E.** Pharmacology and medications for vocational nurses. 2nd ed. Philadelphia: Davis.

b ADVERSE REACTION AND INTERACTIONS

1 **Alsop, J. A.** Adverse drug reactions. Nursing Mirror, 136, 16 Mar 1973, 37–39.

2 **Armstrong-Esther, C. A.** Antibiotics. Agricultural methods [are producing an antibiotic resistant population.] Nursing Times, 71, 16 Jan 1975, 108–110.

3 **Armstrong-Esther, C. A.** Antibiotics. Use or abuse? [Problems created by the indiscriminate use of antibiotics.] Nursing Times, 71, 16 Jan 1975, 107–108.

4 **Blount, M. and Kinney, A. B.** Chronic steroid therapy. [With particular reference to complications and side effects.] American Journal of Nursing, 74 (9), Sep 1974, 1626–1631.

5 **Bosanquet, N.** Doubts about the drug industry. [Criticism on the quality of drugs.] Nursing Times, 71, 12 Jun 1975, 913.

6 **Boyd, E. M.** The safety and toxicity of aspirin. American Journal of Nursing, 71 (5), May 1971, 964–965.

7 **Carney, M. W. P.** Bromism – a clinical chameleon. Nursing Times, 69, 5 Jul 1973, 859–861.

8 **Cooper, P.** Progress in therapeutics. Aspects of drug interaction. 2. Midwife and Health Visitor, 9 (9), Sep 1973, 301–302.

9 **Copeman, P. W. M.** Ill effects of drug treatment on the skin. Nursing Mirror, 138, 12 Apr 1974, 51–54.

10 **Craven, R. F. and others** Anaphylactic shock. [After penicillin injection.] American Journal of Nursing, 72 (4), Apr 1972, 718–721.

11 **Duckworth, D. V.** Drugs in common use and their side effects. Occupational Health, 23 (9), Sep 1971, 300–304.

12 **Dunlop, Sir D.** Drug interactions. [The 1971 Harben Lecture.] Community Health, 4 (1), Jul/Aug 1972, 8–13.

13 **Hatcher, J.** Sensitivity tests: an essential preliminary to antibiotic therapy. Nursing Mirror, 136, 23 Mar 1973, 21–22.

14 **Hill, Sir A. B.** Diseases of treatment. [Committee on the Safety of Drugs.] Public Health, 85 (5), Jul 1971, 197–202.

15 **Johnson, D. A. W.** Psychiatric symptoms produced by drugs. Nursing Mirror, 138, 28 Jun 1974, 72–73.

16 **Johnstone, J.** Drug interactions. Australian Nurses' Journal, 5 (4), Oct 1975, 14–16.

17 **Koprowicz, D. C.** Drug interactions with coumarin derivatives. American Journal of Nursing, 3 (6), Jun 1973, 1042–1044.

18 **L'Estrange Orme, M.** Drug interactions. Nursing Mirror, 134, 26 May 1972, 13–15.

19 **Lambert, M. L.** Drug and diet interactions. American Journal of Nursing, 75 (3), Mar 1975, 402–406.

20 **Lew-Sang, E.** Factors affecting drug action. Australian Nurses' Journal, 4 (10), May 1975, 21–22.

21 **Macaulay, D. B.** Acute anaphylaxis. [After injection.] Nursing Mirror, 139, 12 Jul 1974, 59–60.

22 **Mohney, S.** Some important clues to adverse drug reactions. RN Magazine, 36 (3), Mar 1973, 48–49, 88, 90, 92–93.

23 **O'Reilly, W. J.** Drug interactions. Canadian Nurse, 68 (4), Apr 1972, 47–50.

24 **Pinkey, B.** Psychiatric complications of everyday drugs. Nursing Times, 70, 16 May 1974, 756–757.

25 **Smith, S. E.** Drug therapy 1971. 4. Side-effects. Nursing Times, 67, 15 Apr 1971, 441–442.

26 **Smith, S. E.** How drugs act. 4. Side-effects. Nursing Times, 71, 17 Jul 1975, 1141–1142.

27 **Smith, S. E.** How drugs act. 5. Intolerance, idiosyncrasy and hypersensitivity. Nursing Times, 71, 31 Jul 1975, 1170–1171.

28 **Tobey, L. E. and Covington, T. R.** Antimicrobial drug interaction. American Journal of Nursing, 75 (9), Sep 1975, 1470–1473.

29 **Waters, W. E.** Analgesics and the kidney. [Damage done by phenacetin and other compounds.] Nursing Times, 69, 27 Sep 1973, 1241–1243.

30 **Wood, S. R.** Drug eruptions. [Vascular-type rashes caused by administration of drugs.] Nursing Times, 70, 10 Jan 1974, 40–41.

c DRUG ADMINISTRATION

1 **Alsop, J. A.** Drug control in hospitals. 1. [Shotley Bridge Hospital System.] Nursing Mirror, 136, 9 Mar 1973, 16–20.

2 **American Journal of Nursing** Ideas that work: control system for medication cards. American Journal of Nursing, 71 (11), Nov 1971, 2162.

3 **Bassili, A. R. and McMahon, M. E. A.** Bridging the pharmacy-nursing communications gap: a study at Kingston General Hospital. [Ontario.] Hospital Administration in Canada, 26 (9), Sep 1974, 30, 32–34.

4 **Bennetts, F. E.** Premedication. Nursing Times, 70, 13 Jun 1974, 911–913.

5 **Budd, R.** We changed to unit-dose system. Nursing Outlook, 19 (2), Feb 1971, 116–117.

6 **Danvers, J. N.** Spanner in the works. [Difficulties arising from different views of doctors on right sedation.] Nursing Times, 67, 25 Mar 1971, 364–365.

7 **Ellis, S. and others** Control of drugs in small hospitals. The West Cornwall system. Nursing Times, 68, 16 Mar 1972; Occ. papers, 41–44.

8 **Ford, P. M.** Unit dose drug distribution at ward level. [Experiment at the Hospital for Women at Leeds.] Nursing Times, 69, 27 Sep 1973, 1262–1265.

9 **Frost, D.** Drug administration. 4. Control of drugs in small hospitals. Nursing Times, 69, 2 Aug 1973, 997.

10 **Frost, D.** Drug mistakes in hospitals and ways to prevent them. [Review of two programmed learning booklets issued by Aberdeen to teach their system of drug administration.] Nursing Times, 68, 3 Aug 1972, 978–979.

11 **Greene, R. J.** Drug administration. 2. Drug information at ward level. Nursing Times, 69, 2 Aug 1973, 992–993.

12 **Hayes, M. H.** Pharmacists need nurses – nurses

need pharmacists – patients need both. American Journal of Nursing, 72 (4), Apr 1972, 723–724.

13 Hedley, E. A. and others, editors The prescription and administration of medicines in hospital: a teaching programme for nurse training, based on the Aberdeen Hospitals System. Aberdeen: Waverley Press, 1971. 2 vols.

14 Hopkins, S. J. The widening gap. [Communication between the ward and the pharmacy department.] Nursing Mirror, 136, 26 Jan 1973, 24–25.

15 Lamp The medication void and the need for nursing and pharmacy staff co-operation. Lamp, 32 (8), Aug 1975, 28–30.

16 Librach, I. Return to nursing. 16. Drugs – their administration, action and uses. Nursing Mirror, 133, 10 Sep 1971, 25–31.

17 Mackie, A. M. Prescription drugs to hospital wards – an approach. Australian Nurses' Journal, 2 (3), Sep 1972, 25.

18 Moggach, B. B. Drug administration times should be reexamined. [Revised time schedules put into effect following inservice program reinforced by videotape.] Canadian Nurse, 71 (1), Jan 1975, 17–19.

19 Moir, D. C. Re-evaluation of a method of prescribing drugs in hospital. [Aberdeen General Hospitals Group.] Health Bulletin, 29 (3), Jul 1971, 131–136.

20 Naismith, N. W. Cost effectiveness of a ward pharmacist. UNA Nursing Journal, Jan/Feb 1974, 24–30.

21 Nelson, J. Drug book addiction. [Differences between the control of drugs in hospitals and at home.] Nursing Mirror, 136, 27 Apr 1973, 15.

22 Nursing Mirror Safer drug handling. [Unit-dose dispensing at the Central Hospital, Warwick.] Nursing Mirror, 139, 12 Sep 1974, 55.

23 Nursing Times Prescription in hospital [of barbiturates.] Nursing Times, 71, 18 Sep 1975, 1495–1496.

24 Nursing Times What do we mean by quality control? Nursing Times, 68, 23 Mar 1972, 344–345.

25 Oxford Regional Health Authority The findings of the Committee of Enquiry to investigate the circumstances leading to the death of a three-year old boy at the Horton General Hospital, Banbury, in February 1974. [Mistake in drug dosage.] Nursing Mirror, 139, 9 Aug 1974, 45; Nursing Times, 70, 15 Aug 1974, 1258.

26 Oxfordshire Nursing and Midwives Committee Drug administration. [Booklet on nursing procedures.] Nursing Mirror, 141, Aug 1975, 56–59.

27 Rodman, M. J. Drug therapy today. Dangers of unsupervised medications. RN Magazine, 37 (7), Jul 1974, 51, (8 pages).

28 Schlotfeldt, R. M. Approaches to the study of nursing questions and the development of nursing science. Introduction by Razella M. Schlotfeldt, 484–485. Nursing Research, 21 (6), Nov/Dec 1972, 484–517.

29 Schneiter, L. J. Nurse meets pharmacy technician. Hospitals, 45 (21), 1 Nov 1971, 62, 66, 68, 122.

30 Tank, C. A. Administration of drugs and the role of the nurse. Hospital Administration in Canada, 13 (9), Sep 1971, 28, 30, 56.

d INTRAVENOUS THERAPY

1 American Journal of Nursing I.V. therapy: preventing its hazards. American Journal of Nursing, 74 (11), Nov 1974, 1980–1981.

2 Berger, B. G. Keeping tabs on I.V. fluid intake. RN Magazine, 38 (10), Oct 1975, ICU, 9.

3 Colvin, M. P. and others A safe long-term infusion technique? [System used in the London hospital.] Lancet, 2, 12 Aug 1972, 317–320.

4 Daly, J. M. and others Central venous catherization. American Journal of Nursing, 75 (5), May 1975, 820–824.

5 Donn, R. Intravenous admixture incompatibility. American Journal of Nursing, 71 (2), Feb 1971, 325.

6 Engel, G. Addition of drugs to intravenous fluids. Australian Nurses Journal, 1 (8), Feb 1972, 23–25.

7 Field, E. S. Practical aspects of intravenous infusions. Nursing Mirror, 133, 9 Jul 1971, 31–35; 16 Jul 1971, 30–33.

8 Geolot, D. H. and McKinney, N. P. Administering parenteral drugs. American Journal of Nursing, 75 (5), May 1975, 788–793.

9 Goldberg, L. A. Intravenous additive programme. Nursing Times, 70, 27 Jun 1974, 998–999.

10 Henney, C. R. and Brodlie, P. Problems of administering drugs by intravenous infusion. Nursing Times, 70, 6 Jun 1974, 866–868.

11 Iles, J. E. M. and Newman, M. S. Infusion therapy – problems encountered by nurses. [Survey at the London Hospital.] Nursing Times, 71, 15 May 1975, 767–769.

12 Isler, C. The hidden dangers. I.V. therapy. The case for the I.V. therapist. RN Magazine, 36 (10), Oct 1973, 23, 26–31.

13 Kozma, M. T. and Newton, D. W. Nursing guidelines for in-syringe mixtures. Supervisor Nurse, 6 (8), Aug 1975, 26–27, 31, 33.

14 Lafferty, M. K. 'Don't tell me that drip has run out again' – or 'Whatever happened to that revolutionary intravenous regulator?' [Device to improve intravenous therapy control.] Australian Nurses' Journal, 5 (3), Sep 1975, 30–31.

15 Ledney, D. IV therapy. Bedside Nurse, 4 (8), Aug 1971, 17–20.

16 Masterton, J. P. Intravenous therapy and resuscitation. Australian Nurses' Journal, 3 (2), Aug 1973, 22–25, 42.

17 Meers, P. D. and others Intravenous infusion of contaminated dextrose solution. The Devonport incident. Lancet, 2, 24 Nov 1973, 1189–1192.

18 Mitchell, E. Much ado about something. [Care of intravenous infusions.] Nursing Times, 68, 30 Mar 1972, 367–369.

19 Mutton, C. J. The management of intravenous infusions. Nursing Times, 69, 24 May 1973, 671–672; 69, 31 May 1973, 701–702.

20 Nursing Mirror Infusion therapy and prescription sheet design: a hospital pharmacist's viewpoint. [Reprinted from Pharmaceutical Journal, 1 May 1971.] Nursing Mirror, 133, 23 Jul 1971, 38–39.

21 Plumer, A. L. Principles and practice of intravenous therapy. 2nd ed. Boston: Little, Brown, 1975.

22 RN Magazine A guide to admixture compatibility. 36 RN Magazine, 10, Oct 1973, 32–37; (11), Nov 1973, 36–40; (12), Dec 1973, 32–37.

23 RN magazine How to insert an I.V. step by step. [Mainly illustrations.] RN Magazine, 36 (10), Oct 1973, 24–25.

24 Ross, A. Infusion phlebitis. [Explores the incidence of phlebitis in relation to continuous intravenous infusions.] Nursing Research, 21 (4), Jul–Aug 1972, 313–318.

25 Snider, M. A. Helpful hints on I.V.s. [The technical skills involved in intravenous therapy.] American Journal of Nursing, 74 (11), Nov 1974, 1978–1981.

26 Whyte, B. B. Intravenous fluids – the nurse's view. Nursing Mirror, 134, 21 Jan 1972, 30.

27 Wilmore, D. W. The future of intravenous therapy. American Journal of Nursing, 71 (12), Dec 1971, 2334–2338.

e PATIENT TEACHING AND COMPLIANCE

1 Closson, R. G. and Kikugawa, C. Noncompliance varies with drug class. Study shows that outpatient noncompliance is higher than average in some therapeutic classes, lower in others. Hospitals, 49, 16 Aug 1975, 89–93.

2 Hecht, A. B. Improving medication compliance by teaching outpatients. Nursing Forum, 13 (2), 1974, 112–129.

3 Jones, M. F. and Brown, R. E. 'Home medicines' – two campaigns which highlight the problem of medicine hoarding in the home. [Survey at Hereford and Brighton.] Health Education Journal, 34 (4), 1974, 112–114.

4 Marks, J. and Clarke, M. The hospital patient and his knowledge of the drugs he is receiving. International Nursing Review, 19 (1), 1972, 39–51.

5 Riley, B. B. Medicines – comments on some questions a patient may ask a nurse. Queen's Nursing Journal, 17 (8), Nov 1974, 169–170.

6 Scowen, P. Open forum. Take 27 tablets daily. [Drug prescription for patients at home and hoarding and non-compliance with recommended dosage.] Nursing Mirror, 140, 20 Feb 1975, 71.

7 Stobele, B. How to counsel patients on cortisone. RN Magazine, 38 (7), Jul 1975, 57–60.

8 Wootton, J. Prescription for error. [The necessity of patient education in the use of drugs as shown by a New York hospital survey.] Nursing Times, 71, 5 Jun 1975, 884–886.

f DRUG MISUSE

1 Campaign on the use and restriction of barbiturates 'Too much uncritical use of hypnotic drugs which do not solve any problems.' [Report of a short course for nurses and doctors.] Nursing Times, 71, 25 Sep 1975, 1522.

2 Distasio, C. and Nawrot, M. Methaqualone. Current patterns of abuse of this drug reflect the need for its legal control. American Journal of Nursing, 73 (11), Nov 1973, 1922–1925.

3 Hopkins, S. J. Drug misuse and the law. Nursing Mirror, 138, 12 Apr 1974, 62.

4 Hunter, A. W. A new misuse of drugs laws. Midwives Chronicle, 86, Oct 1973, 320–321.

5 Madden, J. S. Analgesic abuse. [Side effects and misuse by patients.] Nursing Times, 70, 23 May 1974, 795–796.

6 Parliament Misuse of drugs act, 1971. HMSO, 1975.

7 Swaffield, L. Voluntary restraint. [Campaign on the use and restriction of Barbituates.] Nursing Times, 71, 11 Sep 1975, 1440.

g POISONING AND SELF POISONING

1 Baker, J. Survey on suicides and accidental poisoning. Nursing Times, 67, 4 Mar 1971, 258–261.

2 Brown, L. and others Drug overdosage. UNA Nursing Journal, 69, Jul 1971. 8–17.

3 Craft, A. W. Accidental poisoning in children. Nursing Times, 71, 12 Jun 1975, 932–933.

4 Craft, A. W. and Nicholson, A. The management of poisoning in children. Nursing Times, 71, 19 Jun 1975, 977–979.

5 Forrest, J. A. H. Acute poisoning. [Statistics and types of drugs involved in acute poisoning, emergency measures and treatment, and psychiatric aspects.] Nursing Times, 70, 18 Apr 1974, 590–592.

6 Goulding, R. Self-poisoning. Nursing Mirror, 133, 3 Dec 1971, 13–14.

7 Husband, P. Accidental poisoning in childhood. Midwife and Health Visitor, 9 (3), Mar 1973, 81–84.

8 Julyan, M. and Kuzemko, J. A. Accidental poisoning in children: The 'sick family'. [Survey in Peterborough. Conducted by health visitors.] Practitioner, 214, Jun 1975, 813–815.

9 Julyan, M. and Kuzemko, J. A. Parents and their children in accidental poisoning. Practitioner, 208, Feb 1972, 252–253.

10 Kennedy, P. Not another overdose! Nursing Times, 70, 10 Oct 1974, 1566–1567.

11 Kerr, D. N. S. Self poisoning with paracetamol. Nursing Times, 69, 19 Jul 1973, 924–926.

12 Lavington, D. C. Nursing care study. A night to remember. [Admission of patient after an overdose.] Nursing Times, 71, 18 Sep 1975, 1497–1499.

13 Matthew, H. Acute poisoning. Nursing Mirror, 133, 10 Dec 1971, 28–31.

14 Milligan, H. Accidental poisoning and the nurse. Nursing Times, 70, 26 Sep 1974, 1510–1511.

15 Patel, A. R. Attitudes towards self-poisoning. [Study of physicians and senior nurses showing unfavourable attitudes towards patients.] British Medical Journal, 2, 24 May 1975, 426–430.

16 Robertson, A. Medicines can kill. [Report of a Health Education Council campaign against accidental home poisoning.] Queen's Nursing Journal, 18 (2), May 1975, 40–41.

17 Rodman, M. J. Drug therapy today. Poisonings and their treatment. RN Magazine, 35 (11), Nov 1972, 57, 60–64, 67–68, 70.

18 Smith, E. S. Emergency – overdose. Nursing Times, 69, 22 Mar 1973. 370–371.

19 Smith, S. E. How drugs act – 6. Overdosage and poisoning. Nursing Times, 71, 31 Jul 1975, 1220–1221.

20 Thomson, W. Carbon monoxide poisoning. Nursing Times, 67, 3 Jun 1971, 668–669.

21 Townsend, A. Nursing care study. Laura – recovery from an overdose. Nursing Times, 69, 1 Nov 1973, 1446–1448.

22 Tucker, S. M. Kerosene poisoning in children. Mother and Child, 44 (6), Nov/Dec 1972, 9–10.

23 Webster, E. A. Accidental poisoning in children. Health Bulletin, 29 (4), Oct 1971, 214–219.

24 Wilson, P. Nursing care study. Self-administered overdose of imipramine. Nursing Mirror, 141, 4 Sep 1975, 48–49.

25 Wright, N. Acute paracetamol poisoning. Nursing Mirror, 141, 4 Dec 1975, 59–60.

h OXYGEN THERAPY

1 DiPalma, J. R. Drug therapy today. Oxygen as drug therapy. RN Magazine, 34 (8), Aug 1971, 49–51, 53–54.

2 Gaul, A. L. and Hart, G. B. Baromedical nursing combines critical, acute, chronic care. [Hyperbaric oxygen treatment (OHP).] AORN Journal, 21 (6), May 1975, 1038–1047.

3 Gaul, A. L. and others Hyperbaric oxygen therapy. American Journal of Nursing, 72 (5), May 1972, 892–896.

4 Lee, R. M. and Harrison, A. M. Hyperbaric oxygenation. AORN Journal, 21 (6), May 1975, 1048–1053.

5 Mutton, C. J. Oxygen – the need for caution. [It is becoming general practice now that oxygen should be administered only on medical instruction. Not only is the decision to give oxygen a medical decision, but so is the mode of administration and also the flow rate.] Nursing Times, 70, 12 Dec 1974, 1945–1947.

6 Neelon, V. J. and McIntosh, H. D. Hyperbaric oxygenation. 1. Therapeutic benefits. 2. Hazards and implications. Cardio vascular Nursing, 7 (3), May/Jun 1971, 69–72; (4), Jul/Aug 1971, 73–76.

7 Oslick, T. Applied oxygen therapy. RN Magazine, 36 (1), Jan 1973, ICU, 1–2, 4, 6–8.

8 Stark, R. D. and Bishop, J. M. New method of oxygen therapy in the home using an oxygen concentrator. [Rimer-Birlec domiciliary oxygen concentrator in treatment of chronic bronchitis.] British Medical Journal, 2, 14 Apr 1973, 105–106.

59 PAIN

a GENERAL (Includes nursing care)

1 American Journal of Nursing Pain and suffering: a special supplement. American Journal of Nursing, 74 (3), Mar 1974, 489–520.

2 Bowman, M. P. Pain. Nursing Mirror, 136, 5 Jan 1973, 28–29.

3 British Medical Journal Attitude to pain. [Includes comment on Rcn publication 'Information – A prescription against pain'.] British Medical Journal, 3, 2 Aug 1975, 261.

4 British Medical Journal Is your pain really necessary? British Medical Journal, 2, 12 May 1973, 323–324.

5 Cashatt, B. Pain: a patient's view. American Journal of Nursing, 72 (2), Feb 1972, 281.

6 Coleman, V. The algometer: as useful as the thermometer. [For measuring pain.] Nursing Mirror, 141, 17 Jul 1975, 55.

7 Copple, D. What can a nurse do to relieve pain without resort to drugs? Nursing Times, 68, 11 May 1972, 584.

8 Diers, D. and others The effect of nursing interaction on patients in pain. Nursing Research, 21 (5), Sep/Oct 1972, 419–428.

9 Dudley-Hart, F. editor The treatment of chronic pain. Medical and Technical Publishing Co, 1974.

10 Gaumer, W. C. Psychological potentials of chronic pain. Journal of Psychiatric Nursing and Mental Health Services, 12 (5), Sep/Oct 1974, 23–24

11 Goloskov, J. W. and LeRoy, P. L. The evolving role of the nurse and the neurosurgical physician's assistant in the treatment of intractable pain states. Journal of Neurosurgical Nursing, 7 (2), Dec 1975, 107–115.

12 Gowell, E. A. Transactional analysis strategies for dealing with pain. Journal of Psychiatric Nursing and Mental Health Services, 12 (5), Sep/Oct 1974, 25–30.

13 Hayward, J. Information – a prescription against pain. Royal College of Nursing, 1975. (The study of Nursing Care Project Reports Series 2.)

14 Jacox, A. and Stewart, M. Psychosocial contingencies of the pain experience. Iowa University College of Nursing, 1973.

15 Johnson, J. E. and Rice, V. H. Sensory and distress components of pain: implications for the study of clinical pain. Nursing Research, 23 (3), May/Jun 1974, 203–209.

16 Keele, K. D. Pain – how it varies from person to person. Nursing Times, 68, 20 Jul 1972, 890–892.

17 Lloyd, J. W. The problem of pain. District Nursing, 14 (11), Feb 1972, 229–230.

18 McCaffery, M. Nursing management of the patient with pain. Philadelphia: Lippincott, 1972.

19 Melzack, R. The puzzle of pain. Harmondsworth, Penguin Education, 1973. (Penguin science of behaviour series.)

20 Mulcahy, R. A. and Janx, N. Effectiveness of raising pain perception threshold in males and females using a psychoprophylactic childbirth technique during induced pain. Nursing Research, 22 (5), Sep/Oct 1973, 423–427.

21 Physiotherapy Issue on pain. 2 parts. Physiotherapy, 60 (4), Apr 1974, 96–106; (5), May 1974, 128–140.

22 Sambrook, M. A. Pain in the face. Nursing Times, 71, 16 Jan 1975, 97–99.

23 Schultz, N. V. How children perceive pain. Nursing Outlook, 19 (10), Oct 1971, 670–673.

24 Strauss, A. and others Pain: an organizational-work-interactional perspective. [Research into the experience of patients in pain and their interactions with staff.] Nursing Outlook, 22 (9), Sep 1974, 560–569.

b PAIN RELIEF

1 Baskett, P. J. F. The use of Entonox by nursing staff and physiotherapists. [50 per cent nitrous oxide and oxygen contained in a single cylinder for the relief of pain.] Nursing Mirror, 135, 15 Sep 1972, 30–32.

2 Faint, J. Cold comfort – for alleviation of pain. Nursing Mirror, 132, 25 Jun 1971, 32–33.

3 Gill, M. Aspirin, the pain killer. Nursing Care, 6 (5), May 1973, 23–25.

4 Hannington-Kiff, J. G. Pain relief. Heinemann, 1974.

5 Hart, F. D. Control of pain at night. Nursing Times, 69, 3 May 1973, 559–562.

6 Hayden, J. Aspirin – a short review of its history, effects and uses. Queen's Nursing Journal, Sep 1975, 172, 174.

7 Hirskyj, L. Use of entonox in a general hospital. [Inhalational analgesia to relieve pain and discomfort in the accident department and the general wards.] Nursing Times, 67, 21 Oct 1971, 1321–1323.

8 Isler, C. New approach to intractable pain. [A multidisciplinary pain clinic at University Hospital, Seattle.] RN Magazine, 38 (1), Jan 1975, 17–21.

9 Johnson, I. Transcutaneous electrical stimulation. [Use of electricity to relieve pain.] Journal of Neurosurgical Nursing, 7 (2), Dec 1975, 87–90.

10 Keough, G. and Fox, J. L. The neuropacemaker – relief for patients with intractable pain. RN Magazine, 35 (8), Aug 1972, ICU, 1–4.

11 Kerrane, T. A. The Brompton Cocktail. [Analgesic used at the Brompton Hospital following thoracic surgery.] Nursing Mirror, 140, 1 May 1975, 59.

12 Liddell, D. Analgesic on trial: a year's trial in a colliery medical centre has shown Entonox to be a satisfactory light analgesic. Occupational Health, 26 (10), Oct 1974, 396–400.

13 Lipton, S. The relief of intractable pain by cordotomy. Nursing Times, 69, 14 Jun 1973, 755–757.

14 Miles, J. and others Pain relief by implanted electrical stimulators. Lancet, 1, 27 Apr 1974, 777–779.

15 Parkhouse, J. Assessment of relief. Nursing Mirror, 135, 4 Aug 1972, 13–14.

16 Robbie, D. S. The pain clinic. [Efforts to control intractable pain.] Nursing Mirror, 134, 26 May 1972, 33–34.

17 Samarasinghe, J. A series of articles from the Royal Marsden Hospital, London. 4. Clinical evaluation of analgesic drugs. Nursing Mirror, 134, 2 Jun 1972, 18–19.

18 Smith, S. E. Drug therapy, 1971. 10. Drugs and pain. Nursing Times, 67, 30 Sep 1971, 1213–1214.

19 Smith, S. E. How drugs act. 10. Drugs and pain. Nursing Times, 71, 28 Aug 1975, 1379–1380.

20 Swerdlow, M. The pain clinic. British Journal of Clinical Practice, 26 (9), Sep 1972, 403–407.

c TERMINAL AND CANCER PAIN

1 Janzen, E. Relief of pain: prerequisite to the care and comfort of the dying. [St. Christopher's Hospice.] Nursing Forum, 13 (1), 1974, 48–51.

2 Lamerton, R. Care of the dying. 6. The pains of death. Nursing Times, 69, 11 Jan 1973, 56–57.

3 Lloyd, J. W. The role of pain relief in terminal care. Nursing Mirror, 137, 24 Aug 1973, 36–37.

4 McNulty, B. The problem of pain in the dying patient. Queen's Nursing Journal, 16 (7), Oct 1973, 152, 161.

5 Maher, R. M. Cancer pain in relation to nursing care. Nursing Times, 71, 27 Feb 1975, 344–350.

6 Turnbull, F. Pain and suffering in cancer. Canadian Nurse, 67 (8), Aug 1971, 28–30.

7 Twycross, R. G. Diseases of the central nervous system. Relief of terminal pain. [Methods used at St. Christopher's Hospice.] British Medical Journal, 4, 25 Oct 1975, 212–214.

8 Twycross, R. G. The use of narcotic analgesics in terminal illness. [Study of 500 patients admitted to St. Christopher's Hospice with advanced cancer.] Journal of Medical Ethics, 1 (1), Apr 1975, 10–17.

9 Warr, D. On pain of death. [Terminal pain and the administration of drugs.] New Zealand Nursing Journal, 68 (10), Oct 1974, 21–24, Reprinted in Australian Nurses Journal, 5 (1), Jul 1975, 28–31.

60 PRESSURE SORES

1 Barrett, D. and Klibanski, A. Collagenase debridement: a new collagenolytic agent. American Journal of Nursing, 73 (5), May 1973, 849–851.

2 Barton, A. A. and Barton, M. The medical management of pressure sores. Queen's Nursing Journal, 16 (7), Oct 1973, 148–149, 157.

3 Bell, F. and others Pressure sores – their cause and prevention. Nursing Times, 70, 16 May 1974, 740–745.

4 Berecek, K. H. Etiology of decubitus ulcers. Nursing Clinics of North America, 10 (1), Mar 1975, 157–170.

5 Berecek, K. H. Treatment of decubitus ulcers. Nursing Clinics of North America, 10 (1), Mar 1975, 171–210.

6 Carbary, L. J. Bedsores, a real challenge. Nursing Care, 7 (11), Nov 1974, 22–25.

7 Chin, G. Y. Prevention of pressure sores. Nursing Journal of Singapore, 13 (1), May 1973, 48–51.

8 Chin, G. Y. Treatment of pressure sores. Nursing Journal of Singapore, 13 (2), Nov 1973, 124–125, 128.

9 Dawson, R. L. G. Treatment of pressure sores. [Medical and surgical treatment.] Nursing Times, 70, 18 Jul 1974, 1108–1110.

10 Deokali, M. Prevention of pressure sores in spinal paraplegia and tetraplegia. SA Nursing Journal, 38 (4), Apr 1971, 14–18.

11 Denholm, D. H. The hair dryer treatment for decubiti. Canadian Nurse, 70 (3), Mar 1974, 33–34.

12 Di Pirro, E. Surgery: successful treatment for deep decubiti. RN Magazine, 38 (8), Sep 1975, 28–29.

13 Dyson, R. Dealing with bed sores. Nursing Mirror, 133, 30 Jul 1971, 34–35.

14 Dyson, R. The problem – bedsores. The solution – nurse research worker? Why not? Nursing Mirror, 137, 21 Sep 1973, 40–42.

15 Gerson, L. W. The incidence of pressure sores in active hospital treatment. [Study at three hospitals in St. John's Newfoundland.] International Journal of Nursing Studies, 12 (4), 1974, 201–204.

16 Gosnell, D. J. An assessment tool to identify pressure sores. Nursing Research, 22 (1), Jan/Feb 1973, 55–59.

17 Grahame, R. A promising new treatment for pressure sores. [Water immersion bed.] Nursing Times, 68, 20 Jul 1972, 903–904.

18 Grahame, R. The water bed on active service. [The Beaufort-Winchester Flotation Bed, used in the conservative and surgical management of pressure sores.] Nursing Mirror, 139, 2 Aug 1974, 62–63.

19 Greene, R. Ostomy skin barriers for decubitus ulcers. [Karaya powder and other skin barriers used in enterostomal therapy.] Canadian Nurse, 71 (2), Feb 1975, 34–35.

20 Greenfield, R. A. The low air loss bed system. [In the prevention of pressure sores.] Nursing Times, 68, 21 Sep 1972, 1192–1194.

21 Hoffmiller, M. Oxygen therapy: its use in chronic skin ulcers. Journal of Practical Nursing, 23 (5), May 1973, 20–23.

22 Humphreys, C. S. Pressure sores. UNA Nursing Journal, Jan/Feb 1974, 33–35.

23 Isler, C. Decubitus. Old truths and some new ideas. RN Magazine, 35 (7), Jul 1972, 42–45.

24 Johnson, M. L. Problems involved in the prevention of pressure sores. Nursing Mirror, 135, 28 Jul 1972, 39–41.

25 La Rock, K. L. and Hildebrand, A. What to do for the decubitus patient – post-op. RN Magazine, 38 (9), Sep 1975, 31, 36.

26 Lang, C. and McGrath, A. Gelfoam for decubitus ulcers. American Journal of Nursing, 74 (3), Mar 1974, 460–461.

27 Lowthian, P. T. Bedsores – current methods of prevention and treatment. Nursing Times, 67, 29 Apr 1971, 501–503.

28 Macdonald, M. and Rutherford, M. The treatment of bedsores. [A comparison between conventional therapy and a new preparation, Madecassol.] Nursing Times, 69, 11 Oct 1973, 1344.

29 Marshall, R. S. Cold therapy in the treatment of pressure sores. Physiotherapy, 57 (8), Aug 1971, 372–373.

30 Maynes, M. Testing Betadine Aerosol. [Clinical evaluation of a spray for treating pressure sores used at Purdysburn Hospital, Belfast.] Nursing Mirror, 132, 5 Feb 1971, 20.

31 Miller, M. E. and Sachs, M. L. About bedsores: what you need to know to help prevent and treat them. Philadelphia: Lippincott, 1974.

32 Morley, M. H. Decubitus ulcer management – a team approach. Canadian Nurse, 69 (10), Oct 1973, 41–43.

33 Norton, D Research and the problem of pressure sores. Nursing Mirror, 140, 13 Feb 1975, 65–67.

34 Norton, D. Treating pressure sores. [Letter.] Nursing Mirror, 136, 1 Jun 1973, 35–36.

35 Nursing Care Moisturizing and massage of patient skin is a must to prevent decubitus ulcers. Nursing Care, 7, Feb 1974, 26–27.

36 O'Leary, M. Kinetic nursing: a practical means of avoiding and treating decubitus ulceration. World of Irish Nursing, 1 (6), Jun 1972, 117, 119, 121.

37 Pratt, R. The nursing management of acute spinal paraplegia. 3. Prevention of pressure sores and contractures. Nursing Times, 67, 13 May 1971, 567–569.

38 Pratt, R. The nursing management of acute spinal paraplegia. 6. Treatment of established pressure sores. Nursing Times. 67, 3 Jun 1971, 662–663.

39 Rehabilitation The Steeper Co-Ro bed. [For the prevention of pressure sores.] Rehabilitation, no. 89, Apr/Jun 1974, 27.

40 Resio, D. T. and Verhonick, P. J. On the measurement and analysis of clinical data in nursing. [Studies of low and high risk decubitus ulcer patients are used as an example of data analysis.] Nursing Research, 22 (5), Sep/Oct 1973, 388–393.

41 Robertson, C. E. Gel pillow helps prevent pressure sores. Canadian Nurse, 67 (10), Oct 1971, 44–46.

42 Rosenhouse, L. More hospitals use water beds. Nursing Care, 7, Apr 1974, 26–28.

43 Rubin, C. F. and others Auditing the decubitus ulcer problem. [A nine-month study.] American Journal of Nursing, 74 (10), Oct 1974, 1820–1821.

44 Scales, J. T. and Hopkins, L. A. Patient-support system using low-pressure air. [LAL bed which prevents pressure sores and saves nursing time as there is no need to lift the patient.] Lancet, 2, 23 Oct 1971, 885–888.

45 Schetrumpf, J. R. New bed for treating pressure sores. [Thick layer of plastic balls floating on a shallow water bath.] Lancet, 2, 30 Dec 1972, 1399–1400.

46 Torelli, M. Topical hyperbaric oxygen for decubitus ulcers. American Journal of Nursing, 73 (3), Mar 1973, 494–496.

47 Verhonick, P. J. Clinical studies in nursing: models, methods and madness. [Using the prevention of pressure sores as an example.] Nursing Research, 21, Nov/Dec 1972, 490–493.

48 Verhonick, P. J. and Lewis, D. W.

Thermography in the study of decubitus ulcers: preliminary report. Nursing Research, 21 (3), May/Jun 1972, 233–7.

49 Walker, K. A. Pressure sores: prevention and treatment. Butterworths, 1971.

50 Wallace, G. and Hayter, J. Karaya for chronic skin ulcers. [Karaya procedure for decubitus ulcers.] American Journal of Nursing, 74 (6), Jun 1974, 1094–1098; see also Nursing Times, 70, 3 Oct 1974, 1537.

51 Williams, A. A study of factors contributing to skin breakdown. [Decubitus ulcers.] Nursing Research, 21 (3), May/Jun 1972, 238–243.

52 Williams, E. and Hysick, R. M. Gold leaf treatment of decubitus ulcer. Journal of Psychiatric Nursing and Mental Health Services, 12 (5), Sep/Oct 1974, 42–44.

61 NUTRITION AND DIET

a GENERAL (See also Infant Feeding; Elderly)

1 Brereton, P. The professions supplementary to medicine. Dietetics. Nursing Mirror, 141, 6 Nov 1975, 69–72.

2 Cleave, T. L. The saccharine disease. Nursing Times, 70, 15 Aug 1974, 1274–1275.

3 Clegg, D. J. and Sandi, E. Trace elements in food. Canadian Nurse, 69, Feb 1973, 38–42.

4 Coates, M. E. Nutrition and the microbes of the digestive tract. Nursing Times, 71, 23 Jan 1975, 152–153.

5 Cooper, P. The present status of ascorbic acid. [Vitamin C.] Midwife, Health Visitor and Community Nurse, 11 (10), Oct 1975, 346.

6 Council for Professions Supplementary to Medicine. Dietitians Board Dietitions of the future: a report of a working party. The Council, 1975.

7 Davies, J. G. and others Special diets in hospitals; discrepancy between what is prescribed and what is eaten. British Medical Journal, 1, 25 Jan 1975, 200–202.

8 Fawns, H. T. Discovery of vitamin C. James Lind and the scurvy. Nursing Times, 71, 5 Jun 1975, 872–875.

9 Fawns, H. Vitamin B and beriberi. How a random observation in a prison yard led to the discovery, and eventual synthesis of Vitamin B. Nursing Times, 71, 20 Nov 1975, 1870–1873.

10 Feingold, B. F. Hyperkinesis and learning disabilities linked to artificial food flavors and colors. American Journal of Nursing, 75 (5), May 1975, 797–803.

11 Kane, L. T. Canada inside out: surveying the nation's nutrition. Canadian Nurse, 70 (8), Aug 1974, 30–33.

12 Rajapakse, D. A. Beverages and disease – the undiluted truth. Nursing Times, 69, 1 Nov 1973, 1449–1451.

13 Rosenhouse, L. This patient has pica. [Craving for unnatural foods prevalent in children, pregnant women and the elderly.] Nursing Care, 7 (12), Dec 1974, 16–17.

14 Smith, S. E. How drugs act. 7. Vitamins. Nursing Times, 71, 7 Aug 1975, 1256–1257.

15 Snively, W. D. and others Sodium-restricted diet: review and current status. Nursing Forum, 13 (1), 1974, 59–86.

16 Thomas, J. E. The nutritional component of health education. Health Education Journal, 34 (1), 1975, 14–21.

17 Williams, E. R. Making vegetarian diets nutritious. American Journal of Nursing, 75 (12), Dec 1975, 2168–2173.

b COMMUNITY SERVICES

1 Massey-Lynch, M. Dietitian in the practice. Practice Team, (47), Apr 1975, 8, 10.

2 Massey-Lynch, M. The role of the practice-based dietitian [at Maghull, Lancashire.] Queen's Nursing Journal, 17 (9), Dec 1974, 192–193.

3 Robert-Sargeant, S. and Essex-Carter, A. The role of the nutritionist in the community health service. Community Health, 5 (3), Nov/Dec 1973, 137–142.

4 Steven, M. C. The work of nutritionists (dietitians) in community health centres. [Dumbarton Health Centre.] Community Health, 6, Jan–Feb 1975, 199–204.

5 Yorke, R. A. and others The practice based dietitian: a preliminary report on five years' experience. Journal of the Royal College of General Practitioners, 23, Oct 1973, 730–731, 734–735.

c NURSING

1 Anderson, L. and others Nutrition in nursing. Philadelphia: Lippincott, 1972.

2 Beck, M. E. Nutrition and dietetics for nurses. 3rd ed. Churchill Livingstone, 1971. 4th ed., 1975.

3 Blenkiron, C. H. Thought for food. [Control of patients' dietary intake.] Nursing Times, 69, 6 Sep 1973, 1150–1153.

4 Boykin, L. S. Nutrition in nursing. Flushing: Medical Examination Publishing Co, 1975. (Nursing outline series.)

5 Cross, J. E. and Parsons, C. R. Nurse-teaching and goal-directed nurse-teaching to motivate change in food selection behavior of hospitalized patients. Nursing Research, 20 (5), Sep/Oct 1971, 454–458.

6 Dwyer, L. S. and Fralin, F. G. Simplified meal planning for hard-to-teach patients. American Journal of Nursing, 74 (4), Apr 1974, 664–665.

7 Jelliffe, E. P. Nutrition in nursing curricula. [Historical perspective and present day trends.] Journal of Tropical Paediatric and Environmental Health, 20 (3), Jun 1974, 453–456.

8 Johnson, M. Integrating diet therapy in a diploma nursing program: the method developed at Northwest Texas Hospital School of Nursing. New York: National League for Nursing, 1971. (League Exchange, no. 94.)

9 Kurtz, C. Patient nutritional care: a dilemma for the hospital nurse. Journal of the American Dietetic Association, 67 (4), Oct 1975, 367–369.

10 Lapointe, G. A nutritional course for nurses. [At Concordia University, Montreal for qualified nurses.] Canadian Nurse, 71 (1), Jan 1975, 30–31.

11 McCarter, D. Nourishing the solute-sensitive patient. [Nursing care study.] American Journal of Nursing, 73 (11), Nov 1973, 1935–1936.

12 McDaniel, J. M. and Savage, J. R. Diet therapy in the curriculum: survey reveals a decreasing emphasis. Nursing Outlook, 22 (12), Dec 1974, 781–784.

13 McNutt, K. W. Nurses as part of the nutrition team. [Opportunity of the occupational health nurse for providing nutrition education.] Occupational Health Nursing, 23 (4), Apr 1974, 7–11.

d INTRAVENOUS FEEDING

1 Baker, D. I. Hyperalimentation at home. [Long term intravenous therapy carried out at home with the help of a nurse practitioner.] American Journal of Nursing, 74 (10), Oct 1974, 1826–1829.

2 Campbell, M. E. 104 days with Rodney K. [Case history of patient on parenteral hyperalimentation.] RN Magazine, 36 (7), Jul 1973, 34–37.

3 Crooks, P. F. Intravenous feeding and the dietitian. Nutrition, 29 (6), Nov/Dec 1975, 357–365.

4 Deitel, M. Intravenous hyperalimentation. Canadian Nurse, 69 (1), Jan 1973, 38–43.

5 Grant, J. A. The nurse's role in parenteral hyperalimentation. RN Magazine, 36 (7), Jul 1973, 28–33.

6 Grant, J. A. Preventing infection, maintaining flow called primarily nurse's responsibility. [Hyperalimentation.] Hospital Topics, 50 (6), Jun 1972, 94, 98, 100.

7 Humphrey, N. M. and others Parenteral hyperalimentation for children. American Journal of Nursing, 72 (2), Feb 1972, 286–288.

8 Jones, D. Food for thought: a descriptive study of the nutritional nursing care of unconscious patients in general hospitals. Rcn, 1975. (Study of nursing care series, 2 no. 4.) Based on MPhil thesis Surrey University, 1975.

9 Parsa, M. H. and others Central venous alimentation. American Journal of Nursing, 72 (11), Nov 1972, 2042–2047.

10 Persons, C. D. Parenteral nutrition by total intravenous feeding. Australian Nurses' Journal, 3 (4), Oct 1973, 23–27.

11 Soper, R. Catheter care in pediatric hyperalimentation. RN Magazine, 38 (3), Mar 1975, 66–67.

12 Tudor, L. L. Feeding the helpless patient requires a special technique. Nursing Care, 7 (10), Oct 1974, 22–24.

e MALNUTRITION AND DEVELOPING COUNTRIES

1 Bailey, K. V. Malnutrition in the African region. WHO Chronicle, 29 (9), Sep 1975, 354–364.

2 Bailey, K. V. Nutrition and family health [in developing countries]. World of Irish Nursing, 3 (5), May 1974, 76–78.

3 Bengoa, J. M. The problem of malnutrition. WHO Chronicle, 28 (1), Jan 1974, 3–7.

4 Biswas, J. Maternal nutrition. Nursing Journal of India, 64 (6), Jun 1973, 200–201, 204.

5 Brookes, P. Malnutrition – a new approach needed. Nursing Times, 67, 7 Oct 1971, 1237–1239.

6 Calderbank, D. A. Facing the food crisis. Nursing Times, 71, 6 Mar 1975, 366–367.

7 Cross, J. Malnutrition. [In developing countries.] Nursing Times, 68, 21 Dec 1972, 1611.

8 Goodsell, S. Better food for a healthier world. Nursing Mirror, 138, 5 Apr 1974, 47–51.

9 Harding, L. Nursing care study. A losing battle? [Marasmus in twins at St. Luke's Hospital, Msoro, Zambia.] Nursing Mirror, 139, 10 Oct 1974, 72–74.

10 Langesen, M. Child's bangle for the diagnosis of undernutrition. Nursing Journal of India, 66 (8), Aug 1975, 176–177.

11 Latimer, C. Nutrition in the Eastern Solomon Islands. Nursing Mirror, 133, 8 Oct 1971, 40–41.

12 Luker, K. A. A food programme for drought striken Niger. Nursing Times, 71, 6 Mar 1975, 368–370.

13 Morley, D. National nutritional planning [in developing countries]. British Medical Journal, 4, 12 Oct 1974, 85–88.

14 Nkunika, B. Nursing care study. Socio-economic disease. Marasmus among the starving children of the Third World. Nursing Times, 70, 7 Nov 1974, 1752–1753.

15 Nursing Journal of India Issue on nutrition. Nursing Journal of India, 65 (4), Apr 1974, 109–120.

16 Rahimtoola, R. Malnutrition: physical and mental effects on child. Pakistan Nursing and Health Review, 1, 1971. 4–9.

17 World Health Issue on malnutrition. World Health, Feb/Mar 1974, 4–53.

18 World Health Organization Better food for a healthier world. 25 facts about nutrition. Nursing Mirror, 138, 5 Apr 1974, 50–51.

19 WHO Chronicle Nutrition: a review of the WHO programme. 1. WHO Chronicle, 26 (4), Apr 1972, 160–179.

62 REHABILITATION AND THERAPY

a GENERAL

1 Bell, S. J. Rehabilitation pilot scheme. [Rehabilitation unit at the Palmerston North Hospital, New Zealand.] New Zealand Nursing Journal, 66 (12), Dec 1973, 14–16.

2 British Association for Rheumatology and Rehabilitation Symposium on rehabilitation services with particular reference to the future structure of the health service. Rheumatology and Rehabilitation, 12 (4), Nov 1973, 187–194.

3 Central Health Services Council. Standing Medical Advisory Committee Rehabilitation: report of a subcommittee. HMSO, 1972. Chairman: Professor Sir Ronald Tunbridge.

4 China, K. Occupational rehabilitation. [Part played by the occupational health team.] Queen's Nursing Journal, 16 (9), Dec 1973, 200–201.

5 Daniel, J. W. Industrial resettlement of hospital patients. Nursing Times, 69, 18 Oct 1973, 1387–1388.

6 Department of Health and Social Security. Working party on the remedial professions The remedial professions: a report. HMSO, 1973. Chairman: E. L. Macmillan.

7 Drug and Therapeutics Bulletin Convalescence: rehabilitation needs more attention. Drug and Therapeutics Bulletin, 11 (11), 25 May 1973, 43–44.

8 Haupt, F. J. G. A review of rehabilitation. SA Nursing Journal, 61 (13), Jan 1973, 19–24.

9 Joseph, Rt. Hon. Sir K. Strategy for the development of the medical rehabilitation services. Rehabilitation, no. 87, Oct/Dec 1973, 27–35.

10 Kosunen, E. Co-ordination of medical, social, educational and vocational rehabilitation services. Rehabilitation, no. 87, Oct/Dec 1973, 15–17.

11 Lee, R. H. and others Rehabilitation policy: a study of a regional rehabilitation hospital. Hospital and Health Services Review, 70 (10), Oct 1974, 346–350.

12 Lord, D. Towards a national rehabilitation service? [The Tunbridge Report: discussion.] British Hospital Journal and Social Service Review, 82, 11 Nov 1972, 2520–2521.

13 Nichols, P. J. R. Rehabilitation in the reorganized National Health Service. British Journal of Occupational Therapy, 37 (7), Jul 1974, 113–116; Rehabilitation, no. 94, Jul/Sep 1975, 11–18.

14 O'Leary, J. A. Industrial rehabilitation: the specially modified machines installed in the Vauxhall Rehabilitation Centre provide both useful work and remedial exercise for unfit and injured employees. Occupational Health, 26 (10), Oct 1974, 391–395.

15 Preli, C. Rehabilitation: a united effort. Bedside Nurse, 4 (4), Apr 1971, 17–23.

16 Queen's Nursing Journal Issue on rehabilitation. Queen's Nursing Journal, 16 (9), Dec 1973, 197–204.

17 Ramsden, V. J. The ethic. [The ethics of rehabilitation.] Health and Social Service Journal, 84, 27 Jul 1974, 1682.

18 Randle, A. P. H. Rehabilitation and society. [The history of rehabilitation in Great Britain.] Occupational Therapy, 37 (1), Jan 1974, 15–17.

19 Riffle, K. L. Rehabilitation: the evolution of a social concept. Nursing Clinics of North America, 8 (4), Dec 1973, 665–671.

20 Sharman, E. M. The problems of a rehabilitation service. Physiotherapy, 58 (1), 10 Jan 1972, 2–9.

21 Sommerville, J. G. The medical rehabilitation of outpatients. [Medical Rehabilitation Centre, Camden Town.] Community Health, 6 (5), Mar/Apr 1975, 257–261.

22 Sommerville, J. G. Rehabilitation: its background and aims. British Journal of Occupational Therapy, 38 (9), Sep 1975, 193–194.

23 Tapsfield, J. S. The professions supplementary to medicine. Nursing Mirror, 141, 25 Sep 1975, 46–47.

24 Treasure, E. R. The importance of rehabilitation in the changing Health Service. Rehabilitation, no. 87, Oct/Dec 1973, 43–45.

25 Tunbridge, Sir R. E. Priorities for a national rehabilitation service. Rehabilitation, no. 82, Jul/Sep 1972, 7–12.

26 Weiss, M. Current development and trends in rehabilitation in Europe. Rehabilitation, no. 88, Jan/Mar 1974, 46–53.

27 Wreford, B. M. Rehabilitation. Occupational Health, 24 (2), Feb 1972, 39–40.

b NURSING

1 Bernhardt, J. H. The role of the occupational health nurse in employee rehabilitation. Occupational Health Nursing 33(9), Sep 1975, 9–14.

2 Berni, R. and Nicholson, C. The POMR as a tool in rehabilitation and patient teaching. Nursing Clinics of North America, 9 (2), Jun 1974, 265–270.

3 Christopherson, V. A. and others Rehabilitation nursing. New York: McGraw-Hill, 1974.

4 Eriksen, M. K. Changing staff behaviour. [A project to teach nurses the skills required in a rehabilitation unit.] Canadian Nurse, 71 (4), Apr 1975, 39–40.

5 Firth, D. and others The value of health visitors in a rehabilitation unit. Rheumatology and Rehabilitation, 12 (3), Aug 1973, 143–147.

6 Kratz, C. Rehabilitation and the district nurse. [Development of nursing involvement in home rehabilitation.] Queen's Nursing Journal, 18 (1), Apr 1975, 17–18.

7 McMenamin, P. Activities of daily living routine in a ward setting. Occupational Therapy, 34 (6), Jun 1971, 7–10.

8 Malinoski, B. M. Recycle for 'rehab.' [Inservice education in rehabilitation nursing in the Community Nursing Service in Philadelphia.] Journal of Nursing Administration, 4 (1), Jan/Feb 1974, 41–44.

9 Schickedanz, H. and Mayhall, P. D. Restorative nursing in a general hospital. Springfield: Thomas, 1975.

10 Sorenson, L. and Ulrich, P. G. Ambulation guide for nurses. Minneapolis: Sister Kenny Institute, 1974.

11 Spinks, M. Working in a rehabilitation centre. [Social Rehabilitation Centre, West Norwood, London.] Nursing Times, 69, 1 Feb 1973, 162–163.

12 Stryker, R. P. Rehabilitative aspects of acute and chronic nursing care. Philadelphia: Saunders, 1972.

13 Valadez, A. M. and Anderson, E. T. Rehabilitation workshops: change in attitudes of nurses. Nursing Research, 21 (2), Mar/Apr 1972, 132–137.

14 Watrous, W. B. Rehabilitation nurse: counselor and coordinator. Occupational Health Nursing, 21 (12), Dec 1973, 16–18.

15 Wright, V. Rehabilitation and health visitor follow-up. [Attachment of two health visitors to a small rehabilitation unit at Ida Hospital, Leeds.] Nursing Mirror, 136, 19 Jan 1973, 26–27.

c OCCUPATIONAL THERAPY

1 British Association of Occupational Therapists New code of professional conduct. British Journal of Occupational Therapy, 38 (9), Sep 1975, 196.

2 Hagedorn, R. Survey of occupational therapy equipment and techniques. Occupational Therapy, 37 (1), Jan 1974, 11–12.

3 Hutchby, J. P. Community occupational therapy service. Medical Officer, 125, 26 Mar 1971, 161–163.

4 Hutchby, J. P. A community occupational therapy service and its future role. [Buckinghamshire.] Rehabilitation, (76), Jan/Mar 1971, 11–14.

5 Ibbotson, J. Motivation – the occupational therapist's approach. Physiotherapy, 61 (6), Jun 1975, 189–191.

6 Kimmance, K. J. and Chick, J. R. Occupational therapy in the community. Community Medicine, 129 (5), 17 Nov 1972, 111–113; Occupational Therapy, 36 (1), Jan 1973, 33–37.

7 King, J. The professions supplementary to medicine. Occupational therapy. Nursing Mirror, 141, 9 Oct 1975, 70–72.

8 Nixon, Sir C. Occupational therapy in rehabilitation. Queen's Nursing Journal, 16 (9), Dec 1973, 202–204.

9 Nixon, Sir C. The work of the occupational therapist. Health Visitor, 44 (8), Aug 1971, 254–256.

10 Nixon, Sir C. The work of the occupational therapist today. Health Visitor, 46 (7), Jul 1973, 227–228.

11 Paterson, C. F. Occupational therapy and nursing co-operation at Cameron Hospital. Rehabilitation, (80), Jan/Mar 1972, 23–27.

12 Sangoi, M. M. The occupational therapist in a rehabilitation centre. Nursing Journal of India, 44 (8), Aug 1973, 271–272, 289.

13 Watson, L. A. Occupational therapy. SA Nursing Journal, 60 (6), Jun 1973, 25.

d PHYSIOTHERAPY (Includes community services, nursing role)

1 Compton, A. A community physiotherapy service. Queen's Nursing Journal, 16 (9), Dec 1973, 198–199, 219.

2 Compton, A. The physiotherapist in the community. Physiotherapy, 59 (3), Mar 1973, 75–79.

3 Cyriax, J. H. Manipulation – doctor, layman or physiotherapist. Nursing Mirror, 134, 18/25 Feb 1972, 24–27.

4 Dancer, M. E. G. Physiotherapy for community nurses. [Report of course.] District Nursing, 15 (11), Feb 1973, 240–241.

5 Downie, P. A. Physiotherapy and the care of the progressively ill patient. 1. The role of the physiotherapist. [are of the dying patient.] Nursing Times, 69, 12 Jul 1973, 892–893.

6 Downie, P. A. Physiotherapy and the care of the progressively ill patient. 2. The unconscious and bed-ridden patient. [Advice for nurses.] Nursing Times, 69, 19 Jul 1973, 922–923.

7 Downie, P. A. Physiotherapy and the care of the progressively ill patient. 3. Physiotherapy for the paralysed patient. Nursing Times, 69, 26 Jul 1973, 958–959.

8 Duncan, J. T. McN. and Dancer, M. E. J. A three-day course for district nurses on 'simple physiotherapy in the rehabilitation of the housebound patient'. Physiotheraphy, 59 (3), Mar 1973, 81–88.

9 Freedman, G. R. and others Physiotherapy in general practice. Journal of the Royal College of General Practitioners, 25, Aug 1975, 589–591.

10 Furth, S. The professions supplementary to medicine. Physiotherapy. Nursing Mirror, 141, 2 Oct 1975, 52–54.

11 Gaskell, D. Physiotherapy [for cardio-thoracic patients.] Nursing Mirror, 141, 7 Aug 1975, 62–65.

12 Gaskell, D. J. and Webber, B. A. compilers The Brompton Hospital guide to chest physiotherapy. 2nd ed. Oxford: Blackwell, 1973.

13 Hobson, E. P. G. Domiciliary physiotherapy? British Hospital Journal and Social Service Review, 82, 8 Apr 1972, 774.

14 Holmes, J. E. The physical therapist and team care. Nursing Outlook, 20 (3), Mar 1972, 182–184.

15 McLaren, J. B. Analysing a physiotherapy out-patient service. Health and Social Service Journal, 85, 25 Jan 1975, 181–182.

16 Macmillan, C. A. Physiotherapy for the handicapped in the community. Physiotherapy, 60 (8), Aug 1974, 230–231.

17 Norman, P. and others Access by general practitioners to physiotherapy department of a district general hospital. British Medical Journal, 4, 25 Oct 1975, 220–221.

18 Patrick, M. K. Physiotherapy in the community. Physiotherapy, 59 (6), Jun 1973, 180–183.

19 Walsh, R. Physiotherapy and the nurse. [Course of instruction for nurses.] Rehabilitation, no. 80, Jan/Mar 1972, 27–29.

20 Waters, W. H. R. and others A domiciliary physiotheraphy service. Lancet, 1, 25 May 1974, 1033–1034.

21 Waters, W. H. R. and others Organizing a physiotherapy service in general practice. [Three years experience of a domiciliary service.] Journal of the Royal College of General Practitioners, 25, Aug 1975, 576–584.

22 Wilkes, E. Community care. [Trends in community care and their effects upon physiotherapy.] Physiotherapy, 61 (12), Dec 1975, 365–367.

e SPEECH THERAPY (See also Stroke: speech therapy)

1 Bankier, M. The professions supplementary to medicine. Speech therapy. Nursing Mirror, 141, 27 Nov 1975, 61–63.

2 Brown, B. B. Language disorders in children. Public Health, 87 (4), May 1973, 115–118.

3 Department of Education and Science Speech therapy services: report of the Committee. HMSO. Chairman: Professor Randolph Quirk.

4 Ingram, T. T. S. Speech disorders in childhood. 1. Types of speech disorders. Nursing Times, 67, 11 Feb 1971, 171–175.

5 Ingram, T. T. S. Speech disorders in childhood. 2. Slow speech development. Nursing Times, 67, 18 Feb 1971, 205–209.

6 Ison, P. M. Dysphesia. [Problems for the speech therapist and the patient's family.] Rehabilitation, no. 94, Jul/Sep 1975, 45–47.

7 Leche, P. M. The speech therapist and hemiplegia. Physiotherapy, 60 (11), Nov 1974, 346–349.

8 Leutenegger, R. R. Patient care and rehabilitation of communication impaired adults. Springfield; Thomas, 1975.

9 Murrills, G. The Popinjay club. [Symposium on laryngectomy.] Nursing Mirror, 141, 4 Dec 1975, 55–56.

10 Nursing Mirror Investigating voice production. Nursing Mirror, 133, 9 Jul 1971, 40–41..

11 Nursing Mirror Research into childhood aphasia USA training and treatment centre. Nursing Mirror. 132, 2 Apr 1971. 40–41.

12 Owlett, A. Speech rehabilitation. [Symposium on laryngectomy.] Nursing Mirror, 141, 4 Dec 1975, 53–54.

13 Price, S. Speaking proper. [Speech therapy work with children in Hampshire AHA.] Practice Team, (50–51), Jul/Aug 1975, 2, 4.

14 Rackham, K. Residential treatment for children with severe language disorders. Mother and Child, 43 (1), Jan/Feb 1971, 7–9.

15 Rose, F. C. Speech and language disorders in children. Midwife and Health Visitor, 8 (4), Apr 1972, 139–141.

16 Russell, J. The patient's voice: starting from scratch. [Symposium on laryngectomy.] Nursing Mirror, 141, 4 Dec 1975, 56–57.

17 Sanborn, C. J. and others Speech therapy by interactive television. Community Health, 6 (3), Nov–Dec 1974, 134–137.

18 Tait, V. Speaking after laryngectomy. Nursing Mirror, 133, 24 Sep 1971, 22–23.

f ART, MUSIC AND DRAMA THERAPY

1 Alvin, J. A fulfilment in life. [Music and mental handicap.] Nursing Times, 68, 6 Jul 1972, 829–831.

2 Ambrosio, A. Art therapy for the elderly and the disabled. Nursing Care, 8 (8), Aug 1975, 17–18.

3 Andrews, M. Poetry programs in mental hospitals. Perspectives in Psychiatric Care, 8 (1), Jan–Mar 1975, 17–18.

4 Argyle, M. and Cohen, D. The play's the thing. [Improving the social skills of patients at Littlemore Hospital, Oxford.] New Scientist, 60, 27 Dec 1973, 904–906.

5 Bhattacharyya, A. and others Some experiences in sociodrama in a county psychiatric hospital. [St. Crispin Hospital, Northampton. Reprinted from International Journal of Social Psychiatry.] Occupational Therapy, 35 (5), May 1972, 327–332.

6 Boyd, K. and Taylor, A. J. W. Painting in therapy. British Journal of Occupational Therapy, 38 (1), Jan 1975, 3–4.

7 Bright, R. Music in geriatric care. New York: St. Martin's Press, 1972.

8 British Society for Music Therapy Music therapy in the clinical and remedial team. The Society, 1973.

9 Casale, J. The value of psychodrama. [With psychiatric patients.] British Journal of Occupational Therapy, 37 (8), Aug 1974, 136.

10 Clarke, B. and others Sesame. [Psychodrama in rehabilitation of the subnormal.] Nursing Mirror, 133, 20 Aug 1971, 36–38.

11 Cokelet, K. A. The use of remedial drama in an admission unit of a large psychiatric hospital. British Journal of Occupational Therapy, 37 (8), 1974, 135.

12 Colson, J. Drama helps the mentally handicapped. Nursing Times, 68, 20 Apr 1972, 457–459.

13 Colson, J. Music to move to. [For the mentally subnormal.] Nursing Times, 68, 21 Sep 1972, 1189–1191.

14 Cullinan, J. Individual music therapy. [For psychiatric patients.] Nursing Times, 69, 6 Dec 1973, 1634–1635.

15 Cullinan, J. Music and mental handicap. Nursing Times, 68, 6 Jul 1972, 827–828.

16 Disabled Living Foundation and National Council of Social Service Music and the physically handicapped. British Hospital Journal and Social Service Review, 81, 6 Feb 1971, 258–259.

17 Fenwick, A. M. What should he play? Musical instruments in music therapy. [In psychiatric hospitals.] Nursing Times, 68, 26 Oct 1972, 1344–1347.

18 Forrest, C. Music and the psychiatric nurse. Nursing Times, 68, 6 Apr 1972, 410–411.

19 Hope, H. Music has charms to soothe: observations on the effect of relayed background music on patients at Farleigh Hospital, Somerset. [In ward for severely subnormal patients.] Nursing Mirror, 132, 5 Feb 1971, 40–41.

20 Hospitals Art for the patient's sake enhances long-term care facility. Hospitals, 49 (20), 16 Oct 1975, 33–34.

21 Knight, F. E. Developments in music therapy. [Two research projects in a Berlin psychiatric hospital.] British Hospital Journal and Social Service Review, 82, 30 Dec 1972, 2917.

22 Knight, M. R. Music therapy in the psychiatric hospital. New Zealand Nursing Journal, 68 (4), Apr 1975, 20–21.

23 Lerner, A. Poetry therapy. American Journal of Nursing, 73 (8), Aug 1973, 1336–1338.

24 Malcolm, M. Art as a projective technique. [Art therapy with neurotic and psychotic patients.] British Journal of Occupational Therapy, 38 (7), Jul 1975, 147–148.

25 Millin, B. Drama as therapy for the psychopathic personality. Nursing Times, 71, 9 Jan 1975, 69–71.

26 Moore, J. The hospital art centre. [Employment

of an artist at Gogarburn Hospital, for the mentally handicapped, Edinburgh.] Nursing Times, 71, 13 Mar 1975, 407.

27 Nursing Times Through the eyes of a child. An exhibition of art by the mentally handicapped. [Illustrations.] Nursing Times, 70, 19/26 Dec 1974, 1984–1985.

28 Potter, D. Art therapy for the handicapped. [Royal National Hospital for Rheumatic Diseases, Bath.] Nursing Mirror, 138, 26 Apr 1974, 55–57.

29 Priestley, M. Music therapy in one hospital. Nursing Times, 67, 15 Jul 1971, 870—871.

30 Priestley, M. People meeting people. [Music therapy in hospital.] Nursing Times, 68, 30 Nov 1972, 1528–1529.

31 Puttock. D. Dance therapy. Nursing Times, 68, 3 Aug 1972, 960–961.

32 Rollin, H. R. The history of music therapy. History of Medicine, 5 (1), Spring 1973, 15–18.

33 Royston, R. Art as remedial therapy. Health and Social Service Journal, 85, 4 Oct 1975, 2226–2227.

34 Sesame Movement and drama therapy with long-stay schizophrenics. [Sesame research project at Goodmayes Hospital, Ilford.] Occupational Therapy, 34 (12), Dec 1971, 26–27.

35 Sims, L. H. Importance of art to the elderly. Occupational Therapy, 35 (4), Apr 1972, 237–239.

36 Wills, E. Not by word of mouth alone. [Art therapy.] Social Work Today, 4, 23 Aug 1973, 332–334.

SURGERY, ACCIDENTS AND EMERGENCIES

63 SURGERY

a GENERAL

1 Cairney, J. Surgery for students of nursing. 6th ed. Christchurch: Peryer, 1974.

2 Calnan, J. and Martin, P. Development and practice of an autonomous minor surgery unit in a general hospital. [Hammersmith Hospital.] British Medical Journal, 4, 9 Oct 1971, 92–96; Reprinted in NATNews, 9 (5), Oct 1972, 20, 22, 25–26.

3 Harlow, F. W. editor Modern surgery for nurses. 9th ed. Heinemann, 1973.

4 McFarland, J. editor Basic clinical surgery for nurses and medical students. Butterworth, 1973.

5 McWee, A. C. and Browne, M. K. Adult surgery. Heinemann Medical, 1972. (Modern practical nursing series, no. 10.)

6 Moroney, J. Surgery for nurses. 13th ed. Churchill Livingstone, 1975.

7 Nash, D. F. E. The principles and practice of surgery for nurses and allied professions. 5th ed. Arnold, 1973.

8 Shepherd, J. Surgery in the small hospital. NATNews, 9 (1), Feb 1972, 18, 20.

9 Small, J. C. and Morris, J. F. Revision notes for senior nurses. General surgery. Heinemann Medical, 1974.

10 Tracy, G. D. The impact of developments in surgery on nursing in the seventies. Lamp, 29 (3), Mar 1972, 22–24.

b TRANSPLANTS (Includes ethics) (See also Cardiac surgery; Renal transplantation)

1 AORN Journal Worldwide totals for organ transplants. AORN Journal, 21 (4), Apr 1975, 701–702.

2 British Medical Journal. Bar Council report on organ transplants. British Medical Journal, 3, 18 Sep 1971, 716.

3 Calne, B. Y. Transplantation. Journal of Medical Ethics, 1 (2), Jul 1975, 59–60.

4 Dalyell, T. Tissue for transplantation. Journal of Medical Ethics, 1 (2), Jul 1975, 61–62.

5 Demetrius, P. M. Transplantation: the relatives' view. Journal of Medical Ethics, 1 (2), Jul 1975, 71–72.

6 Drug and Therapeutics Bulletin. Transplantation of organs. Drug and Therapeutics Bulletin, 13, 10 Oct 1975, 81–82.

7 General Council of the Bar Report of the Law Reform Committee on the law relating to organ transplantation adopted by the Council on 20 Jul 1971. The Council, 1971.

8 Isler, C. Transplant surgery and its special problems. RN Magazine, 35 (11), Nov 1972, OR 8, 12.

9 Isler, C. The world of transplants. 1. Spare parts for many needs. RN Magazine, 35 (11), Nov 1972, 36–43.

10 Isler, C. The world of transplants. 2. The tissue banks. RN Magazine, 35 (12), Dec 1972, 40–47.

11 Lancet The law of transplantation. Lancet, 2, 25 Aug 1973, 436.

12 Mahoney, J. Ethical aspects of donor consent in transplantation. Journal of Medical Ethics, 1 (2), Jul 1975, 67–70.

13 Thompson, N. Techniques and triumphs of muscle transplantation Nursing Mirror, 136, 25 May 1973, 25–27

c DAY SURGERY

1 Armitage, E. N. and others A day-surgery programme for children incorporating anaesthetic out-patient clinic. [Royal Alexandra Hospital, Brighton.] Lancet, 2, 5 Jul 1975, 21–23.

2 Atwell, J. D. Wessex. Paediatric day-case surgery in Southampton. [Southampton Children's Hospital.] Nursing Times, 71, 29 May 1975, 841–843.

3 Atwell, J. D. and others Paediatric day case surgery. [In Southampton, involving home nursing team attached to unit.] Lancet, 2, 20 Oct 1973, 895–897.

4 Berrill, T. H. A year in the life of a surgical day unit. [At the Coventry and Warwickshire Hospital.] British Medical Journal, 4, 11 Nov 1972, 348–349.

5 Bloomfield, E. Surgical procedures in a health centre. Nursing Times, 69, 8 Mar 1973, 299–301.

6 Dawe, C. L. Outpatient surgery. Australian Nurses' Journal, 3 (2), Aug 1973, 26–28.

7 Department of Health and Social Security and Welsh Office Memorandum on the arrangements for the care of persons attending hospital for surgical procedures as day patients. The Department, 1973. [Issued with Circular HM (73) 32.]

8 Epstein, B. S. and others Outpatient surgery. Guidelines for organization of unit and for selection of patient and surgical procedure. Hospitals, 47 (17), 1 Sep 1973, 80, 82, 84.

9 Honywood, H. Day surgery at Walton Hospital. Practice Team, no. 52, Sep 1975, 11–12.

10 Horohak, I. Outpatient surgery: R.N. role grows with the field. RN Magazine, 38 (7), Jul 1975, 47, 50, 52–56.

11 Imrie, V. J. Short-stay surgery. [Bridgwater General Hospital.] British Hospital Journal and Social Service Review, 82, 21 Oct 1972, 2356–2357.

12 Taylor, D. H. Medical-surgical day care unit. [Short term admission unit at the University of Roch-

ester Medical Center, New York.] American Journal of Nursing, 73 (12), Dec 1973, 2109–2220.

13 Tomalin, C. Waiting lists and day-bed surgery. Health and Social Service Journal, 85, 1 Nov 1975, 2459.

14 Turner, L. M. Day surgery for children. Nursing Times, 71, 2 Oct 1975, 1592–1593.

d ANAESTHESIA

1 Asbury, A. J. Anaesthetics. 1. The tools of the trade. Nursing Times, 69, 4 Oct 1973, 1284–1286.

2 Clark, M. M. Ketalar – a children's anaesthetic. Nursing Times, 69, 8 Mar 1973, 310–311.

3 Coleman, V. The history of anaesthetics. Nursing Mirror, 140, 5 Jun 1975, 63.

4 Corrigan, I. J. Ketamine – a new anesthetic. Canadian Nurse, 68 (4), Apr 1972, 43–44.

5 Devney, A. M. and Kingsbury, B. A. Hypothermia in fact and fantasy. American Journal of Nursing, 72 (8), Aug 1972, 1424–1425.

6 DiPalma, J. R. Drug therapy today. Use of the newer anesthetics. RN Magazine, 36 (7), Jul 1973, 47–59, [8 pages].

7 Drain, C. B. The cigarette smoker: a greater anaesthesia risk. RN Magazine, 38 (7), Jul 1975, OR 8.

8 Drain, C. B. Innovar: a neuroleptic drug. This anesthetic agent provides analgesia during the early post-operative period. American Journal of Nursing, 74 (5), May 1974, 895–896.

9 Hall, K. D. Narcotic anesthesia for cardiovascular surgery. AANA Journal, 43 (1), Feb 1975, 30–38.

10 Hobkirk, J. K. Anaesthetics for nurses. Bailliere Tindall and Cassell, 1971. (Nurses' aids series.)

11 Hopkins, S. J. New anaesthetics. Nursing Mirror, 136, 16 Feb 1973, 34–35.

12 Norris, W. and Campbell, D. A nurse's guide to anaesthetics, resuscitation and intensive care. 6th ed. Edinburgh: Churchill Livingstone, 1975.

13 Pedder, M. Pioneers in anaesthesia. Lamp, 30 (11), Nov 1973, 33–40; (12), Dec 1973, 31–34.

14 Petty, C. Uptake, distribution and excretion of gaseous anesthetics. Journal of the American Association of Nurse Anesthetists, 40 (1), Feb 1972, 21–41.

15 Redden, J. F. and Little, K. Anaesthesia and the Accident Flying Squad: a new anaesthetic machine. [Derby Lipaco Anaesthetic machine used by the Derbyshire Royal Infirmary Accident Flying Squad.] British Medical Journal, 1, 31 Mar 1973, 788–790.

16 Rosenberg, H. Basic concepts and modern trends in anesthesiology. Journal of Practical Nursing, 22 (10), Oct 1972, 18–21, 32, 34.

17 Smith, S. E. Drugs and anaesthesia. Nursing Times, 68, 13 Apr 1972, 447–449.

18 Smith, S. E. How drugs act. 20. Drugs and anesthesia. Nursing Times, 71, 6 Nov 1975, 1780–1781.

19 Swan, H. Clinical hypothermia: its use and accomplishments in surgery. RN Magazine, 37 (4), Apr 1974, OR 16, 18, 22.

e ANAESTHESIA: NURSE'S ROLE

1 AANA Journal A survey of nurse anesthetists, 1975. AANA Journal, 43 (6), Dec 1975, 586–605.

2 Adriani, J. Nurse anesthetists and the law. Journal of the American Association of Nurse Anesthetists, 41 (4), Aug 1973, 307–329.

3 Asbury, A. J. Anaesthetics. 2. The nurse as an assistant. Nursing Times, 69, 11 Oct 1973, 1331.

4 Bakutis, A. R. Assessing the anesthesia patient. AANA Journal, 43 (3), Jun 1975, 255–268.

5 Bakutis, A. R. Nurse anesthetists continuing education review: 700 essay questions and referenced answers. Flushing: Medical Examination Publishing Co., 1975.

6 Davenport, H. T. and Crampton-Smith, A. The nurse in a British department of anaesthetics. NAT-News, 12 (5), Jul 1975, 4.

7 Felton, G. Clinical specialist preparation for the nurse anesthetist. Nursing Outlook, 20 (9), Sep 1972, 597–598.

8 Gunn, I. P. Nurse anesthetist-anesthesiologist relationships: past, present, and implications for the future [in the United States.] AANA Journal, 43, Apr 1975, 129–139.

9 Gunn, I. P. Preparing today's nurse anesthetists to meet contemporary needs: a philosophic and pragmatic approach. AANA Journal, 42 (1), Feb 1974, 25–38.

10 Healey, T. G. Pediatric anesthesia: guidelines for the nurse anesthetist. AANA Journal, 42 (6), Dec 1974, 544–555.

11 Hellewell, J. The nurse's role in anaesthesia. 1. Pre-operative preparation. Nursing Times, 68, 6 Apr 1972, 400–403.

12 Hellewell, J. The nurse's role in anaesthesia. 2. Postoperative care. Nursing Times, 68, 13 Apr 1972, 443–446.

13 Hellewell, J. The nurse's role in anaesthesia. 3. Respiratory failure. Nursing Times, 68, 20 Apr 1972, 467–470.

14 Hellewell, J. The nurse's role in anaesthesia. 4. Cardiac arrest and resuscitation. Nursing Times, 68, 27 Apr 1972, 512–513.

15 Huffman, J. P. The nurse anesthetist and fire prevention. Journal of the American Association of Nurse Anesthetists, 40 (1), Feb 1972, 51–52.

16 McCarthy, R. T. A practice theory of nursing care. [A theory of nursing care of patients who have had spinal anesthesia with regard to the need for catheterisation illustrates how a theory for practice discipline may be developed.] Nursing Research, 21 (5), Sep/Oct 1972, 406–410.

17 Malmuth, D. The nurse anesthetist as a paramedical instructor. Journal of the American Association of Nurse Anesthetists, 41 (4), Aug 1973, 333–337.

18 Mathewson, H. S. The role of the nurse anesthetist in inhalation therapy. Journal of the American Association of Nurse Anesthetists, 40 (1), Feb 1972, 42–44.

19 Modern Hospital Nurse anesthetists: high standards and more surgery help them with acceptance. Modern Hospital, 120, Feb 1973, 70–72.

20 Norris, W. and Campbell, D. A nurse's guide to anaesthetics, resuscitation and intensive care. 6th ed. Edinburgh: Churchill Livingstone, 1975.

21 Parkhouse, J. Anaesthetic department assistants. [Project at the University Hospital of South Manchester to explore the use of trained nurses.] Nursing Times, 68, 14 Sep 1972, 1156–1159.

22 Robertson, P. A. Respiratory care in local anesthesia. AORN Journal, 21 (5), Apr 1975, 797–805.

23 Rosenberg, H. Spinal anesthesia by nurse anesthetists. Journal of the American Association of Nurse Anesthetists, 41 (4), Aug 1973, 330–332.

24 Shaw, B. L. Whither the C.R.N.A.s? Onward and upward. [Nurse Anesthetists.] RN Magazine, 34 (1), Jan 1971, 35–40.

25 Wolf, V. C. Educational objectives. Journal of the American Association of Nurse Anesthetists, 40 (6), Dec 1973, 436–446.

f EQUIPMENT AND DRESSINGS

1 Alsop, J. A. New, neat, non-slip: a bandage that needs no fasteners. [Coban.] Nursing Times, 67, 14 Jan 1971, 48–49.

2 Belkin, N. L. The rationale for re-usables: the other side of the drape. [Disposables in the operating room.] Hospital Topics, 53 (1), Jan/Feb 1975, 45–48, 50–51.

3 Boyle, A. E. Sutureless skin closure. [Using Steri-Strip. A study done at the Royal Hospital for Sick Children, Glasgow.] Nursing Mirror, 134, 16 Jun 1972, 20–21.

4 Broome, W. E. Dressing techniques. Butterworth, 1971. (Nursing in depth series.)

5 Broome, W. E. Hampshire dressing technique [which involves the discontinuation of forceps and the use of sterile gloved hands]. Nursing Mirror, 126, 12 Jan 1973, 12–13.

6 Campbell, A. W. C. Standards in surgical dressings. Health and Social Service Journal, 85, 2 Aug 1975, 1662–1663.

7 Coleman, V. A stitch in time. . . [Selection of sutures.] Nursing Mirror, 140, 26 Jun 1975, 71.

8 Davison, V. Current dressing techniques. Occupational Health, 23 (9), Sep 1971, 287–292.

9 Desmond, S. Some observations on the supply of surgical gauze and associated hospital products. NAT-News, 12 (1), Jan 1975, 5–7.

10 Forrester, J. C. Suture materials and their uses. Nursing Mirror, 140, 16 Jan 1975, 48–57.

11 Harkiss, K. J. editor Surgical dressings and wound healing: proceedings of a symposium. Bradford University Press, 1971.

12 Hayes, H. Revised surgical dressing program. [Recording and controlling of surgical dressing supplies and equipment by nursing staff.] Hospital Progress, 54 (5), May 1973, 104, 106.

13 Hospital Topics Tray system devised for hip surgery. Hospital Topics, 49 (11), Nov 1971, 76–77.

14 Hunt, J. M. The teaching and practice of surgical dressings in three hospitals. Rcn, 1974. (Study of nursing care project series, 1 no. 6.)

15 Johnson, A. Theatre drapes – disposable or re-usable? Nursing Times, 69, 22 Mar 1973, 381–382.

16 Jury, M. Suturing for nurses. Occupational Health, 24 (3), Mar 1972, 75–79.

17 Kendall, A. R. In the cystoscopic suite. A review of old and new equipment. RN Magazine, 34 (2), Feb 1971, 3–6, 9–10.

18 Ker, M. B. Planning a theatre tray service. Nursing Times, 67, 28 Jan 1971, 112–114.

19 Lakie, M. H. and McElroy, A. R. Surgical instruments and dressings: an information service. [Proposal for a regional service staffed by information scientists.] British Medical Journal, 4, 22 Nov 1975, 448–450.

20 Longfield, F. P. and Brimelow, L. A. Emergency trolley. Nursing Times, 67, 20 May 1971, 595–598.

21 McCarville, M. The care and maintenance of surgical instruments. Canadian Hospital, 50 (6), Jun 1973, 14–15.

22 McLeish, J. Hampshire dressing aid. [For use in the community nursing services.] District Nursing, 15 (12), Mar 1973, 263–265.

23 Myers, M. B. Sutures and wound healing. American Journal of Nursing, 71 (9), Sep 1971, 1725–1727.

24 NAT News Surgical dressings in hospital environment. NATNews, 12 (5), Jul 1975, 11.

25 Nursing Mirror Theatre equipment: a review of the latest products for use in operating rooms. Nursing Mirror, 141, 31 Jul 1975, 47–50.

26 Occupational Health Checking surgical dressing techniques. [With reference to the 1961 Rcn report.] Occupational Health, 23 (9), 1971, 293–299.

27 Tarin, D. Wound healing. A diagrammatic and pictorial account. Nursing Times, 69, 30 Aug 1973, 1124–1126.

28 Turner, T. D. and others Swab performance. NATNews, 12 (1), Jan 1975, 8, 14.

29 Turner, T. D. and Brain, K. R. editors Surgical dressings in the hospital environment. Cardiff: UWIST, 1975.

30 Wallace, D. M. The evolution of the cystoscope. Nursing Mirror, 141, 17 Jul 1975, 60–62.

g HAZARDS (Includes pollution and health hazards)

1 Adams, I. Potential hazards of an electro-surgical unit. Hospital Administration in Canada, 13 (7), Jul 1971, 37–38.

2 AORN Journal Federal standards on waste anesthetic gases being prepared. AORN Journal, 20 (6), Dec 1974, 950–951.

3 AORN Journal Waste anesthetic gas suspect as OR health hazard. [Report presented at the annual meeting of the American Society of Anesthesiologists.] AORN Journal, 20 (5), Nov 1974, 754, 756.

4 Ashton, K. Under the influence? [Problem of waste anaesthetic gases in operating theatres.] Nursing Times, 71, 18 Dec 1975, 2006.

5 British Medical Journal Anaesthetists environment. [Occupational hazards with particular reference to inhalation of gases.] British Medical Journal, 1, 15 Feb 1975, 353–354.

6 British Medical Journal Pollution in the operating theatre. [Incidence of spontaneous abortion among married women working in operating theatres and other health hazards.] British Medical Journal, 2, 15 Apr 1972, 123.

7 British Medical Journal Prevention of pollution of operating theatres with halothane vapour by adsorption with activated charcoal. British Medical Journal, 1, 24 Mar 1973, 727–729.

8 Charter, D. Control of electric shock hazards in operating rooms. Canadian Hospital, 48 (2), Feb 1971, 35–36.

9 Corbett, T. H. and Arbor, A. Exposure to anesthetic gases in the operating room. Journal of the American Association of Nurse Anesthetists, 40 (5), Oct 1972, 347–350.

10 Defalque, R. J. Operating room pollution – a menace to the surgical team. AANA Journal, 43 (3), Jun 1975, 294–296.

11 Dobbie, A. K. Accidental lesions in the operating theatre. [Hazards to patients.] NATNews, 11 (9), Dec 1974, 10, 12, 13.

12 Errera, D. W. Anesthesia hazards, O.R. scheduling among topics at Southeastern meeting. Hospital Topics, 51 (6), Jun 1973, 57, 59–61.

13 Gamberale, F. The effect of anesthetic gases on the psychomotor and perceptual functions of anesthetic nurses. Work-Environment–Health, 11 (2), 1974, 108–113.

14 Kernaghan, S. G. Caution: anesthesia may be hazardous to your health. Hospitals, 46 (3), 1 Feb 1972, 143–147.

15 Kernaghan, S. G. Research, regulation turn on waste anesthetics. [Pollution of the operating room and health hazards to staff.] Hospitals, 46 (20), 16 Oct 1972, 152, 154, 156, 158, 160.

16 Knill-Jones, R. P. and others Anaesthetic practice and pregnancy: controlled survey of women anaesthetists in the United Kingdom. Lancet, 1, 17 Jun 1972, 1326–1328.

17 Lancet Anaesthetic bangs. [Explosions in operating theatres.] Lancet, 2, 1 Sep 1973, 489.

18 Lancet Pregnancy and anaesthesia. [Dangers for operating room staff.] Lancet, 2, 26 Jul 1975, 169.

19 Lebourdais, E. The anesthetic threat [to the health of operating room staff. Conclusions and recommendations of a Canadian government committee]. Dimensions in Health Service, 52 (4), Apr 1975, 11.

20 McConnell, M. A. Safety in the operating room. New Zealand Nursing Journal, 65 (10), Oct 1972, 16–17.

21 McWilliams, R. M. Nurses concerned with hazards of waste gases. [Answers to questions from two OR nurses.] AORN Journal, 21 (5), Apr 1975, 857–858, 860.

22 RN Magazine Waste anesthetics implicated anew as OR personnel health hazard. [Results of research undertaken by the American Society of Anesthesiologists.] RN Magazine, 38 (1), Jan 1975, OR 8–9.

23 Spence, A. A. Anaesthetics risk to staff. [A report of the National Association of Theatre Nurses conference on the hazards of working in an operating theatre.] Nursing Times, 70, 31 Oct 1974, 1681.

64 SURGICAL NURSING

a GENERAL AND TEXTBOOKS
(See also Paediatric surgery)

1 Borland, J. General care of the surgical patient. Butterworth, 1972. (Nursing in depth series.)

2 Dupre, A. Aspects of surgical nursing. New Zealand Nursing Journal, 67 (9), Sep 1974, 19–22.

3 Fish, E. J. Surgical nursing. 9th ed. Baillière Tindall, 1974 (Nurses' aids series.)

4 Forrest, J. Foundations of surgical nursing. Arnold, 1974.

5 Fream, W. C. Notes on surgical nursing. Churchill Livingstone, 1971.

6 Ghant, A. D. B. and Napier, M. Factors influencing prediction of surgical in-patient stay. [Survey conducted by the ward sister and the surgeon.] Hospital and Health Services Review, 69 (2), Feb 1973, 52–54.

7 Glenn, F. The elderly as surgical patients. RN Magazine, 37 (6), Jun 1974, 60, (8 pages).

8 Miale, J. E. Caring for the surgical patient. Hospitals, 45 (13), 1 Jul 1971, 72–74.

9 Nursing Clinics of North America Symposium on current surgical nursing. Nursing Clinics of North America, 8 (1), Mar 1973, 105–198.

10 Rains, A. J. H. Surgery in the aged – some reflections and attitudes. [NM Conference Lecture.] Nursing Mirror, 137, 20 Jul 1973, 33–34.

11 Whiteside, J. E. Surgical nursing. 2nd ed. Sydney: Angus and Robertson, 1975.

b PREOPERATIVE AND POSTOPERATIVE CARE (Includes escort nurse, recovery room)

1 Arens, J. Reviews important points in care of patient in recovery room. Hospital Topics, 49 (6), Jun 1971, 83, 87.

2 Asbury, A. J. Recovering the post-anaesthetic patient. Nursing Times, 70, 24 Jan 1974, 106–109.

3 Baker, P. J. Postoperative atelectasis. AANA Journal, 43 (5), Oct 1975, 479–485.

4 Bennetts, F. E. Premedication. Nursing Times, 70, 13 Jun 1974, 911–913.

5 Blackwell, A. K. and Blackwell, W. Relieving gas pains. [Postoperative dysflatulence.] American Journal of Nursing, 75 (1), Jan 1975, 66–67.

6 Civetta, J. M. Recovery room: past, present and future. AORN Journal, 21 (5), Apr 1975, 806–811.

7 Collart, M. E. and Brenneman, J. K. Preventing postoperative atelectasis. American Journal of Nursing, 71 (10), Oct 1971, 1982–1987.

8 Collins, T. 'Recovery-room nursing is a clinical speciality'. RN Magazine, 36 (11), Nov 1973, 43–44, 46, 48, 50.

9 Crowell, D. M. Coded scoring in the recovery room. [A method of evaluating post-operative physical status.] RN Magazine, 35 (10), Oct 1972, OR 30, 32.

10 Drain, C. B. Recovery-room care of the ketamine patient. RN Magazine, 36 (11), Nov 1973, OR 1–2.

11 Ellis, H. Postoperative pulmonary collapse. Nursing Times, 71, 16 Jan 1975, 100–101.

12 Elms, R. R. Recovery room behavior and postoperative convalescence. Nursing Research, 21 (5), Sep/Oct 1972, 390–397.

13 Hill, S. and Fowler, R. Theatre escort service: the escort nurse. [Before and after surgery.] NATNews, 8 (3), Autumn 1971, 38, 41.

14 Hodges, S. A. Patient care in operating theatres. 1. Admission. [Preoperative care.] Nursing Mirror, 134, 28 Apr 1972, 17–19.

15 Hodges, S. A. Patient care in operating theatres. 2. Postoperative care. Nursing Mirror, 134, 5 May 1972, 28–29.

16 Jaffe, B. F. Some causes of postoperative hoarseness. RN Magazine, 37 (6), Jun 1974, ICU 1–2, ICU 4.

17 Johnson, M. Outcome criteria to evaluate postoperative respiratory status: temperature, cough, respiration, and lung condition. American Journal of Nursing, 75 (9), Sep 1975, 1474–1475.

18 Libman, R. H. and Keithley, J. Relieving airway obstruction in the recovery room. American Journal of Nursing, 75 (4), Apr 1975, 603–605.

19 Matthias, A. M. OT transfer system. [Method of transferring patients from their beds to the operating theatre used at Crawley Hospital, Sussex.] Nursing Times, 68, 31 Aug 1972, 1080–1082.

20 Nursing Clinics of North America Symposium on intensive care of the surgical patient. Nursing Clinics of North America, 10 (1), Mar 1975, 1–144.

21 Parsons, M. C. and Stephens, G. J. Postoperative complications: assessment and intervention. [Case study.] American Journal of Nursing, 74 (2), Feb 1974, 240–244.

22 Renfrew, M. and McManus, R. Recovery and reception area. [Stobhill General Hospital, Glasgow.] NATNews, 12 (6), Aug 1975, 13–15.

23 Smith, R. B. and others In a recovery room. Hypoventilation and hypotension. American Journal of Nursing, 73 (1), Jan 1973, 70–73.

24 Smith, S. H. Nil by mouth? A descriptive study of nursing care in relation to pre-operative fasting. Rcn, 1972. (Study of nursing care project reports series, 1 no. 1.)

25 Stillman, H. J. Nursing decisions: experiences in clinical problem solving. A postsurgical patient with leg pain. RN Magazine, 38 (10), Oct 1975, 25–30.

26 Tinker, J. H. and Wehner, R. J. Postoperative recovery and the neuromuscular junction: caring for patients recovering from the effects of neuromuscular blocking agents. American Journal of Nursing, 74 (1), Jan 1974, 74–75.

27 Van Petten, M. Recovery room manual for the small hospital. St. Louis: Catholic Hospital Association, 1974.

28 Winslow, E. H. and Fuhs, M. F. Preoperative assessment for postoperative evaluation. [To assist in planning care.] American Journal of Nursing, 73 (8), 1973, 1372–1374.

29 Wolfer, J. A. Definition and assessment of surgical patients' welfare and recovery: selected review of the literature. Nursing Research, 22 (5), Sep/Oct 1973, 394–401.

c PREOPERATIVE TEACHING AND PATIENT ANXIETY

1 Aiken, L. H. Systematic relaxation to reduce preoperative stress. Canadian Nurse, 68 (6), Jun 1972, 38–42.

2 Bruegel, M. A. Relationship of preoperative anxiety to perception of postoperative pain. Nursing Research, 20 (1), Jan/Feb 1971, 26–31.

3 Canadian Nurse Preadmission patient teaching clinic. [To provide information to groups of elective patients about to have abdominal surgery.] Canadian Nurse, 69 (9), Sep 1973, 39.

4 Crick, E. Patients wait for surgery in 'twilight zone.' [Pre-operative waiting room where nurses can talk to patients.] AORN Journal, 22 (6), Dec 1975, 980, 982.

5 Damsteegt, D. Pastoral roles in presurgical visits. American Journal of Nursing, 75 (8), Aug 1975, 1336–1337.

6 Dirksen, W. S. and Shewchuk, M. G. Preop visits expand the OR nurse's role. [Program of pre- and post operative visiting at the University of Alberta Hospital, Edmonton.] Canadian Nurse, 71 (6), Jun 1975, 27–30.

7 Dumas, R. G. and Johnson, B. A. Research in nursing practice: a review of five clinical experiments. [Psychologically oriented nursing approach to the surgical patient.] International Journal of Nursing Studies, 9 (3), Aug 1972, 137–148.

8 Eisler, J. and others Relationship between need for social approval and postoperative recovery and welfare. Nursing Research, 21 (6), Nov/Dec 1972, 520–525.

9 Ellison, P. V. The pre and post operative visit concept. [Case study.] Nursing Times, 71, 16 Oct 1975; NATN Supplement, iv–vi.

10 Ginsberg, F. and Clarke, B. Providing emotional support is part of OR nurse's job. [Preoperative and postoperative nursing visits.] Modern Hospital, 118 (2), Feb 1972, 118.

11 Graham, L. E. and Conley, E. M. Evaluation of anxiety and fear in adult surgical patients. Nursing Research, 20 (2), Mar/Apr 1971, 113–122.

12 Haven, L. C. and Haven, G. A. Reducing the patient's fear of the recovery room. RN Magazine, 38 (1), Jan 1975, 28–29.

13 Hegyvary, S. T. and Chamings, P. A. The hospital setting and patient care outcomes. [Study of the effects of pre-operative stress, preoperative instructions and the hospital setting on postoperative outcomes.] Journal of Nursing Administration, 5 (3), Mar/Apr 1975, 29–32; (4), May 1975, 36–42.

14 Janis, I. L. Psychological stress: psychoanalytic and behavioral studies of surgical patients. New York: Academic Press, 1974.

15 Kaur, M. and Chua, P. C. Nurse-patient communication in surgery. [Study to show the effectiveness of pre-operative nurse-patient communication to relieve anxiety.] Nursing Journal of Singapore, 15 (1), May 1975, 9–11.

16 Kennedy, M. J. An exploratory study of the responses of the patient to the cancellation of his surgery. International Journal of Nursing Studies, 6 (3), Sep 1969, 121–131.

17 Laird, M. Techniques for teaching pre- and post-opeative patients. American Journal of Nursing, 75 (8), Aug 1975, 1338–1340.

18 Lewis, K. M. Teamwork: a key to better pre-op teaching. [Pre-operative teaching of the patient.] RN Magazine, 37 (5), May 1974, 61–62.

19 Lindeman, C. A. Nursing intervention with the presurgical patient. [Effectiveness of group and individual pre-operative teaching.] Nursing Research, 21 (3), May/Jun 1972, 196–209.

20 Lindeman, C. A. and Aernam, B. V. Nursing intervention with the presurgical patient: effects of structured and unstructured preoperative teaching. Nursing Research, 20 (4), Jul–Aug 1971, 319–332.

21 Lindeman, C. A. and Stetzer, S. L. Effect of preoperative visits by operating room nurses. Nursing Research, 22 (1), Jan/Feb 1973, 4–16.

22 Merkatz, R. and others Preoperative teaching for gynecologic patients. American Journal of Nursing, 74 (6), Jun 1974. 1072–1074.

23 Meyers, B. L. Patients in an O.R. corridor. Can a nurse decrease a patient's anxiety by talking to him in the corridor of the surgical suite?] American Journal of Nursing, 72 (2), Feb 1972, 284–285.

24 Midgley, J. W. and Osterhage, R. A. Effect of nursing instruction and length of hospitalization on postoperative complications in cholecystectomy patients. Nursing Research, 22 (1), Jan/Feb 1973, 69–72.

25 Minckley, B. B. Physiologic and psychologic responses of elective surgical patients: early definite or late indefinite scheduling of surgical procedure. [A study to determine if prolonged waiting time before surgery, affects patients' recovery.] Nursing Research, 23 (5), Sep/Oct 1974, 392–401.

26 Morgan, D. M. Prepared patients make faster surgical recovery. Canadian Hospital, 50 (7), Jul 1973, 45–47.

27 Park, S. Preoperative 'teach-in'. Canadian Nurse, 68 (10), Oct 1972, 38–39.

28 Prsala, H. Admission unit dispels fear of surgery. [Pre-operative teaching.] Canadian Nurse, 70 (12), Dec 1974, 24–26.

29 Ryan, D. W. A questionnaire survey of pre-operative fears. British Journal of Clinical Practice, 29 (1), Jan 1975, 3–6.

30 Sanders, S. An experiment in 'live' theatre. [Use of the pre-operative interview as a learning tool for students.] Australian Nurses' Journal, 5 (6/7), Dec/Jan 1976, 31–32.

31 Saylor, D. E. Understanding presurgical anxiety. AORN Journal, 22 (4), Oct 1975, 624–636, (7 pages).

32 Schmitt, F. E. and Wooldridge, P. J. Psychological preparation of surgical patients. Nursing Research, 22 (2), Mar/Apr 1973, 108–116.

33 Shelter, M. G. Operating room nurses go visiting. [Pre- and post-operative visits by operating room nurses to surgical patients.] American Journal of Nursing, 72 (7), Jul 1972, 1266–1269.

34 Thomas, B. J. Patient-visiting: an expanded role for OR nurses. RN Magazine, 36 (3), Mar 1973, OR 3, 5–6, 8.

65 THEATRE NURSING

a GENERAL

1 AORN Journal Changing role of nurse in OR environment. [Report of a meeting of the American College of Surgeons.] AORN Journal, 21 (1), Jan 1975, 52–53.

2 Association of Operating Room Nurses Operating room. Hospital Topics, 50 (5), May 1972, 47–60.

3 Baxter, B. The 'nurse' in the operating room complex. [Role of nurse as patient's agent.] Nursing Times, 67, 23 Sep 1971, 1190.

4 Brigden, R. J. Operating theatre technique: a textbook for nurses, technicians, operating department assistants, medical students, house surgeons and others associated with the operating theatre. 3rd ed. Edinburgh: Churchill Livingstone, 1974.

5 Campbell, M. H. Theatre routine. Heinemann, 1971. (Modern practical nursing series, no. 2.)

6 Craig, M. As she puts on her mask. [The work of an assistant director of the operating room suite.] AORN Journal, 21 (2), Feb 1975, 223–229.

7 Cranfield, A. B. Theatre nurses handbook. Butterworth, 1972. (Nursing in depth series.)

8 Hadley, B. J. and others O.R. nurses: let's change our image – and our role. Hospitals, 46, 1 May 1972, 100, 104, 106.

9 Hill, S. Working in the operating department in Italy and Greece. NATNews, 11 (4), May 1974, 15–16.

10 Hulme, M. Nursing in the operating theatre. Nursing Mirror, 137, 10 Aug 1973, 30–32.

11 Kit-Ying, H. W. Operating nurse – a distinctive entity. [View of UK operating room nursing by a Hong Kong nurse.] Hong Kong Nursing Journal, (18), May 1975, 33–36.

12 Lawler, J. Theatre sisters on site: a study of Theatre Sisters. Lamp, 31 (2), Feb 1974, 13, 15, 17, 19.

13 Mahomet, A. D. Nursing diagnosis for the OR nurse. AORN Journal, 22 (5), Nov 1975, 709–711.

14 Miller, J. The OR – ivory tower or patient care area? Nursing Clinics of North America, 8 (2), Jun 1973, 349–353.

15 Nolan, M. Team nursing in the OR. American Journal of Nursing, 74 (2), Feb 1974, 272–274.

16 Nolan, M. G. A master nurse clinician for intra-operative care. Nursing Clinics of North America, 10 (4), Dec 1975, 645–653.

17 Nursing Clinics of North America Symposium on perspectives in operating room nursing. Nursing Clinics of North America, 10 (4), Dec 1975, 613–686.

18 Rait, A. The operating department nurse and the acutely ill patient. Nursing Times, 70, 24 Oct 1974, 1651–1653.

19 Richards, S. G. Operating theatres in Europe. Some comparative studies. [Study tour by theatre nurse to EEC countries.] Nursing Times, 69, 22 Feb 1973, 254–257.

20 Ridgeway, S. The new graduate in the O.R. Hospital Administration in Canada, 17 (1), Jan 1975, 18–19, 30.

21 RN Magazine Special issue on operating room nursing. RN Magazine, 36 (3), Mar 1973, 33–47, 96–98.

22 Rogers, P. K. Progress in OR nursing practice. AORN Journal, 21 (7), Jun 1975, 1278, 1280, 1282, 1284, 1286, 1288.

23 Willingham, G. Operating theatre techniques. Heinemann Medical, 1971.

24 Woodcroft, R. Survey into counting precautions in New South Wales operating theatres. Lamp, 29 (12), Dec 1972, 7, 9, 11, 13, 15–19.

b PROFESSIONAL ASPECTS (Includes standards)

1 Association of Operating Room Nurses and American Nurses' Association Division of Medical-Surgical Nursing Practice. Standards of nursing practice: operating room. Kansas City: ANA, 1975.

2 Bosanquet, N. Theatre nurses and Whitehall. [Relationship of nurses and ODAs.] Nursing Times, 70, 24 Oct 1974, 1667–1668.

3 Dinsmore, R. J. OR nurse's liability in needle count. AORN Journal, 20 (6), Dec 1974, 1002–1004.

4 Fehlau, M. T. Implementation of standards of practice. [Published by AORN and the American Nurses Association.] AORN Journal, 22, Nov 1975, 712–718.

5 Lawler, J. Theatre sisters on site. [Research study of the activities and job satisfaction of theatre sisters.] Lamp, 31 (2), Feb 1974, 13, 15, 17, 19; (4), Apr 1974, 31–37.

6 LeBourdais, E. Guideline standards for OR nurse. Dimensions in Health Service, 51 (2), Feb 1974, 45.

7 National Association of Theatre Nurses Codes of practice. NATNews, 12 (4), May/Jun 1975, 10, 12–13.

8 National Association of Theatre Nurses Annual Congress Report. NATNews, 9 (6), Dec 1972.

9 National Association of Theatre Nurses [Annual congress.] Think again theatre nurses urge DHSS, by V. O'Connor. Nursing Times, 69, 18 Oct 1973, 1353.

10 National Association of Theatre Nurses Tenth annual congress. NATNews, 11 (8), Nov 1974, 6–16; Nursing Times, 70, 31 Oct 1974, 1686–1687.

11 National Association of Theatre Nurses Eleventh Annual Congress report – 15–18 Oct. Harrogate. NATNews, 12 (8), Nov 1975, 13–26; NATN Supplement, i–xii; 23 Oct 1975, 1688–1689.
Nursing Mirror, 141, 23 Oct 1975, 43–44; Nursing Times, 71, 16 Oct 1975.

12 Nursing Times Theatre nurses discuss their future. Nursing Times, 67, 4 Nov 1971, 1388–1389.

13 O'Connor, V. A world of its own: the operating department. [Careers in theatre nursing.] Nursing Times, 67, 21 Oct 1971, 1307–1309.

14 Yokes, J. A. Nursing standards measure quality of practice. [For operating room nurses developed by AORN and the American Nurses' Association.] AORN Journal, 20 (6), Dec 1974, 1039–1040, 1042, 1044, 1046.

c EDUCATION AND TRAINING

1 AORN Journal Advice for nurses planning OR inservice programs. AORN Journal, 21 (5), Apr 1975, 763, 766–767.

2 AORN Journal Long-range goal: school to train OR nurses [at AORN Headquarters, Denver]. AORN Journal, 20 (1), Jul 1974, 16.

3 Charter, D. Survey shows how today's nurse gets OR training. [Training of qualified nurses.] Canadian Hospital, 48 (7), Jul 1971, 32.

4 Cowell, R. Behavioural objectives for post basic students in the operating department. NATNews, 12 (5), Jul 1975, 15, 19.

5 Donn, M. C. The training and function integration of the nurse and allied personnel in the operating theatre of the USA. NATNews, 10 (3), Jun 1973, 6–8, 10, 12, 14.

6 Drake, J. Report on operating theatre staff training and conditions in Holland [Study visit.] NATNews, 12 (7) Sep 1975, 24, 26.

7 Drake, J. E. A report on research into training of personnel and staffing of operating theatres in the U.K. NATNews, 11 (3), Apr 1974, 16, 18–19.

8 Finn, B. Post-basic training for theatre nurses. Nursing Mirror, 139, 12 Sep 1974, 78–79.

9 Fish, E. J. Theatre nurse training course. [Recognized by the Joint Board of Clinical Nursing Studies.] Nursing Times, 70, 24 Oct 1974, 1658–1660.

10 Ginsberg, F. and Clarke, B. Training of O.R. nurses lagging behind the need. Modern Hospital, 118 (3), Mar 1972, 128.

11 Griggs, J. OR staff nurse underestimated as educator: role in continuing education. AORN Journal, 21 (4), Mar 1975, 591–592.

12 Joint Board of Clinical Nursing Studies Operating department nursing course for state registered nurses. [Extracts from Joint Board syllabus and handbook.] NATNews, 10 (3), Jun 1973, 24, 26, 38.

13 Morgan, D. M. Effective inservice programming for O.R. nurses. Canadian Hospital, 49 (3), Mar 1972, 39–40, 42–43.

14 Morin, S. Training the new grad nurse in the O.R. [A six month course at Sudbury General Hospital.] Hospital Administration in Canada, 17 (1), Jan 1975, 22, 24–25.

15 National Association of Theatre Nurses Working party report on post-registration theatre courses. NATNews, 8 (3), Autumn 1971, 32, 34, 36.

d MANAGEMENT AND STAFFING

1 AORN Journal AORN survey OR staffing, pay policies. [A survey to establish the ratio of registered nurses to technicians in the United States.] AORN Journal, 22 (3), Sep 1975, 343–349.

2 AORN Journal Do patients need OR staff nurses? AORN Journal, 21(1), Jan 1975, 29–30

3 AORN Journal Moving to a new OR suite causes stress: a case study. AORN Journal, 22(4), Oct 1975, 530–537.

4 AORN Journal Nurse/physician relationship strained. [Study of surgical services in the United States.] AORN Journal, 22 (5), Nov 1975, 811–812.

5 Bramhall, R. Staffing structure in operating rooms in the USA. NATNews, 9 (1), Feb 1972, 15.

6 Central Health Services Council Joint Sub-Committee of the Standing Medical and Standing Nursing Advisory Committees. The organization and staffing of operating departments. HMSO, 1970. Chairman: W. Lewin.

7 Charter, D. How to define and evaluate objectives in the OR. Canadian Hospital, 48 (10), Oct 1971, 36.

8 Cowan, D. The planning of the operating department. SA Nursing Journal, 42 (9), Sep 1975, 5–8.

9 Cox, L. D. Theatre organization under Salmon. Hospital and Health Services Review, 68 (3), Mar 1972, 92–93.

10 Cox, M. P. A layman looks at Lewin. [Reactions of senior theatre staff in the Birmingham area to the Lewin report on theatre staffing.] Nursing Times, 70, 11 Apr 1974, 560–561.

11 Donn, M. C. The training and function integration of the nurses and allied personnel in the operating theatre in the USA. Technic, 20 (5), Oct 1974, 7–11.

12 Dorman, F. D. Study leave in UK. [Impressions of the work and staffing structures of operating theatres.] New Zealand Nursing Journal, 66 (10), Oct 1973, 7–8.

13 Driscoll, J. Establishing, implementing, and enforcing OR policies. AORN Journal, 21 (6), May 1975, 1031–1037.

14 Foster, C. Some thoughts on the staffing of the operating department and the training required. NATNews, 9 (5), Oct 1972, 37–38.

15 Greaves, D. Operating in 'Best Buy' Bury St. Edmunds. [New operating department of the West Suffolk Hospital.] Nursing Times, 70, 24 Oct 1974, 1664–1666.

16 Gruendemann, B. J. and others Nursing audit: challenge to the operating room nurse. Denver: Association of Operating Room Nurses, 1974.

17 Hassell, D. Theatre staffing – a need for change? Nursing Times, 67, 28 Jan 1971; Occ. papers, 13–15.

18 Hoffman, M. A graphic look at OR utilization. [A method of recording operating room usage.] AORN Journal, 23 (3), Sep 1975, 473, 475, 477, 478.

19 Hope, T. Theatre staffing and on call influenced by theatre nurse training. NATNews, 10 (3), Jun 1973, 15.

20 Hull, E. H. Nursing records of patients' operations. American Journal of Nursing, 71 (6), Jun 1971, 1156–1157.

21 Johnson, M. J. Economy in the operating room. Australian Nurses' Journal, 2 (5), Nov 1972, 30–31.

22 Ludwig, D. Winners and losers on the OR team. [Transactional analysis applied to staff relationships in the operating room.] AORN Journal, 20 (1), Jul 1974, 116, 118, 120, 122, 124, 126, 128.

23 Luttman, P. A. OR/RR nursing record improves care. AORN Journal, 22 (6), Dec 1975, 909–912.

24 Maguire, J. M. Changing relationships in the operating theatre. SA Nursing Journal, 42 (9), Sep 1975, 20, 22.

25 Makin, J. S. 'Action' project. [Project carried out by an experienced SEN as part of a pilot scheme in clinical management.] Nursing Mirror, 136, 19 Jan 1973, 31–32.

26 Martin, J. T. An anesthesiologist looks at OR design. AORN Journal, 21 (2), Feb 1975, 259–278, [10 pages].

27 Matthias, M. The operating department team. Nursing Times, 69, 20 Sep 1973, 1232, 1233.

28 National Association of Theatre Nurses The organization and staffing of operating departments. Preliminary comments by National Association of Theatre Nurses. NATNews, 8 (3), Autumn 1971, 8, 10, 14.

29 National Association of Theatre Nurses Staffing operating theatres. [Report of a working party.] NATNews, 11 (1), Jan 1974, 6–10, 12–14.

30 National Association of Theatre Nurses Takeover bid in the operating theatre. [Meeting to discuss Lewin report.] Nursing Times, 67, 14 Oct 1971, 1293.

31 NATNews The PRN scheme and the theatre: impressions on the use of a pool of reserve nurses within operating theatres in the Bromley Area Health Authority. NATNews, 12 (4), May/Jun 1975, 17, 19–20.

32 Organ, C. H. OR nurse, surgeon: common areas of concern. AORN Journal, 22)6), Dec 1975, 898–902.

33 Rait, A. Tomorrow is today. [Organizing the new operating rooms at the Royal Free Hospital.] Nursing Times, 71, 16 Oct 1975, NATN Supplement, i–ii.

34 Raven, K. A. Implications of the Lewin Report on theatre nursing and staffing in general. [8th Annual Congress – Newcastle 1972. Opening Speech.] NATNews. 9 (6), Dec 1972, 14, 17–18.

35 Trouten, F. O.R. nursing past and present – is there a future? Hospital Administration in Canada, 13 (10), Oct 1971, 80–88, [5 pages].

36 Wakeley, J. Nuffield Orthopaedic Centre theatre complex. [The Joseph Trueta complex.] Nursing Times, 70, 24 Oct 1974, 1648–1650.

37 Werry, J. The frightening gap. [Understaffing of operating theatres in New Zealand.] New Zealand Nursing Journal, 68 (2), Feb 1975, 24–26.

38 Wills, M. Communication key topic at Quebec O.R. nurses meeting. Hospital Administration in Canada, 14 (1), Jan 1972, 55.

e OPERATING DEPARTMENT ASSISTANTS

1 Advisory Committee on Ancillary Staff Training The training of operating department assistants.

[Extracts from the report issued by a Working Party of the Advisory Committee on Ancillary Staff Training.] NATNews, 10 (4), Aug 1973, 22, 24.

2 **Charter, D.** The O.R. technician comes of age. Canadian Hospital, 49 (2), Feb 1972, 61.

3 **Davis, H.** You are talking yourselves out of your jobs. [A new paramedical profession for operating department work.] Nursing Times, 68, 14 Sep 1972, 1160.

4 **Department of Health and Social Security** Training of operating department assistants. [Extracts from STM (75) 39.] NATNews, 12 (7), Sep 1975, 12.

5 **Gessner, L.** A short history: the functions and aims of the Association of Operating Room Technicians. Technic, 20 (6), Dec 1974, 4–5.

6 **Good, D. M.** Training theatre technicians: an experiment at Peterborough District Hospital. Nursing Mirror, 132, 22 Jan 1971, 30–31.

7 **Health and Social Service Journal** ODAS and SODAS. [Leading article on operating department assistants.] Health and Social Service Journal, 83, 1 Sep 1973, 1973–1974.

8 **Mitchell, J. and others** Four views on the O.R. nurse and O.R. technician. Hospital Administration in Canada, 14 (5), May 1972, 59–60, 62.

9 **National Association of Theatre Nurses** Some thoughts on the national training of operating department personnel: a provocative document from some members of the Surrey Branch. NATNews, 12 (7), Sep 1975, 17–18.

10 **New South Wales Operating Theatre Association** Technicians. [To relieve the graduate nurse of non-nursing duties in the operating theatre.] Lamp, 29 (6), Jun 1972, 21–22.

11 **Newcomb, R. F.** The surgical assistant – new on the OR team. RN Magazine, 35 (8), Aug 1972, OR 13–16, 20.

12 **Plessis, R. J.** Operating theatre technical assistants: the South African standpoint. SA Nursing Journal, 52 (12), Dec 1975, 27–28, 30.

13 **Roberts, M. and others** Technicians or nurses in the O.R? [The opinions of surgeons.] American Journal of Nursing, 74 (5), May 1974, 906–907.

14 **Roberts, M. and others** Technicians or nurses in the OR? [Three surgeons of Hartford, Connecticut conclude that nurses are needed as well as technicians.] AORN Journal, 20 (3), Sep 1974, 466–467, 470, 472.

15 **Royal College of Nursing** Non-cooperation call to nurses over ODA training. [Report of Rcn conference on the report on the Training of Operating Department Assistants.] Nursing Times, 69, 13 Sep 1973, 1173.

16 **Technic** Lewin report attacked. [Criticism of the job description for Operating Department Assistants.] Technic, 20, Dec 1974, 11.

66 INFECTION AND STERILIZATION

a GENERAL AND INFECTION CONTROL

1 **American Hospital Association** Statement on the danger of bacteria in the water of flower vases in hospitals. AORN Journal, 20 (1), Jul 1974, 8.

2 **Baker, B. H.** Infection control. Bedside Nurse, 5 (10), Oct 1972, 11–13; (11), Nov 1972, 18–21.

3 **British Medical Journal** Carpeting hospital wards. [Leading article on infection risks.] British Medical Journal, 2, 12 Apr 1975, 53.

4 **British Medical Journal** Ward design and cross infection. British Medical Journal, 3, 3 Jul 1971, 5–6.

5 **Butler, H. M.** Infection control. Australian Nurses Journal, 2 (2), Aug 1972, 24–25, 32; UNA Nursing Journal, 70, Jul 1972, 14–16.

6 **Carbary, L. J.** Hospital acquired infections. [Methods of preventing infections.] Nursing Care, 8 (12), Dec 1975, 28–32.

7 **Chewick, S.** Infection control. Infection control demands administrative support. Dimensions in Health Service, 52 (12), Dec 1975, 40–41.

8 **Copping, J. D.** Information and reporting: the basis of infection control. [Guidelines in developing an infection control program.] Hospital Administration in Canada, 17 (4), Apr 1975, 23–24, 26.

9 **De Klerk, M. S.** Theatre discipline in relation to infection control. SA Nursing Journal, 42 (9), Sep 1975, 10, 12.

10 **Dyer, E. D. and Peterson, D. E.** Safe care of IPPB machines: a nurse researcher and microbiologist advise on care of equipment to prevent hospital-acquired infections. American Journal of Nursing, 71 (11), Nov 1971, 2163–2166.

11 **Hnatko, S. I.** The employee health service and infection control [in hospitals]. Dimensions in Health Service, 51 (12), Dec 1974, 11–12.

12 **Hospital Administration in Canada** Infection control recommendations. Hospital Administration in Canada, 17 (9), Sep 1975, 45–46.

13 **Lowbury, E J. L. and others, editors** Control of hospital infection: a practical handbook. Chapman and Hall, 1975.

14 **National League for Nursing** Council of Hospital and Related Institutional Nursing Services. Infection control: papers presented at a workshop . . . New York, March 1975. New York: NLN, 1975.

15 **Neely, J.** Starch granuloma peritonitis. [Dangers of infection from surgical glove powder.] Nursing Mirror, 140, 24 Apr 1975, 62–63.

16 **Newsom, S. W. B.** Contaminated water. [Infection control in hospitals.] Nursing Times, 70, 19 Sep 1974, 1461–1463.

17 **Pilsworth, R.** A regional committee for the control of hospital infection. Health Trends, 4 (3), Aug 1972, 56–58.

18 **Rowland, A. J. and Alder, V. G.** Transmission of infection through towels. Community Medicine, 128, 5 May 1972, 71–73.

19 **Sanderson, P. J.** Hospital acquired infections. 1. Sources and types of infection. 2. Routes of infection. Nursing Times, 71, 19 Jun 1975, 958–960; 26 Jun 1975, 1007–1009.

20 **Selwyn, S.** Changing patterns in hospital infection. Nursing Times, 68, 25 May 1972, 643–646.

21 **Selwyn, S.** Hospital cross infection: a puzzle and its solution. Nursing Times, 68, 1 Jun 1972, 663–666.

22 **Smith, G. and others** Ward design in relation to postoperative wound infection. 3. British Medical Journal, 3, 6 Jul 1974, 13–15.

23 **Smylie, H. G. and others** Ward design in relation to postoperative wound infection. 1 and 2. British Medical Journal, 1, 9 Jan 1971, 67–75.

24 **Taplin, D. and Mertz, P. M.** Flower vases in hospitals as reservoirs of pathogens. Lancet, 2, 8 Dec 1973, 1279–1281.

25 **Williams, R. F.** Hospital infection as a continuing problem. Nursing Times, 70, 8 Aug 1974, 1232–1233.

b INFECTION CONTROL SISTER

1 **Altemeier, W. A.** Conference for nurse epidemiologists held at Ohio State Hospitals. Hospital Topics, 50 (8), Aug 1972, 47–51.

2 **Association for Practitioners in Infection Control** Infection control nurse's problems, role discussed at APIC meeting. Hospital Topics, 52 (4), Apr 1974, 2–3.

3 **Chavigny, K. H.** Nurse epidemiologist in the hospital. American Journal of Nursing, 75 (4), Apr 1975, 638–642.

4 **Connell, A. D.** Controlling operating room related infection in cancer patients. Nursing Clinics of North America, 7 (4), Dec 1975, 667–678.

5 **Finn, B.** Education and training of infection control nurses. [JBCNS Course.] Nursing Times, 71, 13 Feb 1975; Contact, 13–14.

6 **Harte, J. D.** Control of hospital infection: the purpose and functioning of a hospital staff OH department and the overlap with the infection control committee. Occupational Health, 26 (3), Mar 1974, 82–85.

7 **Hollins, V. L.** Duties of an infection control sister in a large general hospital. UNA Nursing Journal, 50, Mar/Apr 1972, 14–15.

8 **Hunt, D.** First in the field: the role of the occupational health nurse in hospital vis a vis the infection and control sister based on the Bedford General Hospital pilot scheme. Nursing Times, 70, 25 Apr 1974, 646–647.

9 **Infection Control Nurses' Association** Contact, (Nos 1–3). Nursing Times, 70, 29 Aug 1974, Supplement, 1–8; 71, 13 Feb 1975, Supplement, 9–16; 71, 11 Sep 1975, Supplement, 17–24.

10 **Kicklighter, L.** The nurse epidemiologist: a vital member of the hospital infection control team. Hospitals, 47 (1), Jan 1973, 48, 52, 54, 56.

11 **O'Connor, V.** Careers in nursing. New clinical specialist – a growing breed. [Infection control sister.] Nursing Times, 67, 14 Oct 1971, 1276–1279.

12 **Parker, M. J.** Infection control nursing education. Nursing Times, 70, 29 Aug 1974, Supplement, 3.

13 **Powell, M.** An environment for wound healing. [The work of the infection-control sister in the Robert Jones and Agnes Hunt Orthopaedic Hospital.] American Journal of Nursing, 72 (10), Oct 1972, 1862–1865.

14 **Robinson, A. M.** Nurse-epidemiologist: key to infection control. RN Magazine, 38 (10), Oct 1975, 63–65, 67.

15 **Stronge, J.** Infection control nurse. Clinical specialist. World of Irish Nursing, 4 (2), Feb 1975, 23.

16 **World of Irish Nursing** Infection control nurses' study day. World of Irish Nursing, 4 (2), Feb 1975, 26–27

c CENTRAL STERILE SUPPLY

1 **British Hospital Journal and Social Service Review** Some new central sterile supply service installations in Great Britain. British Hospital Journal and Social Service Review, 82, 5 Feb 1972, 296–299.

2 **Charrem, G. J.** Central sterile supply. New Zealand Nursing Journal, 66 (1), Jan 1973, 27–30.

3 **Charter, D.** Do we really need a nurse in central service? Canadian Hospital, 48 (7), Jul 1971, 30, 64.

4 **George, J. C. S.** Punch cards in CSSD. NATNews, 9 (4), Aug 1972, 31–32.

5 Health and Social Service Journal Central sterile supply department. Leading opinion. Health and Social Service Journal, 85, 8 Feb 1975, 287.

6 Health and Social Service Journal Central sterile supply departments. [Leading article on the position of the CSSD in the management structure of a hospital.] Health and Social Service Journal, 84, 30 Nov 1974, 2767.

7 Houslop, P. L. CSSD for the Oncological research unit at Fulham Hospital. [Reverse barrier nursing unit.] Health and Social Service Journal, 83, 27 Jan 1973, 201.

8 Jenkins, M. M. CSSD and the nurse. Macmillan Journals, 1971.

9 King, M. J. March to May 1972. An account of the use made of the J & J Travel Award. [CSSD in Nairobi.] NATNews, 9 (5), Oct 1972, 16–17.

10 King, M. One day in the life of a CSSD superintendent. NATNews, 9 (4), Aug 1972, 22, 24.

11 Monty, C. P. and Hayes, C. E. Dust contamination of central sterile supply packs. Nursing Mirror, 137, 10 Aug 1973, 18–19.

12 Napier, E. W. The new CSSD/TSSU at Ninewells. Health and Social Service Journal, 85, 25 Oct 1975, 2392.

13 Sandidge, E. R. Costing CSSD packs. [Based on a study at the Westminster and St. George's Group Hospitals.] British Hospital Journal and Social Service Review, 82, 30 Sep 1972, 2178–2179.

14 Sutterby, J. and Hopkins, E. Introducing a central sterile supply system to a rural community. [Oxfordshire.] Nursing Times, 69, 1 Mar 1973; Occ. papers, 33–35.

15 Warren, M. and Hamilton, P. Administrative problems in the inauguration of a theatre sterile supply service. Hospital and Health Service Review, 70 (2), Feb 1974, 42–43.

d DISINFECTION AND STERILIZATION

1 Adams, M. A. Planning with particular reference to isolation units. Nursing Times, 71, 13 Feb 1975, Contact, 12–13.

2 Alford, D. J. and others Your OR gown: barrier or gateway for bacteria? RN Magazine, 38 (1), Jan 1975, OR 12.

3 Ayliffe, G. A. J. and Gibson, G. L. Antimicrobial treatment of equipment in the hospital. [Suggested methods of sterilizing specific items.] Health and Social Service Journal, 85, 15 Mar 1975, 598–599.

4 Ayliffe, G. A. J. Disinfection of baths and bathwater. Nursing Times, 71, 11 Sep 1975. Contact, 22–23.

5 Basson, R. A. Gamma radiation sterilization [of medical equipment]. SA Nursing Journal, 42 (2), Feb 1975, 27–28.

6 Bateman, P. L. G. The curse of the pharaohs. [Pharoah's Ants in hospitals.] Nursing Times, 70, 9 May 1974, 722–723.

7 British Medical Journal Disinfecting ventilators. Briitsh Medical Journal, 2, 16 Jun 1973, 625.

8 Calder, G. Sterile solutions. Health and Social Service Journal, 83, 4 Aug 1973, 1741–1742, 1744.

9 Cartledge, K. W. An introduction to disinfection. [Historical developments.] Nursing Times, 71, 11 Sep 1975, 1460–1461.

10 Clarke, B. H. Aseptic practice. OR orientation guidelines. [Importance of an orientation programme in the operating room.] Modern Health Care, 3 (2), Feb 1971, 63.

11 Davis, A. E. and Korczynski, M. Hospital disinfection of thermometers. Supervisor Nurse, 6 (3), Mar 1975, 23, 25–27.

12 Erdos, G. and Pecho, Z. The organization of a hospital disinfection system. Hospital, 68 (2), Feb 1972, 45–49.

13 Farrand, R. J. and Williams, A. Evaluation of single use packs of hospital disinfectants. Lancet, 1, 17 Mar 1973, 591–593.

14 Fox, J. A. A system of pre-packed implants sterilized by gamma irradiation. NATNews, 9 (4), Aug 1972, 26–28.

15 Harry, J. Sterilization and prevention of infection in an eye hospital. [Moorfields.] Health and Social Service Journal, 85, 25 Oct 1975, 2393–2395.

16 Holdcroft, A. and others Why disinfect ventilators? Lancet, 1, 3 Feb 1973, 240–241.

17 Huth, M. E. Rationale for OR attire standards [to reduce infection hazards]. AORN Journal, 71 (7), Jun 1975, 1217–1221.

18 Kelsey, J. C. The myth of surgical sterility. Lancet, 2, 16 Dec 1972, 1301–1303.

19 McArthur, B. and others Stopcock contamination in an ICU. [Research carried out by the University of Washington.] American Journal of Nursing, 75 (1), Jan 1975, 96–97.

20 Maurer, I. M. Disinfection and sterilization in domiciliary nursing. District Nursing, 15 (7), Oct 1972, 138, 140–141. Reprinted in Nursing Mirror, 136, 27 Apr 1973, 46–47.

21 Mehaffy, N. L. Rationale for asepsis standards. AORN Journal, 21 (7), Jun 1975, 1213–1216.

22 Mitchell, E. R. Sterilizing cardiac equipment. British Hospital Journal and Social Service Review, 81, 24 Jul 1971, 1492, 1494, 1497.

23 Mitchell, N. J. and Gamble, D. R. Clothing design for operating room personnel. Lancet, 2, 9 Nov 1974, 1133–1136.

24 Northwick Park Hospital and Clinical Research Centre Control of Infection Group. Isolation system for general hospitals. British Medical Journal, 2, 6 Apr 1974, 41–44.

25 Nursing Times Do-it-yourself sterile nursing unit. [Middlesex Hospital.] Nursing Times, 67, 11 Nov 1971, 1393.

26 Public Health Laboratory. Service Board The use of chemical disinfectants in hospitals, by J. C. Kelsey and Isobel M. Maurer. HMSO, 1972.

27 Roberts, R. B. editor Infection and sterilization problems. Boston: Little Brown, 1972.

28 Royal Marsden Hospital The ultimate in isolation? [Advanced leukaemia unit at the Royal Marsden Hospital's Sutton branch, where latest techniques in reverse barrier nursing are used.] Nursing Times, 69, 5 Jul 1973, 855; Nursing Mirror, 137, 14 Sep 1973, 14–17.

29 Sabo, B. Sterilization of anesthesia apparatus. Journal of the American Association of Nurse Anesthetists, 41 (5), Oct 1973, 421–426.

30 South Western Regional Health Authority Notes on disinfection and sterilization. 3rd ed. Bristol: The Authority 1975.

31 Space suit isolator. [A mobile sterile environment for reverse barrier nursing.] Nursing Times, 70, 18 Jul 1974, 1107.

32 Towers, A. and Lidwell, O. System for patient isolation: unidirectional flow ventilation. Nursing Mirror, 135, 28 Jul 1972, 22–23.

33 Trexler, P. C. and others Plastic isolators for treatment of acute leukaemia patients under 'germ-free' conditions. British Medical Journal, 4, 6 Dec 1975, 549–552.

34 United States. National Institutes of Health. Clinical Center Nursing care of patients in the laminar air flow room. Washington: US Dept. of Health, Education and Welfare, 1971.

35 Wells, P. Improving cleanup techniques in the operating room. RN Magazine, 36 (6), Jun 1973, OR 3–4, 6.

36 Woodward, E. M. Plastic bag protection. Nursing Mirror, 133, 6 Aug 1971, 22–23.

e DISINFECTION OF THE SKIN

1 Broome, W. E. and Pallett, F. G. E. Hygienic hands. Nursing Mirror, 133, 30 Jul 1971, 14.

2 Drug and Therapeutics Bulletin Pre-operative disinfectants for surgeons' and nurses' hands. Drug and Therapeutics Bulletin, 11, 7 Dec 1973, 99–100.

3 Drug and Therapeutics Bulletin Preparing the skin for injections and venepuncture. Drug and Therapeutics Bulletin, 10 (19), 15 Sep 1972, 73–74.

4 Fox, M. K. and others How good are hand washing practices? [Study of a random sample of 90 nursing personnel in medical and surgical units.] American Journal of Nursing, 74 (9), Sep 1974, 1676–1678.

5 Infection Control Nurses Association, West Midlands Group Handwashing: surgical wards. Soap and water compared with 70% alcohol. Nursing Times, 70, 29 Aug 1974, Supplement, 4–5.

6 Lewis, M. J. Skin preparation before injection. Nursing Times, 71, 15 May 1975, 786–787.

7 Lilly, H. A. and Lowbury, E. J. L. Disinfection of the skin: an assessment of some new preparations. British Medical Journal, 3, 18 Sep 1971, 674–676.

8 Linton, J. Preparing the operation site. Nursing Times, 70, 4 Jul 1974, Occ. papers, 33–36; 11 Jul 1974, Occ. papers, 37–40; 18 Jul 1974, Occ. papers, 41–43.

9 MacClelland, D. C. Are current skin preparations valid? [A survey of recent literature on pre- and postoperative care including shaving and sterilization.] AORN Journal, 21 (1), Jan 1975, 55–60.

10 Sellers, J. and Newman, J. H. Disinfection of the adult umbilicus for abdominal surgery. Nursing Mirror, 134, 9 Jun 1972, 21–23.

11 Selwyn, S. and Ellis, H. Skin bacteria and skin disinfection reconsidered. British Medical Journal, 1, 15 Jan 1972, 136–140.

67 ACCIDENTS AND EMERGENCIES

a SERVICES (Includes mobile units)

1 Allen, J. R. and others Patient documentation in an accident and emergency department. [A new system introduced at Broadgreen Hospital.] Hospital and Health Services Review, 71, Mar 1975, 84–87.

2 Anthony, M. Accident and Emergency Departments. Australian Nurses' Journal, 1 (5), Nov 1971, 26–28.

3 Barr, E. M. Frenchay Hospital mobile resuscitation unit. Nursing Times, 68, 21 Sep 1972, 1201–1203.

4 Campion, N. A. Patient documentation and records, Accident and Emergency Department. Medical Record, 14 (2), May 1973, 56–57.

5 Clifford, A. H. Gloucestershire's mobile resuscitation units. Health and Social Service Journal, 84, 2 Mar 1974, 480–481.

6 Cullinan, J. Lives of Lincolnshire. [Lincolnshire integrated Voluntary Emergency Services.] Nursing Times, 69, 24 May 1973, 659–660.

7 Davidson, R. G. Paramedics at work. 3. Helicopter rescue. [Helicopter emergency service in Maryland, USA.] Nursing Times, 78, 3 Feb 1982, 193–196.

8 Dunn, A. Bellevue's emergency services. [Bellevue Hospital, Manhattan which combines primary care with emergency services.] Nursing Times, 71, 24 Apr 1975, 642–643.

9 Gray, G. R. GPs and emergency services. [East Riding Voluntary Accident and Emergency Service.] Health and Social Service Journal, 83, 24 Mar 1973, 657–658.

10 Haworth, F. B. Accident and emergency resuscitation trolley [designed and constructed at Northwick Park Hospital for use in the accident and emergency department]. Nursing Times, 70, 9 May 1974, 707.

11 Haworth, F. B. A patient's resuscitation transport trolley. Nursing Times, 70, 19 Sep 1974, 1476–1477.

12 Hoddy, K. The ambulance service – yesterday, today and tomorrow. Community Health, 5 (3), Nov/Dec 1973, 118–123.

13 Little, K. Profile of an accident flying squad. [Operating from Derbyshire Royal Infirmary Casualty Department.] British Medical Journal, 3, 30 Sep 1972, 807–810.

14 McCarrick, H. Air ambulance serving the Western Isles. Nursing Times, 70, 14 Feb 1974, 230–231.

15 Mona, M. Help in a hurry: the crisis clinic. [Outpatient emergency department.] Canadian Nurse, 69 (10), Oct 1973, 35–37.

16 Nursing Times The Midlands. Flying Squad: Derby's accident service. Nursing Times, 70, 12 Sep 1974, 1417.

17 Nursing Times South East. Accident services [at Royal Sussex County Hospital, Brighton, and Kent and Canterbury Hospital, Canterbury.] Nursing Times, 71, 20 Mar 1975, 450–455.

18 Packwood, T. The organization of accident and emergency departments. Health and Social Service Journal, 84, 27 Jul 1974, 1677–1679.

19 Romano, T. and Boyd, D. R. Illinois trauma program. American Journal of Nursing, 73 (6), Jun 1973, 1004–1007.

20 St. Clair Strange, F. G. An area accident service. [East Kent service based in Canterbury.] Royal Society of Health Journal, 93 (1), Feb 1973, 31–35, 49.

21 Snook, R. Accident flying squad. [Of the Bath ambulance service.] British Medical Journal, 3, 2 Sep 1972, 569–574.

22 Squire, P. Ready for tomorrow's needs: the new accident and emergency department at Princess Margaret Hospital, Swindon. Nursing Mirror, 136, 23 Feb 1973, 24–27.

23 Waddell, G. and others Effects of ambulance transport in critically ill patients. British Medical Journal, 1, 15 Feb 1975, 386–389.

b NURSING

1 Anast, G. T. E.R. management, nursing problems discussed at seminars. Hospital Topics, 50 (2), Feb 1972, 41–42, 44.

2 Bolger, M. J. Ambulance accident/emergency courses for nurses. Nursing Mirror, 137, 6 Jul 1973, 12.

3 Cliff, K. S. Accident and emergency care – the role of the nurse. [A study in the Wessex RHB area with a course of training set out as an appendix.] Nursing Times, 70, 19 Sep 1974, 1448–1451.

4 Cosgriff, J. H. Association for ED nurses holds first national meeting. [Emergency Department Nurses Association.] Hospital Topics, 50 (12), Dec 1972, 39–42.

5 Cosgriff, J. H. and Anderson, D. L. The practice of emergency nursing. Philadelphia: Lippincott, 1975.

6 Davis, D. K. and O'Boyle, C. M. Emergency and disaster nursing continuing education review: 425 essay questions and referenced answers. Flushing: Medical Examination Publishing Co, 1975.

7 Goodman, J. Emergency nursing – via helicopter. [Experiences in a critical care course.] RN Magazine, 38 (8), Aug 1975, 58–62, 64.

8 Horoshak, I. The transformation of the ED nurse. 2. Upgrading skills and status. RN Magazine, 38 (8), Aug 1975, 35–38.

9 Jenkins, A. L., editor Emergency department organization and management. St Louis: Mosby, 1975.

10 London, P. S. Return to nursing. 17. Nursing in an accident service. Nursing Mirror, 133, 17 Sep 1971, 25–27.

11 McLeod, K. A. The transformation of the ED nurse. 1. Learning to take the trauma of triage. RN Magazine, 38 (7), Jul 1975, 22–27.

12 Monty, C. P. Accident ... emergency. Nursing Mirror, 133, 24 Dec 1971, 13–15.

13 Morgan, D. M. An instrument for change – policies and procedure in the emergency department. [Procedure manuals.] Canadian Hospital, 49 (1), Jan 1972, 37–39.

14 Morgan, D. M. A pioneer program for the emergency nurse. [Post registration course in Ontario.] Dimensions in Health Service, 51, 13 Mar 1974, 44–47.

15 Morgan, D. M. Special education for emergency nurses. [Formulation of eleven special procedures and the introduction of post basic courses in Ontario.] Dimensions in Health Service, 52 (10), Oct 1975, 10, 12.

16 Nicholls, M. The nurse and accident prevention. New Zealand Nursing Journal, 66 (3), Mar 1973, 4.

17 Nursing Clinics of North America Symposium on emergency nursing. Nursing Clinics of North America, 8 (3), Sep 1973, 375–466.

18 Oliver, W. L. and others Trauma training: expanding the role of ED nurses. [Albany Regional Medical Program. Includes evaluation.] RN Magazine, 38 (9), Sep 1975, OR 9, 10.

19 Rodgers, B. Future trends in A and E nursing. Report ... on the joint conference of the Rcn Accident and Emergency Sub-group and members of the Casualty Surgeon's Association in Plymouth, April 2–5 1975. Nursing Mirror, 140, 10 Apr 1975, 35.

20 Romano, T. Trauma nurse specialist: what trauma nurses do and how they are prepared in the Illinois trauma program. American Journal of Nursing, 73 (6), Jun 1973, 1008–1011.

21 Scott, P. D. Victims of violence. Some understanding of the underlying causes of crimes of violence may help the nurse in her care of the victims. Nursing Times, 70, 4 Jul 1974, 1036–1037.

22 South East Metropolitan Regional Hospital Board Report of a working party set up to advise on the duties and responsibilities of nurses in casualty departments. Croydon: The Board, 1972. Comment in Nursing Times, 68, 25 May 1972, 628.

23 Straub, M. K. Inservice education in the ER. Hospital Topics, 50 (7), Jul 1972, 38–40.

24 Taubenhaus, L. J. Planning today's emergency department. American Journal of Nursing, 72 (11), Nov 1972, 2050–2055.

25 Vickery, D. M. Triage: problem-oriented sorting of patients. Bowie: Brady, 1975.

26 Wagner, M. M. Assessment of patients with multiple injuries. American Journal of Nursing, 72 (10), Oct 1972, 1822–1827.

c PATIENT AND FAMILY
(Includes children)

1 Andersen, M. De.C and Pleticha, J. M. Emergency unit patients' perceptions of stressful life events. [The effect on the patients' subsequent health and assessing patients' readjustment to recent life changes.] Nursing Research, 23 (5), Sep/Oct 1974, 378–383.

2 Birley, J. L. T. Emotional first aid. [Psychiatric problems of casualty patients.] Nursing Times, 69, 6 Dec 1973, 1666.

3 Eggland, E. T. The anxious family in the emergency room. [Nurse's role in care.] Nursing Care, 8 (11), Nov 1975, 28–29, 31–32.

4 Evans, J. and Hawkes, R. Background music in hospital. [Patients reactions to background music in the accident and emergency department of West Hill Hospital, Dartford.] British Hospital Journal and Social Service Review, 82, 18 March 1972, 608–609, 611.

5 Hankoff, L. D. and others Crisis intervention in the emergency room. [Counselling by nurses of emergency room patients.] Nursing Digest, 2 (8), Oct 1974, 11–13.

6 Husband, P. The child with repeated accidents. [A study of children in Nottingham over a six-year period showing accidents resulted from a breakdown in their adjustment to the environment.] Nursing Times, 70, 5 Dec 1974, 1884–1885.

7 Kuenzi, S. H. and Fenton, M. V. Crisis intervention in acute care areas. [Dealing with families and patients in the emergency room setting.] American Journal of Nursing, 75 (5), May 1975, 830–834.

8 Morgan, D. M. At Montreal General. The patient advocate: a new aid for emergency. [Ombudsman to improve communications between patients and the health care team in the emergency department.] Canadian Hospital, 50 (8), Aug 1973, 24–25, 53.

9 Rutter, W. A. Identifying psychiatric and drug-abuse cases in the ED. RN Magazine, 37 (12), Dec 1974, OR 1–2.

10 Severin, N. K. and Becker, R. E. Let psychiatric RNs do ED consultations? [Psychiatric nurses see patients during staff shortages.] RN Magazine, 38 (4), Apr 1975, OR 14, 18.

11 Standen, J. 'Off to casualty again.' [Case study of an 'accident prone' child.] Nursing Times, 70, 5 Dec 1974, 1886–1887.

12 Welnick, J. Are we scaring our patients to death? [Fear in the emergency department.] Nursing Care, 7 (7), Jul 1974, 28–29.

d FIRST AID

1 Atherley, G. R. C. and others Hidden benefits fron first aid. [A research project of the University of Aston, Safety and Hygiene Group.] Occupational Health, 25 (6), Jun 1973, 215–219.

2 Bradley, D. First aid. 1. Main maxims. [Basic first aid.] Nursing Times, 71, 21 Aug 1975, 1322–1324.

3 Bradley, D. First aid. 2. Cardiac and respiratory arrest. Nursing Times, 71, 28 Aug 1975, 1367–1370.

4 Bradley, D. First aid. 3. Haemorrhage and shock. Nursing Times, 71, 4 Sep 1975, 1409–1413.

5 Bradley, D. First aid. 4 and 5. Injuries to bones, joints and muscles. 1–2. Nursing Times, 71, 11 Sep 1975, 1462–1465; 71, 18 Sep 1975, 1502–1504.

6 Bradley, D. First aid. 6. Poisoning, burns and scalds. Nursing Times, 71, 25 Sep 1975, 1542–1545.

7 Bradley, D. First aid. 7. Chest injuries. Nursing Times, 71, 2 Oct 1975, 1582–1584.

8 Cameron, J. D. Changing concepts of first aid. Transactions of the Society of Occupational Medicine, 22 (2), Apr 1972, 52–55.

9 Gardner, A. W. and Roylance, P. J. New essential first aid. Pan, 1972.

10 Hughes, G. O. Need first aid training be dull? Transactions of the Society of Occupational Medicine, 22 (2), Apr 1972, 48–51.

11 Moffat, W. C. First-aid for nurses. Nursing Mirror, 132, 26 Mar 1971, 21–25, 29.

12 Pitman, M. Emergency first aid. 1. Rescue and resuscitation. Nursing Mirror, 132, 2 Apr 1971, 17.

13 Pitman, M. Emergency first aid. 2. Cliff rescue team in action. Nursing Mirror, 132, 9 Apr 1971, 27.

14 St. John Ambulance Association and others First aid manual: the authorized manual of the St. John Ambulance Association and the British Red Cross Society. 3rd ed. Published jointly, 1972.

15 St. John Ambulance Association and Brigade Occupational first aid. 3rd ed. Macmillan, 1973.

16 Tupper, J. M. First aid symposium. Occupational Health, 23 (2), Feb 1971, 51–54.

17 White, D. M. Teaching first aid. Occupational Health, 24 (4), Apr 1972, 109–113.

18 Whyte, S. B. The tragic omission. [Importance of stressing the need to clear air passages in first aid teaching.] Nursing Mirror, 140, 17 Apr 1975, 69.

e HEAD INJURIES

1 Craft, A. W. and others Head injuries in children. British Medical Journal, 4, 28 Oct 1972, 200–203.

2 Hinkhouse, A. Craniocerebral trauma. American Journal of Nursing, 73 (10), Oct 1973, 1719–1722.

3 Hitchcock, E. R. Treatment of head injuries. Nursing Times, 70, 1 Aug 1974, 1193–1195.

4 Jay, S. S. The impact of a boy's head injury on his parents. Maternal-Child Nursing Journal, 4 (1), Spring 1975, 49–56.

5 Jennett, B. Who cares for head injuries? [Continuity of care between different professions involved in acute and recovery stages.] British Medical Journal, 3, 2 Aug 1975, 267–270.

6 Knight, P. N. Rehabilitation of head injuries. Nursing Mirror, 136, 30 Mar 1973, 14–19.

7 Norsworthy, E. Nursing rehabilitation after severe head trauma. American Journal of Nursing, 74 (7), Jul 1974, 1246–1250.

8 Panting, A. and Merry, P. H. The long term rehabilitation of severe head injuries with particular reference to the need for social and medical support for the patient's family. Rehabilitation, (82), Jul/Sep 1972, 33–37.

9 Parsons, L. C. Respiratory changes in head injury. American Journal of Nursing, 71, Nov 1971, 2187–2191.

f HOME ACCIDENTS (Includes children and elderly)

1 Alphey, R. S. and Leach, S. J. Accidental death in the home. [Trends in the number of accidents which lead to death in England and Wales.] Royal Society of Health Journal, 94 (3), Jun 1974, 97–102, 144.

2 Enright, M. J. Nursing care study. Domestic wringer injury. Nursing Miror, 135, 8 Dec 1972, 37–40.

3 Hall, M. H. Hazards to children in the home environment. Community Health, 5 (5), Mar/Apr 1974, 238–245.

4 Hyman, C. A. Accidents in the home to children under two years. A report on a questionnaire. Health Visitor, 47 (5), May 1974, 139–141.

5 Murdock, R. and Eva, J. Home accidents to children under 15 years: survey of 910 cases. British Medical Journal, 3, 13 Jul 1974, 103–106.

6 Nursing Mirror The dark side of the season of goodwill. [Toy safety.] Nursing Mirror, 139, 19 Dec 1974, 46–47.

7 Roberts, J. L. and others Home accidents and health education. Health Education Journal, 33 (2), 1974, 35–45; (3), 1974, 67–78.

8 Shelmerdine, H. R. and Rigby, M. J. Home accident survey. [Results of a year-long survey in Cheshire.] Health and Social Service Journal, 84, 9 Mar 1974, 542–543.

9 Tomiche, F. J. Too many accidents at home. World Health, Feb/Mar 1973, 40–45.

10 Wright, W. J. Accidents in and around the home. Nursing Mirror, 139, 26 Jul 1974, 65–66.

g INJURIES: MISCELLANEOUS (Includes shock)

1 Allen, E. T. Hypothermia: prolonged immersion in cold water. Nursing Times, 70, 12 Dec 1974, 1928–1929.

2 Askew, A. R. Lawn mower injuries. Nursing Times, 70, 4 Jul 1974, 1028–1029.

3 Barron, J. N. Hand injuries and their treatment. Nursing Mirror, 136, 27 Apr 1973, 37–39.

4 Blake, J. Accidental hypothermia in fit young adults. Nursing Mirror, 141, 21 Aug 1975, 46–49.

5 Drug and Therapeutics Bulletin Emergency treatment of accidental hypothermia. Drug and Therapeutics Bulletin, 9 (2), 15 Jan 1971, 5–7.

6 Duffy, B. L. and Kyle, J. W. The stove-in chest. Nursing Times, 71, 3 Jul 1975, 1038–1039.

7 Grimes, O. F. Traumatic injuries of the diaphragm. RN Magazine, 38 (3), Feb 1975, OR 8, 10, 12.

8 Hartley, E. J. Nursing care study. Struck by lightning. Nursing Times, 70, 11 Jul 1974, 1064–1065.

9 Hulme, J. R. The hazards of petrol. Nursing Times, 71, 6 Feb 1975, 224–225.

10 Illingworth, C. and others 200 injuries caused by playground equipment. [Study at the accident and emergency department, Children's Hospital, Sheffield.] British Medical Journal, 4, 8 Nov 1975, 332–334.

11 Keen, G. Chest injuries: a guide for the accident department. Bristol: Wright, 1975.

12 Keen, G. Closed chest injuries. Nursing Mirror, 134, 16 Jun 1972, 14–16.

13 Levy, L. S. Physiological aspects of electric shock. Nursing Times, 71, 11 Sep 1975, 1454–1459.

14 Lloyd, H. M. Nursing care study. Fat embolism following multiple injuries. Nursing Times, 69, 8 Nov 1973, 1490–1492.

15 McIlwraith, G. R. Electric shock. Nursing Times, 71, 22 May 1975, 803–805.

16 Neary, K. The role of the nurse in shock. World of Irish Nursing, 4 (7), Jul 1975, 7.

17 Nicholas, G. G. and Willwerth, B. M. Emergency treatment of neck injuries. RN Magazine, 38 (4), Apr 1975, OR 20, 24.

18 Pagliero, K. M. Chest injuries. 1. Immediate considerations. Nursing Times, 71, 13 Feb 1975, 252–254.

19 Pagliero, K. M. Chest injuries. 2. Specific injuries. Nursing Times, 71, 20 Feb 1975, 296–297.

20 Patten, J. P. Faints and falls. [Nature and causes of sudden loss of consciousness.] Nursing Times, 68, 3 Aug 1972, 967–969.

21 Proctor, H. Stove-in chest. Nursing Mirror, 137, 13 Jul 1973, 20–24.

22 Reep, B. Current concepts concerning the pathophysiology and treatment of shock. Journal of the American Association of Nurse Anesthetists, 41 (3), Jun 1973, 216–218, 223–227.

23 Rowe, N. L. and Beetham, M. D. Maxillofacial injuries – 1. Nursing Times, 67, 26 Aug 1971, 1057–1060.

24 Tharp, G. D. Shock: the overall mechanisms. American Journal of Nursing, 74 (12), Dec 1974, 2208–2211.

25 Westwood, J. Ejection injuries. [Emergency procedures after aircraft accidents.] Nursing Mirror, 141, 10 Jul 1975, 46–49.

26 Wolfgang, G. L. Shoulder surgery: repairing tears of the rotator cuff. RN Magazine, 37 (7), Jul 1974, OR 1–2, 4.

27 Yarington, C. T. The emergency management of facial injuries. Occupational Health Nursing, 22 (6), Jun 1974, 18–21.

h RAPE

1 British Medical Journal Victims of rape. [Leading article.] British Medical Journal, 1, 25 Jan 1975, 171–172.

2 Burgess, A. W. and Holmstrom, L. L. Accountability: a right of the rape victim. [Study to show the attitude of rape victims to professional personnel.] Journal of Psychiatric Nursing and Mental Health Services, 13 (3), May–Jun 1975, 11–16.

3 Burgess, A. W. and Holmstrom, L. L. Crisis and counseling requests of rape victims. Nursing Research, 23 (3), May/Jun 1974, 196–202.

4 Burgess, A. W. and Holmstrom, L. L. The rape victim in the emergency ward. American Journal of Nursing, 73 (10), Oct 1973, 1741–1745.

5 Burgess, A. W. and Holmstrom, L. L. Rape trauma syndrome. Nursing Digest, 3 (3), May–Jun 1975, 17–19.

6 Carbary, L. J. Rape: treating terrified victims. Journal of Practical Nursing, 24 (2), Feb 1974, 20–22.

7 Donadio, B. and White, M. A. Seven who were raped. [The role of the nurse.] Nursing Outlook, 22 (4), Apr 1974, 245–247.

8 Holmstrom, L. L. and Burgess, A. W. Assessing trauma in the rape victim: three new diagnostic categories. American Journal of Nursing, 75 (8), Aug 1975, 1288–1291.

9 Price, V. Rape victims – the invisible patients. [Calgary Rape Crisis Centre.] Canadian Nurse, 71 (4), Apr 1974, 20–34.

10 Williams, C. C. and Williams, R. A. Rape: a plea for help in the hospital emergency room. Nursing Forum, 12 (4), 1973, 388–401.

i RED CROSS AND ST. JOHN'S AMBULANCE BRIGADE

1 Badouaille, M. L. The staff school of the Red Cross in France 1951 to 1971. International Journal of Nursing Studies, 9 (2), Jun 1972, 95–99.

2 Bailey, R. E. Nursing officers . . . not Salmon but St. John. Nursing Times, 67, 29 Apr 1971, 524–525.

3 Bowen, P. G. The flying ambulance. [St. John Air Ambulance Wing.] Health and Social Service Journal, 83, 26 May 1973, 1194–1195.

4 Bryans, A. Competent not merely helpful. [Volunteers in the British Red Cross Society.] Health and Social Service Journal, 84, 13 Jul 1974, 1570–1572.

5 DeMarsh, K. G. Red Cross outpost nursing in New Brunswick. The personal memoirs of an outpost nurse – 25 years later. Canadian Nurse, 69 (6), Jun 1973, 24–27.

6 District Nursing International Red Cross. District Nursing, 15 (4), Jul 1972, 79–81.

7 Philpot, T. Fresh battles for the Red Cross. [First annual Red Cross lecture.] Health and Social Service Journal, 84, 5 Jan 1974, 25.

8 Porritt, Lord The Order of St. John. British Medical Journal, 4, 22 Dec 1973, 722–724.

9 Skeet, M. The work of the professional nurses in a voluntary aid society – you and the Red Cross. Nursing Mirror, 139, 19 Sep 1974, 55–58.

10 Webb, J. The development of first aid. [With reference to Red Cross and St. John's.] Physiotherapy, 57 (8), Aug 1971, 365–369.

11 Williams, M. M. The age of chivalry? [Work of the Order of St. John.] Occupational Health, 27 (11), Nov 1975, 482–483.

12 Williams, W. W. A changing world. [The St. John Ambulance Association.] Health and Social Service Journal, 84, 27 Jul 1974, 1683–1685.

13 Young, P. St. John to the rescue! Nursing Mirror, 139, 12 Sep 1974, 39–40.

j ROAD ACCIDENTS

1 Bagnall, D. Nursing care study – Susie – a road accident victim. Nursing Mirror, 136, 19 Jan 1973, 34–36.

2 Barker, A. Nursing care study. Tommy – road accident victim. Nursing Times, 70, 17 Jan 1974, 82–84.

3 Barnes, T. The emergency treatment of motor vehicle accident casualties. Lamp, 30 (3), Mar 1973, 7–9, 11.

4 Bradley, D. First aid. 8. Road accidents. Nursing Times, 71, 9 Oct 1975, 1622–1624.

5 Brearley, J. Nursing care study. Crash victim with multiple injuries. Nursing Mirror, 137, 2 Nov 1973, 28–33.

6 Brown, W. D. The war on the roads. [A description of one road accident victim.] Nursing Times, 68, 5 Oct 1972, 1243–1244.

7 Craft, A. W. and others Bicycle injuries in children. British Medical Journal, 4, 20 Oct 1973, 146–147.

8 Easton, K. C. Roadside resuscitation. Nursing Mirror, 139, 24 Oct 1974, 68–70.

9 Fawkes, M. A world of shadows. [Case study of the surgical treatment of a road accident victim, resulting in partial sight.] Nursing Times, 70, 26 Sep 1974, 1496–1498.

10 Jolles, K. E. Mothers and babies: how safe in a car? Midwife and Health Visitor, 10 (8), Aug 1974, 238–240.

11 McVittie, C. K. Nursing care study. Multiple fractures caused by a road accident. Nursing Mirror, 141, 21 Aug 1975, 53–55.

12 Pacy, H. First aid for drivers. Canadian Nurse, 69 (7), Jul 1973, 23–26.

13 Pitman, M. Emergency first aid. 3. Road casualties. Nursing Mirror, 132, 16 Apr 1971, 44.

14 Poole, T. Seat belts and the courts. Nursing Mirror, 140, 5 Jun 1975, 66–68.

15 Robinson, W. A. The medical aspects of driving a car. Nursing Times, 69, 11 Jan 1973, 66–67.

16 Snook. R. Crash casualties. Coping with serious injuries. Nursing Times, 69, 18 Oct 1973, 1358–1360.

17 Story, D. A mock disaster on a rural road. A lifelike learning situation for students of nursing was turned into a community exercise. American Journal of Nursing, 72 (12), Dec 1972, 2222–2224.

18 Stroud, M. Nursing care study. Crushed chest injury [due to a car accident]; Nursing Times, 70, 8 Aug 1974, 1226–1228.

k SPORT AND HOLIDAY ACCIDENTS

1 Barber, H. M. Horse sense. [Riding accidents.] Nursing Times, 70, 28 Feb 1973, 322–323.

2 Campbell, I. Exposure and injury on the mountains. NATNews, 8 (1), Spring 1971, 15, 17.

3 Carp, G. Boxing – the hazards and their prevention. [By a doctor who officiates at professional fights.] Nursing Times, 70, 7 Nov 1974, 1738–1740.

4 Drain, C. B. The athletic knee injury. American Journal of Nursing, 71 (3), Mar 1971, 536–537.

5 Frankland, J. C. Caving and cave rescue. Community Health, 7 (2), Oct 1975, 108–114.

6 Hoy, M. A. Sporting times. [Sports Clinic at Brook General Hospital.] Nursing Times, 71, 2 Jan 1975, 36–37.

7 O'Boyle, C. M. Sports injuries in adolescents: emergency care. American Journal of Nursing, 75, Oct 1975, 1732–1739.

8 Physiotherapy Issue devoted to sports injuries. Physiotherapy, 58 (6), Jun 1972, 191–210.

9 Rivers, J. T. Near drowning. Nursing Mirror, 139, 16 Aug 1974, 50–51.

10 Sperryn, P. N. Sports injuries. Physiotherapy, 59 (11), Nov 1973, 354–357.

11 Sperryn, P. N. and Williams, J. G. P. Why sports injuries clinics? British Medical Journal, 3, 9 Aug 1975, 364–365.

12 Thames, T. B. Snakes and snakebites. Occupational Health Nursing, 21 (10), Oct 1973, 25–26, 52.

13 Thrower, R. First aid for riding accidents. Nursing Times, 68, 20 Jul 1972, 900–902.

14 Whitear, M. Venomous fish. [Dangers and precautions.] Nursing Mirror, 141, 21 Aug 1975, 50–52.

15 Wright, W. J. Snakes and snakebite. Nursing Times, 69, 20 Sep 1973, 1222–1223.

68 BURNS AND PLASTIC SURGERY

a GENERAL AND NURSING

1 Archambeault-Jones, C. and Feller, I. Procedures for nursing the burned patient. Ann Arbor: National Institute for Burn Medicine, 1975.

2 Argamaso, R. V. and Argamaso, C. A. Topical sulfamylon-current adjunct in burn therapy. Bedside Nurse, 4 (1), Jan 1971, 22–25.

3 Calleia, P. and Boswick, J. S. A home care nursing program for patients with burns. American Journal of Nursing, 72 (8), Aug 1972, 1442–1444.

4 Clery, A. B. Treatment of burns by split skin grafting. Nursing Times, 70, 5 Dec 1974, 1893–1895.

5 Cooney, B. C. Treatment of burns. District Nursing, 14 (9), Dec 1971, 183–184.

6 Davis, R. W. The burn patient. Bedside Nurse, 4 (6), Jun 1971, 19–23.

7 De Geus, J. J. The burned hand. Nursing Times, 70, 27 Jun 1974, 988–990.

8 Dimick, A. R. Emergency management of acutely burned patients. RN Magazine, 37 (8), Aug 1974, OR 1, (5 pages); 38, Oct 1975, ICU 1–4.

9 Feller, I. and Crane, K. Planning and designing a burn care facility: for better patient care, better research, better teaching. Ann Arbor: Institute for Burn Medicine, 1971.

10 Feller, I. and Jones, C. A. Nursing the burned patient: for teaching better patient care. Ann Arbor: Institute for Burn Medicine, 1973.

11 Gibson, A. Nursing care study. A severely burned patient. Nursing Times, 69, 21 Jun 1973, 791–793.

12 Heron, M. Beds of beads. [Royalaire Fluidizing Bed installed in the Burns Unit of Newcastle General Hospital.] Nursing Times, 68, 12 Oct 1972, 1279–1281.

13 Jacoby, F. G. Nursing care of the patient with burns. St. Louis: Mosby, 1972.

14 Laing, J. E. and Harvey, J. The management and nursing of burns. 2nd ed. English Universities Press, 1971.

15 Law, E. J. New developments in burn care. Journal of Practical Nursing, 21 (10), Oct 1971, 24–25, 46–47.

16 McGranahan, B. C. Nursing care of burn patient. AORN Journal, 20 (5), Nov 1974, 787–793.

17 Megan, B. J. Initial care of the thermally injured. AORN Journal, 20 (5), Nov 1974, 837–838, 840–841, 844.

18 Milward, T. M. The treatment of burns. 1. Initial management. Nursing Times, 67, 18 Nov 1971, 1438–1440.

19 Milward, T. M. The treatment of burns. 2. Skin replacement in burns. Nursing Times, 67, 25 Nov 1971, 1468–1471.

20 Mount Vernon Hospital Burns unit will be first-ever of its kind. [Mount Vernon Hospital, Northwood, Middlesex.] Nursing Times, 67, 4 Nov 1971, 1364.

21 Mount Vernon Hospital New Burns Unit at Mount Vernon Hospital. Nursing Mirror, 138, 19 Apr 1974, 39–41; Nursing Times, 70, 28 Feb 1974, 290.

22 Muir, I. F. K. and Barclay, T. L. Burns and their treatment. 2nd ed. Lloyd-Luke, 1974.

23 Murphy, W. L. Skin coverage for burn injury. AORN Journal, 20 (5), Nov 1974, 794–796, 798–801.

24 Ninman, C. and Shoemaker, P. Human amniotic membranes for burns. American Journal of Nursing, 75 (9), Sep 1975, 1468–1469.

25 Ollstein, R. N. and others Burns and their treatment. Hospital Management, Jan 1971, 22–23, 26–30, 32–34, 39.

26 Ollstein, R. N. and others The burn center concept. Hospital Management, Feb/Mar 1971, 1, 22–26.

27 Phelps, N. Intermittent inhalation in burns dressings. Nursing Times, 68, 3 Aug 1972, 970.

28 Pitman, M. Emergency first aid. 4. Coping with burns. Nursing Mirror, 132, 23 Apr 1971, 46.

29 Rahman, M. M. A preliminary investigation of management information needs in a burns unit. MSC thesis UMIST, Department of Management Services, 1974.

30 Settle, J. A. Outline of the treatment of burns. 1 and 2. Nursing Mirror, 138, 29 Mar 1974, 62–65; 138, 5 Apr 1974, 58–62, 65.

31 Sevitt, S. Reactions to injury and burns and their clinical importance. Heinemann Medical, 1974.

32 Shaw, B. L. Current therapy for burns. RN Magazine, 34 (3), Mar 1971, 33–41.

33 Stinson, V. Porcine skin dressings for burns. American Journal of Nursing, 74 (1), Jan 1974, 111–112.

34 Swartz, E. M. Preventing burn injuries. Journal of Nursing Administration, 3 (1), Jan/Feb 1973, 9–11.

35 Wagner, M. Positioning of burn patients. [Exercises to prevent deformity.] Nursing Care, 7 (8), Aug 1974, 22–25.

36 Wessex Regional Burns Centre [Odstock Hospital.] Nursing Times, 71, 29 May 1975, 844–845.

b CHILDREN

1 Benians, R. C. A child psychiatrist looks at children with burns. Maternal and Child Care, 6, Feb 1970, 215–217, 223–224.

2 Bernstein, N. R. and Quinby, S. Nurse adaption to treating severely burned children. Hospital Topics, 49 (6), Jun 1971, 65–66, 69.

3 Bowden, M. L. and Feller, I. Family reaction to a severe burn. American Journal of Nursing, 73 (2), Feb 1973, 317–319.

4 Elder, A. T. Thinking more deeply. Burns and scalds. Maternal and Child Care, 8, Dec 1971/Jan 1972, 14–16.

5 Keen, J. H. and others Inflicted burns and scalds in children. [Study at Booth Hall Children's Hospital, Manchester.] British Medical Journal, 4, 1 Nov 1975, 268–269.

6 Kunsman, J. Nursing the acutely burned child. Nursing care after primary excision. RN Magazine, 37 (8), Aug 1974, 25–26.

7 Liviskie, S. Definition of body boundaries after burn injury. [In a hospitalized three-year old boy.]

Maternal-Child Nursing Journal, 2 (2), Summer 1973, 101–109.

8 O'Neill, J. A. Continuing care of the acutely burned child. RN Magazine, 37 (9), Sep 1974, 93–94, 97–98, 100, 102, 104, 106.

9 Rosenfield, S. R. Nursing care study. Ruth – victim of electric burns. Nursing Times, 69, 4 Oct 1973, 1289–1291.

10 Settle, J. A. D. Firework burns. Nursing Mirror, 139, 7 Nov 1974, 48–51.

11 Sheehy, E. Nursing the acutely burned child. Primary excision: innovation in pediatric burn care. RN Magazine, 37 (8), Aug 1974, 21–25.

12 Sheehy, E. Pediatric burn care trends. AORN Journal, 20 (5), Nov 1974, 831–832, 834.

13 Smith, J. E. Burns at the Red Cross War Memorial Children's Hospital. S A Nursing Journal, 39 (2), Feb 1972, 23–26, 41.

c PATIENT AND FAMILY

1 Bowden, M. L. and Feller, I. Family reaction to a severe burn. American Journal of Nursing, 73 (2), Feb 1973, 317–319.

2 Davidson, S. P. and Noyes, R. Psychiatric nursing consultation on a burn unit. [Multidisciplinary approach.] American Journal of Nursing, 73 (10), Oct 1973, 1715–1718.

3 Fagerhaugh, S. Y. Pain expression and control on a burn care unit. [Staff's efforts to help patients tolerate pain and the support given by other patients.] Nursing Outlook, 22 (10), Oct 1974, 645–650.

4 Young, K. A. Stigmatization of burn patients. AORN Journal, 20 (5), Nov 1974, 802–808.

d INDUSTRIAL BURNS

1 Browne, T. D. Treatment of acid skin burns. Occupational Health, 26 (6), Jun 1974, 224–228.

2 Cason, J. S. Industrial burns. Nursing Mirror, 138, 12 Apr 1974, 65–68.

3 Howell, R. W. Industrial burns and scalds. [A trial by the British Steel Corporation Medical Service to investigate the comparative healing time of Sofra-Tulle, Carbonet and lanoparaffin tulle dressing.] Nursing Mirror, 140, 13 Feb 1975, 51–54.

4 Occupational Health Acid burns treatment. Occupational Health, 25 (4), Apr 1973, 129–130.

5 Roberts, A. M. OH Congress report. Hydrofluoric acid burns. Occupational Health, 27 (1), Nov 1975, 468–470.

6 Stewart, M. Burn treatment in Bahrain. [In an aluminium smelter.] Occupational Health, 27 (11), Nov 1975, 480–481.

e PLASTIC SURGERY

1 Batsone, J. H. F. External ear reconstruction. Nursing Times, 70, 15 Aug 1974, 1269–1271.

2 Cline, H. L. Expanding frontiers in plastic surgery. Journal of Practical Nursing, 23 (8), Aug 1973, 20–23.

3 David, D. J. Skin grafting. Nursing Times, 68, 23 Nov 1972, 1473–1477.

4 Eckhoff, N. L. Return to nursing. Skin grafting. Nursing Mirror, 133, 20 Aug 1971, 10–11.

5 Hamilton, J. M. Rhytidectomy in the male. [Excision of wrinkles.] RN Magazine, 38 (2), Feb 1975, OR 4, 6.

6 Jackson, I. T. and Macallan, E. S. Plastic surgery and burn treatment. Heinemann Medical, 1971. (Modern practical nursing series, no. 6.)

7 Jennings, S. B. Reconstructive hand surgery. AORN Journal, 21 (1), Jan 1975, 71–76.

8 Kulpa, L. J. and others Restoration of hand function. AORN Journal, 21 (1), Jan 1975, 61–70.

9 Nistor, S. L. Nursing techniques in plastic surgery. Bedside Nurse, 4 (1), Jan 1971, 26–31.

10 Nunis, E. M. Plastic and reconstructive surgery and surgical nursing. Nursing Journal of Singapore, 12 (2), Nov 1972, 65–70.

11 Ollstein, R. N. and others Skin grafting – the burned patient – essentials of nursing care. Journal of Practical Nursing, 21 (11), Nov 1971, 18–22.

12 Poole, M. D. Post-traumatic cosmetic surgery. Queen's Nursing Journal, 17 (2), Feb 1975, 234–236.

13 Rapperport, A. S. Skin grafting technique. AORN Journal, 20 (5), Nov 1974, 852–854.

14 Tempest, M. Correcting facial deformity. Nursing Times, 71, 24 Jul 1974, 1163–1165.

15 Trowbridge, J. E. Caring for patients with facial or intra-oral reconstruction. American Journal of Nursing, 73 (11), Nov 1973, 1930–1934.

16 Tunstall, M. N. Nursing care study. Saddle depression of the nose. [Successful plastic surgery alleviates the condition and benefits the patient psychologically.] Nursing Times, 70, 14 Nov 1974, 1774–1776.

69 DISASTER AND WAR

a DISASTER MANAGEMENT
(Includes bomb incidents)

1 Arena, V. Radiation accidents: what you need to know about them. RN Magazine, 36 (9), Sep 1973, 42–45.

2 Baer, E. Civil disorder: mass emergency of the 70's. American Journal of Nursing, 72 (6), Jun 1972, 1072–1076.

3 Barnes, J. Riders of the cyclone. [Letter describing events at Darwin Hospital after Cyclone Tracy.] Australian Nurses' Journal, 4 (7), Feb 1975, 12, 14–15, 16.

4 Bradley, J. E. A. Nurse management during the bombing crisis in Birmingham. Nursing Times, 71, 24 Jul 1975, 1186–1188.

5 Braverman, S. and Jenks, N. California quake. American Journal of Nursing, 71 (4), Apr 1971, 708–712.

6 British Medical Journal After a bomb. [Leading article.] British Medical Journal, 1, 25 Jan 1975, 172–173.

7 British Medical Journal Disaster planning – fact or fiction? British Medical Journal, 2, 24 May 1975, 406–407.

8 British Medical Journal Moorgate tube train disaster. By members of the medical staff of three London hospitals. British Medical Journal, 3, 27 Sep 1975, 727–731.

9 Caro, D. Major disasters. [Procedures for hospital faced with more than 50 casualties needing treatment.] Lancet, 2, 30 Nov 1974, 1309–1310.

10 Caro, D. and Irving, M. The Old Bailey bomb explosion. Lancet, 1, 23 Jun 1973, 1433–1435.

11 Corneliuson, C. My unforgettable nursing experience. Nursing during the Rapid City flood. Journal of Practical Nursing, 22 (10), Oct 1972, 26–27.

12 Craig, M. I. The role of the theatre during major accidents. [Action plans at the Brook General Hospital, Woolwich.] NATNews, 12 (7), Sep 1975, 20–21.

13 Dopson, L. Bomb scare at the Westminster: lessons from evacuation. Nursing Times, 69, 30 Aug 1973, 1109.

14 Harvey, H. Disaster at Moorgate. Nursing Times, 71, 31 Jul 1975, 1226–1227.

15 Hirst, W. Disaster planning. A guide to the organization of nursing services in the accident and emergency department. Nursing Times, 70, 7 Feb 1974, 186–189.

16 Humphrey, B. and Lim, S. The night of the Birmingham bombs. A personal report on the reception and treatment of casualties. Nursing Mirror, 139, 5 Dec 1974, 34.

17 Jackson, F. E. and others Advances in the treatment of missile wounds of the brain. Nursing Times, 67, 8 Jul 1971, 819–821.

18 Kavalier, F. Bart's staff under pressure after Old Bailey bomb disaster. Nursing Times, 69, 15 Mar 1973, 328.

19 Laube, J. Psychological reactions of nurses in disaster. [Hurricane in Texas.] Nursing Research, 22, Jul/Aug 1973, 343–347.

20 McAlister, E. Intensive care of bomb-blast injuries. Nursing Mirror, 139, 14 Nov 1974, 66–68.

21 Morrow, W. F. K. Blast injuries to the lungs. Nursing Times, 71, 17 Jul 1975, 1136–1137.

22 Newell, P. Nurses at work. Operation disaster. Australian Nurses' Journal, 3 (9), Apr 1974, 16, 18–20.

23 Nursing Mirror Major disasters and plans to deal with them. [For the occupational health nurse.] Nursing Mirror, 138, 28 Jun 1974, 40–41.

24 Nursing Mirror Nightmare. [Emergency care after the Moorgate underground disaster.] Nursing Mirror, 140, 6 Mar 1975, 34.

25 Nursing Times Disaster management. Aftermath – at the scene. [An account by a nurse attending casualties at the site of the Guildford bombing.] Nursing Times, 70, 5 Dec 1974, 1882–1883.

26 Nursing Times Disaster management. At the hospital. SW Thames RHA has assessed the working of its major incident plan: [after the Guildford bombing.] Nursing Times, 70, 5 Dec 1974, 1883.

27 Nursing Times Disaster management. Coping with a catastrophe. [Bomb disasters in Birmingham, Guildford and Woolwich.] Nursing Times, 70, 5 Dec 1974, 1880–1881.

28 Nursing Times Good teamwork at St. George's. [After the bomb explosion at the Hilton Hotel.] Nursing Times, 71, 11 Sep 1975, 1435.

29 Odling-Smee, W. Victim of Belfast's violence. Nursing Times, 69, 6 Sep 1973, 1143–1146.

30 Rutherford, W. H. The injuries of civil disorder [in Ireland]. Community Health, 6 (1), Jul/Aug 1974, 14–21.

31 Sharma, L. Disaster nursing. Nursing Journal of India, 43 (11), Nov 1972, 371, 384.

32 Sharma, L. Nursing preparedness in disaster relief. [Integration into the nursing curriculum.] Nursing Journal of India, 46 (11), Nov 1975, 249–250.

33 Wells, J. H. Don't die through neglect. [Disaster planning.] New Zealand Nursing Journal, 66, May 1973, 16–17, 20–21.

34 Wheeler, J. H. Auckland exercise 'Medaid.' [Civil Defence exercise to assess the role of all nursing, medical and para-medical staff in a disaster.] New Zealand Nursing Journal, 68 (1), Jan 1975, 24–25.

35 Whittall, K. Major disaster procedure: the Birmingham bomb incidents. Nursing Mirror, 141, 24 Jul 1975, 46–49.

36 Zanotelli, P. Civil disaster? These nurses are ready! RN Magazine, 34 (9), Sep 1971, 50–52.

37 Savage, P. E. A. Disaster planning: the use of action cards. British Medical Journal, 3, 1 Jul 1972, 42–43.

b WAR

1 Birch, J. A. Nigeria in peace and war. International Journal of Nursing Studies, 8 (3), Aug 1971, 145–151.

2 Coleman, V. The silver lining. [Medical advances during wartime.] Nursing Mirror, 140, 16 Jan 1975, 71.

3 Compton, C. Y. War injury: identity crisis for young men. Nursing Clinics of North America, 8 (1), Mar 1973, 53–66.

4 Crowe, E. Friends in Nigeria: work done by Quaker Service Team QS1 and QS11 during and after the recent war in Nigeria. Nursing Mirror, 135, 7 Jul 1972, 15–18.

5 Crowe, E. Friends in Nigeria. Nursing Mirror, 135, 14 Jul 1972, 14–17.

6 Crowe, E. Friends in Nigeria: screening for malnutrition in South Eastern State during the recent war in Nigeria. Nursing Mirror, 135, 21 Jul 1972, 26–27.

7 Crowe, E. Friends in Nigeria: smallpox, measles and DPT immunisation programme. Nursing Mirror, 135, 28 Jul 1972, 24.

8 Dworkin, C. A volunteer nurse in Israel. Canadian Nurse, 70 (3), Mar 1974, 30–32.

9 Fraser, M. Psychiatric casualties of war. New Psychiatry, 2 (13), 19 Jun 1975, 12–13.

10 Jones, N. I. 'Someday this will end. . .' [Thoughts of an American army nurse in Vietnam.] American Journal of Nursing, 71 (7), Jul 1971, 1364–1365.

11 Kalter, S. Operating theatre managment in wartime in the fighting area. [Israel.] SA Nursing Journal, 42 (11), Nov 1975, 15–17.

12 McCulloch, G. Why sink a hospital ship? Hospital ships sunk by enemy action in World War II. Nursing Times, 70, 18 Apr 1974, 606–607.

13 Marchesini, E. H. Vietnam veterans are different. [Psychiatric problems.] American Journal of Nursing, 73 (1), Jan 1973, 74–76.

14 Nursing Journal of India Nurses in the army bring cheer to the wounded Jawans. Nursing Journal of India, 63 (1), Jan 1972, 9, 24, 35.

15 Nursing Times In Vietnam – The SCF in action. Nursing Times, 67, 16 Sep 1971, 1158–1159.

16 Ryan, L. Bangla Desh Diary. American Journal of Nursing, 71 (11), Nov 1971, 2158–2161.

17 Ryan, L. Leaves from a nurse's diary. Nursing Journal of India, 62 (9), Sep 1971, 290–291.

18 Sharma, K. J. Target against death: the human tragedies of the Bangla Desh refugee camps. Nursing Journal of India, 62 (9), Sep 1971, 289, 292.

19 Thompson, P. Saving the children in West Bengal. Nursing Times, 68, 8 Jun 1972, 715–716.

20 Toombs, B. J. Death and destruction in Pakistan. Nursing Mirror, 132, 28 May 1971, 18–19.

21 Wright, P. A. Diarrhoea: a specific treatment programme in Palestinian Refugee Camps. Nursing Times, 67, 29 Jul 1971, 915–918.

22 Wright, W. J. Horrors of the A-bomb. Nursing Mirror, 140, 27 Mar 1975, 69–70.

c FORCES NURSING

1 Clark, M. B. Serving with SSAFA in BAOR. [Nursing Sister for Soldiers, Sailors and Airmen's Families Association.] Nursing Mirror, 132, 16 Apr 1971, 40–42.

2 Edmunds, K. Nursing in the Senior Service. Nursing Times, 67, 28 Oct 1971, 1345–1347.

3 Hunt, D. Seventy years on: the QAs past and present. Nursing Mirror, 134, 7 Apr 1972, 13–16.

4 Leitch, M. E. Health visitors to the services. [Work of SSAFA.] Nursing Mirror, 135, 21 Jul 1972, 10–11.

5 Leitch, M. E. Nursing with service families overseas. SSAFA health visitor. District Nursing, 15 (4), Jul 1972, 74–75.

6 Lennon, M. Join the army and see the world. Nursing Times, 67, 4 Nov 1971, 1368–1369.

7 Lockeberg, L. E. The Colonel is a lady – and a nurse. [Director of Nursing, Canadian Armed Forces Medical Service, Lieutenant-Colonel Mary Joan Fitzgerald.] Canadian Nurse, 67 (11), Nov 1971, 23–25.

8 Maslin, M. Pen portraits of people. 1. An army matron. Nursing Mirror, 135, 8 Dec 1972, 16.

9 Morris, M. Mum's Army. [Queen Alexandra's Imperial Military Nursing Service during the Second World War.] Nursing Times, 71, 24 Jul 1975, 1228–1229.

10 O'Connor, V. Nursing link with those men in their flying machines. [Careers in nursing in Princess Mary's Royal Air Force nursing service.] Nursing Times, 67, 11 Nov 1971, 1418–1420.

11 Richards, D. Nursing seven miles up. [The work of RAF Aeromed teams.] Nursing Mirror, 140, 13 Mar 1975, 47–49.

12 Savage, H. K. The role of a QA in a field hospital. Nursing Mirror, 139, 2 Aug 1974, 48–49.

13 Wrennall, M. J. A study of some factors influencing the career decisions of military nurses. MPhil thesis, London Univesity, 1975.

OCCUPATIONAL HEALTH

70 OCCUPATIONAL HEALTH

a GENERAL

1 Atherley, G. R. C. and Booth, R.T. Employee's involvement and health and safety at work. Occupational Health, 27 (5), May 1975, 181–187

2 Briefer, C. Industrial medicine as an instrument of community care. Occupational Health Nursing, 22 (4), Apr 1974, 14–15.

3 Brown, E. M. A focus on the occupational health needs of the non-white worker. Occupational Health Nursing, 23 (3), Mar 1975, 14–16.

4 Brown, J. M. Trends in occupation health health as viewed by management. Occupational Health Nursing, 21 (11), Nov 1973, 7–10.

5 Caplan, P. E. The value of proper evaluation of new products and processes on employee health. Occupational Health Nursing, 21 (3), Mar 1973, 13–15.

6 Duffy, J. C. Trends in occupational health as viewed by the physician. Occupational Health Nursing, 21 (6), Jun 1973, 16–18.

7 Ffrench, G. Occupational health. Lancaster: Medical and Technical Publishing, 1973.

8 French, M. International structure. [Development of the Permanent Commission and International Association on Occupational Health.] Nursing Mirror, 141, 11 Sep 1975, 48–49.

9 Gardner, A. W. and Carter, J. T. Prevention, attribution or blame? The role of health care at work. Community Health, 7 (2), Oct 1975, 79–81.

10 Gauvain, S. Occupational medicine: the response to new challenges. (b) Whither occupational medicine: the response to new challenges. Royal Society of Health Journal, 95 (5), Oct 1975, 246–249.

11 Jones, W. T. Stop stewards' role in OH. Occupational Health, 25 (11), Nov 1973, 417–420.

12 Kolozyn, H. The need to evaluate OH. Occupational Health 27 (4), Apr 1975, 158–159.

13 Muir, J. M. Occupational medicine – past, present and future. [NM conference lecture.] Nursing Mirror, 138, 28 Jun 1974, 58–63.

14 Murray, R. Occupational medicine: the response to new challenges. (a) Occupational health – a personal viewpoint. Royal Society of Health Journal, 95 (5), Oct 1975, 244–246.

15 Murray, R. Production processes and OH. Occupational Health, 26 (7), Jul 1974, 259–267.

16 Nursing Mirror A symposium on occupational health. Nursing Mirror, 141, 11 Sep 1975, 47–67.

17 Occupational Health OH nursing international. [Abstracts of papers presented at the 1975 congress.] Occupational Health, 27 (10), Oct 1975, 426–427.

18 Raffle, P. A. B. The purposes of occupational medicine. British Journal of Industrial Medicine, 32, May 1975, 102–109.

19 Rhoades, R. Industry and disease. Midwife and Health Visitor, 9 (3), Mar 1973, 78–80; (4), Apr 1973, 119–122; (5), May 1973, 151–153.

20 Schilling, R. S. F., editor Occupational health practice. Butterworth, 1973.

21 Schilling, R. S. F. The place of OH in the community. Occupational Health, 27 (10), Oct 1975, 422–425.

22 Swaffield, L. The information gap. [In occupational health.] Occupational Health, 27 (10), Oct 1975, 419–421.

23 University of Aston. Safety and Hygiene Group Can health status be measured? Occupational Health, 25 (3), Mar 1973, 106–107.

24 University of Aston. Safety and Hygiene Group The preventive role of OH. Occupational Health, 25 (4), Apr 1973, 142–143.

25 University of Aston. Safety and Hygiene Group 75 years of progress? [Conditions and treatment in factories 75 years ago.] Occupational Health, 26 (9), Sep 1974, 364–365.

26 Wagner, S. P. Identifying a worldwide resource for nursing education. [The part nurses have played in the development of the Permanent Commission and International Association on Occupational Health.] Occupational Health Nursing, 22 (12), Dec 1974, 12–15.

27 Williams, M. The Permanent Commission. [And International Association on Occupational Health.] Nursing Times, 71, 11 Sep 1975, 1442–1443; Occupational Health, 27 (9), Sep 1975, 378–380.

28 World Health Issue on work and health. World Health, Jul/Aug 1974, 2–40.

b LEGISLATION

1 Department of Employment Protecting people at work: an introduction to the Health and Safety at Work Act 1974. The Department, 1974.

2 Health and Safety Executive List of Statutory Regulations [Relating to the Health and Safety at Work Act.] Occupational Health, 27 (3), Mar 1975, 96–97.

3 Holgate, P. D. Emphasis on consultation: several sections of the Health and Safety at Work Act have specific importance for the OH nurse. Occupational Health 27 (5), May 1975, 200–203.

4 Holgate, P. Health and Safety at work. [Implications of the 1974 Act.] Nursing Mirror, 140, 17 Apr 1975, 39–40; Physiotherapy, 61 (5), May 1975, 150–151.

5 Janner, G. Health and Safety at Work Act: it's impact on you. Health and Social Service Journal, 85, 7 Jun 1975, 1200–1201.

6 Occupational Health Provisions of the Bill. The Health and Safety at Work Bill. Occupational Health, 26 (6), Jun 1974, 210–213.

7 Orriss, H. D. Industrial health service. [Consultative proposals.] Health and Social Service Journal, 83, 8 Sep 1973, 2050.

8 Parliament Health and Safety at Work Act 1974. HMSO, 1974.

9 Simpson, W. Occupational medicine: the response to new challenges. (c) The Health and Safety at Work etc. Act 1974. Royal Society of Health Journal, 95 (5), Oct 1975, 249–242, 263.

10 University of Aston. Safety and Hygiene Group Limitations defined. [The Health and Safety at Work Bill.] Occupational Health, 26 (4), Apr 1974, 136–137.

11 Wakelin, E. N. Health and Safety at Work. (a) Aspects of the Act affecting the local authority as the enforcement authority. Royal Society of Health Journal, 95 (6), Dec 1975, 309–312.

12 Whincup, M. A duty of reasonable care. [The duty of employers to ensure safety under 1974 Act.] Occupational Health, 27 (5), May 1975, 188–196.

13 Whincup. M. Employers' liability. Occupational Health, 25 (12), Dec 1973, 463–468.

14 Whincup, M. Practitioners' duties. [Legal position of occupational health service staff.] Occupational Health, 27 (4), Apr 1975, 147–154.

15 Whincup, M. Responsibility for safety: the four guidelines. Occupational Health, 26 (1), Jan 1974, 19–22.

c SERVICES

1 Alston, R. OH in Europe – 1. The UK. [Gillette industries, Reading.] Occupational Health, 27 (1), Jan 1975, 7–12.

2 Devine, J. OH – a backyard service? [Integration of industrial health service with reorganized health service.] Occupational Health, 24 (6), Jun 1972, 200–202.

3 Gauvain, S. Recent developments in occupational medical services. Journal of the Society of Occupational Medicine, 25 (3), Jul 1975, 78–85.

4 Hill, R. N. With one eye on the accounts: group occupational health services today. Transactions of the Society of Occupational Medicine, 22 (1), Jan 1972, 24–29.

5 Occupational Health Encouraging results. [Summary of annual reports of West Midlands Industrial Health Service, Bedford General hospital OHS and Slough.] Occupational Health, 26 (2), Feb 1974, 40–41.

6 Pollitt, W. A. OH in a county authority. [Cheshire County Council.] Occupational Health, 25 (2), Feb 1973, 50–54.

7 **Ross, D.** A medical record system. [Babcock & Wilcox Medical Service.] Occupational Health, 27 (12), Dec 1975, 516–523.

8 **Stewart, D.** Group services. [Work of the seven independent group occupational health services in the UK] Nursing Mirror, 141, 11 Sep 1975, 54–56.

9 **Sullivan, M. P.** Licence to work? [Personal views on ways of improving occupational health services.] Occupational Health, 27 (9), Sep 1975, 395–397.

10 **Swaffield, L.** Local authority OH services. [Conference report.] Occupational Health, 27 (12), Dec 1975, 524–528.

11 **Swaffield, L.** The Midlands. Industrial health in the West Midlands. Nursing Times, 70 (7), 12 Sep 1974, 1422–1423.

12 **University of Aston. Safety and Hygiene Group** Putting Robens into practice. Occupational Health, 25 (9), Sep 1973, 342–344.

13 **Welsh Council** Occupational health service in Wales. The Council, 1974.

d EMPLOYMENT MEDICAL ADVISORY SERVICE

1 **British Medical Journal** E.M.A.S. gets going. [Summary of the first report.] British Medical Journal, 3, 23 Aug 1975, 449–450.

2 **Davies, T. A. L.** Employment Medical Advisory Service. Health Trends, 5 (3), Aug 1973, 45–47.

3 **Employment Medical Advisory Service** Case histories. [Adapted from the EMAS report to show the range of work.] Occupational Health, 27 (9), Sep 1975, 374–377.

4 **Employment Medical Advisory Service** EMAS. Consumer opinions. Occupational Health, 27 (9), Sep 1975, 370–373.

5 **Employment Medical Advisory Service** Two year report. [Summary.] Occupational Health, 27 (9), Sep 1975, 364–367.

6 **Gauvain, S.** EMAS – a pioneer service. [Interview with Suzette Gauvain.] Occupational Health, 27 (9), Sep 1975, 368–369.

7 **Gracey, M.** Employment Medical Advisory Service. British Journal of Industrial Medicine, 30 (1), Jan 1973, 92–94.

8 **Neild, F. G.** Employment Medical Advisory Service. Community Health, 6 (5), Mar/Apr 1975, 279–285.

9 **Orriss, H. D.** Employment Medical Advisory Services. Nursing Mirror, 139, 7 Nov 1974, 71–72.

10 **Public Health** Enter E.M.A.S. [Employment Medical Advisory Service.] Public Health, 87 (3), Mar 1973, 53–56.

11 **Society of Occupational Medicine** Health and safety at work. Discussion of the Robens Committee Report and the Employment Medical Advisory Service. Journal of the Society of Occupational Medicine, 23 (1), Jan 1973, 27–28.

e ROBENS REPORT

1 **Atherley, G.** Robens: a question of balance. Occupational Health, 24 (8), Aug 1972, 277–281.

2 **Browne, R. C.** Safety and health at work: the Robens Report. British Journal of Industrial Medicine, 30 (1), Jan 1973, 87–91.

3 **Committee on Safety and Health at Work** Report, 1970–72. HMSO, 1972, Cmnd 5034. Chairman: Lord Robens.

4 **Jones, W. T.** Robens: the error of equating safety with health. Community Medicine, 128 (16), 4 Aug 1972, 376–377.

5 **Lloyd, P. V.** A breath of fresh air, but. . . The Rcn comments on the health aspects of the Robens report. Occupational Health, 24 (9), Sep 1972, 308–309.

6 **McKie, D.** Robens: reinforcement needed? Community Medicine, 128 (15), 28 Jul 1972, 350.

7 **Macmillan, Rt. Hon. M.** Safety and health at work. [Speech given at TUC Conference on the Robens Report.] Rehabilitation, 86, Jul/Sep 1973, 31–36.

8 **Murray, R.** Robens: the nettle Robens failed to grasp. Occupational Health, 24 (8), Aug 1972, 275–276.

9 **Occupational Health** Reaction to Robens. Occupational Health, 24 (10), Oct 1972, 349.

10 **Occupational Health** Robens. Sweeping changes to involve workers in safety. [Summary of the Robens report on Safety and Health at Work.] Occupational Health, 24 (8), Aug 1972, 269–274.

11 **Royal College of Nursing** Rcn evidence to Robens Committee. Occupational Health, 23 (4), Apr 1971, 124–125.

12 **Society of Occupational Medicine** Committee on safety and health at work. Evidence of the Society of Occupational Medicine. Transactions of the Society of Occupational Medicine, 21 (2), Apr 1971, 43–46.

f SERVICES OVERSEAS

1 **Hamilton, M.** Relationship between OH and other services. [Summary of reports from different countries on the integration of occupational health and other medical services.] Occupational Health, 27 (11), Nov 1975, 471–473.

2 **Izmerov, N.** Workers in the USSR. Health comes first. World Health, Jul/Aug 1974, 22–25.

3 **Kavoussi, N.** Industrial health in Iran. Occupational Health, 25 (10), Oct 1973, 381–384.

4 **May, C. R.** OH practice in Canada. Occupational Health, 26 (2), Feb 1974, 49–51.

5 **Occupational Health Nursing** Results of occupational injuries and illnesses survey. [US Department of Labor, Bureau of Labor Statistics Report.] Occupational Health Nursing, 21 (8), Aug 1973, 38–40.

6 **Radwanski, D.** Occupational health services in Nigeria. International Nursing Review, 19 (3), 1972, 283–288.

7 **Rehtanz, H.** The organization of occupational safety in the German Democratic Republic. International Labour Review, 112, Dec 1975, 419–429.

8 **Ringer, J. H.** The development of an emergency medical program in industry. Occupational Health Nursing, 23 (9), Sep 1975, 20–22.

9 **Steinfeld, J. L.** Occupational health and safety programs of HEW – a progress report. Occupational Health Nursing, 21 (3), Mar 1973, 16–19.

10 **University of Aston. Safety and Hygiene Group** Labour protection in USSR. Occupational Health, 26 (10), Oct 1974, 401–403.

11 **Whincup, M.** Accident compensation in NZ. Occupational Health, 26 (8), Aug 1974, 311–316.

g ENVIRONMENT AND ERGONOMICS

1 **Bretten, P.** Ergonomics. Principles of posture. Occupational Health, 25 (6), Jun 1973, 209–214;

designing for man. Occupational Health, 25 (7), Jul 1973, 260–262.

2 **Bretten, P.** Ergonomics. [Role of ergonomics in promoting safety and health.] Physiotherapy, 61 (5), May 1975, 146–149.

3 **Brown, M. L.** The quality of the work environment. [Implications of the Occupational Safety and Health Act.] American Journal of Nursing, 75 (10), Oct 1975, 1755–1760.

4 **Butler, A.** Environmental survey: close examination of the working conditions in a small department. Occupational Health, 25, Sep 1973, 332–335.

5 **Department of Employment** Lifting and carrying. HMSO 1972. (Health and Safety at Work, no. 1).

6 **Hamilton, M.** OH congress session. Ergonomics. Occupational Health, 27 (10), Oct 1975, 428–430.

7 **Hayne, C.R.** Ergonomics – the scientific study of men at work. Physiotherapy, 59 (10), Oct 1973, 321–325.

8 **Karvonen, M. J.** Ergonomics – a young technology: fitting the job to the worker. World Health, Jul/Aug 1974, 30–35.

9 **Karvonen, M. J.** Shop floor ergonomics. Occupational Health, 25 (3), Mar 1973, 103–104.

10 **Orriss, H.** Taking the misery out of work. [Activities of the Department of Employment's Work Research Unit in improving work environment and job satisfaction.] Nursing Mirror, 140, 19 Jun 1975, 54–55.

11 Quality of working life: a new steering group. Occupational Health, 25 (7), Jul 1973, 248–249.

12 **Roshchin, A. V.** Protection of the working environment. International Labour Review, 110 (3), Sep 1974, 235–249.

13 **Singleton, W. T.** Introduction to ergonomics. Geneva: World Health Organisation, 1972.

14 **Snook, S. H. and Ciriello, V. M.** Maximum weights and work loads acceptable to female workers. Occupational Health Nursing, 22 (8), Aug 1974, 11–20.

15 **WHO Chronicle** Health hazards in the working environment. WHO Chronicle, 27 (9), Sep 1973, 344–346.

16 **Wicks, D.** Case history. Humidifier contamination. Occupational Health, 25 (8), Aug 1973, 310–313.

17 **Widgery, J.** Colour choice. [Colour in the working environment.] Occupational Health, 25 (9), Sep 1973, 336–338.

h INDUSTRIAL INJURIES AND ACCIDENTS

1 **Bagley, C. R. and Richardson, D. M.** Treatment of industrial injury: hospital or OH service? [Study of hospital treated accidents in the Brighton area.] Occupational Health, 27 (4), Apr 1975, 140–146.

2 **Blyghton, A.** Industrial injuries benefit. Occupational Health, 26 (3), Mar 1974, 80–81.

3 **Harries, A. J. and West, R. R.** Accidents and their management at two casualty units. [Comparison of hospital and factory units.] Journal of the Society of Occupational Medicine, 25 (3), Jul 1975, 95–98.

4 **Jenkins, J. H.** Case study. An industrial accident. [Severely lacerated right hand.] Nursing Times, 70, 30 May 1974, 834–835.

5 **Occupational Health** Tutorial. Electrical injuries. Occupational Health, 27 (3), Mar 1975, 105–107.

6 **Poole, F. T.** Abnormal result of treatment.

[Employer's liability.] Occupational Health, 26 (2), Feb 1974, 55–57.

7 Poole, F. T. Establishing liability. [Employers' liability in accident cases.] Occupational Health, 27 (4), Apr 1975, 160–161.

8 Poole, F. T. Injury compensation. Occupational Health, 27 (3), Mar 1975, 115–116.

9 Poole, F. T. Injury on employers' premises. Occupational Health, 25 (11), Nov 1973, 424–425.

10 Ross, D. S. and Bamber, L. Cost of accidents. [An investigation carried out at Babcock and Wilcox.] Occupational Health, 27 (2), Feb 1975, 49–56.

11 University of Aston. Safety and Hygiene Group Accident investigation systems. Occupational Health, 27 (3), Mar 1975, 110–113.

i MENTAL HEALTH AND STRESS

1 Ennals, Rt. Hon. D. Why ignore mental health? [The case for a national occupational mental health service.] Occupational Health, 25 (1), Jan 1973, 14–17.

2 Ferguson, D. A study of neurosis and occupation. British Journal of Industrial Medicine, 30 (2), Apr 1973, 187–198.

3 Guest, D. and Williams, R. How home affects work. [Family pressures' effect on a worker's attitude.] New Society, 23, 18 Jan 1973, 114–117.

4 Hines, J. Mental illness in industry. Personnel Management, 6 (4), Apr 1974, 38–40.

5 Hunt, C. OH congress paper. Stress and the young worker. Occupational Health, 27 (10), Oct 1975, 441–443.

6 Martin, R. W. Human behaviour in the work situation. Nursing Mirror, 140, 27 Mar 1975, 72–73.

7 South London Industrial Mission Windows on work. The stained glass windows at Christchurch in Blackfriars Road, London, headquarters of the South London Industrial Mission, with nine full time chaplains visiting people in their places of work. Occupational Health, 27 (8), Aug 1975, 333–335.

8 Spry, W. B. Recognizing mental disorder. [This may begin with an examination of the work setting to detect early signs.] Occupational Health, 27 (6), Jun 1975, 238–240.

9 Taylor, R. Stress at work. New Society, 30, 17 Oct 1974, 140–143.

j NOISE AND HEARING LOSS

1 Department of Employment and Productivity Code of practice for reducing the exposure of employed persons to noise. HMSO 1972.

2 Hamilton, M. OH Congress session. Noise and vibration. Occupational Health, 27 (11), Nov 1975, 474–476.

3 Murray, R. Medico-legal aspects of noise. [Reprinted from Applied Ergonomics.] Occupational Health, 25 (2), Feb 1973, 55–59.

4 Occupational Health Benefit for hearing loss. Occupational Health, 25 (12), Dec 1973, 449–450.

5 Occupational Health Workers' choice. [Description of a new combined ear defence and music system used at Benson International Factory, Stroud.] Occupational Health, 26 (12), Dec 1974, 474.

6 Rosenhouse, L. Noise. Nursing Care, 7 (11), Nov 1974, 26–28.

7 Russell, S. Personal hearing protection. Occupational Health, 25 (12), Dec 1973, 460–462.

8 Selwyn, N. Deafness litigation. Occupational Health, 25 (9), Sep 1973, 339–341.

9 Selwyn, N. Why so few deafness cases? [Law relating to occupational deafness.] Occupational Health, 25 (8), Aug 1973, 296–297.

10 University of Aston. Safety and Hygiene Group Education by example? [The wearing of hearing protectors in industry.] Occupational Health, 26 (5), May 1974, 182–183.

11 University of Aston. Safety and Hygiene Group Machinery noise control. Occupational Health, 26 (2), Feb 1974, 52–53.

12 Wreford, B. M. Prevention and noise. [Application of preventive principles to problems of noise.] Nursing Mirror, 141, 11 Sep 1975, 57–59.

k SAFETY

1 Bell, J. A. Sewer safety. Occupational Health, 25 (1), Jan 1973, 20–21.

2 Butler, A. Prevention of specific hazard. Occupational Health, 26 (6), Jun 1974, 220–223.

3 Craig, A. Health and Safety Officer. [Experience of an occupational health nurse appointed to this post.] Occupational Health, 25 (8), Aug 1973, 301–302.

4 Forssman, S. P. M. The teaching of occupational health and safety. WHO Chronicle, 27 (4), Apr 1973, 149–152.

5 Harvey, B. H. The right to work in safety. [Work of the Factory Inspectorate.] Occupational Health, 24 (10), Oct 1972, 350–351.

6 Hewitt, P. J. The rationale of safety assessment. Occupational Health, 27 (7), Jul 1975, 293–295.

7 McMichael, A. J. An epidemiologic perspective on the identification of workers at risk. Occupational Health Nursing, 23 (1), Jan 1975, 7–11.

8 Nursing Times Watchdogs on safety. [Leading article on the Factory Inspectorate.] Nursing Times, 70, 5 Dec 1974, 1873.

9 Occupational Health High time for expansion [of the factory inspectorate]. Occupational Health, 26 (11), Nov 1974, 419.

10 Poole, F. T. Safe scaffolding. Occupational Health, 26 (9), Sep 1974, 366–367.

11 Sprackling, G. H. Health and Safety at Work. (b) Aspects of safety in the building industry. Royal Society of Health Journal, 95 (6), Dec 1975, 312–315, 321.

12 University of Aston. Safety and Hygiene Group Design for machinery safety. Occupational Health, 27 (1), Jan 1975, 24–26.

13 University of Aston. Safety and Hygiene Group Exhaust ventilation. Occupational Health, 27 (7), Jul 1975, 303–305.

14 University of Aston. Safety and Hygiene Group Finishes under fire. Occupational Health, 25 (10), Oct 1973, 386–387.

15 University of Aston. Safety and Hygiene Group Letter to the Chairman [of the Health and Safety Commission]. Occupational Health, 26 (11), Nov 1974, 444–446.

16 University of Aston. Safety and Hygiene Group Management must act. [Safety organization.] Occupational Health, 25 (11), Nov 1973, 422–423.

17 University of Aston. Safety and Hygiene Group Motivation and propaganda. [Safety propaganda and posters.] Occupational Health, 26 (3), Mar 1974, 92–95.

18 University of Aston. Safety and Hygiene Group Personal protection. Occupational Health, 27 (2), Feb 1975, 71–74.

19 University of Aston. Safety and Hygiene Group A policy on hazard control. Occupational Health, 25 (1), Jan 1973, 23–24.

20 University of Aston. Safety and Hygiene Group Problems in measuring safety. Occupational Health, 25 (6), Jun 1973, 227–228.

21 University of Aston. Safety and Hygiene Group Protective clothing. Occupational Health, 26 (7), Jul 1974, 268–270.

22 University of Aston. Safety and Hygiene Group Risk taking. Occupational Health, 25 (8), Aug 1973, 306–307.

23 University of Aston. Safety and Hygiene Group Safety. Accident attitudes. Occupational Health, 27 (8), Aug 1975, 330–332.

24 University of Aston. Safety and Hygiene Group Safety audits [to identify areas of safety where improvements are needed]. Occupational Health, 26 (12), Dec 1974, 494, 497.

25 University of Aston. Safety and Hygiene Group Safety economics. Occupational Health, 27 (11), Nov 1975, 488–490.

26 University of Aston. Safety and Hygiene Group The safety policy. Occupational Health, 27 (5), May 1975, 212–216.

27 University of Aston. Safety and Hygiene Group Splendid isolation. [Isolation of electric machinery from all voltage when not in use.] Occupational Health, 27 (10), Oct 1975, 451–452.

28 University of Aston. Safety and Hygiene Group Targets set for training. [Safety training.] Occupational Health, 25 (7), Jul 1973, 263–264.

29 University of Aston. Safety and Hygiene Group Under-reporting of accidents. Occupational Health, 26 (1), Jan 1974, 16–17.

30 University of Aston. Safety and Hygiene Group Ventilation systems. Occupational Health, 26 (8), Aug 1974, 320–322.

71 OCCUPATIONAL HEALTH NURSING

a GENERAL AND UNITED KINGDOM

1 Barnard, J. M. The links with community nursing. [Similar health goals of occupational health nurses, health visitors and district nurses.] Nursing Mirror, 141, 11 Sep 1975, 65–67.

2 Brown, G. What makes an OH nurse? [Research suggests that personality factors play an important part in determining the success and job satisfaction of an OH nurse.] Occupational Health, 25 (12), Dec 1973, 451–457.

3 D'Ardenne, D. The role of the occupational health nurse in industry. Community Health, 6 (6), May–Jun 1975, 326–329.

4 Durston, V. OH nurses as initiators. [The extending role of the nurse. Abridged version of Rcn Congress address.] Occupational Health, 26 (4), Apr 1974, 123–128.

5 French, M. The nurse's role in prevention and treatment. Occupational Health Nursing, 21 (2), Feb 1973, 15–17.

6 Green, M. D. Changing attitudes [towards nursing, and in particular towards occupational health nursing]. Occupational Health, 26 (5), May 1974, 175–178.

7 Hamilton, J. A derisory start. [A trade unionist's view of how the skill of OH nurses is being wasted.] Occupational Health, 24 (5), May 1972, 155.

8 Hammond, G. Letter from the chairman of the OH Section of the Rcn to Lord Halsbury. Occupational Health, 26 (11), Nov 1974, 425–426.

9 Hammond G. The nurse's contribution to health and safety at work. Physiotherapy, 61 (5), May 1975, 144–145.

10 Harrison, E. Occupational health nursing. Nursing Mirror, 138, 26 Apr 1974, 83–84.

11 Holgate, P. D. Practical implications of standard OH nursing practice. Occupational Health, 23 (5), May 1971, 155–162.

12 Jarman, B. Occupational health nursing. 1. What it is all about. Nursing Mirror, 136, 2 Feb 1973, 21–22.

13 Jarman, B. Occupational health nursing. 2. The occupational health nurse and the employer. Nursing Mirror, 136, 9 Feb 1973, 28.

14 King's Fund Centre Responsibilities of nurses within the Salmon structure for occupational health and counselling: report of a meetings held on 6 March and 11 September 1972. The Centre, 1972.

15 Lane, R. E. Twenty-fifth anniversary [of the Journal Occupational Health]. Occupational Health, 26 (1), Jan 1974, 7–9.

16 Lloyd, P. Development in the UK. [Emphasising the role of the Rcn in promoting occupational health nursing.] Nursing Mirror, 141, 11 Sep 1975, 50–52.

17 Lloyd, P. V. The need for professional organization in occupational health nursing. Occupational Health Nursing, 21 (2), Feb 1973, 9–11.

18 Lloyd, P. No experience necessary? Varying standards of occupational health nursing. Occupational Health, 24 (8), Aug 1972, 288–289.

19 Lloyd, P. OH nurse advisers and managers on the cheap. [Analysis of an Rcn salary survey.] Occupational Health, 27 (8), Aug 1975, 324–329.

20 Lloyd, P. Where does the OH nurse fit in? [with the implications of the Health and Safety at Work Act 1974.] Occupational Health, 27 (5), May 1975, 197–199.

21 Permanent Commission and International Association on Occupational Health, Nursing subcommittee Report: on the nurse's contribution to the health of the worker 1971–1973. Report no. 2: education of the nurse. The Commission, 1974.

22 Radwanski, D. and Pearson, J. C. G. Occupational health nursing in Scotland. Transactions of the Society of Occupational Medicine, 22 (4), Oct 1972, 122–125.

23 Ross, D. S. and Maccoll, E. Recruiting an OH nurse: analysis of a number of advertisements for OH post has emphasised the need for dissemination of information among employers about the speciality. Occupational Health, 27 (5), May 1975, 206–209.

24 Royal College of Nursing An occupational health nursing service: a handbook for nurses and employers. Rcn, 1975.

25 Royal College of Nursing Occupational health nursing structure. Revised ed. Rcn, 1971.

26 Royal College of Nursing Occupational health section 1952–1973: 21st anniversary and annual conference at the Royal Society of Medicine 23–24 November, 1973. Rcn, 1973.

27 Slaney, B. The need for professional identification in occupational health nursing. Occupational Health Nursing, 21 (5), May 1973, 19, 33.

28 Williams, M. M. The third decade: the history of the Rcn Occupational Health Section. Occupational Health, 26 (1), Jan 1974, 10–15.

29 Wreford, B. M. Occupational Health Conference Royal College of Nursing 1971. Occupational Health, 24 (2), Feb 1972, 56–59.

b UNITED STATES

1 American Association of Industrial Nurses Guide for the development of functions and responsibilities in occupational health nursing. Revised ed. New York: American Association of Industrial Nurses, 1975.

2 American Association of Industrial Nurses Issue giving papers from the 23rd AAIN Annual President's meeting with the theme 'AAIN action line for '76.' Occupational Health Nursing, 23, Dec 1975, 9–36.

3 American Association of Industrial Nurses Objectives of an occupational health nursing service. New York: The Assocation, 1971.

4 American Association of Industrial Nurses Standards for evaluating an occupational health nursing service. New York: The Association, 1975. Reprinted in Occupational Health Nursing, 23 (11), Nov 1975, 26–34.

5 Ashley, J. A. Reforms in nursing and health care: industrial nurses can lead the way. Occupational Health Nursing, 23 (6), Jun 1975, 11–14.

6 Bartel, C. K. The nurse practitioner in industry. [Experiences on an advanced course for occupational health nurses and subsequent employment in an expanded role.] Occupational Health Nursing, 23 (8), Aug 1975, 7–14.

7 Bill, S. A. Current and future trends of occupational health nursing. Occupational Health Nursing, 21 (12), Dec 1973, 9–11.

8 Bill, S. A. A glimpse into AAIN's past. Occupational Health Nursing, 23 (12), Dec 1975, 20–22.

9 Brown, M. L. The occupational health nurse: a new perspective. In Zenz, C. Occupational medicine: principles and practical applications. Chicago: Year Book Medical Publishers, 41–59, 1975.

10 Brown, M. L. Trends for the future of occupational health nursing. Occupational Health Nursing, 21 (8), Aug 1973, 7–11.

11 Cannavo, J. J. The industrial nurse's role in occupational safety. Occupational Health Nursing, 22 (2), Feb 1974, 7–9.

12 Cipolla, J. A. and Collings, G. H. Nurse clinicians in industry. American Journal of Nursing, 71 (8), Aug 1971, 1530–1534.

13 Copeland, M. E. What the consultant nurse can do for industry and the industrial nurse. Occupational Health Nursing, 21 (8), Aug 1973, 18.

14 Curtis, M. The nurse as an occupational health worker. Occupational Health Nursing, 21 (10), Oct 1973, 7–10.

15 Dingman, R. Occupational health nursing: tomorrow? or tomorrow! Occupational Health Nursing, 21 (6), Jun 1973, 9–15.

16 Doona, M. E. Professional judgement and the occupational health nurse. Occupational Health Nursing, 23 (10), Oct 1975, 18–20.

17 Ede, L. Legal aspects of occupational mental health nursing. Occupational Health Nursing, 21 (1), Jan 1973, 12–27.

18 Ellingson, H. V. Industrial diseases and the industrial nurse. Occupational Health Nursing, 23 (2), Feb 1975, 7–11.

19 Ford, L. C. Opportunities and obstacles in occupational health nursing. Occupational Health Nursing, 21 (7), Jul 1973, 9–14.

20 Hausman, D. M. Community health nursing includes occupational health nursing experience. Occupational Health Nursing, 21 (11), Nov 1973, 11–12.

21 Lacey, D. W. and Healey, J. T. Strategies for assessing and improving the utilization of occupational health nurses. Occupational Health Nursing, 22 (8), Aug 1974, 21–27.

22 Marino, R. A. AAIN salute to Bicentennial 1776–1976. [Brief history of the American Association of Industrial Nurses.] Occupational Health Nursing, 23 (9), Sep 1975, 23.

23 Martin, F. A. The state consultant. [The work of an occupational health nursing consultant in evaluating the provision of services.] Occupational Health Nursing, 23 (2), Feb 1975, 14–15.

24 Murchinson, I. A. Law – an element of quality control in occupational health nursing practice. [The effect of the increasing independence of the nursing profession from medical supervision.] Occupational Health Nursing, 22 (11), Nov 1974, 9–14.

25 Murphy, A. J. The nurse and employee health – efficiency and stability. Occupational Health Nursing, 22 (3), Mar 1974, 7–20, 47.

26 Popiel, E. S. Principles and concepts of occupational health nursing. Occupational Health Nursing, 21 (9), Sep 1973, 23–25.

27 Rost, J. New opportunity for occupational health nursing. [Public relations.] Occupational Health Nursing, 23 (12), Dec 1975, 12–14.

28 Siegel, M. A. Involved or not involved. [Ways in which the OH nurse may be involved in a changing society's needs.] Occupational Health Nursing, 23 (4), Apr 1975, 18–20.

29 Stiens, W. L. The expanded roles of the occupational health nurse. Occupational Health Nursing, 23 (8), Aug 1975, 18–21.

30 Talbot, D. Cultural lag and occupational health nursing. [Social change and the survival of occupational health nursing.] Occupational Health Nursing, 23 (10), Oct 1975, 11–15.

31 Talbot, D. M. Social change and occupational health nursing. Occupational Health Nursing, 22 (4), Apr 1974, 7–13.

32 Taylor, J. Genesis of the nurse practitioner role. [Formal nurse practitioner program at the University of Colorado for occupational health nurses.] Occupational Health Nursing, 23 (8), Aug 1975, 15–17.

33 United States Department of Health, Education and Welfare. Health Services and Mental Health Administration Fundamentals of occupational health nursing practice. Cincinnati: The Department, 1972.

34 United States. Department of Labor, Occupational Safety and Health Administration The occupational nurse. Washington, the Department, 1972. (Careers in safety and health.)

c OVERSEAS COUNTRIES

1 Alston, R. OH in Europe. 2 France. [Gillette Industries, Annecy.] Occupational Health, 27 (2), Feb 1975, 57–59.

2 Alston, R. OH in Europe. 3. Germany. [Gillette Industries, West Berlin.] Occupational Health, 27 (3), Mar 1975, 102–104.

3 Alston, R. OH in Europe. 4. Italy. [Gillette Industries, Milan.] Occupational Health, 27 (4), Apr 1975, 156–157.

4 Alston, R. OH in Europe. 5, Spain. [Gillette Industries, Seville.] Occupational Health, 27 (5), May 1975, 217–218.

5 Alston, R. OH in Europe. 6 comparisons. [A comparison of nurses in Gillette Industries in Europe shows the UK nurse has a wider range of duties.] Occupational Health, 27 (6), Jun 1975, 248–252.

6 Ann, M. H. Occupational health – a new challenge. [In Singapore.] Nursing Journal of Singapore, 13 (2), Nov 1973, 75–77.

7 Asogwa, S. E. The role of the nurse in tropical industries. Nigerian Nurse, 7 (3), Jul-Sep 1975, 18–20.

8 Frische, G. A. and Glass, W. I. Occupational health nursing. [Progress over last 50 years in New Zealand.] New Zealand Nursing Journal, 68 (3), Mar 1975, 4–6.

9 Sanchez, Z. M. Unity in diversity. [Aims and objectives of occupational health nursing in the Philippines.] Philippine Journal of Nursing, 44 (2), Apr–Jun 1975, 82–84.

10 Stewart, M. OH nurse in Bahrain. Occupational Health, 26 (3), Mar 1974, 86–91.

11 Zionzee, D. R. The occupational health nurse and how people at work make use of her presence, and her response to this. Lamp, 30 (11), Nov 1973, 7, 9, 11, 13.

d EDUCATION AND TRAINING

1 American Association of Industrial Nurses AAIN statement on continuing education. New York: The Association, 1975. Also in Occupational Health Nursing, 23 (10), Oct 1975, 21–25.

2 Amundsen, M. A. and Appelbaum, J.J. An in-service continuing education and expanded role program for occupational health nurses. Occupational Health Nursing, 23 (7), Jul 1975, 10–13.

3 Ashworth, E. Training course. [Personal experience of the occupational health nursing course at the Rcn.] Nursing Mirror, 141, 11 Sep 1975, 53.

4 Bamford, M. Addition to Briggs? [Training of for basic occupational health nursing incorporated within the Briggs recommendations.] Occupational Health, 26 (12), Dec 1974, 490–491.

5 Courtenay, I. The beginning of occupational health nursing graduate education at the University of North Carolina. Occupational Health Nursing, 21 (5), May 1973, 20–21.

6 De Tournay, R. Continuing education – professional responsibility or governmental regulation? Occupational Health Nursing, 23 (6), Jun 1975, 7–10.

7 Holgate, P. D. Industry-based training for occupational health nurses. [Evening course at Ford Motor Company.] Nursing Mirror, 140, 17 Apr 1975, 46–49.

8 Holgate, P. D. Statutory qualifications? [For occupational health nursing.] Occupational Health, 27 (1), Jan 1975, 13–19.

9 Holgate, P. D. and others OH congress paper. Day-release as a scheme of study [leading to an Rcn certificate in occupational health nursing.] Occupational Health, 27 (10), Oct 1975, 434–440. See also report in NursingTimes, 71, 25Sep 1975, 1523.

10 Holloway, M. The Indiana Academy of occupational health nursing. Occupational Health Nursing, 21 (9), Sep 1973, 26–28.

11 Keller, M. J. Nursing education and the occupational health setting. [Learning opportunities for nursing students.] Occupational Health Nursing, 22 (1), Jan 1974, 14–18.

12 Klutas, E. M. The occupational health nurse views future needs in continuing education. What do we want? Where do we get it? Occupational Health Nursing, 21 (9), Sep 1973, 9–15.

13 Ognjevic, I. OH nurses need post graduate education. Occupational Health, 24 (4),Apr 1972, 115–117.

14 Parsons, R. Occupational health nursing education in New South Wales, 1949–1975. Lamp, 32 (1), Jan 1975, 5, 7, 9, 11, 13.

15 Slaney, B. Nursing sub-committee report. Education for Occupational Health Nursing. Occupational Health Nursing, 21 (2), Feb 1973, 20–22.

e SPECIAL ASPECTS OF ROLE

1 Burkeen, O. E. The role of the occupational health nurse in performing health examinations. Occupational Health Nursing, 21 (5), May 1973, 22–26.

2 Campbell, J. and others The role of the occupational health nurse in redundancy. Occupational Health Nursing, 21 (2), Feb 1973, 12–14.

3 Cosin, L. Z. Industrial gerontology. [The older worker in industry.] Rehabilitation no. 92, Jan–Mar 1975, 39–43.

4 Hawkins, G. M. Counselling: the nurse's role. Occupational Health, 25 (6), Jun 1973, 223–226.

5 Healey, J. T. A counselling program in industry. [A training program for occupational health nurses at Western Electric using videotapes.] Occupational Health Nursing, 23 (1), Jan 1975, 12–13.

6 Hotch, W. A shot in the arm. [A programme of health education in a Massachusetts factory.] Occupational Health Nursing, 20 (8), Aug 1972, 9–12.

7 Howard, L. S. Counselling in occupational health nursing. Occupational Health Nursing, 20 (4), Apr 1972, 7–8.

8 Neill, A. M. Safety and the industrial nurse. New Zealand Nursing Journal, 66 (2), Feb 1973, 13–14.

9 Occupational Health Health interviews. [Pre-employment, in-service and special health examinations.] Occupational Health, 27 (9), Sep 1975, 381–384.

10 Pretty, P. L. A health education project for a group of middle aged men. [Project at the Sun Printers done in co-operation with the occupational health nursing staff.] Health Education Journal, 33 (1), 1973, 10–11.

11 Reznikoff, P. A. Safety, management and nursing. Occupational Health Nursing, 22 (6), Jun 1974, 26–27, 37.

12 Stevenson, E. A study of the needs and problems of workers 65 years of age and over. Occupational Health Nursing, 21 (2), Feb 1973, 18–19.

13 Weintraub, M. The role of industrial nurses in improving patients' adherence to therapeutic plans. Occupational Health Nursing, 23 (5), May 1975, 16–17.

14 Zionzee, D. R. Services to people at work: medical, welfare and counselling. [Nursing services.] Lamp, 32 (6), Jun 1975, 9, 11.

72 OCCUPATIONAL HEALTH IN HEALTH SERVICES

1 American Hospital Association Guidelines on tuberculosis control programs for hospital employees. Hospitals, 49 (13), 1 Jul 1975, 57–60.

2 Bedford Group Hospital Management Committee Bedford General Hospital occupational health service: reports 1–7. The Committee, 1967–1974.

3 Bedford Hospital Success of a project – seven years of staff occupational health at Bedford General. A final report on the findings of research. Nursing Mirror, 141, 18 Sep 1975, 36; Nursing Times, 71, 18 Sep 1975, 1480.

5 Bryan, M. Is hospital a dangerous place to work in? [Extracts from a research document 'Health and Safety of Hospital Personnel'.] Australian Nurses' Journal, 4 (7), Feb 1975, 36–38.

5 Clark, L. OH service in hospital. [Airedale Hospital, Keighley.] Occupational Health, 25 (10), Oct 1973, 376–380.

6 Department of Health and Social Security Occupational health centre for hospital staff: a design guide. DHSS, 1973.

7 Farrant, E. M. The occupational health service at the Middlesex Hospital, London. Nursing Mirror, 140, 1 May 1975, 46–49.

8 French, G. E. Centre Lunch talk. Occupational health [in the reorganized NHS]. Health and Social Service Journal, 85, 1 Nov 1975, 2451.

9 Gale, R. C. A hospital occupational health service. Nursing Times, 68, 30 Mar 1972, 373–374; 6 Apr 1972, 415–416.

10 Grant, N. Who is liable? [Progress of health and safety legislation in the NHS.] Nursing Times, 71, 18 Sep 1975, 1484–1485.

11 Hamilton, M. Services of NRPB [Radiological Protection Board.] Occupational Health, 27 (7), Jul 1975, 296–299.

12 Hammond, G. Aiming for a healthy hospital. [Occupational health services in hospitals.] Grace Hammond talks to Michael Bangs. Nursing Times, 70, 25 Apr 1974, 643–644.

13 Harrington, J. M. Medical laboratory safety. Occupational Health, 25 (11), Nov 1973, 411–416.

14 Harte, J. D. Bedford Staff Occupational Health Department. British Hospital Journal and Social Service Review, 82, 1 Jan 1972, 22–23.

15 Harte, J. D. Hospital staff occupational health department. Nursing Mirror, 139, 6 Sep 1974, 53–55.

16 Harte, J. D. Occupational health services for health authority and local authority staff. (c) Occupational health for area health authority staff. Royal Society of Health Journal, 94 (6), Dec 1974, 292–295.

17 Harte, J. D. Support of mentally ill hospital staff. Occupational Health, 26 (9), Sep 1974, 346–351.

18 Horton Psychiatric Hospital Who nurses the nurses? One positive answer. [Staff health service at Horton Psychiatric Hospital, Epsom.] Nursing Mirror, 134, 16 Jun 1972, 31–32.

19 Hospital and Health Services Review An occupational health department. [Editorial on the Salford group of hospitals occupational health scheme.] Hospital and Health Services Review, 71 (3), Mar 1975, 79.

20 Hunt, D. OH in the National Health Service. Nursing Mirror, 141, 11 Sep 1975, 62–65.

21 Jenkins, C. Health in hospitals: a service for NHS employees. Nursing Times, 70, 25 Apr 1974, 616–617.

22 Lampwick, D. 'Tis not enough to help the feeble up. . .' [The inadequacy of occupational health services for NHS staff.] Nursing Mirror, 140, 30 Jan 1975, 67–68.

23 Lancet Tuberculosis in hospital staff. [Leading article.] Lancet, 1, 10 Mar 1973, 525–526.

24 Laycock, J. Occupational health and hazards in the health service. [The development, objectives and particular problems of a hospital occupational health service.] Community Health, 4 (3), Nov/Dec 1972, 142–148.

25 Lord, D. Occupational health and management. [Fifth report of Bedford Hospital Occupational Health Service.] Health and Social Service Journal, 83, 21 Apr 1973, 913, 915.

26 Lunn, J. A. The health of staff in hospitals. Heinemann, 1975.

27 Lunn, J. A. Hospital hazards. Practitioner, 210, Apr 1973, 490–499.

28 McLauchlan, G. P. Occupational health in an integrated health service [for local authority employees based on experience in the City of Exeter.] Health and Social Service Journal, 84, 15 Jun 1974, 1335–1336.

29 Manchester Area Health Authority. Central District. Occupational Health Service Report on the first year's work. 1 Jan to 31 Dec, 1974. Manchester AHA, 1974.

30 Mellish, J. M. Occupational health nursing in the hospital setting. SA Nursing Journal, 13 (1), Jan 1975, 7.

31 Monard, P. and others The care of the health of hospital staff: a survey of hospital occupational health services in England and Wales, with appendices. TUC Centenary Institute of Occupational Health, 1974. [2 vols.]

32 Moore, W. K. S. Occupational health services for health authority and local authority staff. (a) The purpose and practice of occupational health services. Royal Society of Health Journal, 94 (6), Dec 1974, 286–288.

33 Murray, R. Occupational health in the NHS. British Hospital Journal and Social Service Review, 81, 13 Nov 1971, 2369.

34 Nursing Times An Act witn no substance. [Effect of Health and Safety at Work Act on hospital occupational services.] Nursing Times, 71, 10 Apr 1975, 553.

35 Royal Society of Medicine. Section of Occupational Medicine Occupational health services in hospitals. Proceedings of the Royal Society of Medicine 65, May 1972, 447–466.

36 Salford Hospital Management Committee. Occupational Health Department Report on first year's work of the occupational health scheme. [1 Oct, 1972 to 30 Sep, 1973.] The Committee, 1973.

37 Shaw, C. H. Occupational health services for health authority and local authority staff. (b) Occupational health in local government. Royal Society of Health Journal, 94 (6), Dec 1974, 289–292.

38 Slaney, B. M. The work of the occupational health nurse in the National Health Service. District Nursing, 14 (7), Oct 1971, 143–144.

39 Swaffield, L. Waiting for guidance. [Implications of the Health and Safety at Work Act for NHS staff.] Nursing Times, 71, 10 Apr 1975, 560–561.

40 United States Department of Health Education and Welfare. National Institute of Occupational Safety and Health Hospital occupational health services study. The Department, 1975–1976. 7 vols.

41 Watson, E. Occupational health in the NHS. [Lecture given at the Rcn OH section annual conference.] Nursing Mirror, 141, 3 Jul 1975, 72–73.

42 World Health Organization Manual of radiation protection in hospitals and general practice. Geneva: WHO, 1975. 3 vols.

73 OCCUPATIONAL HEALTH, SPECIAL AREAS

a AGRICULTURE

1 Elliott, C. K. Rural medicine: a new skill for the practice team in the countryside. Nursing Times, 141, 17 Jul 1975, 46–49.

b ASBESTOS

1 Brookes, P. Asbestos and cancer: findings of international meeting in Lyons. Nursing Times, 69, 18 Jan 1973, 95.

2 Gasson, E. Asbestos in industry. [Including the role of the occupational health nurse.] Occupational Health, 26 (8), Aug 1974, 298–306; (9) Sep 1974, 353–362.

3 Hamilton, M. OH congress session. Asbestos. Occupational Health, 27 (10), Oct 1975, 431–433.

4 Lee, G. Asbestos-based and other industrial materials. Concern over health problems and development of alternative materials. Occupational Health, 26 (12), Dec 1974, 484–487.

5 Lewinsohn, H. C. Health hazards of asbestos: a review of recent trends. Journal of the Society of Occupational Medicine, 24 (1), Jan 1974, 2–10.

6 Poole, F. T. A strict interpretation: the obligations imposed by the Asbestos Regulations. Occupational Health, 26 (10), Oct 1974, 404–405.

7 Shield, A. C. Deadly asbestos. Australian Nurses' Journal, 5 (3), Sep 1975, 33–34.

c CHEMICAL INDUSTRY

1 Carter, R. L. and Roe, F. J. C. Chemical carcinogens in industry. Journal of the Society of Occupational Medicine, 25 (3), Jul 1975, 86–94.

2 Farr, E. M. HCN (hydrogen cyanide) and cyanides: a guide for nurses. Occupational Health, 27 (8), Aug 1975, 336–338, 341.

3 Forde, J. P. Case history. Xylene affected platelet count. Occupational Health, 25 (11), Nov 1973, 429–433.

4 Hartigan, R. L. Emergency care of chemical injuries in industry. Occupational Health Nursing, 21 (12), Dec 1973, 12–15.

5 Henning, H. F. Labelling for safety: a standard system for dangerous chemical substances. Occupational Health, 25 (10), Oct 1973, 370–374.

6 Occupational Health Tutorial. Toxic gases and vapours. Occupational Health, 26 (11), Nov 1974, 428–437.

7 Ross, D. S. Case history. Acute acetone intoxication. Occupational Health, 27 (3), Mar 1975, 120–124.

8 Seagle, E. F. Ozone as an occupational health hazard. Occupational Health Nursing, 21 (8), Aug 1973, 14–17.

9 Smith, D. C. Handling isocyanates safely. Occupational Health, 25 (3), Mar 1973, 92–96.

10 University of Aston. Safety and Hygiene Group The limitations of TLVs. [Concentration of toxic substances in air – threshold limit values.] Occupational Health, 27 (6), Jun 1975, 263–265.

d METAL INDUSTRY

1 Hamilton, M. Hazards of plutonium. Occupational Health, 26 (12), Dec 1974, 475–477.

2 Kipling, M.D. Hard metal disease. Occupational Health, 25 (4), Apr 1973, 131–134.

3 Ross, D. S. Lead fumes affected welders: case history. Occupational Health, 25 (4), Apr 1973, 146–149.

6 Ross, D. S. Routine medicals for welders. Occupational Health, 26 (12), Dec 1974, 478–483.

5 Ross, D. S. Tracing Doig's welders: the first stage of a follow-up study of the health of a group of welders originally examined in 1944. Occupational Health, 26 (11), Nov 1974, 442–443.

6 Ross, D. S. Vibration stress. [Among templet makers.] Occupational Health, 24 (10), Oct 1972, 372–374.

7 Ross, D. S. Welders wanted: a follow-up study. Occupational Health, 25 (10), Oct 1973, 375.

8 Ross, D. S. Welders' metal fume fever. [A survey of workers at Babcock & Wilcox.] Journal of the Society of Occupational Medicine, 24 (4), Oct 1974, 125–129.

9 Tutorial, Hazards of welding. Occupational Health, 27 (2), Feb 1975, 60–65. Erratum: (3), Mar 1975, 95.

10 Welding Institute and Royal College of Nursing Assessing hazards of welding fumes. [One day seminar.] Occupational Health, 27 (5), May 1975, 176–177.

11 Williams, D. The role of the occupational health nurse in the lead-using industry. SA Nursing Journal, 42 (2), Feb 1975, 15–16.

e MINING

1 Bryan, A. The evolution of health and safety in mining. Ashire Publishing, 1975.

2 Hodgson, G. A. Skin diseases of coal miners in Britain with special reference to the history of changes in mining. Journal of the Society of Occupational Medicine, 25 (2), Apr 1975, 66–71.

3 Horton, E. Blood on the coal: treating the victims of a pit disaster. Nursing Times, 69, 1 Nov 1973, 1436–1438.

4 McCarrick, H. Miners prefer women. [A colliery medical centre in South Wales run by a nursing officer.] Nursing Times, 69, 1 Mar 1973, 286–288.

5 Richards, R. C. Miners' health. Occupational Health, 26 (10), Oct 1974, 387–390; (11), Nov 1974, 438–441.

6 Richardson, J. Focus on care of the men who cut the coal. Nursing Week, 13, 17 Jan 1974, 6–7.

f OIL INDUSTRY

1 British Medical Association. Scottish Council Report of the working party on the medical implications of oil related industry. Edinburgh: The Association, 1975. Condensed in British Medical Journal, 3, 6 Sep 1975, 576–580.

2 British Medical Journal High pressure medicine. [Problems of divers working under pressure in the North Sea.] British Medical Journal, 4, 6 Dec 1975, 541–542.

3 Gray, R. M. Dysbarism – a relatively new medical emergency. [Decompression sickness.] Nursing Mirror, 140, 30 Jan 1975, 44–46.

4 Gunn, A. D. G. Safety in the North Sea. Nursing Times, 70, 12 Dec 1974, 1924–1925.

5 Hamilton, M. Health hazards in compressed air.

[Current research and future plans discussed at a conference.] Occupational Health, 27 (6), Jun 1975, 258, 261–262.

6 McMillan, A. North sea oil – what will be the price? [The socio-economic implications of the industry with possible effects on health.] Nursing Times, 70, 12 Dec 1974, 1922–1923.

7 Miller, J. N. Caisson disease. [Decompression sickness.] District Nursing, 14 (7), Oct 1971, 140–142.

8 Occupational Health Voluntary code for tankers. Occupational Health, 27 (8), Aug 1975, 323.

9 Swaffield, L. Plumbing the shallows. [Comments on the BMA's Scottish Council report. 'The medical implications of oil related industry'.] Occupational Health, 27 (10), Oct 1975, 446–450.

10 University of Aston. Safety and Hygiene Group Pressure vessel dangers. Occupational Health, 25 (5), May 1973, 182–183.

g STUDENT HEALTH

1 Betts, S. 'Just a headache.' [Experiences of a college nurse.] Nursing Times, 71, 7 Aug 1975, 1261.

2 Blaine, G. B. and McArthur, C. C. Emotional problems of the student. 2nd ed. Butterworths, 1971.

3 Cauthery, P. Student health. Priory Press, 1973. [Care and welfare library.]

4 Chantry-Price, A. An insight into university health nursing. Nursing Times, 68, 21 Dec 1972, 1609–1610.

5 Edmonds, O. P. Examinations – an occupational hazard of University students. [Analysis over six years of attendance at Manchester University Health Centre for examination strain.] Journal of the Society of Occupational Medicine, 25 (4), Oct 1975, 135–138.

6 Edmonds, O. P. Health hazards on the campus. [Particular reference to workshops and laboratory staff.] Occupational Health, 24 (12), Dec 1972, 435–438.

7 Edmonds, O. P. Pyschological upsets at a University Institute of Science and Technology. Transactions of the Society of Occupational Medicine, 20 (4), Oct 1970, 140–142.

8 Fox, R. Today's students. (c) Suicide among students and its prevention. Royal Society of Health Journal, 91 (4), Jul/Aug 1971, 181–183.

9 Fulford, R. C. and Roberts, N. G. Hospital university student health service. [Seven-year experiment involving the University of West Florida and Baptist Hospital, Pensacola.] Hospitals, 49 (2), 16 Jan 1975, 52–54.

10 Gunn, A. D. G. Students under stress. New Society, 17, 25 Mar 1971, 485–487.

11 Gunn, A. D. G. Today's students. (a) Students' health. Royal Society of Health Journal, 91 (4), Jul/Aug 1971, 175–179.

12 Hallett, C. P. Community health services in a college of further education. Public Health, 88 (3), Mar 1974, 105–120.

13 Honywood, H. Comprehensive care for students: the Reading University health service. Practice Team, no. 47, Apr 1975, 2,4, 6–7.

14 Humphreys, D. Careers extraordinary. Handling university health. Nursing Times, 68, 27 Apr 1972, 506–508.

15 Journal of the Royal College of General Practitioners Student health services – general practice or not? [Editorial.] Journal of the Royal College of General Practitioners, 23, Feb 1973, 77–79.

16 MacKenzie, N. Psychiatric nursing care in a university. [Sussex University.] Nursing Mirror, 134, 28 Jan 1972, 30–31.

17 Malleson, N. Pre-examination strain: treatment of tension in the over-anxious student. Nursing Times, 70, 16 May 1974, 735–736.

18 Manderson, W. G. and Sclare, A. B. Mental health problems in a student population. Health Bulletin, 31 (5), Sep 1973, 233–239.

19 Millar, D. A bird's-eye view of student health. Community Health, 5 (5), Mar/Apr 1974, 259–263.

20 Moyer, P. J. and Conover, B. J. The new style of campus nursing. American Journal of Nursing, 70 Sep 1970, 1900–1903.

21 Parkes, M. The nurse as a counsellor. [In a university health service.] Nursing Times, 69, 1 Feb 1973, 156.

22 Pashley, B. W. and Shepherd, A. M. Staff and student perceptions of a student health service. [Survey at Hull University.] Journal of the Royal College of General Practitioners, 25, Nov 1975, 845–851.

23 Ripley, G. D. Student health service at a college of further education. Journal of the Royal College of General Practitioners, 22, Mar 1972, 169–171.

24 Royal College of Nursing University and college health nursing structure. Rcn, 1974.

25 Still, R. J. Student problems (problems of student health). Health Education Journal, 32 (2), 1973, 36–40.

26 Stordy, B. J. University students – their food and nutrition intake. Nutrition, 27 (4), Aug 1973, 262–266.

27 Student mental health and the general practitioner. Drug and Therapeutics Bulletin, 13 (25), 5 Dec 1975, 99–100.

28 Vaughan, H. W. British Student Health Association. Occupational Health, 22 (5), May 1970, 158–159.

29 Watson, E. The University of Reading health service. District Nursing, 14 (7), Oct 1971, 139–150.

30 Woodmansey, A. C. Pyschotherapy in the student health service. Lancet, 1, 29 May 1974, 1122–1123.

h TRANSPORT, TRAVEL AND SPORT

1 Bateman, S. C. Physiological aspects of jet travel. Occupational Health, 24 (1), Jan 1972, 3–10.

2 Bergin, K. G. The medical problems of space flight. Nursing Times, 67, 1 Jul 1971, 787–789.

3 Brigstocke, H. Nurses break the ice: nurses aboard an icebreaker in the Arctic. Canadian Nurse, 70 (4), Apr 1974, 38–41.

4 Browning, D. Accident department on wheels. [International Grand Prix Medicine Services Unit.] Nursing Times, 71, 2 Jan 1975, 32–34.

5 Bruton, D. M. Taking good care of ground crew. Occupational Health, 25 (3), Mar 1973, 97–102.

6 Conroy, R. T. W. L. Jet travel and circardian rhythms. Nursing Times, 68 (13), 30 Mar 1972, 370–372.

7 Crockford, G. W. Buoyancy suits for fishermen. Occupational Health, 25 (8), Aug 1973, 288–295.

8 Cullinan, J. Racecouse nurses. Nursing Times, 67, 21 Jan 1971, 69–71.

9 Farrell, B. L. and Allen, M. F. Physiologic/psychologic changes reported by USAF female flight nurses during flying duties. Nursing Research, 22 (1), Jan/Feb 1973, 31–36.

10 Foley, M. F. Air travel for patients. American Journal of Nursing, 73 (6), Jun 1973, 1020–1023.

11 Follow the sun – the nurse's life afloat. [Nursing on a cruise ship.] Nursing Times, 71, 16 Jan 1975, 92–93.

12 Fowke, L. The Cunard group health service. Nursing Mirror, 137, 2 Nov 1973, 41–45.

13 Hamilton, M. OH Congress session. Shift work. [Summary of three papers on locomotive driving.] Occupational Health, 27 (11), Nov 1975, 477–479.

14 Hutchison, A. The health of seafarers. 1. Historical background and present situation. WHO Chronicle, 29 (10), Oct 1975, 387–392.

15 Kelson, M. Supporting life in space. Nursing Times, 70, 20 Jun 1974, 943–946.

16 Kirby, K. Weekend flight nurse. Occupational Health Nursing, 20 (5), May 1972, 11.

17 Mason, J. K. Disease of aircrew as a cause of aircraft accidents. Community Health, 6 (2), Sep/Oct 1974, 62–67.

18 Nursing Mirror Nurses in space. NASA's research project for candidates for the space shuttle. [Mainly illustrations.] Nursing Mirror, 139, 23 Aug 1974, 48–50.

19 O'Connor, V. Careers extraordinary. Life on the ocean wave. [A ship's nurse.] Nursing Times, 68, 8 Jun 1972, 721–723.

20 Preston, F. S. The ups. . . and downs. . . of supersonic travel. Nursing Times, 70, 20 Jun 1974, 938–942.

21 Rich, V. Safety in space. [Safety problems in the Soyuz/Apollo mission.] Occupational Health, 27 (9), Sep 1975, 362–363.

22 Starr, D. S. Health care at Toronto International Airport. Canadian Nurse, 69 (2), Feb 1973, 32–37.

23 Tomaszunas, S. The health of seafarers. 2. International aspects. WHO Chronicle, 29 (10), Oct 1975, 393–396.

24 Turner, A. C. Motion sickness and travellers' diarrhoea. Nursing Mirror, 134, 7 Jan 1972, 31–33.

25 World Health On the great waters. [Health services for seamen.] World Health, Jul/Aug 1973, 31–46.

26 Wreford, J. Executives at risk? [Coronary thrombosis in a shipping department.] Occupational Health, 26 (2), Feb 1974, 42–46.

i OTHER AREAS

1 Hall-Patch, E. OH in the food industry. Nursing Mirror, 141, 11 Sep 1975, 60–61.

2 Haynes, M. Careers in nursing. A job with a difference. [Work of an occupational health nurse in a motor company.] Nursing Times, 67, 30 Sep 1971, 1215–1217.

3 Hunter, W. J. Medical aspects of work in the food industry. Community Health, 7 (2), Oct 1975, 83–85.

4 Jarman, B. Post office nursing. Occupational health service. Nursing Mirror, 140, 19 Jun 1975, 56–58.

5 Kilburn, K. H. and others Byssinosis: matter from lint to lungs. [The hazard of plant particles in lint to textile workers.] American Journal of Nursing, 73 (11), Nov 1973, 1952–1956.

6 Lockeberg, L. E. All in the day's work . . . an occupational health nurse in a large department store in Toronto shares some highlights of her work. Canadian Nurse, 69 (6), Jun 1973, 33–36.

7 McLean, A. and Clarke, A. C. W. V. Atomic safety. Occupational Health, 25 (5), May 1973, 171–175.

8 Nursing Mirror Post Office nursing. A day in the life of. . . Nursing Mirror, 140 (23), 19 Jun 1975, 58–59.

9 Nursing Times In the money. Industrial nursing at the Royal Mint. Nursing Times, 69, 1 Mar 1973, 289–291.

10 Pelmear, P. L. Vibration white finger. Occupational Health, 26 (8), Aug 1974, 307–310.

PSYCHIATRY

74 PSYCHIATRIC SERVICES

a PSYCHIATRIC SERVICES AND MENTAL HEALTH

1 Beattie, N. R. Community mental health: the preventive aspects. Community Health, 4 (1), Jul–Aug 1972, 2–7.

2 Binitie, A. The importance of mental health in the society. Nigerian Nurse, 6 (1), Jan/Mar 1974, 42, 44–46.

3 Boorer, D. All our yesterdays is theme at NAMH conference. Come back Enoch, all is forgiven. Nursing Times, 69, 22 Mar 1973, 388–389.

4 Bush, M. T. and others The meaning of mental health: a report of two enthnoscientific studies. [Defined by the central city resident and psychiatric-mental health professional.] Nursing Research, 24 (2), Mar–Apr 1975, 130–131, 138.

5 Carstairs, G. M. Mental health – what is it? [Reprinted from World Health, May 1973.] Psychiatric Nursing and Mental Health Services, 12 (1), Jan/Feb 1974, 37–42.

6 Clark, J. Conference report. Who's afraid of integration? [Conference on interdisciplinary collaboration in the field of mental health held at the Tavistock Institute.] Nursing Times, 69, 23 Aug 1973, 1104.

7 Dalzell-Ward, A. J. Mental health – a physiological model. Community Health, 6 (5), Mar/Apr 1975, 286–291.

8 Ennals, D. Health of mind matters most. Health Visitor, 44 (7), Jul 1971, 230–231.

9 Evang, K. International trends. Mental health – public health. Journal of Psychiatric Nursing and Mental Health Services, 13 (4), Jul/Aug 1975, 47–49.

10 Jacobson, S. R. A study of interprofessional collaboration [in mental health projects.] Nursing Outlook, 2 (12), Dec 1974, 751–755.

11 Kahn, J. H. Mental health and family life. World Health, Feb/Mar 1973, 8–15.

12 Munday, B. A fair deal for the mentally ill. British Hospital Journal and Social Service Review, 82, 30 Sep 1972, 2181–2182.

13 Priest, R. G. Towards better psychiatric services. Nursing Mirror, 139, 16 Aug 1974, 69–72.

14 Sampson, G. Mental health. British Hospital Journal and Social Service Review, 82, 16 Dec 1972, 2811–2812.

15 Shearer, A. Passing the buck. [White Paper – Better services for the mentally ill.] New Society, 34, 23 Oct 1975, 214.

16 Smith, D. L. Wild land: a mental health resource to enrich human existence, as the world becomes more urban and technological. Canadian Nurse, 70 (6), Jun 1974, 20–22.

17 Welsh, R. R. Positive mental health. New Zealand Nursing Journal, 69 (9), Sep 1975, 6–8.

18 Welsh Hospital Board Care of the mentally handicapped, mentally ill and the elderly: a final report of the survey team concerning action already taken, the on-going commitment, major problems. Cardiff: The Board, 1974.

19 Wertheim, E. S. Positive mental health, western society and the family. Social Psychiatry, 21 (4), Winter 1975, 247–255.

20 Wilting, J. The mentally healthy person. Canadian Journal of Psychiatric Nursing, 15 (5), Sep–Oct 1974, 13–14.

21 World Health Issue on mental health. World Health, Oct 1974, 3–35.

b LEGISLATION

1 Brennan, K. S. W. Legal aspects of community psychiatry. Community Health, 5 (3), Nov/Dec 1973, 169–174.

2 Brennan, K. S. W. Psychiatry and the law. Nursing Times, 69, 22 Nov 1973, 1570–1571.

3 French, C. W. Notes on the Mental Health Act 1959. 2nd ed. Shaw, 1971.

4 Gostin, L. O. A human condition: the Mental Health Act from 1959 to 1975. Observations, analysis and proposals for reform. Mind, 1975.

5 Harrison, P. Compulsory psychiatry. [Reform of the Mental Health Act.] New Society, 28, 16 May 1974, 377–379.

6 Jacob, J. The Mental Health Act explained: edited by Denise Winn. Mind/National Association for Mental Health, 1975.

7 Nursing Mirror Mental Health Act amended. [Mental Health (Amendment) Act 1975.] Nursing Mirror, 141, 11 Sep 1975, 35.

8 Philpot, T. Lord Shaftesbury and the reform of the Lunacy Laws. Nursing Mirror, 137, 2 Nov 1973, 15–16.

9 Venables, H. D. S. A guide to the law affecting mental patients. Butterworth, 1975.

10 Whitehead, J. A. Mental illnesses, human rights and the law. Nursing Mirror, 137, 21 Sep 1973, 22–23, 30.

c COMMUNITY SERVICES

1 Bennett, D. H. Community psychiatry. Community Health, 5 (2), Sep/Oct 1973, 58–64.

2 Brook, A. Mental health in the community: some aspects of inter-professional co-operation. Community Medicine, 129, 15 Dec 1972, 213–215.

3 Brook, P. and Cooper, B. Community mental health care: primary team and specialist services. Journal of the Royal College of General Practitioners, 25, Feb 1975, 93–98, 103–110.

4 Cawley, R. and McLachlan, G., editors Policy for action: a symposium on the planning of a comprehensive district psychiatric service. Oxford University Press for the Nuffield Provincial Hospitals Trust, 1973.

5 Denham, J. Community psychiatry and the health service. (One service – now or never!) Public Health, 86 (2), Jan 1972, 53–56.

6 Durlong, R. B. Community psychiatry. Health and Social Service Journal, 83, 19 May 1973, 1137–1138.

7 Ebie, J. C. An experimental multi-disciplinary social casework Centre. [Craigmillar Health, Welfare and Advice Centre, Edinburgh. Staff includes health visitors, a psychiatrist and social workers.] Community Health, 3 (6), May/Jun 1972, 277–284.

8 French, C. W. Evaluation of a community mental health service [in Bedfordshire.] Social Work Today, 2, 17 Jun 1971, 22–26.

9 Hulme, J. R. The town of Geel – legend and reality. [A town in Belgium where 4000 mentally ill live within the community.] Nursing Mirror, 141, 4 Dec 1975, 64–65.

10 Kahn, J. H. A pioneer scheme in community mental health. Nursing Mirror, 132, 12 Feb 1971, 33–35, 39.

11 McNally, D. J. Whither mental health? [The value of community psychiatric care should be proved before existing facilities are curtailed or abolished.] Nursing Mirror, 135, 24 Nov 1972, 36–37.

12 Mair, H. Community mental health services. Public Health, 86 (2), Jan 1972, 73–78.

13 Mitchell, R. Advances in psychiatry. Institutional psychiatry v. community psychiatry. Nursing Times, 70, 14 Nov 1974, 1769–1771.

14 Robinson, W. A. Mental health and the community. [Report of conference on the effect of the NHS reorganization on community mental health and Social Services.] Nursing Times, 68, 16 Nov 1972, 1452.

15 Smith, E. The Isis Centre. [Centre in Oxford for treatment of psychiatric patients in the community staffed by a multidisciplinary team.] Nursing Times, 68, 11 May 1972, 561–563.

16 Whitehead, C. E. St. Columba-Emmanuel Centre. [For those experiencing mental stress.] Queen's Nursing Journal, 16 (8), Nov 1973, 185–186.

17 Ziman, D. Unwanted neighbours. [Report of a conference at the Hospital Centre on the problems of community care for the mentally sick and handicapped.] British Hospital Journal and Social Service Review, 82, 9 Sep 1972, 2013–2015.

d OVERSEAS COUNTRIES

1 Bailly-Salin, P. The 'sectorization' of comprehensive psychiatric services in France. Journal of Psychiatric Nursing and Mental Health Services, 11 (5), Sep/Oct 1973, 42–43.

2 Carter, F. M. Community mental health services in the USSR. Nursing Outlook, 20 (3), Mar 1972, 164–168.

3 Coleman, W. Mental health in British Honduras. Nursing Times, 69, 17 May 1973, 652–653.

4 Davis, A. J. Psychiatric problems and services in Kenya. International Nursing Review, 22 (1), Jan/Feb 1975, 25–27.

5 Feldman, S. and Goldstein, H. H. Community mental health centres in the United States; an overview. International Journal of Nursing Studies, 8 (4), Dec 1971, 247–255.

6 Hess, G. Impressions of mental health service delivery systems in Finland, Poland, Soviet Russia and Czechoslovakia. International Journal of Nursing Studies, 8 (4), Dec 1971, 223–233.

7 Hunter, D. Organizational problems in community psychiatric programs. Canadian Journal of Psychiatric Nursing, 16 (3), May/Jun 1975, 8–11.

8 Lego, S. The community mental health system: is it an improvement over the old system? Perspectives in Psychiatric Care, 8 (3), Jul–Sep 1975, 105–112.

9 Lowery, B. J. and Janulis, D. Community mental health and the unanswered questions. Perspectives in Psychiatric Care, 11 (1), Jan/Mar 1973, 26–28.

10 Luiz, H. A. Community psychiatry. [Components of an effective service.] SA Nursing Journal, 42 (3), Mar 1975, 26–27.

11 Mehryar, A. and Khajavi, F. Some implications of a community mental health model for developing countries. International Journal of Social Psychiatry, 21 (1), Winter–Spring 1974, 45–51.

12 Murray, J. E. Failure of the community mental health movement. American Journal of Nursing, 75 (11), Nov 1975, 2034–2036.

13 Roscher, C. I. Community care with special emphasis on psychiatric community care. SA Nursing Journal, 38 (8), Aug 1971, 31–33, 25.

14 Serebrjakova, Z. N. Preventive aspects of the comprehensive psychiatric service in the USSR. Journal of Psychiatric Nursing and Mental Health Services, 11 (5), Sep/Oct 1973, 43–44.

15 Segall, A. Community mental health: some problems in measurement. Canadian Journal of Psychiatric Nursing, 16 (4), Jul/Aug 1975, 6–7.

16 WHO Chronicle Mental health services in the developing countries. WHO Chronicle, 29 (6), Jun 1975, 231–235.

17 Woods, W. J. Community psychiatry. Australian Nurses' Journal, 4 (10), May 1975, 28–31.

e PSYCHIATRIC SOCIAL WORK

1 Cooper, B. and others An experiment in community mental health care. [A social worker attached to a group practice.] Lancet 2, 7 Dec 1974, 1356–1358.

2 Lee, W. E. Society at work. Conflict of model. [Conflict between trained social workers and medical and nursing staff in a psychiatric hospital.] New Society, 25, 23 Aug 1973, 457–458.

3 Miles, A. Social workers in psychiatric hospitals. Social Work Today, 2, 10 Feb 1972, 2–6.

4 Oram, E. V. Social work departments in psy-

chiatric hospitals. Health and Social Service Journal, 84, 22 Jun 1974, 1393–1394.

5 Orriss, H. D. Is psychiatric social work suffering under Seebohm? Nursing Times, 71, 10 Apr 1975, 584–585.

6 Tod, E. D. M. and Gordon, H. A new role for psychiatric social workers in general practice. Medical Officer, 125 (20), 14 May 1971, 255–256.

75 PSYCHIATRIC NURSING

a TEXTBOOKS

1 Altschul, A. Psychiatric nursing. 4th ed. Bailliere Tindall, 1973. (Nurses aids series.)

2 Chapman, A. H. and Almeida, E. M. The interpersonal basis of psychiatric nursing. New York: Putnam, 1972.

3 Crawford, A. L. and Buchanan, B. B. Psychiatric nursing: a basic manual. 4th ed. Philadelphia: Davis, 1974.

4 Dreyer, S. and others A guide to nursing management of psychiatric patients. St Louis: Mosby, 1975.

5 Evans, F. M. C. Psychosocial nursing: theory and practice in hospital and community and mental health. New York: Macmillan, 1971.

6 Fowlie, H. C. Psychiatry in comprehensive nursing. Collins, 1972.

7 Gibson, J. Psychiatry for nurses. 3rd ed. Oxford: Blackwell, 1971.

8 Kalman, M. E. and Davis, A. J., editors New dimensions in mental health psychiatric nursing. 4th ed. New York: McGraw-Hill, 1974.

9 Kyes, J. J. and Hofling, C. K. Basic psychiatric concepts in nursing. 3rd ed. Philadelphia: Lippincott, 1974.

10 Longhorn, E. Psychiatric care and conditions. Aylesbury: H.M. & M. 1975. (Nursing modules series.)

11 Maddison, D. and others. Psychiatric nursing. 4th ed. Edinburgh: Churchill Livingstone, 1975.

12 Manfreda, M. L. Psychiatric nursing. 9th ed. Philadelphia: Davis, 1973.

13 Mereness, D. A. & Taylor, C. M. Essentials of psychiatric nursing. 9th ed. St. Louis: Mosby, 1974.

14 Roberts, T. A handbook for psychiatric nurses. Bristol: Wright, 1971.

15 Robinson, A. M. Working with the mentally ill. 4th ed. Philadelphia: Lippincott, 1971.

16 Robinson, L. Psychiatric nursing as a human experience. Philadelphia: Saunders, 1972.

17 Saxton, D. F. and Haring, P. W. Care of the patient with emotional problems: a textbook for practical nurses. St. Louis: Mosby, 1971.

18 Sheahan, J. Essential psychiatry for nurses: a guide to important principles for nurses and laboratory technicians. Lancaster Medical and Technical Publishing, 1973.

19 Sim, M. Guide to psychiatry. 3rd ed. Edinburgh: Churchill Livingstone, 1974.

20 Sim, M. and Gordon, E. B. Basic psychiatry. 2nd ed. Edinburgh: Churchill Livingstone, 1972.

b GENERAL

1 Campbell, W. Nursing practice at John Connolly Hospital. Nursing Times, 67, 18 Nov 1971, 1427–1429.

2 Chase, L. G. The visiting professional. [An American nurse spends five weeks at Dingleton Hospital.] Nursing Outlook, 19 (5), May 1971, 322–324.

3 Cheadle, A. J. Statistical ratings for psychiatric patients. [A rating scale to assess progress, developed at St. Wulstan's Hospital, Malvern.] Nursing Times, 71, 24 Jul 1975, 1182–1185.

4 Cox, A. Group nursing at Stratheden. Nursing Mirror, 132, 19 Mar 1971, 33–35.

5 Dalton, M. H. Psychiatric nursing moves forward. [Symposium at St. James's Hospital, 'A new look at psychiatry.'] Nursing Mirror, 141, 30 Oct 1975, 35.

6 Gibson, J. Open forum. Nurse – or not? Nursing Mirror, 132, 11 Jun 1971, 31.

7 Harries, C. J. Rethinking psychiatric nursing care. Nursing Mirror, 133, 23 Jul 1971, 13–16.

8 Hobson, K. Nurse, teacher, or social therapist? Nursing Times, 67, 7 Jan 1971, 28.

9 Macpherson, E. L. R. Does 'care' cure? [In psychiatric nursing.] Nursing Times, 67, 2 Sep 1971, 1087–1088.

10 Marriner, E. J. Why become a psychiatric nurse? Nursing Mirror, 134, 10 Mar 1972, 24.

11 Morris, M. and Rhodes, M. Guidelines for the care of confused patients. American Journal of Nursing, 72 (9), Sep 1972, 1630–1633.

12 Nichol, G. A mental nursing tradition is born in Coventry. Nursing Times, 68, 29 Jun 1972, 810–811.

13 Nickless, G. N. Assessment within the psychiatric hospital. Nursing Mirror, 132, 2 Apr 1971, 38–39.

14 Pounds, V. A. Cinderella's debut: the past five years have proved fruitful in improving the status of psychiatric nurses and the standards of their hospitals. Nursing Times, 68, 22 Jun 1972, 787.

15 Ross, G. Student's choice: the team system in operation at St. Crispin Hospital, Northampton. Nursing Mirror, 133, 29 Oct 1971, 15–16.

16 Sharpe, D. Things have changed. [Changes over the past 15 years in psychiatric hospitals and psychiatric nursing.] Nursing Mirror, 134, 24 Mar 1972, 21–23.

17 Swanson, M. G. and Woolson, A. M. A new approach to the use of learning theory with psychiatric patients. Perspectives in Psychiatric Care, 10 (2), Jun 1972, 55–68.

18 Towell, D. Understanding psychiatric nursing: a sociological study of modern psychiatric nursing practice. Rcn, 1975 (Research series.) Based on a PhD thesis, Cambridge University, 1973.

19 Wallace, C. M. Psychiatrists versus nurses. Nursing Mirror, 134, 7 Jan 1972, 8–9.

c OVERSEAS COUNTRIES

1 American Nurses' Association Professional development in psychiatric and mental health nursing. Kansas City: ANA, 1975.

2 Asuni, T. Psychiatric nursing as seen from the point of view of a psychiatrist. Nigerian Nurse, 4 (3), Jul/Sep 1972, 12, 14–15, 19.

3 Bazley, M. Commonwealth, scholarship study. [Of psychiatric nursing.] New Zealand Nursing Journal, 64 (8), Aug 1971, 4–6.

4 Bazley, M. Psychiatric nursing in New Zealand. International Journal of Nursing Studies, 10 (2), May 1973, 103–108.

5 Boughton, J. A. and Alchin, S. The psychiatric nurse – a professional stereotype? Australian Nurses' Journal, 3 (5), Nov 1973, 34–35, 45.

6 Dasler, K. A. Advances in psychiatric nursing. New Zealand Nursing Journal, 66 (6), Jun 1973, 16–17, 20.

7 Davis, A. J. Psychiatric problems and services in Kenya. International Nursing Review, 22 (1), Jan/Feb 1975, 25–27.

8 Ganzevoort, J. New tasks for psychiatric nurses. [Work in a socio-therapeutic community in the Netherlands.] International Nursing Review, 22 (4), Jul/Aug 1975, 109–112.

9 Gedan, S. This I believe . . . about psychiatric nursing practice. Nursing Outlook, 19 (8), Aug 1971, 534–536.

10 Grant, R. and Sanford, N. The way it will be: psychiatric nursing in the United States. International Nursing Review, 20 (2), Mar/Apr 1973, 47–48.

11 Hortling, E. Psychiatric nursing and nursing education in Finland. International Journal of Nursing Studies, 9 (4), Nov 1972, 185–192.

12 Irish Nurses' Organization INO memorandum to working party on psychiatric nursing services. Irish Nurses Journal, 4 (5), May 1971, 8–10.

13 Kappelmuller, I. I. Psychiatric nursing in Austria. International Journal of Nursing Studies, 10 (2), May 1973, 87–93.

14 Lee, L. P. N. A. C. – Twenty-two years of progress. [Psychiatric Nurses Association of Canada.] Canadian Journal of Psychiatric Nursing, 13 (2), Mar/Apr 1972, 8–11.

15 Muscat, J. The care of the mentally ill, and psychiatric nursing in Malta. International Journal of Nursing Studies, 10 (1), Jan 1973, 43–52.

16 Sekamaganga, T. N. A nurse in Tanzania. [Psychiatric nursing services.] Journal of Psychiatric Nursing and Mental Health Services, 13 (3), May/Jun 1975, 37–39.

17 Sekamaganga, T. N. A nurse in Tanzania: how a developing country has been able to adapt some modern methods of care for mental patients. World Health, Oct 1974, 12–15.

18 Sharma, G. C. and Dubay, B. L. Personality of the psychiatric male and female nurses – a comparative study. Nursing Journal of India, 46 (11), Nov 1975, 257–258.

19 Simmons, S. M. Psychiatric nursing in Connecticut. Nursing Times, 71, 19 Jun 1975, 984–985.

20 Stockdale, P. Psychiatric nursing – what is it? UNA Nursing Journal, 2, Mar/Apr 1974, 19.

21 Traux, C. B. Towards effective psychiatric nursing: the beginning of self-learning. Canadian Journal of Psychiatric Nursing, 6 (6), Nov/Dec 1972, 8–13.

22 Turner, P. An optimistic look at psychiatric nursing. New Zealand Nursing Journal, 66 (3), Mar 1973, 17.

d ATTITUDES

1 Brink, P. J. Role distance: a manoeuver in nursing. [Nurses' inappropriate behaviour at a daily conference in a psychiatric unit.] Nursing Forum, 11 (3), 1972, 323–332.

2 Burton, D. A. Nursing attitudes to mental illness: a questionnaire study of the effectiveness of a three month's psychiatric course. MA thesis, Leicester University, 1974.

3 Caulfield, J. The nurse and the patient – the need to examine objectively our attitudes and behaviour towards psychiatric patients. Nursing Mirror, 139, 10 Oct 1974, 48.

4 Clark, C. C. Tactics for counteracting staff apathy and hopelessness on a psychiatric unit. Journal of Psychiatric Nursing and Mental Health Services, 13 (3), May–Jun 1975, 3–5.

5 Distefano, M. K. and Pryer, M. W. Effect of brief training on mental health knowledge and attitudes of nurses and nurses' aides in a general hospital. Nursing Research, 24 (1), Jan/Feb 1975, 40–42.

6 Fabrega, H. and Brouse, S. Semantic and stylistic features of nursing students' knowledge of mental illness. Nursing Research, 20 (4), Jul/Aug 1971, 352–356.

7 Frost, M. Institutionalization of mental nurses. British Hospital Journal and Social Service Review, 82, 5 Feb 1972, 301–302.

8 Godejohn, C. J. and others Effect of simulation gaming on attitudes toward mental illness. [An investigation of student nurses' attitudes.] Nursing Research, 24 (5), Sep–Oct 1975, 367–370.

9 Hall, J. N. Nurses' attitudes and specialized treatment settings: an exploratory study. [Use of attitude scales to select students for work on a behaviour modification ward.] British Journal of Social and Clinical Psychology, 13 (3), Sep 1974, 333–334.

10 Harries, C. J. Nursing preference in psychiatric hospitals. [Preference for particular wards and particular patients.] Nursing Times, 68, 25 May 1972, Occ. papers, 81–84.

11 Holmes, G. R. and others Nursing students' attitude changes toward psychiatric patients. [Research study of students assigned to three different treatment settings.] Journal of Psychiatric Nursing and Mental Health Services, 13 (3), May/Jun 1975, 6–10.

12 McCarthy, C. L. and others Nurses' attitudes and expectations toward psychiatric patients with multiple readmissions. Nursing Research, 22 (5), Sep/Oct 1973, 427–431.

13 Meyer, L. M. Comparison of attitudes toward mental patients of junior and senior nursing students and their university peers. Nursing Research, 22 (3), May/Jun 1973, 242–245.

14 Nursing Times A time of isolation: an indictment of attitudes towards mental illness through the eyes of a general nurse. Nursing Times, 71, 10 Apr 1975, 590–591.

15 Rickelman, B. L. Reactions of staff to psychiatric patients. Nursing Forum, 13 (2), 1974, 147–156.

16 Swain, H. L. Nursing students' attitudes towards mental illness. Nursing Research, 22 (1), Jan/Feb 1973, 59–65.

17 Thomas, N. W. Attitudes to mental illness. [Survey carried out among the general public, university students and nursing students by the John Conolly/Rubery Hill Hospitals Training School.] Nursing Times, 70, 7 Mar 1974, 350–351.

18 Walsh, J. E. Instruction in psychiatric nursing, level of anxiety, and direction of attitude change toward the mentally ill. Nursing Research, 20 (6), Nov/Dec 1971, 522–529.

e ROLE

1 Bowling, T. Nursing care study: the changing role of the psychiatric nurse. Nursing Mirror, 139, 19 Jul 1974, 85–86.

2 Christie, L. S. Conflicting needs and concepts in psychiatric hospitals. [The importance to the work of the psychiatric nurse.] Nursing Times, 71, 18 Dec 1975, 2036–2037.

3 Davis, M. K. Intrarole conflict and job satisfaction on psychiatric units: [with particular reference to nurses' expectations of involvement in decision making.] Nursing Research, 23 (6), Nov–Dec 1974, 482–488.

4 Fraser, D. and Cormack, D. The nurse's role in psychiatric institutions. 1. [Studies showing deficiencies in nurse/patient interaction.] Nursing Times, 71, 18 Dec 1975, Occ. papers, 125–127.

5 Fraser, D. and Cormack, D. The nurse's role in psychiatric institutions. 2. [Considers the constraints placed upon the psychiatric nurse by various factors which limit the development of her therapeutic potential.] Nursing Times, 71, 25 Dec 1975, Occ. papers, 129–132.

6 Golden, K. The role of the psychiatric nurse. Report from the I.M.A. Conference. World of Irish Nursing, 1 (8), Aug 1972, 159–160.

7 Larson, M. L. From psychiatric to psychosocial nursing. Nursing Outlook, 21 (8), Aug 1973, 520–523.

8 McIvor, D. L. Psychiatric nurses provide leadership. [A psychologist's view of psychiatric nurses.] Canadian Journal of Psychiatric Nursing, 16 (6), Nov/Dec 1975, 7.

9 Sedgwick, R. Nursing's contribution to social psychiatry; a holistic approach to personhood. [Nurse's role in preventive psychiatricy.] International Nursing Review, 22 (6), Nov/Dec 1975, 177–180.

10 Talent, N. and others An expanded role for psychiatric nursing personnel: psychological evaluation and interpersonal care. Journal of Psychiatric Nursing and Mental Health Services, 10 (3), May/Jun 1974, 19–23.

f CLINICAL NURSE SPECIALIST

1 Armacost, B. and others A group of 'problem patients'. [Group meetings between nurses and patients, led by a psychiatric nurse consultant.] American Journal of Nursing, 74 (2), Feb 1974, 289–292.

2 Bermosk, L. Students learn to negotiate for role and demonstrate skill as group. [Training of clinical specialists in psychiatric nursing for work in an interdisciplinary mental health team.] Journal of Psychiatric Nursing and Mental Health Services, 11 (5), Sep/Oct 1973, 16–19.

3 Colbert, L. The psychiatric nurse clinical specialist works with nursing service. Journal of Psychiatric Nursing, 9 (4), Jul–Aug 1971, 21–22.

4 Denny, E. D. The clinical specialist: a role model for students during their psychiatric experience. Journal of Psychiatric Nursing, 10 (3), May/Jun 1972, 14–17.

5 Hanson, E. T. Nurse practitioners in ambulatory psychiatric care. Nursing Clinics of North America, 8 (2), Jun 1973, 313–323.

6 Henrion, R. P. At which level does the psychiatric clinical specialist practice? [The role of the psychiatric clinical nurse specialist.] Journal of Psychiatric Nursing and Mental Health Services, 12 (3), May/Jun 1974, 14–18.

7 McElroy, E. and Narciso, A. Clinical specialist in the community mental health program. Journal of Psychiatric Nursing, 9 (1), Jan/Feb 1971, 19–23, 26.

8 Mesnick, J. Clinical nurse specialists: seeing the forest and the trees. [Work of a internal health clinical nurse specialist.] Canadian Journal of Psychiatric Nursing, 16 (5), Sep–Oct 1975, 7–9.

9 Rodgers, J. A. The clinical specialist as a change agent. Journal of Psychiatric Nursing and Mental Health Services, 12 (6), Nov–Dec 1974, 5–9.

10 Schuler, S. and Campbell, L. B. The theme is change. [A head nurse and a psychiatric nurse clinical specialist act as nurse leaders in an organizational change in a psychiatric unit.] Journal of Psychiatric Nursing and Mental Health Services, 12 (4), Jul/Aug 1974, 15–22.

11 Stachyra, M. Self-regulation through certification: a rationale for certification of clinical specialists in psychiatric mental health nursing. Perspectives of Psychiatric Care, 11 (4), Oct/Dec 1973, 148–154.

12 Stafford, L. F. The clinical specialist in the geographic unit system. [The role of the psychiatric clinical nurse specialist in a hospital unit.] Journal of Psychiatric Nursing and Mental Health Services, 11 (6), Nov/Dec 1973, 22–25.

13 Termini, M. and Hauser, M. J. The process of the supervisory relationship [in the preparation of graduate students for the role of clinical nurse specialist.] Perspectives in Psychiatric Care, 11 (3), Jul/Sep 1973, 121–125.

14 Whitehead, J. A. Clinical responsibility and its proper reward. [An investigation into a clinical role for senior psychiatric nurses.] Nursing Mirror, 134, 21 Apr 1972, 42.

g EDUCATION AND TRAINING

1 Aitken, J. and others Improving general nurse training by psychiatric secondment. Nursing Times, 70, 27 Jun 1974, Occ. papers, 29–32.

2 Andrews, J. Teaching psychiatric nursing. [Rcn conference.] Nursing Mirror, 133, 24 Sep 1971, 12–13.

3 Arje, F. B. and others, editors Psychiatric-mental health nursing: 1500 multiple choice questions and referenced answers. 3rd ed. Flushing: Medical Examination Publishing Co, 1972. (Nursing Examination review book no 2.)

4 Bhattacharya, A. Examining in psychiatric nursing. Nursing Times, 70, 8 Aug 1974, 1237–1239.

5 Budge, U. V. Psychiatric nursing needs. [Letter commenting on the proposals for psychiatric training outlined in Briggs.] Nursing Mirror, 139, 5 Dec 1974, 42–43.

6 Cormack, D. Clinical teaching in a psychiatric hospital. Nursing Times, 68, 5 Oct 1972, 1261–1262; 12 Oct 1972, 1289–1290.

7 Damant, M. Community training for mental nurses. [Scheme in Leicestershire.] Health and Social Service Journal, 85, 8 Mar 1975, 547.

8 Darcy, P. T. Practical learning for psychiatric nurses. Nursing Mirror, 140, 5 Jun 1975, 61–62.

9 Darwin, E. J. An opportunity for married women. [Views of students on an experimental scheme of part-time training in psychiatric nursing for married women at Netherne Hospital.] Nursing Times, 69, 13 Dec 1973, 1696–1697.

10 Frost, M. SRNs' dilemma in psychiatry. [SRNs' reactions to psychiatric training.] Nursing Mirror, 134, 19 May 1972, 42–43.

11 Kenworthy, N. The new intermediate examination in mental nursing: a descriptive evaluation. Nursing Times, 68, 17 Aug 1972, Occ. papers, 129–132.

12 McIntegart, J. P. Learning and the psychiatric nurse. [In-service training at unit level at Exe Vale Hospital.] Nursing Mirror, 137, 28 Sep 1973, 12–13, 27.

13 Nursing Times Teaching psychiatric nursing. Nursing Times, 67, 30 Sep 1971, 1226.

14 Nursing Times Training the psychiatric nurse of the future. [Post registration RMN training recently started at St. Luke's-Woodside Hospital.] Nursing Times, 69, 15 Mar 1973, 346–348.

15 O'Hare, B. and Ragg, W. Working with small groups. 1. Foreword. 2. Sensitivity training in a conventional mental hospital. [Inservice training at Downshire Hospital.] Nursing Times, 68, 28 Sep 1972, Occ. papers, 153–156.

16 Pattemore, J. C. Assessing the psychiatric student. Nursing Times, 68, 7 Dec 1972, 1560–1561.

17 Reavley, W. and Winkley, J. C. A training programme for assessors. Nursing Times, 67, 30 Sep 1971, Occ. papers, 153–154.

18 Roberts, T. Advice to assessors: a pattern for psychiatric examination assessors. Nursing Mirror, 132, 5 Feb 1971, 16–17.

19 Roberts, M. Untangling the confusing: the differing needs and training necessary in the specialised fields of mental illness and mental handicap. Nursing Times, 70, 3 Oct 1974, 1555.

h EDUCATION AND TRAINING: OVERSEAS COUNTRIES

1 Adams, J. A quantitative follow up study of nursing student reactions to an interactional group experience. Journal of Psychiatric Nursing, 10 (5), Sep/Oct 1972, 11–14.

2 Adams, J. Student evaluation of an interactional group experience. Journal of Psychiatric Nursing, 9 (4), Jul–Aug 1971, 28–36. Follow up study, 9 (6), Nov/Dec 1971, 17–20.

3 Anderson, C. J. and Sainato, H. K. Ward based hospital in-service education for psychiatric nurses. Washington: National Institute of Mental Health, 1972.

4 Balgopal, P. R. Variations in sensitivity training groups. Perspectives in Psychiatric Care, 11 (2), Apr/Jun 1973, 80–86.

5 Bolzoni, N. J. and Geach, P. Premature reassurance: a distancing maneuver. [How the instructor can help students communicate with psychiatric patients.] Nursing Outlook, 23 (1), Jan 1975, 49–51.

6 Burr, J. C. Where the nurse is the treatment. [Education of psychiatric nurses and aspects of psychiatric training with general nurse training.] Australian Nurses Journal, 4 (2), Aug 1974, 31–33, 47.

7 Cowell, D. The practice of nursing. Psychiatric care. [Future training of psychiatric nursing as seen by the 'Goals in nursing education' report.] Australian Nurses' Journal, 5 (3), Sep 1975, 9–12.

8 Davidhizar, R. H. Stress patients: a new dimension in psychiatric nursing education. Perspectives in Psychiatric Care, 11 (3), Jul/Sep 1973, 129–131.

9 Deloughery, G. W. and others Teaching organizational concepts to nurses in community mental health. Journal of Nursing Education, 8 (1), Jan 1974, 8–14.

10 Farnsworth, J. Camp: Computer and me, psychotherapeutically. [The feasibility of using computer programs in psychiatric nursing education.] Journal of Nursing Education, 13 (4), Nov 1974, 26–29.

11 Geach, B. The problem solving technique: as taught to psychiatric students. Perspectives in Psychiatric Care, 12 (1), Jan/Mar 1974, 9–12.

12 George, I. V. H. Sister tutors' refresher course [in psychiatric nursing.] Nursing Journal of India, 52 (8), Aug 1971, 255, 277.

13 Habeeb, M. C. and others Experiential teaching. [eight-week course in psychiatric nursing.] American Journal of Nursing, 71 (8), Aug 1971, 1568–1571.

14 Kamp. M. and Burnside, I. M. Computer-assisted learning in graduate psychiatric nursing. Journal of Nursing Education, 13 (4), Nov 1974, 18–25.

15 Mealey, A. R. and Peterson, T. L. Self-actualization of nursing students resulting from a course in psychiatric nursing. Nursing Research, 23 (2), Mar/Apr 1974, 138–143.

16 Navin, H. L. Psychiatric nursing education at a 'General'. Australian Nurses' Journal, 1 (8), Feb 1972, 31–32.

17 Nelson, K. J. and Hesbacher, P. Sensitivity training in psychiatric nursing: evolution and evaluation of a student group experience. Journal of Psychiatric Nursing, 10 (5), Sep/Oct 1972, 21–26.

18 Padilla, E. and Goldston, S. E. Nurses and mental health training in schools of public health in the United States. International Nursing Review, 20 (3), May/Jun 1973, 82–84.

19 Palmer, I. S. and Borofsky, R. B. Boston University School of Nursing. Graduate program in psychiatric nursing. Perspectives in Psychiatric Care, 10 (5), Dec 1972, 232–235.

20 Price, J. L. and others Value assumptions in humanistic psychiatric nursing education. Perspectives in Psychiatric Care, 12 (2), Apr/Jun, 64–69.

21 Reischel, H. J. Nurse education in mental health, Victoria: past, present and future. UNA Nursing Journal, 2, Mar/Apr 1974, 14–17.

22 Sauber, S. R. and Campbell, J. Psychiatric nursing: facilitating the development of a helping person. [A social psychological model of learning.] Journal of Psychiatric Nursing and Mental Health Services, 12 (4), Jul/Aug 1974, 23–27.

23 Smith, E. F. B. Teaching group therapy in an undergraduate curriculum. Perspectives in Psychiatric Care, 11 (2), Apr/Jun 1973, 704.

24 Spitz, H. and Saddock, B. J. Small interactional groups in the psychiatric training of graduate nursing students. Journal of Nursing Education, 12 (2), Apr 1973, 6–13.

25 Strong, P. G. Psychiatric nurse education in Finland. [National Florence Nightingale Memorial Committee Scholarship study tour.] Nursing Mirror, 141, 30 Oct 1975, 71–73.

i MANAGEMENT AND STAFFING

1 Adamson, G. The organisation of a ward in a psychiatric hospital. Social Service Quarterly, 47 (2), Oct/Dec 1973, 55–59, 66.

2 Boyle, M. A. Will the charge nurse ever change her spots? [Extension of her role after release from non-nursing duties.] Australian Nurses' Journal, 4 (10), May 1975, 36–38.

3 Cheadle, J. Three weeks in the life of a psychiatric charge nurse. [Work study.] Nursing Mirror, 133, 22 Oct 1971, 39–42.

4 Christie, L. S. Researching staffing needs in psychiatric hospitals. Nursing Times, 70, 28 Nov 1974, 1870–1871.

5 Cormack, D. F. S. A descriptive study of the work of the charge nurse in acute admission wards of psychiatric hospitals. MPhil thesis, Edinburgh University, 1975. Reported in Nursing Mirror, 141, 24 Jul 1975, 57.

6 Fenn, M. F. Consultation – the road to change. [The integration of male and female patients in a psychiatric hospital.] Nursing Mirror, 135, 11 Aug 1972, 40–41.

7 Frost, M. Giving and taking reports in psychiatric hospitals. Nursing Times, 67, 7 Jan 1971, 7–9.

8 Frost, M. Psychiatric patients at night. [Observations made in a 15-bed mixed psychiatric unit within a general hospital.] Nursing Times, 70, 2 May 1974, 658–659; 9 May 1974, 708–709.

9 Hadley, R. D. and others The SEN in the psychiatric hospital. Nursing Mirror, 139, 30 Aug 1974, 65–68.

10 Lynch, C. C. Management of nursing care on a psychiatric service. Nursing Clinics of North America, 8 (2), Jun 1973, 293–303.

11 Mercer, A. D. A model for nursing cost: for long stay psychiatric wards based on degree of ambulance. [Research survey.] Hospital and Health Services Review, 71 (6), Jun 1975, 194–195.

12 Moores, B. Nursing expenditure variables in mental illness and mental subnormality hospitals. Nursing Times, 68, 9 Nov 1972, Occ. papers, 177–180.

13 Noble, M. A. Organizational structure, ideology and personality in psychiatric nursing. Journal of Psychiatric Nursing, 9 (4), Jul/Aug 1971, 11–17.

14 Ride, T. Psychiatric patients at night. [The work of the psychiatric nurse on night duty.] New Psychiatry, 1, 17 Oct 1974, 10–11.

15 Seager, J. H. C. Modernizing night administration in a psychiatric hospital. [Shelton Hospital, Shrewsbury.] Nursing Times, 69, 4 Jan 1973, Occ.papers, 1–4.

16 Sharpe, D. Multidisciplinary management – a psychiatric nurse's view. [The work of a professional executive.] Nursing Mirror, 140, 23 Jan 1975, 73–74.

17 South West Metropolitan Regional Hospital Board Developing the role of she SEN: a staffing experiment in a psychiatric hospital. The Hospital Board, 1972.

18 Taylor-Brown, N. Salmon in a psychiatric hospital group 7. The link with domestic services. Nursing Mirror, 132, 1 Jan 1971, 38–39.

19 Willer, B. and Stasiak, E. Automated nursing notes in a psychiatric institution. Journal of Psychiatric Nursing, 11 (2), Mar/Apr 1973, 27–29.

j NURSE PATIENT RELATIONSHIP

1 Altschul, A. T. Patient-nurse interaction: a study of interaction patterns in acute psychiatric wards. Edinburgh: Churchill Livingstone, 1972. (University of Edinburgh Department of Nursing Studies, Monograph 3.) Based on 'Measurement of patient-nurse interaction in relation to in-patient psychiatric treatment.' MSc (Soc Sci) thesis, Edinburgh University, 1968.

2 Altschul, A. T. Relationships between patients and nurses in psychiatric wards. International Journal of Nursing Studies, 8 (3), Aug 1971, 179–186.

3 Bleazard, R. An approach to psychiatric nursing. A therapeutic relationship between the nurse and the psychiatric patient requires full acceptance of the patient as a person. Nursing Times, 71, 16 Oct 1975, 1654–1656.

4 Briggs, P. F. Specialising in psychiatry: therapeutic or custodial? [Constant supervision in a one-to-one relationship.] Nursing Outlook, 22 (10), Oct 1974, 632–635.

5 Burkett, A. D. A way to communicate [with psychiatric patients by using games and pictures]. American Journal of Nursing, 74 (12), Dec 1974, 2185–2187.

6 Cheadle, J. The rejected patient. Nursing Times, 67, 21 Jan 1971, 81–84.

7 De Cangas, J. P. C. The science of nursing. [The patient as a person.] Canadian Journal of Psychiatric Nursing, 16 (2), Mar–Apr 1975, 6–7.

8 Fanning, V. L. and others Patient involvement in planning own care: staff and patient attitudes. Journal of Psychiatric Nursing, 10 (1), Jan/Feb 1972, 5–8.

9 Francis, N. Teamwork in action. [Staff and patient partnership at Cassel Hospital, Richmond, Surrey.] New Psychiatry, 2, 14 Aug 1975, 16–17.

10 Frost, M. 'Acting out' in psychiatric patients. Nursing Times, 67, 13 May 1971, 573–574.

11 Hall, B. A. Socializing hospitalized patients into the psychiatric sick role. Perspectives in Psychiatric Care, 8 (3), Jul–Sep 1975, 123–129.

12 Horton, L. What will happen to Mr. Lang? [The effect on a patient brought out of his lethargy by a nursing student, when that student has to leave him?] Canadian Nurse, 69 (5), May 1973, 39–40.

13 Johnson, M. N. and Olatawura Cross-cultural psychotherapy. [Nurse-client relationship between a West African and a nurse educated in America.] International Journal of Nursing Studies, 12 (2), Jul 1975, 95–105.

14 Journal of Psychiatric Nursing Aspects of the Petrie test in psychiatric patients. Journal of Psychiatric Nursing, 11 (2), Mar/Apr 1973, 15–16.

15 Klingbeil, A. Toward an understanding of the behaviours of persons experiencing mental health problems. Jamaican Nurse, 12 (3), Dec 1972, 28–30.

16 Leonard, C. V. Patient attitudes toward nursing interventions [in a psychiatric hospital.] Nursing Research, 24 (5), Sep–Oct 1975, 335–339.

17 Leslie, J. A. Nurse-patient therapy. [A case study.] Nursing Times, 70, 15 Aug 1974, 1272–1273.

18 McFarland, G. K. and Apostoles, F. E. The nursing history in a psychiatric setting: adaptions to a variety of nursing care patterns and patient populations. Journal of Psychiatric Nursing and Mental Health Services, 13 (4), Jul/Aug 1975, 12–17.

19 Mansfield, E. Empathy: concept and identified psychiatric nursing behaviour. [Interactions between a psychiatric nurse and six patients were videotaped and rated on the Truax Accurate Empathy Scale.] Nursing Research, 22 (6), Nov/Dec 1973, 525–530.

20 Marshall, J. C. and Feeney, S. Structured versus intuitive intake interview. [Admission interviews with patients in mental hospitals.] Nursing Research, 21 (3), May/Jun 1972, 269–272.

21 Munsadia, I. D. Therapeutic effects of nurse patient relationships. Health Bulletin, 29 (2), Apr 1971, 73–78.

22 Oravan, S. K. Patients help plan nursing care. [The effectiveness of involving psychiatric patients in their own care.] Canadian Nurse, 68 (9), Sep 1972, 46–48.

23 Putten, T. V. The psychiatric nurse as the guardian of the ward atmosphere. Psychiatric Nursing and Mental Health Services, 12 (1), Jan/Feb 1974, 18–21.

24 Reuell, V. M. Nurse-managed care for psychiatric patients. [Motivating patients to take care of themselves.] American Journal of Nursing, 75 (7), Jul 1975, 1156–1157.

25 Roberts, T. Learning to understand. [Psychiatric nurses need to be particularly sensitive to the patient's motivation.] Nursing Mirror, 141, 28 Aug 1975, 63.

26 Speakman, J. My name is John. . . [Communication between staff and patients in psychiatric hospitals.] Nursing Mirror, 140, 1 May 1975, 65–66.

27 Spitzer, S. P. and Volk, B. A. Altercasting the difficult patient. American Journal of Nursing, 71 (4), Apr 1971, 732–735.

k PSYCHIATRIC CARE IN PHYSICAL ILLNESS

1 Brooks, P. W. A psychiatric liaison service in a general hospital. [Referrals to the Psychiatric Department from other wards in the Western General Hospital, Edinburgh.] Health Bulletin, 32 (1), Jan 1974, 23–27.

2 Burch, J. W. and Meredith, J. L. Help with problem patients: nurses as the core of a psychiatric team. [Patients having psychiatric problems in addition to physical illness.] American Journal of Nursing, 74 (11), Nov 1974, 2037–2038.

3 Cohen, R. G. Providing emotional support for the seriously ill. [Support provided by a psychiatric clinical nurse-specialist.] RN Magazine, 37 (10), Oct 1974, 62–64, 66, 68, 70.

4 Grace, M. J. The psychiatric specialist and medical – surgical patients. American Journal of Nursing, 74, Mar 1974, 481–483.

5 Joynes, V. A. Psychiatric nursing advisory service: results of six months' pilot study. [Service for general wards and accident and emergency department at Guy's Hospital.] Nursing Times, 70, 6 Jun 1974, 882–883.

6 Lindenberg, R. E. The need for crisis intervention in hospitals: as a part of total care, hospitals should treat the psychological crises that often accompany physical illness. Hospitals, 46 (1), 1 Jan 1972, 52–55, 110.

7 Zahourek, R. and Morrison, K. Help with problem patients: mental health nurses as consultants to staff nurses. [A psychiatric nurse consultation service in Denver provides help for general hospitals.] American Journal of Nursing, 74 (11), Nov 1974, 2034–2036.

76 PSYCHIATRIC NURSE THERAPIST

a GENERAL

1 Baker, R. The chronic psychiatric patient – a new hope for treatment? [Use of operant conditioning.] Nursing Times, 68, 14 Sep 1972, 1161–1163.

2 Boorer, D. Conference report. . . the biggest breakthrough since chlorpromazine? [Conference on 'The Psychiatric Nurse as Therapist'.] Nursing Times, 69, 3 May 1973, 585.

3 Chesser, E. S. and Robertson, J. R. Behaviour therapy. 1. The behavioural approach. Nursing Times, 71, 24 Jul 1975, 1168–1169.

4 Connolly, J. The psychiatric nurse as therapist. 5. The psychiatric nurse and the adult neurotic. Nursing Times, 69, 27 Sep 1973, Occ. papers, 153–156.

5 Connolly, T. Nursing care study. Peter – a response to behaviour modification. Nursing Times, 71, 6 Feb 1975, 217–218.

6 Graveling, B. and others Relax and recover. [Relaxation classes and behaviour therapy conducted by nurses at Hellesdon Hospital, Norwich.] Nursing Times, 68, 10 Aug 1972, 996–998.

7 Gray, M. Behaviour modification in a long-term psychotic ward. [Rewards for good behaviour.] Nursing Times, 68, 4 May 1972, 540–541.

8 Haffner, C. Psychiatric nurse as therapist. [Correspondence.] British Medical Journal, 3, 8 Sep 1973, 545.

9 Hall, J. N. and Rosenthall, G. The psychiatric nurse as therapist. 3. Operant treatment of the long-term patient. Nursing Times, 69, 6 Sep 1973; 13 Sep 1973, Occ. papers, 143–148.

10 Hallam, R. S. The training of nurse-therapists. Nursing Mirror, 140, 8 May 1975, 48–50.

11 Kiernan, C. The psychiatric nurse as therapist. 4. Behaviour modification and the nurse. Nursing Times, 69, 20 Sep 1973, Occ. papers, 149–152.

12 Langworthy, S. A token economy experiment. [Warlingham Hospital.] Health and Social Service Journal, 84, 11 May 1974, 1046–1047.

13 Love, M. J. Behaviour therapy. Nursing Times, 67, 23 Sep 1971, 1180–1182.

14 McArdle, M. A nurse-therapist's viewpoint. Nursing Mirror, 140, 8 May 1975, 55–56.

15 McArdle, M. Treatment of a phobia. [Case study of treatment by a psychiatric nurse therapist.] Nursing Times, 70, 25 Apr 1974. 637–639.

16 Macilwaine, H. Behaviour therapy. 3. Home treatment of a patient by a ward staff nurse. Nursing Times, 71, 7 Aug 1975, 1250–1251.

17 Marks, I. Introduction and overview. [Symposium on the psychiatric nurse-therapist.] Nursing Mirror, 140, 8 May 1975, 46–48.

18 Marks, I. The psychiatric nurse as therapist: developments and problems. Introduction. Nursing Times, 69, 30 Aug 1973, Occ. papers, 137–138.

19 Marks, I. M. and others Nurse therapists in behavioural psychotherapy. [Training of five RMN's at the Maudsley Hospital.] British Medical Journal, 3, 19 Jul 1975, 144–148.

20 Marks, I. M. and others Psychiatric nurse as therapist. British Medical Journal, 3, 21 Jul 1973, 156–160.

21 Marks, I. M. and others The psychiatric nurse as therapist. 1. An advanced nursing role. Nursing Mirror, 136, 2 Mar 1973, 21.

22 Morrice, J. K. The psychotherapeutic role of the nurse. Nursing Times, 71, 9 Oct 1975, 1634–1635.

23 Nursing Mirror A symposium on the psychiatric nurse-therapist: a new form of clinical nurse specialist from the Institute of Psychiatry, Maudsley Hospital, London. Nursing Mirror, 140, 8 May 1975, 46–64.

24 Nursing Times The psychiatric nurse as therapist: collected papers based on addresses given at the conference organized by the British Association for Behavioural Pscyhotherapy. Macmillan Journals, 1973.

25 Ojo, J. Habit training – a critical analysis. [Re-education of the long-stay psychiatric patient.] Nursing Times, 69, 4 Oct 1973, 1282–1283.

26 Peck, D. F. The psychiatric nurse as therapist. 1. An agent of behaviour change. Nursing Times, 69, 30 Aug 1973, Occ. papers, 139.

27 Rosenthall, G. and others The chronic psychiatric patient – a new hope for treatment? A study of operant conditioning – 2. Nursing Times, 68, 21 Sep 1972, 1182–1185.

28 Saunders, W. M. and Miller, A. Occupational therapy versus operant conditioning techniques in the treatment of long term psychiatric patients. British Journal of Occupational Therapy, 38 (5), May 1975, 103–107.

29 Tatlow, A. Behaviour therapy. 2. A training for nurses. [Domiciliary treatment.] Nursing Times, 71, 31 Jul 1975, 1212–1213.

30 Tatlow, A. Behaviour therapy – 4. Treatment of multiple problems. Nursing Times, 71, 14 Aug 1975, 1299–1300.

b OVERSEAS COUNTRIES

1 Agras, W. S., editor Behaviour modification: principles and clinical applications. Boston: Little Brown, 1972.

2 Anderson, C. J. and Sainato, H. K. Use of videotape feedback as a psychotherapeutic nursing approach with long-term psychiatric patients; a pilot study. Nursing Research, 22 (6), Nov/Dec 1973, 507–515.

3 Berni, R. and Fordyce, W. E. Behaviour modification and the nursing process. St. Louis: Mosby, 1973.

4 Branson, H. K. The nurse's role in behaviour modification. Nursing Care, 8 (12), Dec 1975, 21–23.

5 Carignan, T. Self-motivation and self-control in operant conditioning. [Nurses as primary change agents.] Perspectives in Psychiatric Care, 12 (1), Jan/Mar 1974, 36–41.

6 Closurdo, J. S. Behavior modification and the nursing process. Perspectives in Psychiatric Care, 8 (1), Jan–Mar 1975, 25–36.

7 Freitas, L. and Johnson, L. Behavior modification approach in a partial day treatment center. [San Diego, California.] Journal of Psychiatric Nursing and Mental Health Services, 13 (2), Mar–Apr 1975, 14–18.

8 Gedan, S. and others The nurse therapist: a staff nurse position which emphasizes clinical practice. Journal of Psychiatric Nursing, 11 (1), Jan/Feb 1973, 18–23.

9 Graff, H. and others Nurses as multiple therapists. Journal of Psychiatric Nursing, 11 (1), Jan/Feb 1973, 15–17.

10 Gralnick, A. and D'Elia, F. A social nursing-therapy service: concept and development [at High Point Hospital, Port Chester, New York.] International Journal of Social Psychiatry, 20 (1/2) Spring/Summer 1974, 1–7.

11 Johnson, W. G. and Groves, L. The token economy: a challenge to nursing. Journal of Psychiatric Nursing, 10 (3), May/Jun 1972, 10–13.

12 LeBow, M. D. Behaviour modification: a significant method in nursing practice. New Jersey: Prentice-Hall, 1973. (Scientific foundations of nursing practice series.)

13 Lego, S. Nurse psychotherapists: how are we different? Perspectives in Psychiatric Care, 11 (4), Oct/Dec 1973, 144–147.

14 Long, E. Y. and others Token economy programme in Singapore: report of a trial. Nursing Journal of Singapore, 13 (2), Nov 1973, 103–109.

15 Luiz, H. A. and Hotz, P. B. Psychotherapy training for nurses: a nursing necessity. S A Nursing Journal, 42 (8), Aug 1975, 8–9.

16 Marcus, A. M. and others Primary therapist project on an inpatient psychiatric unit. Canadian Nurse, 71 (9), Sep 1975, 30–33.

17 Martin, G. L. Behaviour modification to develop self control. Canadian Journal of Psychiatric Nursing, 56 (6), Nov/Dec 1975, 8–10.

18 Meldman, M. J. and others Patients' responses to nurse-psychotherapists. American Journal of Nursing, 71 (6), Jun 1971, 1150–1151.

19 Moscado, B. A. The psychiatric nurse as outpatient psychotherapist. Journal of Psychiatric Nursing and Mental Health Services, 13 (5), Sep/Oct 1975, 28–30.

20 Raeburn, J. and Soler, J. Behavior therapy approach to psychiatric disorder. Canadian Nurse, 67 (10), Oct 1971, 36–38.

21 Randolph, G. T. Experiences in private practice. [A nurse's experiences as a psychotherapist.] Journal of Psychiatric Nursing and Mental Health Services, 13 (6), Nov/Dec 1975, 16–19.

22 Redmond, G. T. A study of modification of socially acceptable eating behavior. [Using techniques of social approval and a token system.] Perspectives in Psychiatric Care, 11 (3), Jul/Sep 1973, 126–128.

23 Ujhely, G. B. The nurse as psychotherapist: what are the issues? Perspectives of Psychiatric Care, 11 (4), Oct/Dec 1974, 155–160.

24 Vidoni, C. The development of intensive positive countertransference feelings in the therapist toward a patient. American Journal of Nursing, 75 (3), Mar 1975, 407–409.

25 Williams, C. Behaviour modification for nurses: work schedule and manual Revised ed. Lew Hospital, Bromsgrove the author, 1974.

26 Wood, D. D. and others The nurse as therapist: assertion training to rehabilitate the chronic mental patient. Journal of Psychiatric Nursing and Mental Health Services, 13 (4), Jul/Aug 1975, 41–46.

c CRISIS INTERVENTION

1 Aguilera, D. C. and Messick, J. M. Crisis intervention: theory and methodology. 2nd ed. St. Louis: Mosby, 1974.

2 Ambury R. G. Crisis intervention in family and adolescent care. Nursing Mirror, 135, 17 Nov 1972, 33–35.

3 Birley, L. J. T. Emotional first aid. [Psychiatric casualty service at the Maudsley Hospital.] Nursing Times, 69, 6 Dec 1973, 1666.

4 Donner, G. J. Parenthood as a crisis: a role for the psychiatric nurse. Perspectives in Psychiatric Care, 10 (2), Jun 1972, 84–87.

5 Frederick, C. J. The role of the nurse in crisis intervention and suicide prevention. Journal of Psychiatric Nursing, 11 (1), Jan/Feb 1973, 27–31.

6 Grier, A. M. and Aldrich, C. K. The growth of a crisis intervention unit under the direction of a clinical specialist in psychiatric nursing. Perspectives in Psychiatric Care, 10 (2), Jun 1972, 73–83.

7 Lieb, J. and others The crisis team: a handbook for the mental health professional. Hagerstown, Maryland: Harper & Row, 1973.

8 McKenzie, D. J. Training for crisis therapy. Australian Nurses' Journal, 4 (9), Apr 1975, 24–27.

9 Mazzola, R. and Jacobs, G. B. Helping the patient and the family deal with a crisis situation. Journal of Neurosurgical Nursing, 6 (2), Dec 1974, 85–88.

10 Messick, J. M. Crisis-intervention concepts: implications for nursing practices. Journal of Psychiatric Nursing, 10 (5), Sep/Oct 1972, 3–5.

11 Mindham, R. H. S. and others A psychiatric casualty department. [Maudsley Hospital.] Lancet, 1, 26 May 1973, 1169–1171.

12 Navel, E. Crisis intervention: the nurses' role. Nursing Care, 6 (2), Feb 1973, 24–27.

13 Nursing Clinics of North America Symposium on crisis intervention. Nursing Clinics of North America, 9 (1), Mar 1974, 1–96.

14 Resnik, H. L. P. and others, editors Emergency psychiatric care: the management of mental health crises. Bowie: Charles Press Publishers, 1975.

15 Sheahan, J. First aid in mental distress. 1. Mental functions. Nursing Times, 67, 16 Dec 1971, 1559–1560.

16 Sheahan, J. First aid to mental distress. 2. Thinking and intelligence. Nursing Times, 67, 23 Dec 1971, 1608–1609.

17 Sheahan, J. First aid in mental distress. 3. Emotion and personality. Nursing Times, 67, 30 Dec 1971, 1638–1639.

18 Sheahan, J. Principles of relieving mental distress. Nursing Times, 68, 13 Jan 1972, 60–61.

19 Sheahan, J. Psychiatric emergencies. Occupational Health, 26 (6), Jun 1974, 214–219.

20 Sheahan, J. Signs of mental distress. Nursing Times, 68, 6 Jan 1972, 28–29.

21 Sheahan, J. Some states of mental distress. Nursing Times, 68, 20 Jan 1972, 94–95.

22 Shields, L. Crisis intervention: implications for the nurse. Journal of Psychiatric Nursing and Mental Health Services, 13 (5), Sep/Oct 1975, 37–42.

23 Smiley, O. R. and Smiley, C. W. The community health nurse and crisis intervention. [The successful management of the crisis situation.] International Nursing Review, 21 (5), Sep/Oct 1974, 151–152.

24 Wallace, M. A. and Fanning, V. L. Organization of emergency services: the crisis nurse in the community mental health center. Journal of Psychiatric Nursing and Mental Health Services, 11 (4), Jul/Aug 1973, 6–12.

d FAMILY THERAPY

1 Barry, M. P. Feedback concepts in family therapy. Perspectives in Psychiatric Care, 10 (4), Oct/Nov 1972, 183–189.

2 Cacciatore, E. W. Conjoint therapy as an adjunct to individual therapy. Journal of Psychiatric Nursing, 11 (2), Mar/Apr 1973, 19–24.

3 Haller, L. L. Family systems theory in psychiatric intervention. [Treatment of the family as a whole by a psychiatric nurse clinical specialist.] American Journal of Nursing, 74 (3), Mar 1974, 462–463.

4 Harrow, A. A nursing approach to multiple family group therapy. In Association for the Psychiatric Study of Adolescents. Proceedings of the fifth annual conference, Edinburgh, 1970. The Association, 1971.

5 Hartmann, K. and Bush, M. Action-oriented family therapy. [Role playing and home sessions.] American Journal of Nursing, 75, Jul 1975, 1184–1187.

6 Henrion, R. P. Family nurse therapist: a model of communication. Journal of Psychiatric Nursing and Mental Health Services, 12 (6), Nov–Dec 1974, 10–13.

7 Hill, S. The nurse as a family therapist. [With descriptions of sessions with two families.] Canadian Nurse, 70 (9), Sep 1974, 30–32.

8 Lynch, M. and others Family unit in a children's psychiatric hospital. [Unit concentrating on the psychotherapy of family problems at Park Hospital, Oxford.] British Medical Journal, 2, 19 Apr 1975, 127–129.

9 Macdonald, J. M. The emotional cripple – a family problem. [Nursing care study.] Nursing Times, 70, 14 Feb 1974, 236–237.

10 Monea, H. P. A family in trouble. [A case study of a family in conjoint family therapy.] Perspectives in Psychiatric Care, 12 (4), Oct–Dec 1974, 165–170.

11 Saper, B. Patients as partners in a team approach. [Family therapy involving psychiatrists, nurses, activity therapists and patients at Forest Hospital, Des Plaines, Illinois.] American Journal of Nursing, 74 (10), Oct 1974, 1844–1847.

12 Travers, J. Naylands – families in a therapeutic community. [Naylands Family Unit, Northampton, develops social experience for complete families in need of help.] Nursing Times, 71, 6 Mar 1975, 391–392.

e GROUP THERAPY

1 Beard, M. T. and Scott, P. Y. The efficacy of group therapy by nurses for hospitalized patients. Nursing Research, 24 (2), Mar/Apr 1975, 120–124.

2 Greenfield, R. C. Trial by fire: rites of passage into psychotherapy groups. [Problem of introducing new members to a group.] Perspectives in Psychiatric Care, 12 (4), Oct–Dec 1974, 152–156.

3 Janosik, E. H. A pragmatic approach to group therapy. Journal of Psychiatric Nursing, 10 (4), Jul/Aug 1972, 7–11.

4 Jones, M. J. D. Project alternative: the road away from isolation. [Therapeutic social groups for long-term psychiatric patients.] Canadian Nurse, 71 (2), Feb 1975, 25–27.

5 King, P. D. Life cycle in the "Tavistock Study Group." [Mental health professionals participate in group therapy.] Perspectives in Psychiatric Care, 8 (4), Oct/Dec 1975, 180–184.

6 Klingbeil, S. A. and Alvandi, O. M. Concepts of transactional analysis and anxiety with persons in crisis. [A study to compare different approaches to group therapy.] Journal of Psychiatric Nursing and Mental Health Services, 13 (6), Nov/Dec 1975, 5–10.

7 Light, N. The 'chronic helper' in group therapy. Perspectives in Psychiatric Care, 11 (3), Jul/Sep 1974, 129–134.

8 McGrew, W. L. and Jensen, J. L. A technique for facilitating therapeutic group interaction. Journal of Psychiatric Nursing, 10 (4), Jul/Aug 1972, 18–21.

9 McLaughlin, F. E. and White, E. Small group functioning under six different leadership formats. Nursing Research, 22 (1), Jan/Feb 1973, 37–54.

10 Marram, G. D. Coalition attempts in group therapy – indicators of inclusion and group cohesion problems. Journal of Psychiatric Nursing, 10 (3), May/Jun 1972, 21–23.

11 Marram, G. D. Latent content and covert group forces in therapy with acute psychiatric patients. Journal of Psychiatric Nursing and Mental Health Services, 9 (2), March/April 1971, 24–27.

12 Matheson, W. E. Group therapy as theatre. Journal of Psychiatric Nursing and Mental Health Services, 13 (5), Sep/Oct 1975, 16–19.

13 Matheson, W. E. Which patient for which therapeutic group. Journal of Psychiatric Nursing and Mental Health Services, 12 (3), May/Jun 1974, 10–13.

14 Mims, F. H. The need to evaluate group therapy. Nursing Outlook, 19 (12), Dec 1971, 776–778.

15 Rouslin, S. Relatedness in group psychotherapy. Perspectives in Psychiatric Care, 11 (4), Oct/Dec 1973, 165–171.

16 Rynveld, J. Towards self-discovery. [Experiences of group therapy.] Mind and Mental Health Magazine, Aut 1972, 31–33.

17 Ward, J. T. The sounds of silence: group psychotherapy with non-verbal patients. Perspectives in Psychiatric Care, 12 (1), Jan/Mar 1974, 13–19.

18 Woodcock, E. and others The blackboard and care plan – nursing treatment tools. [Group therapy in which patient's therapeutic needs are made more visible to himself and the group.] Journal of Psychiatric Nursing, 10 (6), Nov/Dec 1972, 15–17.

77 COMMUNITY PSYCHIATRIC NURSING

a UNITED KINGDOM

1 Altschul, A. T. A multidisciplinary approach to psychiatric nursing. [Experiment at Dingleton Hospital, involving staff, patients and the community.] Nursing Times, 69, 19 Apr 1973, 508–511.

2 Bryant, J. and Sandford, F. Psychiatric nursing in the community. [Student nurses spending some time with the Moorhaven Hospital, nursing after care scheme.] Nursing Mirror, 134, 2 Jun 1972, 37, 39.

3 Cole, E. J. Community psychiatric nursing course. [At Chiswick Polytechnic.] Nursing Mirror, 132, 14 May 1971, 16.

4 Greaves, G. M. Community psychiatric nursing. British Hospital Journal and Social Service Review, 82, 7 Oct 1972, 2239–2240.

5 Haque, G. Psychosocial nursing in the community. Nursing Times, 69, 11 Jan 1973, 51–53.

6 Hartie, M. Community nursing care study. A social outcast. [The problems of a psychiatric patient after discharge into the community.] Nursing Times, 72, 9 Sep 1976, 1392–1394.

7 Henderson, J. G. and Leven, B. The role of the psychiatric nurse in domiciliary treatment service. 1. The treatment team and clinical operation of the service. Nursing Times, 69, 11 Oct 1973, 1334–1336.

8 Henderson, J. G. and others The role of the psychiatric nurse in domiciliary treatment service. 2. An examination of the patients. Nursing Times, 69, 18 Oct 1973, 1377–1378.

9 Henderson, J. G. and others The role of the psychiatric nurse in domiciliary treatment service. 3. Illustrative case histories. Nursing Times, 69, 25 Oct 1973, 1418–1419.

10 Hunter, P. Community psychiatric nursing in Britain: an historical review. International Journal of Nursing Studies, 2, Dec 1974, 223–233.

11 Kavalier, F. A rebellious community nurse. [Betty Stobie, Dingleton Hospital's community nurse in the Berwickshire area.] Nursing Times, 68, 5 Oct 1972, 1252–1254.

12 Leopoldt, H. and others A critical review of experimental psychiatric nurse attachment scheme in Oxford. Practice Team, no. 39, Aug 1974, 2, 4–6.

13 Leopoldt, H. GP attachment and psychiatric domiciliary nursing. [An experimental scheme at Oxford.] Nursing Mirror, 140, 13 Feb 1975, 82–84.

14 Leopoldt, H. Psychiatric community nursing. Health and Social Service Journal, 83, 3 Mar 1973, 489–490.

15 Leopoldt, H. The role of the psychiatric community nurse in the therapeutic team. Nursing Mirror, 138, 19 Apr 1974, 70–72.

16 Leopoldt, H. and Hurn, R. Towards integration. [An experiment in psychiatric domiciliary nursing in a group practice attachment.] Nursing Mirror, 136, 1 Jun 1973, 38–42.

17 Llewellyn, E. M. Community psychiatric nursing. Midwife and Health Visitor, 10 (1), Jan 1974, 7–9.

18 MacDonald, D. J. Psychiatric nursing in the community. [Dingleton Hospital.] Nursing Times, 68, 20 Jan 1972, 80–83.

19 McDonald, R. Behavioural psychotherapy in a domiciliary setting. [Symposium on the psychiatric nurse-therapist.] Nursing Mirror, 140, 8 May 1975, 57.

20 MacDonald, D. J. Psychiatric nursing in the community. [Dingleton Hospital.] Nursing Times, 68, 20 Jan 1972, 80–83.

21 Maisey, M. A. Hospital based psychiatric nurse in the community. [A survey.] Nursing Times, 71, 27 Feb 1975, 354–355.

22 Mandelson, M. and Stevens, D. W. Community psychiatry at Park Day Hospital. Nursing Times, 68, 15 Jun 1972, 733–734.

23 Maxwell, A. The health visitor's role in community psychiatry. Nursing Mirror, 139, 7 Nov 1974, 74–76.

24 Moore, J. H. Planning comprehensive care. [Psychiatric team of nurses and social workers at Moorhaven Hospital.] Practice Team, no. 30/31. Nov/Dec 1973, 2–5.

25 Moss, A. C. Nursing care study. Community psychiatric nursing. Nursing Mirror, 135, 4 Aug 1972, 26–29.

26 Nickerson, A. Psychiatric community nurses in Edinburgh. Nursing Times, 68, 9 Mar 1972, 289–291.

27 Parkes, C. M. Interdisiciplinary collaboration in the field of mental health. Report of a conference. [The health visitor's view briefly expressed by June Clark.] Journal of the Royal College of General Practitioners, 24, Jan 1974, 77–80;

28 Parnell, J. W. Psychiatric nursing in the community. Queen's Nursing Journal, 27 (2), May 1974, 36–38.

29 Sclare, A. B. The district nurse and community mental health. Nursing Times, 67, 2 Sep 1971, 1080–1082.

30 Sharpe, D. Role of the community psychiatric nurse. Nursing Mirror, 141, 16 Oct 1975, 60–62.

31 Sladden, S. Hospital based community psychiatric nursing service. [Summary of research study.] Nursing Mirror, 141, 24 Jul 1975, 56.

32 Stewart, M. and others Psychiatric nurse in the community. [Home visiting project by community psychiatric nurses at Ailsa Hospital, Ayrshire.] Nursing Mirror, 139, 5 Jul 1974, 84.

33 Stickle, E. A. The district nursing sister and community psychiatry. Based on a talk given at a symposium at Sunnyside Royal Hospital, Montrose, in November 1973. Nursing Mirror, 139, 31 Oct 1974, 63–65.

34 Stobie, E. G. and Hopkins, D. H. G. Crisis intervention. A psychiatric community nurse in a rural area. [Dingleton Hospital.] Nursing Times, 68, 26 Oct 1972; 2 Nov 1972, Occ. papers, 169–172.

35 Wallace, J. G. and others The Darlington experiment: by, with and for the community. Nursing Times, 68, 23 Nov 1972, Occ. papers, 185–188.

36 Warren, J. Long-acting phenothiazine injections given by psychiatric nurses in the community. (Harrison Hospital, Dorchester.) Nursing Times, 67, 9 Sep 1971, Occ. papers, 141–143.

b OVERSEAS COUNTRIES

1 Bagley, C. and Evan-Wong, L. The community psychiatric nurse's role and potential interest in psychiatric nursing in teenagers making career choice decisions. [Report of research.] International Journal of Nursing Studies, 10 (4), Dec 1973, 271–277.

2 Bayer, M. A nurse–catalyst in rural community mental health. [Experiences in the United States.] Australian Nurses' Journal, 3 (11), Jun 1974, 33–35.

3 Bayer, M. Psychiatric nursing care in a community hospital. RN Magazine, 37 (11), Nov 1974, 71–72, 74, 76, 78, 80, 82.

4 Bell, J. and Tarnopolski, M. P. Transition to the community: the role of the psychiatric nurse. Canadian Journal of Psychiatric Nursing, 16 (2), Mar/Apr 1975, 10–11.

5 Copping, J. A. The challenge of community psychiatric nursing. SA Nursing Journal, 42 (8), Aug 1975, 22–23.

6 Crow, N. The multifaceted role of the community mental health nurse. Journal of Psychiatric Nursing, 9 (3), May/Jun 1971, 28–31.

7 Deloughery, G. W. and others Consultation and community organization in community mental health nursing. Baltimore: Williams and Wilkins, 1971.

8 Dowling, I. The nurse's role in a community health education programme. 2. World of Irish Nursing, 2 (10), Oct 1973, 181, 183.

9 Dulaney, P. E. and Woods, J. Patient neighbor: a dilemma of the community mental health nurse. Journal of Psychiatric Nursing and Mental Health Services, 13 (4), Jul/Aug 1975, 18–21.

10 Frank, D. The process of implementing the nurse's role in a neighbourhood center. [The community mental health nurse.] Journal of Psychiatric Nursing and Mental Health Services, 12 (2), Mar/Apr 1974, 33–38.

11 Hess, G. Between two worlds. [Community mental health nursing in the USA.] International Journal of Nursing Studies, 8 (1), Feb 1971, 37–46.

12 Hicks, C. F. and others Progress in community mental health nursing: is role diffusion ending? Journal of Psychiatric Nursing and Mental Health Services, 9 (2), Mar/Apr 1971, 28–29.

13 Hildebrandt, D. E. and Davis, J. M. Home visits: a method of reducing the pre-intake dropout rate. [Visits by psychiatric nurses prior to the scheduled hospital appointment.] Journal of Psychiatric Nursing and Mental Health Services, 13 (5), Sep/Oct 1975, 43–44.

14 Howard, L. A. and Baker, F. Ideology and role function of the nurse in community mental health. Nursing Research, 20 (5), Sep/Oct 1971, 450–454.

15 Keener, M. L. The public health nurse in mental health follow-up care. Nursing Research, 24 (3), May/Jun 1975, 198–201.

16 Lindberg, H. G. Community health nursing in the changing mental scene. Journal of Nursing Administration, 3, Nov/Dec 1973, 41–44.

17 Morgan, A. J. and Moreno, J. W. The practice of mental health nursing: a community approach. Philadelphia; Lippincott, 1973.

18 Santopietro, M. C. and Rozendal, N. A. Teaching primary prevention in mental health. [Outline of a course teaching intervention with high risk members of the community to prevent psychiatric illness.] Nursing Outlook, 23 (12), Dec 1975, 774–777.

19 Subhadra, V. The public health nurse in mental health programme. Nursing Journal of India, 65 (9), Sep 1974, 233–234.

20 Williams, R. Teamwork: the key to community psychiatric nursing. Canadian Journal of Psychiatric Nursing, 15 (4), Jul/Aug 1974, 15, 17.

21 Zahourek, R. Nurses in a community mental health center: functions, competencies and satisfactions. Nursing Outlook, 19 (9), Sep 1971, 592–595.

78 PSYCHIATRIC HOSPITALS

a GENERAL

1 Andrews, J. Less ignored – but still impoverished. [Psychiatric hospitals.] Nursing Times, 68, 17 Feb 1972, 217–219.

2 Bavin, J. Who minds. [Environment of psychiatric hospitals.] Nursing Mirror, 132, 7 May 1971, 20–23.

3 Boorer, D. Are mental hospitals doomed? [Meeting of National Association of Chief and Principal Nursing Officers.] Nursing Times, 67, 13 May 1971, 584–585.

4 Borowska, E. and others Evaluation of a night hospital service. [Supplementing the treatment given in a psychiatric ward of the Royal Edinburgh Hospital.] Health Bulletin, 31 (5), Sep 1973, 247–251.

5 Bushnell, M. E. Phasing out a state mental hospital. Journal of Psychiatric Nursing, 11 (1), Jan/Feb 1973, 5–8.

6 Christie, L. S. Are mental hospitals really necessary? Nursing Mirror, 140, 20 Feb 1975, 69–70.

7 Coffey, M. Hospital services for the mentally ill. Nursing Mirror, 134, 23 Jun 1972, 12–14.

8 Coleman, A. D. The planned environment in psychiatric treatment: a manual for ward design. Springfield, Illinois: Thomas, 1971.

9 Dean, D. J. Are psychiatric hospitals doomed? Nursing Mirror, 132, 19 Feb 1971, 12–13.

10 Dean, D. J. Concern for care. [HM (71) 97. Memorandum on hospital services for the mentally ill.] Nursing Times, 68, 13 Jan 1972, 62–63.

11 De Maria, W. The mental health simplex. [State psychiatric hospitals in New South Wales.] Lamp, 30 (5), May 1973, 33–35.

12 Department of Health and Social Security Hospital services for the mentally ill. HMSO, 1971.

13 Estello, O. Notes on the mental hospital. Nursing Mirror, 136, 29 Jun 1973, 9–10.

14 Harkin, J. P. Mental hospitals – have they a future? Nursing Times, 69, 15 Feb 1973, 209–210.

15 McBrien, M. Projecting the image. [Of a psychiatric hospital by means of public relations.] Nursing Mirror, 134, 4 Feb 1972, 30–32.

16 Magu, J. G. The role of the psychiatric hospital. Kenya Nursing Journal, 4 (2), Dec 1975, 41–42, 45.

17 Masters, A. What went wrong. . . ? [Problems of psychiatric hospitals.] Nursing Times, 68, 17 Feb 1972, 220–221.

18 Wertheimer, A. Co-ordination or chaos – the rundown of psychiatric hospitals. Royal Society of Health Journal, 95 (3), Jun 1975, 136–138, 163.

19 Wilcox, F. Boredom in long-stay hospitals. [Based on visits to seven hospitals for mental illness, seven hospitals for the mentally handicapped and 36 geriatric hospitals all in Scotland.] Nursing Mirror, 139, 31 Oct 1974, 71–72.

20 Young, J. J. and Golding, A. M. B. The need to communicate. [Communication between consultants and staff.] Nursing Times, 70, 11 Apr 1974, 566–567.

21 Zeal, B. The anti-therapeutic community. [The closed door psychiatric hospital.] Nursing Times, 71, 9 Jan 1975, 79.

b DAY HOSPITALS

1 Aime, D. Philosophy and structure of a day treatment center. Journal of Psychiatric Nursing and Mental Health Services, 11 (4), Jul/Aug 1973, 27–30.

2 Burch, J. W. and Siassi, I. How effective is a one-day-a-week community psychiatric service? Perspectives in Psychiatric Care, 11 (1), Jan/Mar 1973, 29–32.

3 Carney, M. W. P. Adelphi House: a day hospital. Nursing Times, 67, 11 Feb 1971, 176–178.

4 Cohen, S. Community care of the mentally ill. [Day Centres.] Nursing Mirror, 134, 7 Jan 1972, 17–20.

5 Freeman, H. and others A survey of psychiatric

day care in Salford. Community Medicine, 128, 26 May 1972, 143–146.

6 Gath, D. H. and others Whither psychiatric day care? A study of day patients in Birmingham. British Medical Journal, 1, 13 Jan 1973, 94–98.

7 Hassall, C. and others Psychiatric day-and care in Birmingham. British Journal of Preventive & Social Medicine, 26 (2), May 1972, 112–120.

8 Henschen, R. S. Learning impulse control through day care. Perspectives in Psychiatric Care, 9 (5), Sep/Oct 1971, 218–224.

9 Janzen, S. A. Psychiatric day care in a rural area. American Journal of Nursing, 74 (12), Dec 1974, 2216–2217.

10 Kinsella, T. E. The day hospital as part of a psychiatric service. SA Nursing Journal, 39 (3), Mar 1972, 23–24, 34.

11 Moore, J. H. and O'Brien, T. Day care services in Plymouth. [Psychiatric services at Plymouth Nuffield Clinic.] Practice Team, no. 52, Sep 1975, 6, 8–9.

12 Orbach, C. E. and Aldrige, E. E. A follow-up survey of the post-treatment adaption of former day hospital patients. Journal of Psychiatric Nursing and Mental Health Services, 11 (6), Nov/Dec 1973, 5–13.

13 Williamson, F. Day hospital in a troubled community. [Alexander Gardens Day Hospital, Belfast.] Nursing Times, 68, 28 Dec 1972, 1638–1641.

14 World Health Organization. Regional Office for Europe Trends in psychiatric care: day hospitals and units in general hospitals: report on a symposium. . . . Copenhagen: WHO, 1971.

c INDIVIDUAL HOSPITALS

1 Bethlem Royal Hospital and the Maudsley Hospital. [Articles about the new ward combining the disciplines of neurology and psychiatry.] Nursing Times, 69, 6 Dec 1973, Supplement, 1–8.

2 Coleshill — Stafford, J. 'Residents as individuals'. [Coleshill Hospital, Birmingham.] Nursing Mirror, 134, 28 Apr 1972, 42–46.

3 Colney Hatch — Pearsall, R. History of Colney Hatch. Nursing Mirror, 133, 5 Nov 1971, 40.

4 Dingleton — Jones, M. Psychiatry and change. [Experiences at Dingleton Hospital compared with work at Fort Logan Mental Health Center, Denver, Colorado.] Nursing Times, 68, 7 Dec 1972, 1547–1550.

5 Doncaster Long-term care in Doncaster. The new Loversall Hospital together with the psychiatric unit of Doncaster Royal Infirmary provides the area with a complete service. Nursing Mirror, 134, 14 Apr 1972, 24–25.

6 Fulbourn — Whiteley, E. The evolution and progress of a psychiatric hospital. [Fulbourn Hospital.] Health and Social Service Journal, 83, 3 Nov 1973, 2556–2558.

7 Garth Angharad — Ziman, D. Trust and love for psychopaths. [Open unit treatment with increased freedom for patients at Garth Angharad Hospital, Denbigh.] Health and Social Service Journal, 83, 25 Aug 1973, 1929–1930.

8 John Connolly — Campbell, W. Nursing practice at John Connolly Hospital. Nursing Times, 67, 18 Nov 1971, 1427–1429.

9 John Connolly — Campbell, W. and Thomson, L. B. Part of the community: John Connolly Hospital. Nursing Times, 68, 23 Nov 1972, 1486–1489.

10 Napsbury — Department of Health and Social Security Report of the professional investigation into medical and nursing practices on certain wards at Naps-

bury Hospital, nr. St. Albans. HMSO, 1973. Chairman: R. R. Bomford.

11 Nunsuch — Mihordin, R. J. The Nunsuch handbook: a psychiatric staff handbook for mental health teams at the Nunsuch Mental Center. Perspectives in Psychiatric Care, 11 (3), Jul/Sep 1974, 126–128.

12 Prestwich — Whitehead, A. and others Prestwich overcomes the problems. Nursing Mirror, 132, 29 Jan 1971, 25–27.

13 St. George's — Headland, R. H. Forging links. [As part of a campaign to educate the public in modern psychiatric care. St. George's Hospital, Morpeth make a film of the hospital.] Nursing Times, 71, 7 Aug 1975, 1266–1267.

14 St. James' — Nursing Mirror Psychiatric services in Wessex. St. James' Hospital, Portsmouth. Nursing Mirror, 133, 20 Aug 1971, 27–29.

15 Whittingham — Department of Health and Social Security Committee of Inquiry into Whittingham Hospital. Report. Cmnd 4861. HMSO, 1972. Chairman: Sir Robert Payne.

16 Whittingham — Boorer, D. Whittingham: reform into action. British Hospital Journal and Social Service Review, 82, 20 May 1972, 1102.

17 Whittingham — Greaves, J. and others Current attitudes at Whittingham. British Hospital Journal and Social Service Review, 82, 8 Jul 1972, 1508–1509.

18 Whittingham Hospital and Health Services Review, 68 (3), Mar 1972, 75–77.

d THERAPEUTIC COMMUNITY

1 Burkitt, P. A. The concept of a therapeutic community. Course held at the Henderson Hospital, Sutton. Nursing Times, 71, 9 Jan 1975, 75–78.

2 Calnan, T. Whose agent? A re-evaluation of the role of the psychiatric nurse in the therapeutic community. Perspectives in Psychiatric Care, 10 (5), Dec 1972, 210–219.

3 Cooke, R. Fragmentation and conflict in a therapeutic community. [Henderson Hospital.] Social Work Today, 6, 18 Sep 1975, 364–365.

4 Heales, K. Taking off the labels. [Greenwoods therapeutic community.] Nursing Times, 71, 1 May 1975, 698–700.

5 Heath, P. J. A long-stay therapeutic community. Lancet, 1, 12 Jun 1971, 1231–1232.

6 Inn, T. J. The role of the psychiatric nurse in the therapeutic community. Nursing Journal of Singapore, 12 (2), Nov 1972, 87–89.

7 Kincheloe, M. Democratization in the therapeutic community. Perspectives in Psychiatric Care, 11 (2), Apr/Jun 1973, 75–79.

8 Latham, R. and de Freyne-Martin, T. G. The Phoenix Unit. [Administration in a specialised unit at Littlemore Hospital, Oxford, run on the lines of a therapeutic community.] Nursing Mirror, 137, 27 Jul 1973, 22–24.

9 Leone, D. and Zahourek, R. 'Aloneness' in a therapeutic community. [Psychiatric patients living alone.] Perspectives in Psychiatric Care, 12 (2), Apr/Jun 1974, 60–63.

10 Mitchell, R. Advances in psychiatry. The therapeutic community v. traditional psychiatry. Nursing Times, 70, 21 Nov 1974, 1810–1812.

11 Nickless, G. Therapeutic teams and their patients: a major relocation exercise. [Scheme at Herrison Hospital, Dorset.] Nursing Mirror, 140, 20 Mar 1975, 78–80.

12 Pond, D. A. The therapeutic community. Occupational Therapy, 37 (5), May 1974, 73.

13 Royston, R. Therapeutic communities revisited. [Conference organized by the Richmond Fellowship.] Health and Social Service Journal, 85, 10 May 1975, 1061.

14 Sanders, R. M. The role of the social therapist in a therapeutic community. [With particular reference to Henderson Hospital, Surrey and Dingleton Hospital, Melrose.] Nursing Times, 69, 20/27 Dec 1973, 1746–1747.

15 Sharp, V. Social control in the therapeutic community. Farnborough: Saxon House, 1975.

16 Taylor, A. J. W. A therapeutic community. [Adaptation of the therapeutic community in a general hospital to improve patient care.] New Zealand Nursing Journal, 68 (5), May 1975, 24–26.

e PSYCHIATRIC UNITS IN GENERAL HOSPITALS

1 Ben-Arie, O. The acute psychiatric unit in a general hospital; with special reference to Groote Schuur. SA Nursing Journal, 42 (3), Mar 1975, 28–29.

2 Frank, S. The place of a psychiatric unit in a general hospital. British Journal of Occupational Therapy, 37 (5), May 1974, 71–72.

3 Frost, M. This is progress in psychiatry. [Psychiatric unit in a general hospital.] Nursing Mirror, 132, 26 Feb 1971, 42–43.

4 Grover, E. and Gormly, E. F. A study of a psychiatric walk-in clinic in a general hospital. Hospital Progress, 53 (11), Nov 1972, 70–72, 74, 84.

5 Hill, O. W. Psychiatry in the general hospital. Nursing Mirror, 138, 10 May 1974, 54–57.

6 Hurst, T. W. Psychiatric units attached to general hospitals. [A meeting at the King's Fund Centre examining problems of incorporation.] Health and Social Service Journal, 85, 23 Aug 1975, 1854.

7 Kidd, C. B. and Zorbas, A. From out-group to in-group. The introduction of a psychiatric unit to a general hospital. International Journal of Social Psychiatry, 17 (2), Spring 1971, 101–110.

8 Raphael, Winifred Just an ordinary patient: a preliminary survey of opinion on psychiatric units in general hospitals. King Edward's Hospital Fund for London, 1974. See also Kings Fund Centre Conference. Nursing Times, 70, 5 Dec 1974, 1978.

9 Vitale, J. H. and others Small group method on a general hospital nursing unit. Journal of Psychiatric Nursing and Mental Health Services, 11 (3), May/Jun 1973, 9–12.

10 Whitehead, T. and Barry, J. The psychiatric hospital in transition. [Disappearance of the large psychiatric hospital and the transition to general and community hospitals.] Health and Social Service Journal, 84, 11 May 1974, 1038.

11 Williams, P. The district general hospital psychiatric unit and the mental hospital – some comparisons. University Hospital of Wales, Psychiatric Unit compared with Whitchurch Hospital, Cardiff.] British Journal of Preventive and Social Medicine, 28 (2), May 1974, 140–145.

f PATIENTS' VIEWS AND WELFARE (Includes physical illness)

1 Adam, I. Who minds . . . [about the quality of life of people in hospital]. [With particular reference to long-stay psychiatric patients.] Nursing Mirror, 132, 14 May 1971, 33–35.

2 Bouchier, M. L. Personal space and chronicity in the mental hospital. [Effect of restriction of space on the behaviour of psychiatric patients.] Perspectives in Psychiatric Care, 9 (5), Sep/Oct 1971, 206–210.

3 Boxall, B. J. A patients' affairs department. [Graylingwell Hospital, Chichester.] Hospital, 67 (9), Sep 1971, 311–314.

4 British Medical Journal Freedom in hospital. [Editorial discussing NAMH Publication, 'Patients' rights'.] British Medical Journal, 3, 11 Aug 1973, 307–308.

5 British Medical Journal The patient's view. [Of psychiatric hospitals.] British Medical Journal, 3, 7 Jul 1973, 5–6.

6 Burgess, A. C. and Burns, J. Why patients seek care. [Study conducted in the pscyhiatric unit of a general hospital to find out patients' views.] American Journal of Nursing, 73 (2), Feb 1973, 314–316.

7 Canadian Journal of Psychiatric Nursing A patient's view: a candid interview. Canadian Journal of Psychiatric Nursing, 16 (2), Mar/Apr 1975, 8–9.

8 Cannings, W. H. and Vahey, P. G. Casualties to patients: a research project carried out in a psychiatric hospital. Nursing Mirror, 133, 16 Jul 1971, 17–21.

9 Chastko, H. E. and others Patients' posthospital evaluations of psychiatric nursing treatments. Nursing Research, 20 (4), Jul– Aug 1971, 333–338.

10 Cheadle, J. A place of one's own at the table. [A study of patients taking their places at meals carried out at St. Wulstan's Hospital, Malvern.] Nursing Times, 67, 7 Oct 1971, 1258–1259.

11 Crockett, H. Fulbourne Hospital – a patient's view. [Recovery from a nervous breakdown.] Nursing Times, 70, 18 Apr 1974, 603–604.

12 Doyle, M. C. Rabbit: therapeutic prescription. [A study to investigate the value of pets in psychiatric wards.] Perspectives in Psychiatric Care, 8 (2), Apr/Jun 1975, 79–82.

13 Florer, R. M. The key of hope. [Chronic mentally ill patients.] Nursing Mirror, 135, 11 Aug 1972, 32.

14 Frost, M. Advice to psychiatric patients. Nursing Times, 68, 23 Nov 1972, 1478.

15 Frost, M. Early warnings. Physical illness in the psychiatric and geriatric patient. Nursing Times, 67, 25 Feb 1971, 235–236.

16 Gray, J. C. Come on in – the water's fine. [Student nurse spends a week in a psychiatric ward as a aptient.] Nursing Mirror, 133, 24 Sep 1971, 16.

17 Hofford, E. C. Patients as people. [Reactivation and resocialisation of a group of long-stay patients.] Nursing Times, 70, 15 Aug 1974, 1283–1285.

18 Hollander, D. and Bendhem, T. A lifetime in hospital: what is it like to spend 50 years of your life in a mental hospital? A man of 75 tells his own story. New Society, 32, 22 May 1975, 465–467.

19 Lewis, T. The patient is responsible. [A nurse questions the way in which personal decisions are made for patients and describes changes in attitude at Whitchurch Hospital, Cardiff.] Nursing Times, 71, 13 Mar 1975, 434–435.

20 Loughran, J. M. Mental welfare in Scotland: the work of the Mental Welfare Commission. [Welfare of patients in psychiatric hospitals.] Nursing Times, 70, 14 Feb 1974, 218–219.

21 McCreadie, R. G. Clinical and social aspects of a non-geriatric long-stay psychiatric unit. [Gartnavel Royal Hospital, Glasgow.] Health Bulletin, 31 (6), Nov 1973, 300–306.

22 McGlennon, J. West Park hospital bank. Health and Social Service Journal, 84, 6 Jul 1974, 1500.

231 Mathers, J. Custodial or residential care for the long-stay patient? Lancet, 1, 22 Apr 1972, 894–895.

24 Mayhew, C. and others Life in a psychiatric ward. Health Service Journal, 25 (1), Jan 1972, 5–6.

25 Merchant, T. Mind Kept in the background. Drawing on his own experience as an in-patient, the author suggests some simple ways of making life in hospital more beneficial. Mind and Mental Health Magazine, Autumn 1972, 47–48.

26 Mitchell, R. G. Visiting time and the psychiatric nurse: the extra hour. Nursing Times, 69, 20 Sep 1973, 1234–1235.

27 National Association for Mental Health Crossing the borderline. [4 members of the Mind Campaign's experiences as in-patients in mental hospitals.] Nursing Mirror, 133, 8 Oct 1971, 10–11.

28 National Association for Mental Health Patients' rights: the mentally disordered in hospital. The Association, 1973. (Mind report no. 10.)

29 Nevill, E. C. N. and others A study of long stay patients in a mental hospital. [Bexley Hospital.] Community Medicine, 126, 29 Oct 1971, 241–242.

30 Oram, E. V. Money problems of psychiatric patients. Nursing Mirror, 140, 17 Apr 1975, 57–58.

31 Raphael, W. and Peers, V. Practical results of surveys. [Response of Graylingwell Hospital, Chichester and Netherne Hospital, Coulsdon to King's Fund survey on psychiatric hospitals.] Health and Social Service Journal, 83, 2 Jun 1973, 1254, 1256.

32 Raphael, W. and Peers, V. Psychiatric hospitals viewed by their patients. King Edward's Hospital Fund for London, 1972.

33 Robinson, G. C. and Owen, J. No one told me to. [Institutionalized patients and staff attitudes.] Nursing Outlook, 22 (3), Mar 1974, 182–183.

34 Sanders, R. All play and no work. . . [A survey taken at the West Park Hospital, Epsom, reveals the problems of boredom in long stay hospitals.] New Psychiatry, 1 (4), 31 Oct 1974, 10–11.

35 Scottish Hospital Centre Patients' clothes and valuables in long-stay hospitals. [Summary of a survey carried out by the Scottish Hospital Centre.] Health and Social Service Journal, 84, 30 Nov 1974, 2777.

36 Shamsie, S. J. and Titus, A. L. Evaluation of a treatment centre by its clients. [Mental health centre, Toronto.] Hospital Administration in Canada, 17 (6), Jun 1975, 58–60.

37 Skuse, D. H. Attitudes to the psychiatric outpatient clinic. [Interviews with fifty patients.] British Medical Journal, 3, 23 Aug 1975, 469–471.

38 Trott, C. Personal clothing for patients: a further report on the scheme at Graylingwell Hospital. Hospital and Health Service Review, 68 (1), Jan 1972, 11–12.

39 Unwin, F. T. Cruelty in psychiatric hospitals. Nursing Times, 69, 12 Jul 1973, 894.

40 Vandyk, N. D. A patient's perspective. [Point of view of a disturbed person.] District Nursing, 15 (5), Aug 1972, 94–96.

41 Weddell, M. Physical medicine in psychiatry – can we cope? [Survey of psychiatric admissions showing high incidence of physical illness.] Nursing Times, 67, 8 Jul 1971, Occ. papers, 105–106.

42 Wilcox, F. Boredom in long-stay hospitals. [Based on visits to seven hospitals for mental illness, seven hospitals for the mentally handicapped, and 36 geriatric hospitals all in Scotland.] Nursing Mirror, 139, 31 Oct 1974, 71–72.

g SPECIAL HOSPITALS, SECURE UNITS, LOCKED WARDS

1 Bowden, P. Liberty and psychiatry. [Lack of adequate facilities for mentally abnormal offenders.] British Medical Journal, 4, 11 Oct 1975, 94–96.

2 Bright, S. Communication on all levels. [Visit to Carstairs special security hospital.] Nursing Times, 71, 8 May 1975, 716–717.

3 British Medical Journal Secure hospital units. British Medical Journal, 3, 27 Jul 1974, 215–216.

4 Craft, M. J. and others, editors Lost Souls services for mentally abnormal offenders. A report of the proceedings of a working party. King Edward's Hospital Fund for London, 1975. (Mental handicap papers 7.)

5 Department of Health and Social Security Regional Security Unit Design Guidelines. DHSS, 1975.

6 Department of Health and Social Security Security in NHS hospitals for the mentally ill and mentally handicapped. DHSS, 1971. HSC (16) 61.

7 Department of Health and Social Security Working Party on Security in NHS Psychiatric Hospitals. Revised report. DHSS, 1974. Chairman: Dr. J. E. Glancy.

8 Hinton, J. Development of objective behaviour rating scales for use by nurses on patients in special hopitals. Special Hospitals Research Unit, 1975. (Special hospitals research report, no. 13.)

9 Home Office and Department of Health and Social Security Committee on Mentally Abnormal Offenders. Report. HMSO, 1975. Chairman: Lord Butler of Saffron Waldren.

10 Institute of Mental Subnormality 'Security is a frame of mind'. Training essential for secure unit staff – PNO. [Conference on violent patients.] Nursing Times, 71, 10 Apr 1975, 556.

11 Lancet Dangerous offenders. Lancet, 2, 1 Nov 1975, 856–858.

12 Lester, J. Carstairs believes in tomorrow. [State Hospital – a maximum security psychiatric hospital.] Nursing Mirror, 140, 24 Apr 1975, 39–41.

13 McLean, E. K. Prison and humanity. [Psychiatric services at Grendon high security prison, Buckinghamshire, observed by the author acting as a casual member of the psychiatric staff for three weeks.] Lancet, 1, 1 Mar 1975, 507–511.

14 Martin, A. The Butler report. Nursing Times, 71, 18 Dec 1975, 2007.

15 Nursing Times Special role for nurses in secure units. [Comments on the Butler committee report.] Nursing Times, 71 9 Oct 1975, 1604.

16 Oxford Regional Hospital Board Report of a working party on individuals requiring security. Oxford: The Board, 1971.

17 Pritchard, J. Integrating the special hospitals. Community Medicine, 129 (19), 23 Feb 1973, 387–389.

18 Rampton Hospital Rampton Hospital study day. Putting Rampton on the map, by P. Dack./Nursing/ Nursing Mirror, 140, 13 Feb 1975, 40–41, by A. Dunn. Behind bars. Nursing Times, 71, 13 Feb 1975, 244.

19 Rampton Hospital Special hospital. [Rampton

Hospital.] Health and Social Service Journal, 85, 22 Mar 1975, 658–659.

20 Scott, P. D. Solutions to the problem of the dangerous offender. British Medical Journal, 4, 14 Dec 1974, 640–641.

21 Teeling-Smith, G. Society at work. Locked wards. [Procedures for compulsory detention under the Mental Health Act 1959.] New Society, 23, 22 Feb 1973, 416–417.

22 Wiltshire, S. S. and Kreinbrook, S. B. Disturbed wards – do we need them? [A study to investigate the value of special 'disturbed wards' in psychiatric hospitals.] Journal of Psychiatric Nursing and Mental Health Services, 13 (5), Sep/Oct 1975, 24–27.

23 Winch, J. Medicine and the law. Broadmoor nurse's conviction quashed. Lancet, 1, 25 Jan 1975, 233.

h VIOLENCE

1 Allison, C. and Bale, R. A hospital policy for the care of patients who exhibit violent behaviour. [Policy at St. James' Hospital, Portsmouth, based on the recent NAMH document.] Nursing Times, 69, 22 Mar 1973, 375–377.

2 Bale, R. and Allison, C. Disturbed behaviour in a psychiatric hospital. [Progress of the use of 'incident forms' at St. James' Hospital, Portsmouth, to examine violent behaviour.] Nursing Times, 71, 8 May 1975, 743–745.

3 Brailsford, D. S. Psychiatric hospitals. A further viewpoint. [Factors related to violent and unpredictable behaviour.] Nursing Times, 69, 2 Aug 1973, 1001–1003.

4 Brailsford, D. S. and Stevenson, J. Factors related to violent and unpredictable behaviour in psychiatric hospitals. Nursing Times, 69, 18 Jan 1973, Occ. papers, 9–11.

5 British Medical Journal Dangerous patients. British Medical Journal, 1, 23 Mar 1974, 527.

6 British Medical Journal Death of a nurse. [Editorial comment on the incident at Tooting Bec.] British Medical Journal, 4, 22 Nov 1975, 425.

7 British Medical Journal Violence against nurses. [Investigations in Sweden and New Zealand.] British Medical Journal, 4, 21 Oct 1972, 129–130.

8 British Medical Journal Violence in hospitals. British Medical Journal, 3, 21 Aug 1971, 443.

9 Budge, U. V. Pathways of persuasion. [Physical restraint of mental patients.] Nursing Mirror, 133, 8 Oct 1971, 12.

10 Coffey, M. Violence in institutions. Nursing Mirror, 134, 14 Apr 1972, 36–37; 21 Apr 1972, 44–45.

11 Frost, M. Violence in psychiatric patients. Nursing Times, 68, 15 Jun 1972, 748–749.

12 Harries, C. J. Disturbed behaviour. Report of a day symposium at Fulbourn Hospital, Cambridge, 5 July 1973. Nursing Times, 70, 16 May 1974, 748–750.

13 Harrington, J. A. Hospital violence. Nursing Mirror, 135, 21 Jul 1972, 12–13; 135, 28 Jul 1972, 32–33.

14 Hope, H. F. Nursing care study. Trigger factors. [Violence in a mentally handicapped patient.] Nursing Mirror, 137, 20 Jul 1973, 43.

15 Horton Hospital Report by the examination team. [An investigation into the problem of violent patients in a psychiatric hospital.] The Hospital, 1974.

16 Hospital Attacks on hospital staff and others.

[Criminal Injuries Compensation Board.] Hospital, 67 (9), Sep 1971, 323–324.

17 James, D. J. Practical care of the aggressive patient. [Mentally subnormal.] Nursing Times, 68, 26 Oct 1972, 1352–1353.

18 Jones, K. Violence and the mentally handicapped. [The difficulties faced by nurses who care for violent patients.] New Society, 27, 31 Jan 1974, 247–249.

19 Kavalier, F. The violent patient. HMC publishes new guidelines. [South Birmingham HMC.] Nursing Times, 69, 24 May 1973, 656.

20 Lancet Violent patients. Lancet, 1, 20 Mar 1971, 587.

21 Lion, J. R. Restraining the violent patient. Journal of Psychiatric Nursing, 10 (2), Mar/Apr 1972, 9–11.

22 Lyon, M. G. Safety in the psychiatric field. [Risks to the psychiatric nurse.] New Zealand Nursing Journal, 66 (4), Apr 1973, 35.

23 McArthur, C. H. Nursing violent patients under security restrictions. Nursing Times, 68, 13 Jul 1972, 861–863.

24 National Association for Mental Health A guide to good practice: guidelines for the care of patients who exhibit violent behaviour in mental and mental subnormality hospitals. Mental Health, Spring 1971, 32–35. Summary and comment in Nursing Mirror, 133, 9 Jul 1971, 15–16; Nursing Times, 67, 15 Apr 1971, 449–450.

25 Nursing Times Code on violence. [Editorial.] Nursing Times, 70, 7 Mar 1974, 329.

26 Nursing Times Reasonable force. A barrister looks at the implications of a recent Queen's Bench decision. [The conviction of a Broadmoor nurse for assault on a patient.] Nursing Times, 71, 13 Feb 1975, 245.

27 Penningroth, P. E. Control of violence in a mental health setting. American Journal of Nursing, 75 (4), Apr 1975, 606–609.

28 Reid, J. A. Controlling the fight/flight patient. Canadian Nurse, 69 (10), Oct 1973, 30–34.

29 Royal College of Psychiatrists and Royal College of Nursing. Psychiatric Section The care of the violent patient. The Colleges, 1972.

30 South Birmingham Hospital Management Committee Guidelines for the management of violent patients: an official policy statement. The Committee, 1974.

31 South Birmingham Hospital Management Committee Guidelines for the management of violent patients for nurses in training. The Committee, 1974.

32 South East Metropolitan Regional Hospital Board Guidelines for handling violent patients in psychiatric hospitals and violence in casualty, accident and emergency departments. The Board, 1973.

33 South West Thames Regional Health Authority An inquiry into the circumstances leading to the death of Mr. Daniel Carey at Tooting Bec Hospital, on 2nd August 1974. The Health Authority, 1975. Comment in Nursing Times, 71, 20 Nov 1975, 1837.

34 Strong, P. G. Aggression in the general hospital. [Disturbed behaviour of patients.] Nursing Times, 69, 8 Feb 1973, Occ papers, 21–24.

35 Whitehead, T. Violence in psychiatric hospitals. World Medicine, 9 (21), 17 Jul 1974, 41–42.

i VOLUNTEERS

1 Collins, A. The role of the volunteer in mental health. [Activities of the Association for Mental Health

in Gloucestershire.] Social Service Quarterly, 45 (3), Jan/Mar 1972, 95–96.

2 Ennals, D. Turning sympathy into action. [Mind campaign for volunteers in the mental health service.] Health and Social Service Journal, 83, 27 Oct 1973, 2486–2487; Health Visitor, 46 (9), Sep 1973, 309.

3 Fell, J. H. Young ambassadors. [Residential weekend . . . Whalley.] Nursing Mirror, 132, 18 Jun 1971, 36–37.

4 Gilvary, K. Toc H volunteers make their mark. [Barrow Psychiatric Hospital, Bristol.] Nursing Times, 71, 12 Jun 1975, 944–945.

5 Hoare, J. H. and McKay, J. Volunteer workers at The Towers Leicester. Nursing Times, 66, 17 Sep 1970, 1189–1191.

6 King, C. The quiet revolution. [Volunteers in psychiatric hospitals.] Mind and Mental Health Magazine, Spring 1973, 41–46.

7 Kings fund Centre Young volunteers in mental health. [King's Fund project.] British Hospital Journal and Social Service Review, 82, 28 Oct 1972, 2413–2414.

8 Matthews, D. G. Sixth-formers and the psychiatric hospitals. Nursing Times, 66, 15 Oct 1970, 1343.

9 Nursing Times On being a volunteer – by one of them. [During nurses' strike at Highcroft Hospital.] Nursing Times, 70, 15 Aug 1974, 1259.

10 Nursing Times Volunteer or staff? [Volunteers in psychiatric hospitals.] Nursing Times, 71, 17 Jul 1975, 1149.

11 Owen, A. and Gordon, G. A willingness to be involved. [Student volunteers at Farleigh.] Mind and Mental Health Magazine, summer 1972, 30–35.

12 Phillips, M. Nursing MAN power. [Use of male university students as psychiatric assistants.] Canadian Nurse, 71 (12), Dec 1975, 23–25.

13 Sharpe, D. The befrienders. [Scheme at Warlingham Park Hospital.] Nursing Times, 69, 10 May 1973, 603–604.

79 PSYCHIATRIC DISORDERS

a GENERAL AND PSYCHIATRY

1 Haupt, F. J. G. Historical survey of psychiatry. 1. SA Nursing Journal, 41 (1), Jan 1974, 16–19.

2 Lipsedge, M. Early detection of mental disorders. Occupational Health, 25 (7), Jul 1973, 254–259.

3 Mitchell, R. Advances in psychiatry. Medical model v. social model. [Two different concepts about the nature of mental disorder.] Nursing Times, 70, 28 Nov 1974, 1851–1853.

4 Mitchell, R. Advances in psychiatry. 8. Organic disorders. Nursing Times, 70, 15 Aug 1974, 1276–1278.

5 Nursing Mirror Mental illness – it can be lived with. [By a former mental patient.] Nursing Mirror, 137 13 Jul 1973, 17–18.

6 Ripley, G. D. Early detection of mental illness. District Nursing, 15 (12), Mar 1973, 266–267.

b SOCIAL ASPECTS

1 Brandon, S. Psychiatric illness in women. Nursing Mirror, 134, 21 Jan 1972, 17–18.

2 D'Orban. P. T. Baby stealing. British Medical Journal, 2, 10 June 1972, 635–639.

3 Gibbens, T. C. N. and others Mental health

aspects of shop lifting. British Medical Journal, 3, 11 Sep 1971, 612–615.

4 Hunter, J. The problem of baby stealing. Social Work Today, 4, 26 Jul 1973, 266–268.

5 Sheahan, J. Long term mental disorder and family stress. Nursing Mirror, 141, 11 Dec 1975, 66–68.

6 Stillman, P. New town blues. [The incidence of psychiatric illness in Crawley.] Nursing Times, 71, 9 Jan 1975, 50–51.

7 Walshe-Brennan, K. S. Football hooliganism. [Social factors and psychiatric causes.] Nursing Mirror, 141 13 Nov 1975, 46–49.

c DRUG THERAPY AND TREATMENT

1 Ballinger, B. R. and Ramsay, A. C. The 'As required' prescription in psychiatric in-patients. [Study undertaken at Royal Dundee Liff Hospital and Maryfield Hospital, Dundee.] Health Bulletin, 32 (3), May 1974, 96–99.

2 Burke, F. J. Physical treatments in psychiatry. Nursing Times, 70, 30 May 1974, 825–827.

3 Cannicott, S. M. Unilateral electro-convulsive therapy. Nursing Times, 70, 18 Jul 1974, 1116–1117.

4 Cohen, R. EST + Group therapy = improved care. [Electroshock.] American Journal of Nursing, 71, Jun 1971, 1195–1198.

5 Dembicki, E. L. Psychiatric drugs and trends. Journal of Psychiatric Nursing and Mental Health Services, 13 (2), Mar/Apr 1975, 36–37.

6 Fitzgerald, R. G. and Long, I. Seclusion in the treatment and management of severely disturbed manic and depressed patients. Perspectives in Psychiatric Care, 11 (2), Apr/Jun 1973, 59–64.

7 Greene, R. J. Drug administration. 2. Drug information at ward level. Nursing Times, 69, 2 Aug 1973, 992–993.

8 Greene, R. J. and others Drug administration. 3. Drug administration in psychiatric hospitals. Nursing Times, 69, 2 Aug 1973, 994–996.

9 Kilgalen, R. K. Hydrotherapy – is it all washed up? Journal of Psychiatric Nursing, 10 (6), Nov/Dec 1972, 3–6.

10 Kline, N. S. and Davis, J. M. Psychotropic drugs. American Journal of Nursing, 73 (1), Jan 1973, 54–62.

11 O'Dwyer, M. Electro-convulsive therapy. Nursing Times, 69, 15 Mar 1973, 352–353.

12 Shaw, D. M. Lithium in the treatment of depressive orders. Nursing Mirror, 141, 2 Oct 1975, 62–63.

13 Sheahan, J. Drug administration. 1. Drug administration in psychiatric hospitals. Nursing Times, 69, 2 Aug 1973, 991.

14 Smith, S. E. Drug therapy 1972. 11. Drugs and the mental state. Nursing Times, 68, 10 Aug 1972, 1001–1002.

15 Smith, S. E. How drugs act. 26. Drugs and the mental state. Nursing Times, 71, 18 Dec 1975, 2030–2031.

16 Todd, J. J. The use of drugs in psychiatry. District Nursing, 14 (8), Nov 1971, 165–167.

17 Tredgold, R. F. Effects of leucotomy on personality. Nursing Mirror, 137, 10 Aug 1973, 39–40.

18 Ventura, M. S. A look at restraining practices and the use of psychotropic drugs. Journal of Psychiatric Nursing and Mental Health Services, 12 (3), May/Jun 1974, 3–9.

d ANOREXIA NERVOSA

1 Baldwin, W. Anorexia nervosa. Nursing Times, 71, 23 Jan 1975, 134–135.

2 Bruch, H. Eating disorders: obesity, anorexia nervosa and the person within. Routledge, 1973.

3 Day, S. Dietary management of anorexia nervosa. Nutrition, 28 (5), 1974, 289–295.

4 Drug and Therapeutics Bulletin The management of anorexia nervosa. Drug and Therapeutics Bulletin, 13, 6 Jun 1975, 45–46.

5 Hext, M. and Murchland, A. Adolescent anorexia nervosa: the patient: an approach. Journal of Psychiatric Nursing, 10 (6), Nov/Dec 1972, 18–23.

6 Joynes, V. Nursing care study. Anorexia nervosa [treated by operant conditioning]. Nursing Mirror, 138, 22 Mar 1974, 84–86.

7 Kalucy, R. S. Anorexia nervosa: a nursing challenge. Nursing Mirror, 136, 23 Mar 1973, 11–16.

8 Kalucy, R. S. Anorexia nervosa – some aspects of nursing management. Nursing Times, 69, 18 Jan 1973, 76–79.

9 King, D. A. Anorexic behavior: a nursing problem. Journal of Psychiatric Nursing, 9 (3), May/Jun 1971, 11–17.

10 Melton, J. H. A boy with anorexia nervosa. American Journal of Nursing, 74 (9), Sep 1974, 1649–1651.

11 Schmidt, M. P. W. and Duncan, B. A. B. Modifying eating behavior in anorexia nervosa. Operant conditioning. American Journal of Nursing, 74 (9), Sep 1974, 1646–1648.

e DEPRESSION

1 Banks, S. A. Nursing care study. Agitated depression. Nursing Times, 69, 27 Sep 1973, 1250–1251.

2 Bishop, S. Nursing care study. Depression. Nursing Times, 71, 2 Oct 1975, 1567–1569.

3 Crary, W. G. and Crary, G. C. Depression. American Journal of Nursing, 73 (3), Mar 1973, 472–475.

4 Cropper, C. F. J. A disease called depression. Nursing Times, 69, 30 Aug 1973, 1122–1123.

5 Fricker, R. and O'Dwyer, M. Depression refractive to treatment. Nursing Times, 67, 1 Jul 1971, 794–797.

6 Frost, M. Depression – the mental 'cold'. Nursing Mirror, 137, 5 Oct 1973, 46–47.

7 Frost, M. Playing it by ear. A case of psychotic depression. Nursing Times, 68, 6 Jul 1972, 838.

8 Hardial, M. Treatment of depression. Nursing Times, 69, 31 May 1973, 703–706; 7 Jun 1973, 741–743.

9 Kicey, C. A. Catecholamines and depression: a physiological theory of depression. American Journal of Nursing, 74 (11), Nov 1974, 2018–2020.

10 Lyons, D. G. Nursing care study. Endogenous depression. Non-co-operation. Nursing Mirror, 139, 17 Oct 1974, 93–94.

11 McEvoy, P. Nursing care study. Reactive depression in a psychopathic personality. Nursing Times, 69, 26 Apr 1973, 539–540.

12 Maxson, K. W. Assuming the patient role. [A personal experience of depression.] Perspectives in Psychiatric Care, 11 (3), Jul/Sep 1974, 119–122.

13 Mitchell, R. Advances in psychiatry. 3. Depression. Nursing Times, 70 11 Jul 1974, 1085–1087.

14 Mitchell, R. Advances in psychiatry. 6. Manic depression. Nursing Times, 70, 1 Aug 1974, 1199–1201.

15 Schapira, K. The masks of depression. Nursing Mirror, 140, 19 Jun 1975, 46–48.

16 Shaw, D. M. Lithium in the treatment of depressive disorders. Nursing Mirror, 141, 2 Oct 1975, 62–63.

17 Swanson, A. R. Communicating with depressed persons. Perspectives in Psychiatric Care, 8 (2), Apr/Jun 1975, 63–67.

18 Weeks, P. Abnormal emotional reaction in an adolescent. [Case study of patient suffering from depression.] Nursing Times, 69, 8 Nov 1973, 1485–1487.

f FEAR, PHOBIAS, ANXIETY, STRESS

1 Bradley, M. E. Nursing care study. Treatment of a phobic condition. [Agoraphobia.] Nursing Times, 71, 19 Jun 1975, 964–967.

2 Connolly, J. and Hallam, R. S. The psychiatric nurse – turned therapist. 2. Phobias. Nursing Mirror, 136, 9 Mar 1973, 24–25, 35.

3 Connolly, J. and Hallam, R. S. The psychiatric nurse as a therapist. 3. Obsessions. Nursing Mirror, 136, 16 Mar 1973, 25–26.

4 Hartie, A. Phobia of bees and wasps. Nursing Times, 71, 27 Mar 1975, 488–491.

5 Hawkrigg, J. J. Agoraphobia. [Research project in Rochdale, using behaviour therapy techniques.] Nursing Times, 71, 14 Aug 1975, 1280–1282; 21 Aug 1975, 1337–1338.

6 Lewis, A. Phobia: a private experience. Journal of Psychiatric Nursing, 11 (2), Mar/Apr 1973, 30–32.

7 Lindley, P. Nurse-therapists at work: six case studies. 1. Pigeon phobia. [Symposium at Maudsley Hospital.] Nursing Mirror, 140, 8 May 1975, 58.

8 McArdle, M. Nurse therapists at work: six case studies. 2. Agoraphobia complicated by alcoholism. [Symposium at Maudsley Hospital.] Nursing Mirror, 140, 8 May 1975, 59–60.

9 McArdle, M. Treatment of a phobia. [Case study by a psychiatric nurse therapist.] Nursing Times, 70, 25 Apr 1974, 637–639.

10 McDonald, R. Nurse-therapists at work: six case studies. 3. Social phobia. [Symposium at Maudsley Hospital.] Nursing Mirror, 140, 8 May 1975, 60–61.

11 McEvoy, P. Phobia in an inadequate personality: nursing care study. Nursing Times, 69, 5 Apr 1973, 455–457.

12 Marshall, W. K. Clomipramine intravenous drip: treatment of obsessional and phobic anxiety states. Nursing Times, 68, 16 Nov 1972, 1448–1449.

13 Melville, J. Social phobia. [Treatment of agoraphobia and the work done by the Open Door.] New Society, 25, 5 Jul 1973, 25–26.

14 Mitchell, J. Advances in psychiatry. 1. Anxiety. Nursing Times, 70, 27 Jun 1974, 991–993.

15 Mitchell, R. Advances in psychiatry. 4. Obsessions. Nursing Times, 70, 18 Jul 1974, 1113–1115.

16 O'Connor, P. J. Fear of flying. District Nursing, 14 (10), Jan 1972, 207–208.

17 Orwin, A. and Duffy, T. Blood phobia. Nursing Mirror, 134, 16 Jun 1972, 25–26.

18 Priestman, C. Frank – a long-stay patient. [Obsessional behaviour.] Nursing Times, 70, 12 Sep 1974, 1418–1419.

19 **Ramsay, M.** Nurse-therapists at work: six case studies. 4. Obsessive-compulsive disorder. [Symposium at Maudsley Hospital.] Nursing Mirror, 140, 8 May 1975, 61–62.

20 **Stern, R. S.** Treatment of common phobias. District Nursing, 14 (10), Jan 1972, 206, 208.

21 **Thompson, E.** The road to independence from agoraphobia. Queen's Nursing Journal, 16 (11), Feb 1974, 252–253.

22 **Wallace, C. M.** Looking at psychiatry. 2. Nursing the obsessional-compulsive patient. [Case history.] Nursing Mirror, 136, 4 May 1973, 36–37.

23 **Watson, J. P.** Phobic disorders. 1. Clinical aspects. Nursing Mirror, 134, 3 Mar 1972, 22–23.

24 **Watson, J. P.** Phobic disorders. 2. Management. Nursing Mirror, 134, 10 Mar 1972, 32–35.

25 **Watson, J. P.** The treatment of anxiety. Nursing Mirror, 138, 17 May 1974, 72–73.

26 **Williamson, F.** The fourth is freedom from fear. [A study of 13 patients with phobias in the Alexandra Gardens Day Hospital, Belfast.] Nursing Times, 70, 28 Nov 1974, 1840–1845.

g PERSONALITY DISORDERS

1 **Birkett, M.** Nursing care study. Hysterical personality. Nursing Mirror, 136, 20 Apr 1973, 33–34.

2 **Bond, D.** Osmondmania: physiology of hysteria. [Teenage hysteria at a pop concert.] Nursing Times, 70, 7 Feb 1974, 176–177.

3 **Brennan, K. S. W.** Personality and behaviour disorders. Nursing Times, 67, 17 Jun 1971, 731–733.

4 **Carbary, L. J.** Helping the hysteric. Nursing Care, 8 (5), May 1975, 24–26, 28.

5 **Frost, M.** Playing it by ear. Kathy, a girl with hysterical personality. Nursing Times, 68, 29 Jun 1972, 809.

6 **Loh, S. F.** Nursing care study. A psychopathic personality. Nursing Times, 71, 4 Sep 1975, 1406–1408.

7 **MacArthur, C. H.** Nursing patients with personality disorders. Nursing Times, 67, 2 Dec 1971, 1494–1495.

8 **Mitchell, R.** Advances in psychiatry. 2. Hysteria. Nursing Times, 70, 4 Jul 1974, 1030–1032.

9 **Mitchell, R.** Advances in psychiatry. 5. Personality disorders. Nursing Times, 70, 25 Jul 1974, 1153–1155.

10 **Nicholas, D. H.** Nursing care study. Jane. Coping with hysteria. Nursing Times, 70, 4 Jul 1974, 1023–1024.

11 **O'Connell, B. A.** Psychopathic disorder. Nursing Mirror, 140, 26 Jun 1975, 51–53.

12 **Orr, J.** James – a psychopath. [A case study.] Nursing Times, 70, 12 Dec 1974, 1932–1933.

13 **Wallace, C. M.** Looking at psychiatry. 1. Nursing the hysterical patient. [Case history.] Nursing Mirror, 136, 27 Apr 1973, 40–41.

h SCHIZOPHRENIA

1 **Affleck, J. W. and Forrest, A. D.** A comprehensive treatment service for schizophrenics. Health Bulletin, 29 (4), Oct 1971, 203–205.

2 **Anderson, N. P.** Suicide in schizophrenia. Perspectives in Psychiatric Care, 11 (3), Jul/Sep 1973, 106–112.

3 **Beard, M. T. and others** Effects of sensory stimulation and remotivation on schizophrenic persons. Journal of Psychiatric Nursing, 10 (2), Mar/Apr 1972, 5–8.

4 **Bickford, J. A. R.** Schizophrenia. Nursing Times, 69, 21 Jun 1973, 794–796. [Reprinted from Practitioner, January 1973.]

5 **Bradbury, A.** Why psychotherapy for schizophrenics? A reply to Monica Frost. Nursing Times, 67, 13 May 1971, 588–589.

6 **Canadian Journal of Psychiatric Nursing** Three articles on schizophrenia. Canadian Journal of Psychiatric Nursing, 14 (2), Mar/Apr 1973, 3–9, 11–14.

7 **Cliffe, M. J.** The nurse as a behavioural engineer. [Rehabilitation of a psychiatric patient by a nurse who reinstated speech in a chronic schizophrenic.] Nursing Times, 70, 5 Sep 1974, 1396–1397.

8 **Cloud, E. D.** The plateau in therapist-patient relationships. [Psychotherapeutic treatment of chronic schizophrenics.] Perspectives in Psychiatric Care, 10 (3), 1972, 112–121.

9 **Cohen, R. G.** Anxiety as a manifestation of associated drives and events in a female schizophrenic patient, [including nursing implications]. Journal of Psychiatric Nursing and Mental Health Services, 11 (3), May/Jun 1973, 16–21.

10 **Cooper, P.** Progress in therapeutics. Drugs for schizophrenia. Midwife and Health Visitor, 10 (5), May 1974, 129.

11 **Creighton, P.** Nursing care study. Mary – a paranoid schizophrenic. Nursing Times, 70 23 May 1974, 803.

12 **Cullen, M.** A 'General' meets a schizophrenic. [A case study.] Australian Nurses' Journal, 4 (5), Nov 1974, 39–40.

13 **Davies, A. L.** The use of chlorpromazine in schizophrenia. Nursing Times, 69, 13 Dec 1973, 1694–1695.

14 **De Falco, M. L.** The rehospitalization of discharged schizophrenic patients. Perspectives in Psychiatric Care, 8 (3), Jul/Sep 1975, 130–135.

15 **Diamond, R.** The archetype of death and renewal in 'I never promised you a rose garden.' [Book by Hannah Green – a Schizophrenic.] Perspectives in Psychiatric Care, 8 (1), Jan/Mar 1975, 21–24.

16 **Emery, R. H.** Schizophrenic with malformations. [Case study which illustrates congenital malformation as a cause of schizophrenia.] New Zealand Nursing Journal, 68 (10), Oct 1974, 15–17.

17 **Field, W. E. and Ruelke, W.** Hallucinations and how to deal with them. [In schizophrenia.] American Journal of Nursing, 73 (4), Apr 1973, 638–640.

18 **Forrest, A. and Affleck, J., editors** New perspectives in schizophrenia. Edinburgh: Churchill Livingstone, 1975.

19 **Frost, M.** Schizophrenia. 1. Diagnosis and prognosis. Nursing Times, 71, 27 Feb 1975, 328–332.

20 **Frost, M.** Schizophrenia. 2. Psycho-analytical and other opinions. Nursing Times, 71, 6 Mar 1975, 386–387.

21 **Frost, M.** Schizophrenia. 3. Delusions and hallucinations: an account of two teaching sessions with student nurses. Nursing Times, 71, 13 Mar 1975, 431–433.

22 **Frost, M.** Schizophrenia. 4. Aggressives and natural isolates. Nursing Times, 71, 20 Mar 1975, 471–475.

23 **Frost, M.** Schizophrenia. 5. Physical treatments and drugs. Nursing Times, 71, 27 Mar 1975, 506–507.

24 **Frost, M.** Schizophrenia. 6. Acute schizophrenia. Nursing Times, 71, 3 Apr 1975, 542–544.

25 **Frost, M.** Schizophrenia. 7. Group treatment of the acute and chronic patient. Nursing Times, 71, 10 Apr 1975, 587–589.

26 **Frost, M.** Schizophrenia and psychotherapy. Nursing Times, 67, 11 Mar 1971, 297–298. See reply under Bradbury, A.

27 **Frost, M.** Treatment for schizophrenics. [Need for occupational therapy.] Health and Social Service Journal, 83, 8 Sep 1973, 2049.

28 **Geach, B. and White, J. C.** Emphatic resonance: a countertransference phenomenon [in nurses who work intensively with chronic schizophrenic patients]. American Journal of Nursing, 74 (7), Jul 1974, 1280–1285.

29 **Gowardman, M.** Token economy in chronic schizophrenia. [A scheme at Kingseat Hospital, Papakura.] New Zealand Nursing Journal, 68 (11), Nov 1974, 22–24.

30 **Jensen, J. L. and McGrew, L.** Leadership techniques in group therapy with chronic schizophrenic patients. Nursing Research, 23 (5), Sep/Oct 1974, 416–420.

31 **Johnson, H.** Nursing care study. Alice – a case of schizophrenia. Nursing Times, 70, 21 Mar 1974, 420–423.

32 **Kelleher, M. J.** Reappraisal of nurse's role in the treatment of schizophrenia. [Development of clinical and therapeutic skills in the light of recent advances in treatment.] International Journal of Nursing Studies, 2 (4), Dec 1974, 197–202.

33 **Knight, S. W. and Donlon, P. T.** The successful management of 'refractory' ambulatory schizophrenic patients [by a psychiatric nurse therapist]. Journal of Psychiatric Nursing and Mental Health Services, 12 (1), Jan/Feb 1974, 3–6.

34 **Kroah, J.** Strategies for interviewing in language and thought disorders. [Communication patterns of the schizophrenic.] Journal of Psychiatric Nursing and Mental Health Services, 12 (2), Mar/Apr 1974, 3–9.

35 **McEvoy, P.** Hebephrenic schizophrenia. Nursing Times, 69, 21 Jun 1973, 797–798.

36 **Mitchell, R.** Advances in psychiatry. 7. Schizophrenia. Nursing Times, 70, 8 Aug 1974, 1234–1236.

37 **Moffit, A. J.** Helping schizophrenics to help themselves. [The good effects of team nursing in reducing violence.] Nursing Times, 70 11 Apr 1974, 553–554.

38 **Nakagawa, H. and others** Fallacies in schizophrenia. Nursing Research, 23 (5), Sep/Oct 1974, 410–415.

39 **Nicholson, T. E.** Saving time and money. [Change over from trifluoperazine (Stelazine) tablets or syrup to the Spansule preparation for chronic schizophrenic patients.] Nursing Times, 68, 20 Jul 1972, 893–895.

40 **Nistor, S. L.** Mountains of the mind. [A case of paranoid schizophrenia.] Nursing Care, 6 (3), Mar 1973, 22–27.

41 **Pickford, J. A. R.** Schizophrenia. Nursing Mirror, 141, 28 Aug 1975, 49–50.

42 **Pochtman, G. A.** Disturbances in object relations in a chronic schizophrenic patient. Perspectives in Psychiatric Care, 8 (1), Jan/Mar 1975, 13–16.

43 **Rachman, S.** Schizophrenia: a look at Laing's views. New Society, 24, 26 Apr 1973, 184–186.

44 **Spire, R. H.** Photographic self-image confrontation. [By a nurse clinician in patients with schizophrenia.] American Journal of Nursing, 73 (7), Jul 1973, 1207–1210.

45 Stephens, D. A. Aspects of schizophrenia in the elderly. Nursing Mirror, 138, 26 Apr 1974, 52–54.

46 Stewart, B. M. Biochemical aspects of schizophrenia. American Journal of Nursing, 75 (12), Dec 1975, 2176–2179.

47 Walker, E. Nursing care study. Paranoid schizophrenia. Nursing Mirror, 138 (6), 26 Apr 1974, 86–87.

48 Weeks, P. Pamela – a paranoid schizophrenic. Nursing Times, 70, 5 Sep 1974, 1388–1390.

49 Wilson, H. S. and Ranks, J. Deciphering a schizophrenic's disguised communication: a task for clinical supervisory conference. International Journal of Nursing Studies, 8 (1), Feb 1971, 15–28.

50 Woolley, E. Nursing care study. Arthur – a case for integration? [A withdrawn and uncommunicative catatonic schizophrenic.] Nursing Mirror, 139, 7 Nov 1974, 78–79.

51 World Health Organization Schizophrenia: a multinational study. A study of the initial evaluation phase of the International Pilot Study of Schizophrenia. Geneva: WHO, 1975. (Public health papers no. 63.)

i SCHIZOPHRENIA: FAMILY AND COMMUNITY

1 Benington, H. R. Long acting phenothiazine in psychiatric practice [so that schizophrenics may remain in the community]. Nursing Mirror, 133, 26 Nov 1971, 28–29.

2 British Medical Journal Looking after schizophrenics. [The run down of mental hospitals, and the lack of care in the community.] British Medical Journal, 2, 4 May 1974, 236–237.

3 Cheer, C. Living with schizophrenia. [Results of a survey among relatives to assess adequacy of available services.] Social Work Today, 6, 3 Apr 1975, 2–7.

4 Creer, C. and Wing, J. Schizophrenia at home. Institute of Psychiatry, 1974.

5 Frost, M. Relatives of schizophrenic patients. [The role of the health visitor in their support.] Midwife and Health Visitor, 10 (2/3), Feb/Mar 1974, 56–57.

6 Frost, M. Schizophrenia. 8. From hospital to community. Nursing Times, 71, 17 Apr 1975, 623–627.

7 Giggs, J. High rates of schizophrenia among immigrants in Nottingham. Nursing Times, 69, 20 Sep 1973, 1210–1212.

8 Hare, E. H. Social class and schizophrenia. Nursing Mirror, 136, 23 Feb 1973, 37–38.

9 Hiep, A. A viable programme for schizophrenic out-patients. Australian Nurses' Journal, 4 (8), Mar 1975, 29–31, 42.

10 Leff, J. P. The maintenance treatment of schizophrenia. Nursing Mirror, 137, 7 Sep 1973, 26–27.

11 Morritt, C. Long-acting phenothiazines and schizophrenia. Nursing Mirror, 138, 12 Apr 1974, 57–59.

12 National Schizophrenia Fellowship Schizophrenia. Surbiton: The Fellowship, 1975.

13 Pringle, J. Living with schizophrenia. Mind and Mental Health Magazine, Spring 1972, 15–20.

14 Procter, T. Rehabilitation of the long-stay schizophrenic. Nursing Mirror, 139, 26 Sep 1974, 57–59.

15 Smith, N. The tangled web: my son – a schizophrenic. [By a nurse.] Johnson Publications, 1975.

16 Wing, J. editor Schizophrenia from within. Surbiton: National Schizophrenia Fellowship, 1975.

j SLEEP DISORDERS

1 Albert, I. R. and Albert, S. E. Penetrating the mysteries of sleep and sleep disorders. RN Magazine, 37 (8), Aug 1974, 36–39.

2 Chamarette, N. P. Dreams. 1. Dreams – their therapeutic usage. Nursing Times, 71, 6 Feb 1975, 208–209.

3 Chamarette, N. P. Dreams. 2. Why do we dream? Nursing Times, 71, 13 Feb 1975, 249–251.

4 Chamarette, N. P. Dreams. 3. Therapy by dream analysis. Nursing Times, 71, 20 Feb 1975, 312–313.

5 Fass, G. Sleep, drugs and dreams. American Journal of Nursing, 71 (12), Dec 1971, 2316–2320.

6 Guilleminault, C. Sleep apnoea – insomnia. [Study in a sleep laboratory.] Nursing Times, 70, 31 Oct 1974, 1708–1709.

7 Jenkins, J. B. and Spensley, J. Electrosleep therapy. Nursing Times, 67, 21 Oct 1971, 1310–1312.

8 Martin, I. C. A. Some therapeutic concepts of sleep. Nursing Times, 71, 9 Oct 1975, 1611–1614.

9 Norris, C. M. Restlessness: a nursing phenomenon in search of meaning. [An investigation by a nurse clinician.] Nursing Outlook, 23 (2), Feb 1975, 103–107.

10 Parkes, J. D. Narcolepsy. Nursing Times, 71, 5 Jun 1975, 881–883.

11 Robin, I. G. Snoring. Nursing Times, 69, 21 Jun 1973, 788–790.

12 Smith, S. E. Drugs and sleep. Nursing Times, 67, 7 Oct 1971, 1248–1249.

13 Smith, S. E. How drugs act. 11. Drugs and sleep. Nursing Times, 71, 4 Sep 1975, 1417–1418.

14 Williams, D. H. Sleep and disease. American Journal of Nursing, 71 (12), Dec 1971, 2321–2334.

k SUICIDE

1 Bagley, C. Evaluating suicide prevention agencies. [With special reference to the Samaritans.] Community Medicine, 129 (7), 1 Dec 1972, 159–162.

2 Bahra, R. J. The potential for suicide. American Journal of Nursing, 75 (10), Oct 1975, 1782–1788.

3 Day, G. H. Suicide – a need for sympathy. Nursing Times, 67, 7 Oct 1971, 1235–1236.

4 Delbridge, P. M. Identifying the suicidal person in the community. Canadian Nurse, 70 (11), Nov 1974, 14–17.

5 Fox, R. The suicide drop – why? [Statistical changes since the Second World War and preventive measures such as the formation of the Samaritans.] Royal Society of Health Journal, 95 (1), Feb 1975, 9–13, 20.

6 Lavina The Samaritans: a nurse's impressions. Nursing Mirror, 134, 31 Mar 1972, 26–27.

7 Midwife, Health Visitor and Community Nurse Time to listen. [The work of the Samaritans Organization.] Midwife, Health Visitor Community Nurse, 11 (1), Jan 1975, 20–21.

8 Nursing Times The Samaritans. Nursing Times, 70, 10 Oct 1974, 1570–1571.

9 Poulos, J. The geriatric suicide. Bedside Nurse, 4 (7), Jul 1971, 24–26.

10 Stevens, B. J. A phenomenological approach to understanding suicidal behavior. Journal of Psychiatric Nursing, 9 (5), Sep/Oct 1971, 33–35.

11 Vollen, K. H. and Watson, C. G. Suicide in relation to time of day and day of week. American Journal of Nursing, 75 (2), Feb 1975, 263.

12 Westercamp, T. M. Suicide. American Journal of Nursing, 75 (2), Feb 1975, 260–262.

l SUICIDE: NURSING CARE AND ATTITUDES

1 Bray, D. E. Good night nurse . . . and goodbye. . . [Nursing intervention in suicide.] Journal of Practical Nursing, 25 (12), Dec 1975, 16–17, 32.

2 Chapman, M. Movement therapy in the treatment of suicidal patients. Perspectives in Psychiatric Care, 9 (3), May/Jun 1971, 119–122.

3 Clemmons, P. K. The role of the nurse in suicide prevention. Journal of Psychiatric Nursing, 9 (1), Jan/Feb 1971, 27–30.

4 Cunningham, R. What do nurses do to help patients who attempt suicide? [An exploratory study of public health nurses.] Canadian Nurse, 71 (1), Jan 1975, 27–29.

5 Floyd, G. J. Nursing management of the suicidal patient. Journal of Psychiatric Nursing and Mental Health Services, 13 (2), Mar/Apr 1975, 23–26.

6 Frost, M. Counselling the suicidal patient. Nursing Mirror, 139 (1), 5 Jul 1974, 74–75.

7 Heath, M. 'Quiet cries'. Can I help? Will you listen? [Suicidal patient.] Nursing Care, 6 (4), Apr 1973, 26–30.

8 Leonard, C. V. Treating the suicidal patient: a communication approach. Journal of Psychiatric Nursing and Mental Health Services, 13 (2), Mar/Apr 1975, 19–22.

9 Moreton, K. Nursing care study. Keith – a treatment problem. [After attempted suicide.] Nursing Times, 71, 10 Jul 1975, 1097–1100.

80 PSYCHIATRIC REHABILITATION

a REHABILITATION (See also Art, music and drama therapy)

1 Barnes, M. A chance to live again. [Experiences at Kingsley Hall used by the Philadelphia Association for Psychotherapeutic Work.] Nursing Times, 71, 24 Apr 1975, 660–661.

2 Barnes, R. Helping institutionalized patients back to life outside hospital. [A community project in Salford.] Community Medicine, 129, 20 Oct 1972, 566–567.

3 Bennett, D. H. Rehabilitation in psychiatry. Occupational Therapy, 36 (4), Apr 1973, 290–291.

4 British Medical Journal Rootless wanderers. [Leading article on the effects of the run-down of mental hospitals and the plight of discharged patients.] British Medical Journal, 3, 7 Jul 1973, 1–2,

5 Britten, C. S. The function of a half-way house within a long-stay ward. International Journal of Social Psychiatry, 20 (1/2), Spring/Summer 1974, 78–79.

6 Christie, H. A. Fulbrook – the crossroads? [Fulbrook Ward, Littlemore Hospital, used as a centre for the assessment of rehabilitation potential in long term psychiatric patients.] Nursing Mirror, 136, 6 Apr 1973, 25–27.

7 Cox, A. Group nursing in ward 5. [Assessment after two years of a scheme of nursing involving intensive rehabilitation of long stay patients at Stratheden Hospital.] Nursing Mirror, 136, 2 Feb 1973, 39–41.

8 Cresdee, D. B. Something to look forward to.

[Summer holidays for the mentally ill.] Nursing Times, 68, 6 Jul 1972, 851–852.

9 Dix, J. M. The forgotten patient. [Follow-up care for discharged patient.] Journal of Psychiatric Nursing, 10 (5), Sep/Oct 1972, 15–17.

10 Dowker, E. M. A beauty salon in a psychiatric hospital. [High Royds Hospital, Menston, Yorks.] Nursing Mirror, 140, 23 Jan 1975, 59–61.

11 Erickson, D. Psychiatric rehabilitation: a discussion of alternatives. Canadian Journal of Psychiatric Nursing, 14 (6), Nov/Dec 1973, 8–12.

12 Gray, J. C. The considerate campers: camping holiday for long-stay psychiatric patients. Nursing Mirror, 135, 25 Aug 1972, 12–14.

13 Harrison, P. The careless community. [Provisions made for patients discharged from psychiatric hospitals.] New Society, 24, 28 Jun 1973, 742–745.

14 Holkar, I. M. Rehabilitation of long stay psychiatric patients. Nursing Journal of India, 63 (2), Feb 1972, 47, 58.

15 Holland, E. Change – rehabilitation in psychiatric nursing. New Zealand Nursing Journal, 69 (9), Sep 1975, 24–25.

16 Jansson, D. P. Return to society: problematic features of the re-entry process. Perspectives in Psychiatric Care, 8 (3), Jul/Sep 1975, 136–142.

17 Leavitt, M. The discharge crisis: the experience of families of psychiatric patients. Nursing Research, 24 (1), Jan/Feb 1975, 33–40.

18 Leins, J. A. The psychiatric nurse in rehabilitation – a continuing role. Canadian Journal of Psychiatric Nursing, 14 (1), Jan/Feb 1973, 4–5.

19 Lucas, R. Rehabilitation of the psychiatric patient. Queen's Nursing Journal, 16 (10), Jan 1974, 234, 242.

20 Morgan, K. E. Their rightful place: rehabilitation into the community for long-stay patients. Nursing Mirror, 136, 26 Jan 1973, 18–19.

21 Murray, E. W. Mental illness: is rehabilitation worth the effort? [Benefits for the mentally ill in hospital compared with the community.] Nursing Mirror, 139, 2 Aug 1974, 64–65.

22 Newnham, W. H. A comprehensive psychiatric rehabilitation programme: [at the Towers Hospital, Leicester]. Rehabilitation, no. 88, Jan/Mar 1974, 9–16.

23 Oldham, A. J. P. Rehabilitation of the mentally ill. Theme – rehabilitation within the future structure of psychiatric services in England. Rehabilitation, no. 80, Jan/Mar 1972, 37–39.

24 Payne, J. Restored to life. [The work of St. Wulstan's Hospital, Malvern, in psychiatric rehabilitation.] Mind and Mental Health Magazine, Autumn 1972, 2–8.

25 Penn, V. A helping hand. [Shopping trip for mentally disturbed patients.] Nursing Times, 68, 14 Sep 1972, 1169.

26 Price, J. and Vincent, P. Program evaluation: what to ask before you start. [Using follow-up service for discharged mental patients as an example.] Nursing Outlook, 24 (2), Feb 1976, 84–86.

27 Royston, R. Psychiatric rehabilitation: apathy to self-assertion. [The work of the Psychiatric Rehabilitation Association.] Health and Social Service Journal, 84, 7 Dec 1974, 2831.

28 Smith, G. Institutional dependence is reversible. [Scheme at the Old Manor Hospital, Salisbury, where psychiatric patients are discharged to live with families in the community.] Social Work Today, 6, 16 Oct 1975, 426–428.

29 Tibbenham, L. S. A new beginning. [Rehabilitation of the long-stay chronic psychiatric patient at Hellesdon Hospital, Norwich.] Nursing Mirror, 135, 29 Dec 1972, 22–23.

30 Wilk, R. A. Dingleton's phased rehabilitation programme. Nursing Mirror, 134, 11 Feb 1972, 35–37.

31 Wills, P. Rehabilitation: clinical and occupational. Occupational Therapy, 36 (4), Apr 1973, 292–296.

32 Wing, J. K. Principles of rehabilitation of the mentally ill. Occupational Therapy, 36 (4), Apr 1973, 285–289.

b GROUP HOMES AND HOSTELS

1 Anstice, E. Half way home. [Work of the Richmond Fellowship.] Nursing Times, 69, 25 Jan 1973, 129–131.

2 Barnes, R. Group homes and social networks. [For discharged mental patients.] Health and Social Service Journal, 83, 14 Jul 1973, 1587–1588.

3 Bates, M. and Tylden, E. Stepping stones in psychiatry. [The Stepping Stones Club, a pioneer day-care centre at Bromley Hospital.] Social Service Quarterly, 48 (1), Jul/Sep 1974, 172–174.

4 Boucherat, N. From hospital to home. [Hostel for discharged psychiatric patients run by Hertfordshire County Council.] Social Work Today, 3, 22 Mar 1973, 13–17.

5 Creighton, P. A home of their own. [A group home for selected psychiatric patients at St. Francis Hospital, Haywards Heath.] Nursing Times, 70, 23 May 1974, 804–805.

6 Crighton, D. Half-way hostel. [Stoke-on-Trent.] Health and Social Service Journal, 83, 22 Sep 1973, 2185.

7 Hall, M. E. A patients' commune in Paddington. [Communal living accommodation for psychiatric patients at Paddington Day Hospital.] British Hospital Journal and Social Service Review, 82, 16 Dec 1972, 2813–2814.

8 Johnstone, T. and Presly, A. S. Psychiatric out-patients: some observations of a follow-up group. Nursing Times, 68, 24 Feb 1972, 228–230.

9 Leopoldt, H. It is for them to say. [Opinion survey of group-home residents.] Rehabilitation, no. 84, Jan/Mar 1973, 43–45.

10 Leopoldt, H. and others Selection for group-home living. [Guidelines for assessing psychiatric in-patients for group home living used at the Littlemore Hospital, Oxford.] Nursing Mirror, 139, 5 Dec 1974, 58–62.

11 Leopoldt, H. and Hurn, R. J. Thorncliffe House. [A psychiatric half-way house which became a day-care centre and out patient clinic.] Health and Social Service Journal, 85, 2 Aug 1975, 1671–1672.

12 Mind and Mental Health Magazine [Experimental housing project for mental patients run by the Norfolk and Norwich Association for Mental Health.] Mind and Mental Health Magazine, Autumn 1971, 10–15.

13 Moore, J. Half-way houses – then what? [Richmond Fellowship conference which demonstrated the need for research into therapeutic communities.] Nursing Times, 71, 24 Apr 1975, 640–641.

14 Prosser, J. Half-way at Hill House. [Mental after-care hostel in Elstree.] British Hospital Journal and Social Service Review, 82, 1 Jan 1972, 27–28.

15 Psychiatric Rehabilitation Association Nicholas

House: an exercise in residential care of the mentally ill. The Association, 1972.

16 Rice, B. and Walker, D. L. Starting a group home [for psychiatric patients in Gloucester]. Health and Social Service Journal, 84, 13 Jul 1974, 1557–1558.

17 Whitehead, J. A. Boarding out since St. Dymphna. [The schemes at Severalls Hospital and Brighton.] Nursing Times, 67, 16 Dec 1971, 1555–1558.

c WORK THERAPY AND EMPLOYMENT

1 Breary, G. and Milne, J. Workers' group. [Group formed at Rees House Day Hospital, Croydon, Surrey, to help psychiatric patients find employment.] Occupational Therapy, 36 (7), Jul 1973, 412–413.

2 Craib, H. G. Rehabilitation in psychiatric hospitals: a review of industrial therapy. Nursing Mirror, 140, 30 Jan 1975, 58–59.

3 Davies, M. H. The rehabilitation of psychiatric patients at an industrial therapy unit outside the hospital. [Birmingham Industrial Therapy Association Factory.] International Journal of Social Psychiatry, 18 (2), Summer 1972, 120–126.

4 Early, D. F. Sheltered groups in open industry: a new approach to training and to employment. [The Industrial Therapy Organization, Bristol.] Lancet, 1, 21 Jun 1975, 1370–1373.

5 Health and Social Service Journal Self help in psychiatry. [Industrial education unit of PRA Plastics – set up by the Psychiatric Rehabilitation Association.] Health and Social Service Journal, 83, 10 Mar 1973, 538–539, 541.

6 Kerr, W. S. Employment of the mentally ill. Nursing Times, 69, 22 Mar 1973, Occ. papers, 45–48.

7 Mantus, L. On finding a job. [The problems of a person with a history of mental illness.] Mind and Mental Health Magazine, Autumn 1972, 9–12.

8 Moores, B. Work therapy. [For patients in mental hospitals.] Health and Social Service Journal, 83, 7 Apr 1973, 791–792.

9 Sclafani, M. The institutional milieu as a work environment. Journal of Psychiatric Nursing, 11 (2), Mar/Apr 1973, 17–18.

10 Toombs, K. Industrial therapy at Friern Hospital. Nursing Times, 69, 1 Feb 1973, 137–138.

11 Troman, F. Task force. [Work therapy in Mayo Unit, a long-stay rehabilitation unit at Littlemore Hospital, Oxford.] Nursing Mirror, 138, 29 Mar 1974, 79–80.

81 MENTAL HANDICAP

a GENERAL AND SERVICES

1 Andrews, J. Better services for the mentally handicapped. Nursing Mirror, 133, 22 Oct 1971, 9–10.

2 Andrews, J. Breaking the bounds. [Second annual congress of the Association of Professions for the Mentally Handicapped.] Nursing Mirror, 140, 1 May 1975, 41–42.

3 Association of Professions for the Mentally Handicapped Better services – the realities. Proceedings of the Association's first annual congress, 15–18 July 1974. The Association, 1974.

4 Association of Professions for the Mentally Handicapped Conference studies care of mentally handicapped. Multi-disciplinary approach needed. British

Journal of Occupational Therapy, 38 (9), Sep 1975, 205–206.

5 Bone, M. and others Plans and provision for the mentally handicapped. Allen & Unwin, 1972. (National Institute for Social Work Training series no. 23.)

6 Bosanquet, N. The back wards. [Comment on 'Opening the door' by Dr. Kathleen Jones.] Nursing Times, 71, 11 Sep 1975, 1441.

7 Bosanquet, N. Talking point. New hope for the handicapped. Nursing Times, 71, 6 Mar 1975, 364–365.

8 British Journal of Mental Subnormality [Editorial on the setting up of the 'National Development Group' and 'Development Team' by the DHSS.] British Journal of Mental Subnormality, 21, Jun 1975, 1–2.

9 Castle, B. Four point plan for mental handicap services. [Reported by P. Dack.] Nursing Mirror, 140, 6 Mar 1975, 40.

10 Clarke, M. and Clarke, A. D. B. Mental deficiency: the changing outlook. 3rd ed. Methuen, 1974. (Manuals of modern psychology.)

11 Department of Health and Social Security and Welsh Office Better services for the mentally handicapped. HMSO, 1971.

12 Dutton, G. Assessment of mental handicap. Health and Social Service Journal, 84, 18 May 1974, 1110–1111.

13 Forrest, A. and others, editors New perspectives in mental handicap. Edinburgh: Churchill Livingstone, 1973.

14 Gorman, V. Mental handicap – what should be the priorities? Health and Social Service Journal, 85, 20 Sep 1975, 2096.

15 Gunzberg, H. C., editor Advance in the care of the mentally handicapped. British Society for the Study of Mental Subnormality, distributed by Baillière Tindall, 1973.

16 Gunzburg, H. C. Subnormality – an integrated service. Nursing Mirror, 132, 5 Mar 1971, 34–38.

17 Hallas, C. H. The care and training of the mentally handicapped. 5th ed. Bristol: Wright, 1974.

18 Heaton-Ward, W. A. Mental subnormality: subnormality and severe subnormality. 4th ed. Bristol: Wright, 197.

19 Hills, M. Someone is asking us: an action research project conducted through the King Edward's Hospital Fund for London, involving fieldworkers from different disciplines, is attempting to improve the co-ordination of the services for the mentally handicapped. Nursing Times, 67, 9 Sep 1971, 1119–1120; 16 Sep 1971, 1148–1149.

20 Jones, A. W. Challenges of severe and profound mental retardation. Health and Social Service Journal, 84, 22 Jun 1974, 1397.

21 Jones, K. Opening the door: a study of new policies for the mentally handicapped. Routledge and Kegan Paul, 1975. (International Library of Social Policy.)

22 Kekstadt, H. and Primrose, D. A. A. Mental subnormality. Heinemann, 1973. (Modern practical nursing series, no. 15.)

23 King's Fund Centre Strategies for profound mental handicap. The Fund, 1972. (Mental handicap papers, 1.)

24 Kirman, B. H. Mental handicap: a brief guide. Crosby: Lockwood Staples, 1975.

25 Kirman, B. H. and Bicknell, J. Mental handicap. Edinburgh: Churchill Livingstone, 1975.

26 Kushlick, A. The future for the mentally handicapped. Health and Social Service Journal, 83, 17 Mar 1973, 606–609.

27 Labour Party Labour's plans for the mentally handicapped: a national service? Nursing Times, 70, 4 Jul 1974, 1018–1019.

28 MacCarthy, J. S. Change in subnormality care. Nursing Times, 67, 16 Sep 1971, Occ. papers, 145–147.

29 McLachlan, G., editor Approaches to action: a symposium on services for the mentally ill and handicapped. Oxford University Press (for Nuffield Provincial Hospitals Trust), 1972. (Occasional hundreds, no. 5.)

30 Madeley, B. R. A host of new ideas: physical needs of the mentally handicapped. Nursing Mirror, 132, 15 Jan 1971, 28–29.

31 Malin, N. A. An investigation into the facilities for the care, training and education of the mentally handicapped and into the expressed attitudes of staff towards clients . . . MPhil thesis CNAA (Paisley College of Technology), 1975.

32 National Development Group for the Mentally Handicapped Mental handicap planning together. Revised ed. The Group, 1975.

33 Office of Health Economics Mental handicap. The Office, 1973. (Studies on current health problems no. 47.)

34 O'Toole, R. New deal for mentally handicapped. British Hospital Journal and Social Service Review, 82, 29 Jul 1972, 1678.

35 Pilkington, T. L. Mental handicap in perspective. Nursing Times, 68, 29 Jun 1972, 804–806.

36 Pilkington, T. L. A new deal for the mentally handicapped. Hospital and Health Services Review, 71 (1), Jan 1975, 9–12.

37 Pilkington, T. L. Public and professional attitudes to mental handicap. Public Health, 87 (3), Mar 1973, 61–66.

38 Royal College of Nursing and Mind 'One foot in the community.' [Report of an Rcn conference 'Sharing Care' which considered the roles of professionals in caring for the mentally handicapped.] Nursing Times, 71, 20 Mar 1975, 444; Nursing Mirror, 140, 20 Mar 1975, 36.

39 Royal College of Psychiatrists Better services for the mentally handicapped: teach-in. Nursing Times, 67, 21 Oct 1971, 1324.

40 Segal, S. S., compiler Mental handicap: a select annotated bibliography. Slough: National Foundation for Educational Research in England and Wales, 1972.

41 Shapiro, A. Modern approach to mental handicap and its historical development. Nursing Times, 67, 18 Feb 1971; 25 Feb 1971, Occ. papers, 25–31.

42 Sheahan, J. Towards security: meeting the needs of the mentally handicapped. Nursing Times, 71, 10 Jul 1975, 1110–1111.

43 Shearer, A. An ark for survival. [L'Arche – an international movement for the mentally handicapped.] New Society, 31, 13 Mar 1975, 650–651.

44 Shearer, A. Mental handicap. [International League of Societies for the Mentally Handicapped conference.] New Society, 33, 25 Sep 1975, 699.

45 South-East Metropolitan Regional Hospital Board and Spastics Society The mentally handicapped today. Nursing Mirror, 132, 8 Jan 1971, 10–11.

46 Taylor, J. B. [Reorganization.] White elephant land. [Progress of mental handicap provision since reorganization.] Nursing Times, 71, 3 Apr 1975, 534–536.

47 Tizard, J. Mental handicap 1947–1972: a review of policies progress and problems. Community Medicine, 129 (10), 22 Dec 1972, 235–237.

48 Tizard, J. Research into services for the mentally handicapped: science and policy issues. British Journal of Mental Subnormality, 18 (1), Jun 1972, 6–17.

b OVERSEAS COUNTRIES

1 Cruickshank, W. The USA scene. [Services for the mentally handicapped.] Health and Social Service Journal, 83, 1 Dec 1973, 2809.

2 Goodworth, M. D. Holland can show us how to care for the subnormal. Occupational Therapy, 35 (9), Sep 1972, 667–668.

3 Kings Fund Centre Mental handicap and normalization. [Comparison of care of subnormal in Scandinavia and Britain.] Nursing Times, 67, 28 Jan 1971, 122–123; Hospital, 67 (2), Feb 1971, 59–60; British Hospital Journal and Social Service Review, 81, 6 Mar 1971, 416–417.

4 Lambo, T. A. Services for the mentally handicapped in Africa. Royal Society of Health Journal, 93 (1), Feb 1973, 20–23, 56.

5 Lee, L. Canadian facilities for the mentally retarded. 'Much being done, much left to do.' Canadian Journal of Psychiatric Nursing, 13 (5), Sep/Oct 1972, 4–7.

6 Nicolausson, U. Provisions for the mentally handicapped in Sweden. Royal Society of Health Journal, 93 (1), Feb 1973, 24–28.

7 Shearer, A. Danish services for the retarded. British Hospital Journal and Social Service Review, 82, 29 Jan 1972, 251.

8 Strong, P. G. Services for the mentally handicapped in Scandinavia. Nursing Mirror, 141, 18 Sep 1975, 64–67.

c COMMUNITY CARE

1 Andrews, J. The experts report. [A review of 'Buildings for mentally handicapped people'.] Nursing Times, 67, 1 Jul 1971, 809–811.

2 Bagnall, N. A Steiner village. [Village community for the mentally handicapped at Bolton, Yorkshire.] New Society, 27, 13 Sep 1973, 643–644.

3 Bayley, M. Mental handicap and community care: a study of mentally handicapped people in Sheffield. Routledge and Kegan Paul, 1973.

4 Blair, P. Accommodation for Sheffield's mentally handicapped. [Programme for developing residential and day care.] Health and Social Service Journal, 85, 26 Apr 1975, 942–943.

5 Blair, P. Mental handicap provision. [Report of the Architects of the Norton housing scheme, Sheffield presented to the DHSS.] Health and Social Service Journal, 85, 3 May 1975, 1004–1005.

6 Browne, R. A. Symposium of the 'hospitalized' patient in the community. 1. The needs of patients in subnormality hospitals if discharged to community care. British Journal of Mental Subnormality, 17 (1), Jun 1971, 7–24.

7 Caddell, J. and others Guardianship programme in a mental subnormality hospital. [Scheme at Bryn-y-Neuadd Hospital, North Wales, whereby patients living in boarding houses attend the hospital each day.] Nursing Times, 69, 1 Mar 1973, 265–267.

8 Craft, M. and others Small group homes for subnormals: the range of care offered in Denbighshire. Social Work Today, 4, 21 Mar 1974, 791–793.

9 Crawford, D. Community care and the mentally

handicapped. [Consequences of phasing out hospitals for the mentally handicapped.] Nursing Times, 68, 8 Jun 1972, 713–714.

10 Cullinan, J. New wine into old bottles. [Village community for mentally subnormal at Brentwood, Essex.] Nursing Times, 68, 27 Apr 1972, 493–496.

11 Davis, E. F. Caring for the mentally handicapped. [Home Farm Trust.] Social Service Quarterly, 46 (3), Jan/Mar 1973, 96–98.

12 Department of Health and Social Security Buildings for mentally handicapped people: a report. HMSO, 1971.

13 Edwardson, W. J. Rehabilitation in the community. Aim for mentally handicapped at Calderstones Hospital, Blackburn. Nursing Mirror, 135, 1 Dec 1972, 47–51.

14 Elliott, J. and Bayes, D. Room for improvement: a better environment for the mentally handicapped. King Edward's Hospital Fund for London, 1972.

15 Forbes, P. Caring for the mentally handicapped. [Village community for mentally handicapped people at Blackerton, Devon.] Social Service Quarterly, 46 (1), Jul/Sep 1972, 16–19.

16 Francklin, S. Homes for mentally handicapped people. Campaign for the Mentally Handicapped, 1974. (CMH discussion papers, no. 4.)

17 Gibson, J. Greenacres. [Family unit for the mentally handicapped.] British Hospital Journal and Social Service Review, 81, 2 Oct 1971, 2028–2029.

18 Gunzburg, H. C. The physical environment of the mentally handicapped. 8 – '39 steps' leading towards normalized living practices in living units for the mentally handicapped. British Journal of Mental Subnormality, 19, Dec 1973, 91–99.

19 Gunzburg, H. C. The physical environment of the mentally handicapped. 9. The search for a home environment. [Project in the design of Wordsley Mental Handicap Unit – House.] British Journal of Mental Subnormality, 20 (1), Jun 1974, 28–42.

20 Harbert, W. B. Hostels for mentally handicapped adults. Health and Social Service Journal, 84, 21 Sep 1974, 2164–2165.

21 Jones, A. W. Group homes for the mentally subnormal. Health and Social Service Journal, 83, 13 Jan 1973, 93–94.

22 Kings Fund Centre Outside the walls. [Conference on caring for the mentally handicapped in the community.] Health and Social Service Journal, 85, 19 Jul 1975, 1537; Nursing Times, 71, 3 Jul 1975, 1032.

23 Marais, E. Cast adrift. [The discharge of the mentally handicapped into the community.] New Society, 25, 9 Aug 1973, 335–336.

24 Nellist, A. I. Building for the mentally handicapped. [This should be less institutional, more human, personal and domestic in size and atmosphere.] Health and Social Service Journal, 84, 14 Dec 1974, 2883–2884.

25 Nursing Mirror Villas for the mentally handicapped [at Witham and Colchester]. Nursing Mirror, 141, 3 Jul 1975, 69.

26 Pascoe, F. E. A community service for the mentally handicapped. Mother and Child, 43 (3), May/Jun 1971, 11–14.

27 Pilkington, T. L. Some family and community aspects of mental handicap. Community Medicine, 127 (11), 17 Mar 1972, 143–144.

28 Quinn, M. and others Community accommodation for the mentally handicapped. British Journal of Mental Subnormality, 20, Dec 1974, 86–89.

29 Robinson, W. A village for the mentally handicapped. Blackerton. Nursing Times, 69, 19 Jul 1973, 932–934.

30 Simpson, W. H. The physical environment of the mentally handicapped. 7. Homes for the mentally handicapped – South-west Wales. British Journal of Mental Subnormality, 19, Jun 1973, 48–53.

31 Slater, H. Community care for the mentally frail. Social Work Today, 2 (6), 17 Jun 1971, 3–8.

32 Smiley, C. The integration of the mentally handicapped: the Kingston pilot project. International Journal of Health Education, 16 (3), 1973, 199–204.

33 Webster, C. Housing the mentally handicapped – is money the answer? Nursing Mirror, 136, 8 Jun 1973, 15.

34 Welsh Hospital Board Houses for the handicapped. [Welsh Hospital Board arrangements.] Health and Social Service Journal, 83, 24 Mar 1973, 674.

35 White, T. Priorities for the mentally handicapped in the community. [National Society for Mentally Handicapped Children conference.] Nursing Mirror, 140, 5 Jun 1975, 51–52.

36 Williams, C. E. Symposium on the 'hospitalized' patient in the community. 3. A study of the patients in a group of mental subnormality hospitals. British Journal of Mental Subnormality, 17 (1), Jun 1971, 29–41.

d HOSPITALS

1 Arenillas, L. Emptying subnormality hospitals. British Hospital Journal and Social Service Review, 81, 18 Dec 1971, 2666–2667.

2 Brown, J. Ward 99. [The author's work as a nursing assistant in a hospital for the mentally handicapped.] Nursing Times, 68, 17 Feb 1972, 197–201.

3 Dainty, K. Individual patients' clothing involving budgetary control 1970/71. [Mentally handicapped patients at Glenfrith Hospital, Leicester.] Nursing Times, 67, 25 Nov 1971, Occ. papers, 185–187.

4 Department of Health and Social Security Hospital building for the mentally handicapped: a background to design. The Department, 1973. (Design bulletin, no. 1.)

5 Fryd, J. Consumer report on subnormality hospitals. Maternal and Child Care, 7, Sep 1971, 78–80.

6 Jenkins, T. D. M. 'But for the grace. . . .' the long stay hospitals, mental handicap. South East Metropolitan Regional Hospital Board, 1973.

7 Jones, K. The media and hospital scandals. [The gap between the Government's recommendations for mental handicap provision and what is practicable.] Health and Social Service Journal, 85, 25 Jan 1975, 173.

8 Kay, J. Institutions: an acceptable face. [Pilot investigation on measures to avoid the institutionalization of the inmates.] Health and Social Service Journal, 84, 10 Aug 1974, 1802–1803.

9 Kerr, G. Personal view. [On how to improve hospitals for the mentally subnormal.] British Medical Journal, 3, 30 Sep 1972, 822.

10 Kings Fund Centre Decentralization of large hospitals: mental handicap conference. Nursing Mirror, 132, 26 Mar 1971, 13–14; Hospital, 67 (4), Apr 1971, 129–130.

11 Nursing Times What is your score? [Hospitals for the mentally handicapped, including Southampton, Birmingham and Harperbury.] Nursing Times, 70, 17 Oct 1974, 1604–1607; 24 Oct 1974, 1676–1677; 31 Oct 1974, 1698–1701.

12 Primrose, D. A. The changing pattern of admission to a mental deficiency hospital. [Royal Scottish National Hospital, Larbert.] Health Bulletin, 32 (5), Sep 1974, 213–215.

13 Rowe, D. The effort of a more stimulating environment on the behaviour of a group of severely subnormal adults. [At Harmston Hall Hospital, Lincolnshire.] British Journal of Mental Subnormality, 20 (1) (38), Jun 1974, 6–13.

14 Scottish Health Services Council Standing Medical Advisory Committee and Standing Nursing and Midwifery Advisory Committee. The staffing of mental deficiency hospitals. Edinburgh: HMSO, 1970. Chairman: I. R. C. Batchelor.

15 Stacey, M. Mental handicap: deployment of resources. [Large hospitals should be run down in favour of small units.] Health and Social Service Journal, 85, 19 Apr 1975, 885–886.

16 Stoke Park Student Nurses Do hospitals meet the needs of subnormality? [Letter from student nurses of the Stoke Park Group of Hospitals in Bristol asking for a 'complete reappraisal of the methods of care for the mentally subnormal and Government policy on such care.' Followed by discussion with student nurses.] Nursing Times, 68, 22 Jun 1972, 764–766.

17 Sylvester, P. E. The long-stay hospital – a modern concept. [Greenacres, a residential unit for adults and children at St. Lawrence's Hospital, Caterham.] Nursing Mirror, 136, 18 May 1973, 34–37.

e INDIVIDUAL HOSPITALS

1 Abbeyfields A new residential hospital for the mentally handicapped. [Mainly illustrations.] Nursing Mirror, 139, 17 Oct 1974, 72–73.

2 Brockhall Another hospital enquiry. [Summary of the report of the enquiry into standards of patient care at Brockhall Hospital.] Hospital and Health Services Review, 71 (2), Feb 1975, 41.

3 Bryn-y-Neuadd — Craft, M. J. Hospital with a purpose. British Hospital Journal and Social Service Review, 81, 14 Aug 1971, 1654–1656.

4 Coldeast Hospital — Amsden, A. L. Anatomy of achievement. What the nurses did and are doing. Nursing Times, 67, 3 Jun 1971, 670–673.

5 Coldeast Hospital Design Team The physical environment of the mentally handicapped. 11. From ward to living unit. A pilot scheme in reshaping the mental subnormality hospital. [Coldeast Hospital, Hampshire.] British Journal of Mental Subnormality, 17, Jun 1971, 54–65.

6 Earls House, Durham — Hay, D. N. New hospital – new patterns of care. Nursing Times, 67, 16 Sep 1971, 1150–1151.

7 Earls House — Kerr, G. Caring for the mentally handicapped: theory and practice. [Creating a therapeutic environment.] Nursing Mirror, 137, 19 Oct 1973, 16–19.

8 Ely Hospital The first stage in the redevelopment of a hospital for the mentally handicapped. Hospital, 67 (9), Sep 1971, 318–319.

9 Essex Hall Living space. [Essex Hall Hospital, Colchester for the elderly mentally handicapped. Mainly illustrations.] Nursing Times, 71, 5 Jun 1975, 870–871.

10 Farleigh Hospital Committee of Inquiry Report. HMSO, 1971. Chairman: Tasker Watkins.

11 Farleigh Hospital Hospital, 67 (5), May 1971, 143–144.

12 Farleigh — Owen, A. S. Innocent? Guilty? Or

just plain vulnerable? One nurse's view of a court of inquiry and its sequel. Health Services, 25 (6), Jun 1972, 8–9.

13 Fieldhead Village at Fieldhead. Domestic concept of site of new hospital for mentally handicapped. Nursing Mirror, 136, 19 Jan 1973, 37–39.

14 Gogarburn — Forrest, A. D. Edinburgh's care for the subnormal. [Based on Gogarburn Hospital.] British Hospital Journal and Social Service Review, 81, 16 Oct 1971, 2140–2141.

15 Grove Park — Semrock, R. Aspects of mental handicap. [Living in small family units at Grove Park Hospital, London.] Nursing Times, 70, 5 Dec 1974, 1909–1911.

16 Ida Darwin Focus on Ida Darwin. Purpose built hospital for mentally handicapped at Fulbourn, Cambridge. Nursing Mirror, 135, 29 Sep 1972, 29–31.

17 Leavesden — Sprince, H. V. The physical environment of the mentally handicapped. 6. An Architect's approach to the design of a patients' club. [Leavesden Hospital.] British Journal of Mental Subnormality, 18 (2), Dec 1972, 108–112.

18 Leavesden — Wertheimer, A. Cared for and caring. [Family grouping experiment at Leavesden Hospital.] Mind and Mental Health Magazine, Spring 1972, 39–43.

19 Little High Wood — Hunt, T. P. Little High Wood – lessons of training. [In the care of the mentally handicapped.] British Hospital Journal and Social Service Review, 81, 6 Nov 1971, 2308–2309.

20 Little High Wood — Meehan, J. The long-stay hospital – a modern concept. [Little High Wood, Brentwood Group Hospital, Essex.] Nursing Mirror, 136, 25 May 1973, 38–40.

21 Meanwood Park — Spencer, D. A. Redevelopment of a hospital for mentally handicapped. [Meanwood Park, Leeds.] Nursing Times, 70, 25 Jul 1974, 1172–1173.

22 Meanwood Park — Spencer, D. A. What is your score? A check list for hospitals for the mentally handicapped. [Compiled at Meanwood Park Hospital, Leeds, and covers services and provisions affecting all aspects of patient care.] Nursing Times, 68, 16 Nov 1972, 1450–1451.

23 Monyhull Hospital – Multi-disciplinary Working Party The physical environment of the mentally handicapped. V-Ward design and ward programme. British Journal of Mental Subnormality, 18, Jun 1972, 48–57.

24 South Ockendon — Bosanquet, N. Talking point. After Ockendon. Nursing Times, 70, 30 May 1974, 818–819.

25 South Ockendon – Committee of Inquiry into South Ockendon Hospital Report to the House of Commons, 13 May 1974. HMSO, 1974. Chairman: J. Hampden Inskip.

26 South Ockendon — Ross, H. The South Ockendon report – a deeply disturbing document. Nursing Mirror, 138, 24 May 1974, 38–39.

27 Stoke Park Assessment unit for the mentally subnormal. Nursing Times, 68, 13 Apr 1972, 425–427.

f NURSING

1 Bangs, M. Serving and caring. [Report of an Rcn conference discussing the Briggs recommendations for the mentally handicapped.] Nursing Times, 71, 30 Jan 1975, 166.

2 Bury, M. Life on yellow ward. [Daily life on a ward for the severely subnormal, and the attitudes of the nurses towards subnormality.] New Society, 28, 2 May 1974, 249–250.

3 Bush, T. E. C. Pause for thought. [Nursing the mentally subnormal.] Nursing Mirror, 139, 12 Sep 1974, 56.

4 Forrest, A. Nurse's role in the hospital for the mentally handicapped. Nursing Mirror, 134, 16 Jun 1972, 48–49.

5 Gault, A. R. An operational research study of mental subnormality nursing. MSC thesis, Strathclyde University Department of Operational Research, 1973.

6 Gibson, J. and French, T. Nursing the mentally retarded. 3rd ed. Faber, 1971.

7 Hughes, D. L. Camels or thoroughbreds? An enquiry into professional ethics and the role of the professional within the subnormality service. Nursing Mirror, 141, 21 Aug 1975, 67–68.

8 Hume, P. J. Perspectives in nursing the mentally handicapped. World of Irish Nursing, 4 (6), Jun 1975, 6–7.

9 Humphries, S. R. The role of the community nurse concerned with after care. [Mentally handicapped patients in residential homes.] Nursing Times, 69, 26 Apr 1973, 537–538.

10 Jacobs, A. M. Critical nursing behaviours in the care of the mentally retarded. International Nursing Review, 20 (4), Jul/Aug 1973, 117–122.

11 Jones, K. Nursing attitudes [to the mentally handicapped]. In Opening the door: a study of new policies for the mentally handicapped. Routledge, 1975. Chapter 4, 67–95.

12 King's Fund Centre Perspective of the Brigg's report: a discussion paper on the future role and training of subnormality nurses, and their relationship with residential care staff. The Fund, 1973. (Mental Handicap papers no. 4).

13 Lee, H. and Farrell, P. Mental health practitioner? [Problems of wastage among mental handicap nurses and a possible solution.] Nursing Times, 71, 6 Nov 1975, 1789–1790.

14 Lockett, R. W. Assessment of patients' dependency. In relation to nurse staffing levels in a hospital group caring for the mentally handicapped. Nursing Times, 68, 13 Apr 1972, Occ. papers, 57–60.

15 McMillan, A. A punch drunk profession. [Nurses in mental handicap.] Nursing Times, 70, 22 Aug 1974, 1314.

16 Mental deficiency nursing [Letter from a group of Scottish nurses.] British Medical Journal, 3, 4 Sep 1971, 582–583.

17 Milner, F. Duties of a divisional night officer. [In a mental subnormality hospital.] Nursing Mirror, 132, 11 Jun 1971, 34–35.

18 Mitchell, B. The slow progress of change. [Progress in mental handicap nursing.] New Psychiatry, 2 (13), 19 Jun 1975, 16–17.

19 O'Shea, M. C. The challenge to subnormality nursing. Nursing Times, 68, 23 Mar 1972, 354–355.

20 O'Toole, R. Nurse or educator? [Role of the nurse in the field of mental subnormality.] Nursing Mirror, 135, 15 Dec 1972, 15–16.

21 O'Toole, R. Where should the NO's office be? [In the individual unit or centrally situated, with particular reference to subnormality hospitals.] Nursing Mirror, 133, 3 Dec 1971, 17–18.

22 Paton, X. and Stirling, E. Frequency and type of dyadic nurse-patient verbal interactions in a mental subnormality hospital. [Observational study.] International Journal of Nursing Studies, 11 (3), Sep 1974, 135–144.

23 Poidevin, D. Le A medical nursing staff discussion group in a mental deficiency hospital. Health Bulletin, 30 (2), Apr 1972, 139–146.

24 Rogers, P. J. Caring for the mentally handicapped: the role of the nurse. Nursing Times, 67, 4 Mar 1971, 265–267.

25 Shoesmith, E. Rating abilities and handicaps: an examination of the SPI and SSL scales for mental handicap. [Kushlick Scales.] Community Health, 7 (2), Oct 1975, 101–105.

26 Strong, P. G. and Sandland, E. T. Subnormality nursing in the community. [Survey of opinion among senior nurses in mental handicap.] Nursing Times, 70, 7 Mar 1974, 354–356.

27 Thomas, D. A new caring profession. [Is it necessary? Need of the mentally handicapped.] Nursing Times, 69, 26 Jul 1973, 969–972.

28 Ticktum, R. F. The role of the RNMS in caring. Nursing Times, 68, 8 Jun 1972, 725.

29 Toogood, R. J. The potential development index: a method of assessing staff requirements in wards and other units for the mentally handicapped. Kidderminster: Institute of Mental Subnormality, 1974.

30 Tuckwell, P. Mental handicap. [Comment on the membership of the committee of inquiry into the nursing and care of the mentally handicapped.] New Society, 33, 28 Aug 1975, 476.

31 Tyne, A. Images of the mentally handicapped. [Report of a recent study.] Nursing Mirror, 140, 26 Jun 1975, 70–71.

32 Wakeley, J. Mental subnormality nursing [in Great Britain]. Supervisor Nurse, 6 (6), Jun 1975, 4.

g NURSING EDUCATION AND TRAINING

1 Hay, D. N. Training to care for the mentally handicapped. Nursing Mirror, 133, 17 Dec 1971, 8.

2 Haynes, M. Teaching mental retardation nursing. [Introduction into the curriculum at the University of Tennessee, Memphis.] American Journal of Nursing, 75 (4), Apr 1975, 626–628.

3 Hegarty, J. Passing on assessment skills to charge nurses. [A project in a subnormality hospital training charge nurses to complete progress assessment charts.] Nursing Mirror, 141, 4 Dec 1975, 62–63.

4 Holt, R. The first of the few . . ? [Nurse/teacher experimental course in mental subnormality at Greaves Hall Hospital and Preston Polytechnic.] Nursing Mirror, 138, 26 Apr 1974, 80.

5 Kelly, S. One man's version of mental handicap training. [Reorganization of training with nine special training colleges and a six year course.] Nursing Mirror, 141, 11 Sep 1975, 37.

6 Lewis, K. C. Interdisciplinary education in mental retardation. [Result of a study tour in the USA.] Nursing Mirror, 139, 30 Aug 1974, 48–50.

7 Roberts, M. Untangling the confusing: the differing needs and training necessary in the specialized fields of mental illness and mental handicap. Nursing Times, 70, 3 Oct 1974, 1555.

8 Royal College of Nursing Rcn seeks government assurance on mental handicap qualification. Nursing Times, 71, 27 Feb 1975, 321.

9 Strong, P. G. The training of care assistants in Denmark [for the mentally handicapped]. Nursing Times, 71, 4 Dec 1975, 1956–1958.

h TREATMENT (Includes behaviour therapy)

1 Barker, P. Handicapped by preconceptions: the need for basic independence training for the profoundly retarded. [Operant conditioning project conducted by nurses.] Nursing Mirror, 141, 20 Nov 1975, 66–68.

2 Barker, P. Handicaps in perspective. [An operant conditioning project teaching basic skills in self-feeding and toiletting to four profound retardates.] Nursing Mirror, 141, 27 Nov 1975, 65–67.

3 British Journal of Mental Subnormality Symposium on the treatment of behavioural problems. British Journal of Mental Subnormality, 18 (2), Dec 1972, 66–93.

4 Clarke, A. D. B. and Clarke, A. M., editors Mental retardation and behavioural research: study group held at the University of Hull under the auspices of the Institute for Research into Mental Retardation. Edinburgh: Churchill Livingstone, 1973.

5 Cortazzi, D. and Baquer, A. Action learning: a guide to its use for hospital staff based on a pilot study in co-ordination in hospitals for the mentally handicapped. Kind Edward's Hospital Fund for London, 1972.

6 Cumming, D. Motivating the mentally subnormal [at Lynebank Hospital, Dunfermline]. Nursing Mirror, 132, 26 Mar 1971, 42–45.

7 Davies, M. It's my week for the doll. [Token economy.] Nursing Times, 71, 30 Jan 1975, 184–186.

8 Eaton, P. and Brown, R. I. The training of mealtime behaviour in the subnormal. British Journal of Mental Subnormality, 20 (39), Dec 1974, 78–85.

9 Edmunds, R. and Smith, D. L. A leap with LIP. [Life Enrichment Activation programme for long-stay patients which increased the amount of professional nursing time given to patients.] Canadian Nurse, 71 (4), Apr 1975, 25–28.

10 Evans, E. Nursing care study. Training a severely subnormal person. Nursing Times, 71, 6 Mar 1975, 374–375.

11 Hogg, J. Behaviour modification in mental handicap. Royal Society of Health Journal, 95 (6), Dec 1975, 277–281.

12 Institute of Mental Subnormality Behaviour modification: proceedings of the conference, Lea Castle Hospital, Bromsgrove, 14 March, 1973. Kidderminster: The Institute, 1973.

13 Jackson, M. W. Teaching self-help skills to the mentally handicapped using behaviour modification techniques. Kidderminster: Institute of Mental Subnormality, 1974.

14 Lewin, C. From hospital to hostel via tokens. Kidderminster: Institute of Mental Subnormality, 1974.

15 MacKay, D. N. Evaluation of tranquillizers with subnormal patients, Nursing Mirror, 133, 30 Jul 1971, 17–18; 133, 6 Aug 1971, 32–33; 133, 13 Aug 1971, 34–37.

16 Martin, G. L. Behavior modification to develop self control. Canadian Journal of Psychiatric Nursing, 16 (6), Nov/Dec 1975, 8–10.

17 Pantall, J. Training project for hospitals for the mentally handicapped 1970–1974. Manchester Business School, 1974.

18 Paton, X. and Petrusev, B. The stimulation of verbal skills in the high grade mentally retarded patient: a nurse administered treatment procedure. International Journal of Nursing Studies, 11 (2), Jul 1974, 119–126.

19 Pounds, V. A. Taming of the shrew. [The treatment in hospital of subnormal patients with severe behaviour problems.] Nursing Times, 69, 18 Jan 1973, 94–95.

20 Roos, P. Human rights and behavior modification. Nursing Digest, 3 (2), Mar/Apr 1975, 48–49.

21 Sandow, S. A study of informal approaches to the treatment of self-injurious behaviour in the severely subnormal. British Journal of Mental Subnormality, 21, Jun 1975, 10–17.

22 Taylor, J. B. Training the mentally handicapped patient. Nursing Mirror, 133, 17 Dec 1971, 9.

23 Tierney, A. J. Toilet training: a report of an evaluation of the implementation of an experimental behaviour modification programme. Nursing Times, 69, 20/27 Dec 1973, 1740–1745.

i REHABILITATION AND RECREATION

1 Barker, E. M. Daily living skills for mentally handicapped adults. Occupational Therapy, 34 (11), Nov 1971, 20–26.

2 Beverley, M. G. Rehabilitation. [A multidisciplinary programme for patients in subnormality hospital in Colchester.] Nursing Times, 71, 7 Aug 1975, 1258–1260.

3 British Journal of Mental Subnormality Symposium on preparing for life in the open community. British Journal of Mental Subnormality, 21 (2), Dec 1975, 61–83.

4 Colson, J. Recreational therapy. [For subnormal patients.] British Hospital Journal and Social Service Review, 82, 6 May 1972, 997–998.

5 Deacon, J. Tongue tied: fifty years of friendship in a subnormality hospital. National Society for Mentally Handicapped Children, 1974. (Subnormality in the seventies, no. 8.)

6 Goodwin, K. P. Maud – getting her hat straight. [The rehabilitation of a mentally handicapped woman.] Nursing Times, 70, 24 Jan 1974, 110–111.

7 King's Fund Centre Adult education for mentally handicapped people. The Centre, 1975. (Mental handicap papers, no. 6.)

8 Lamont, J. Afloat on the Broads. [Eight mentally and physically handicapped people.] Nursing Times, 69, 19 Apr 1973, 498–502.

9 Lucas, M. H. Educational approach to mental retardation. UNA Nursing Journal, 2, Mar/Apr 1974, 20–21.

10 Murray, M. Rehabilitating the mentally subnormal. 1. Occupational and social training. Nursing Mirror, 132, 8 Jan 1971, 32–33.

11 Murray, M. Rehabilitating the mentally subnormal. 2. Social training of higher potential subnormals. Nursing Mirror, 132, 15 Jan 1971, 44–45.

12 Nursing Mirror Aldingbourne adventure camp. For patients of Manor Hospital, Epsom. Nursing Mirror, 137, 26 Oct 1973, 20–21.

13 Nursing Mirror Calderstones' 73 club is swinging! [A club for mentally handicapped patients at Whalley, Blackburn.] Nursing Mirror, 137, 20 Jul 1973, 36–39.

14 Paton, X. Teaching the mentally retarded to read: some personal experiences. Book Trolley, 3 (5), Mar 1972, 9–11.

15 Robinson, W. Sport and recreation for the mentally and physically handicapped. Nursing Times, 69, 12 Jul 1973, 895–897.

16 Robinson, J. R. Why mentally subnormal patients fail in outside employment. Nursing Times, 67, 5 Aug 1971, 953–954.

17 Solly, K. A philosophy of leisure in relation to the retarded. National Society for Mentally Handicapped Children, 1975. (Publications for parents and professionals.)

18 Taylor, J. B. Training the mentally handicapped patient. Nursing Mirror, 133, 17 Dec 1971, 9.

19 Ziman, D. Libraries for mentally handicapped readers. [Report of King's Fund Seminar.] Health and Social Service Journal, 83, 17 Nov 1973, 2689.

j SEX

1 British Journal of Mental Subnormality Point of view. [Sex education and the mentally handicapped.] British Journal of Mental Subnormality, 19 (1), Jun 1973, 3–6.

2 David, H. P. and Linder, M. A. Family planning for the mentally handicapped. WHO Bulletin, 52 (2), 1975, 155–161.

3 De La Cruz, F. F. and La Veck, G. D., editors Human sexuality and the mentally retarded. Butterworth, 1973.

4 Department of Health and Social Security Sterilisation of children under 16 years of age: discussion paper. The Department, 1975.

5 Enby, G. Let there be love: sex and the handicapped. Elek, Pemberton, 1975.

6 Gilderdale, S. Society at work. Research attitudes. [A study of a group of female patients in subnormality hospitals who have had children.] New Society, 20, 25 May 1972, 411–412.

7 Jones, A. W. Subnormality and sexual relations. British Hospital Journal and Social Service Review, 82, 12 Aug 1972, 1801.

8 Katz, G., editor Sexuality and subnormality: a Swedish view. National Society for Mentally Handicapped Children, 1972.

9 Lee, G. W. and Katz, G. Sexual rights of the retarded: two papers reflecting the international point of view. National Society for Mentally Handicapped Children, 1974.

10 Shearer, A. A right to love? A report on public and professional attitudes towards the sexual and emotional needs of handicapped people. Spastics Society and National Association for Mental Health, 1972.

11 Smiley, C. W. Sterilization and therapeutic abortion counselling for the mentally retarded. International Journal of Nursing Studies, 10 (2), May 1973, 137–140; Journal of Psychiatric Nursing and Mental Health Services, 10 (3), May/Jun 1974, 24–26.

k VOLUNTEERS

1 Boorer, D. Why the mentally handicapped need voluntary help. Nursing Times, 67, 26 Aug 1971, 1055–1056.

2 Burn, C. D. Society at work. Breaking the ice. [An experiment at 4 hospitals for the mentally handicapped to create individual and personal contact between volunteers and the handicapped.] New Society, 30, 19 Dec 1974, 756–757.

3 Elliott, J. The role of the voluntary agency in mental handicap. Health and Social Service Journal, 85, 5 Apr 1975, 760–761; Nursing Mirror, 141, 17 Jul 1975, 73–75.

4 Kings Fund Centre Voluntary work with the mentally handicapped. [Report of a conference.] Health and Social Service Journal, 85, 25 Jan 1975, 180.

DISEASES AND TREATMENT

82 CANCER

a GENERAL

1 British Medical Journal General knowledge of cancer. British Medical Journal, 4, 18 Nov 1972, 381–382.

2 British Medical Journal Informing the public about cancer. British Medical Journal, 3, 19 Jul 1975, 119–120.

3 Brookes, P. 'War games' against cancer. [Workshop organized by the International Agency for Research on Cancer.] Occupational Health, 27 (11), Nov 1975, 484.

4 Davison, R. L. Cancer, and education for life. Community Health, 4 (6), May/Jun 1973, 315–319.

5 Davison, R. L. Cancer and the nurse's social role. [Health education.] Nursing Times, 69, 10 May 1973, 601–602.

6 Fitzpatrick, G. Cancer detection: a responsibility for every nurse. Nursing Care, 8 (1), Jan 1975, 9.

7 Grant, A. S. and Davison, R. L. Questions behind the answers: what people really want to know about cancer. [Study carried out by the Manchester Regional Committee on Cancer.] International Journal of Health Education, 18 (2), 1975, 109–118.

8 Isler, C. The fatal choice – cancer quackery. RN Magazine, 37 (9), Sep 1974, 55–59.

9 Marie Curie Memorial Foundation Cancer group discusses national attitudes and needs. [Marie Curie Memorial Foundation symposium – cancer and the nation.] Nursing Times, 71, 22 May 1975, 794; Nursing Mirror, 140, 5 Jun 1975, 36.

10 Mould, R. F. Statistics and cancer. [Use of statistics in showing incidence treatment success and survival rates.] Nursing Times, 71, 17 Jul 1975, 1122–1133.

11 Raven, R. W. Cancer prevention – recent encouragement in preventive measures. (b) Cancer prevention – the key of control. Royal Society of Health Journal, 92 (6), Dec 1972, 287–291.

12 Sellwood, R. A. Screening, diagnosis and surgical management [of cancer, Nursing Mirror Forum '75]. Nursing Mirror, 141, 9 Oct 1975, 53–54.

13 Thornes, D. Cancer research: a personal view of maintenance therapy to prevent recurrence. Nursing Mirror, 140, 22/29 May 1975, 60–61.

14 Wakefield, J. Public education about cancer. British Hospital Journal and Social Service Review, 81, 27 Feb 1971, 374–375.

15 Winner, A. The Ringberg Clinic at Rottach-Egern. Nursing Times, 67, 11 Mar 1971, 281–282.

16 World Health Issue on international control of cancer. World Health, Nov 1975, 3–31.

b NURSING

1 Barckley, V. Work study program in cancer nursing. Nursing Outlook, 19 (5), May 1971, 328–330.

2 Boore, J. The planning of nursing care [of the cancer patient. Nursing Mirror, Forum 75]. Nursing Mirror, 141, 9 Oct 1975, 59–62.

3 Boorer, D. Nursing in Australia. 2. Buying time. Victoria's cancer clinic: a nursing ideal. Nursing Times, 70, 23 May 1974, 806–807.

4 Browning, M. H. and Lewis, E. P., compilers Nursing and the cancer patient. New York: American Journal of Nursing Co., 1973.

5 Capra, L. G. The care of the cancer patient. Heinemann Medical, 1972.

6 Copen, P. The terminal cancer patient. [Nursing care study.] Nursing Care, 6 (5), May 1973, 27–30.

7 Cox, S. A course in oncology. [Discussion of the aspects of oncology that might usefully be included in a course for post-certificate nurses.] Queen's Nursing Journal, 17 (4), Jul 1974, 77–78.

8 Cox, S. A review of cancer nursing services in North America. [Report of a study tour.] Nursing Mirror, 141, 25 Sep 1975, 66–68.

9 Deeley, T. J. and others A guide to oncological nursing. Churchill Livingstone, 1974.

10 Dixon, T. Care of the cancer patient – a personal view. Queen's Nursing Journal, 17 (12), Mar 1975, 259–260.

11 George, M. M. Long-term care of the patient with cancer. Nursing Clinics of North America, 8 (4), Dec 1973, 623–631.

12 Heusinkveld, K. B. Cues to communication with the terminal cancer patient. Nursing Forum, 11 (1), 1972, 105–113.

13 Jones, S. J. Working in cancer research: a nurse research assistant working on the problem of lung cancer explains her job. Nursing Times, 70, 5 Dec 1974, 1903–1905.

14 Klagsbrun, S. C. Communications in the treatment of cancer. American Journal of Nursing, 71 (5), May 1971, 944–948.

15 Lee, R. M. International symposium on cancer nursing [at the Memorial Sloan-Kettering Cancer Centre]. AORN Journal, 22 (6), Dec 1975, 987–998; 992–996, 1000, 1002–1003.

16 Mary St. Andrew, Sister Understanding cancer. 2. The nurse's relationship with the patient. Nursing Times, 71, 8 May 1975, 736–737.

17 Nursing Mirror Standards of care. 2. Care of the patient with cancer. [Papers from Nursing Mirror, Forum 75.] Nursing Mirror, 141, 9 Oct 1975, 53–66.

18 Sainsbury, M. J. and Milton, G. W. The nurse in a cancer ward. Medical Journal of Australia, 2, 1975, 911–913.

19 Sosamma, V. K. Cancer, its treatment and nursing care. Nursing Journal of India, 63 (2), Feb 1972, 49–50, 55.

20 Shepardson, J. Team approach to the patient with cancer. American Journal of Nursing, 72 (3), Mar 1972, 488–491.

21 Stewart, B. M. Living with cancer. [Experience of a nurse working in a cancer clinic.] Nursing Forum, 13 (1), 1974, 52–58.

22 Thornton, M. The giving of care [to the cancer patient. Nursing Mirror, Forum 75]. Nursing Mirror, 141, 9 Oct 1975, 62–63.

23 Tiffany, R. Cancer education and training. [With special reference to the JBCNS course at the Royal Marsden Hospital and the concept of the clinical specialist.] Nursing Mirror, 141, 14 Aug 1975, 66–68.

24 Van Lier, M. A. A nursing care study. [Of inoperable cancer.] New Zealand Nursing Journal, 67 (5), May 1974, 20–23.

c THERAPY

1 Baker, J. W. Recent advances in radiotherapy. Nursing Mirror, 140, 2 Jan 1975, 24–27.

2 Bruya, M. A. and Madeira, N. P. Cancer update. Stomatitis after chemotherapy. American Journal of Nursing, 75, Aug 1975, 1349–1352.

3 Cole, M. P. Other methods of the treatment of cancer. [Nursing Mirror, Forum 75.] Nursing Mirror, 141, 9 Oct 1975, 54–59.

4 Dickerson, W. T. Nutrition and the cancer patient. Nursing Mirror, 134, 23 Jun 1972, 17–19; 30 Jun 1972, 33–35; 7 Jul 1972, 39–40.

5 Fowler, J. F. A new tool for cancer research. [Radiotherapy developments at Mount Vernon Hospital.] Nursing Mirror, 141, 10 Jul 1975, 40–42.

6 Golden, S. Cancer chemotherapy and management of patient problems. Nursing Forum, 14 (3), 1975, 278–303.

7 Hellmann, K. Cancer chemotherapy today. Nursing Times, 70, 11 Apr 1974, 547–548.

8 Hendrickson, F. R. and Browning, D. Radiotherapy treatment for cancer: guidelines for nursing care. Journal of Practical Nursing, 22 (2), Feb 1972, 18–20, 34.

9 Hopkins, S. J. A new dawn in cancer therapy? Nursing Mirror, 132, 5 Feb 1971, 14.

10 Jansson, J. The relationship of radiotherapy and surgery for the treatment of cancer. Lamp, 30 (7), Jul 1973, 31–41.

11 Kay, J. J. George's dilemma. [Patient's decision to undergo radiotherapy treatment.] Nursing Times, 69, 15 Nov 1973, 1538–1539.

12 Lees, A. W. Cancer treatment in the 1970s: the development of oncology centres. Queen's Nursing Journal, 17 (1), Apr 1974, 7–9.

13 McCarthy, S. Cancer complicated in growth, treatment. AORN Journal, 21 (4), Apr 1975, 706–707; 710–711.

14 Mary St. Andrew, Sister Understanding cancer. 1. Cancerous growth and types of treatment. Nursing Times, 71, 1 May 1975, 690–692.

15 Mathai, S. Radiotherapy for cancer patients. Nursing Journal of India, 64 (2), Feb 1973, 46, 48.

16 Price, L. A. Drug treatment of cancer. 1. Current status and future prospects. 2. Some psychological aspects. Nursing Times, 68, 9 Nov 1972, 1411–1413.

17 Prosnitz, L. R. Treatment for malignant disease. RN Magazine, 34 (3), Mar 1971, 42–47.

18 Silverstein, M. J. and Morton, D. L. Cancer immunotherapy. American Journal of Nursing, 73 (7), Jul 1973, 1178–1181.

19 Smith, S. E. Drugs and cancer. Nursing Times, 68, 27 Jul 1972, 927–929.

20 Smith, S. E. How drugs act. 23. Drugs and cancer. Nursing Times, 71, 27 Nov 1975, 1910–1911.

21 Sugden, B. M. Nutrition in malignant disease. Nursing Mirror, 132, 11 Jun 1971, 19, 23.

22 Teitelbaum, A. C. Intra-arterial drug therapy. [In the treatment of cancer.] American Journal of Nursing, 72 (9), Sep 1972, 1634–1637.

23 Windeyer, B. Modern trends in the treatment of malignant disease. Nursing Mirror, 135, 28 Jul 1972, 12–15.

d PATIENT AND FAMILY (Includes home care)

1 Atherton, E. The small blue note book. [Written by a patient suffering from advanced carcinoma of both lungs.] Nursing Times, 69, 4 Oct 1973, 1299–1300.

2 Barckley, V. Caring for the cancer patient at home. Journal of Practical Nursing, 24 (10), Oct 1974, 24–27.

3 Buehler, J. A. Cancer update. What contributes to hope in the cancer patient? American Journal of Nursing, 75 (8), Aug 1975, 1353–1356.

4 Hannan, J. F. Talking is treatment, too. Cancer patients want to find meaning in their disease and are eager to share their experiences to help other patients. American Journal of Nursing, 74 (11), Nov 1974, 1991–1992.

5 Harris, J. I have cancer. [Thoughts of a person with cancer.] Nursing Mirror, 138, 31 May 1974, 71–72.

6 Kratz, C. R. Community care [of the cancer patient. Nursing Mirror, Forum 75]. Nursing Mirror, 141, 9 Oct 1975, 64–66.

7 Lord, E. A. My crisis with cancer. [The personal feelings of a nurse who had cancer.] American Journal of Nursing, 74 (4), Apr 1974, 647–649.

8 McIntosh, J. Processes of communication, information seeking and control associated with malignant disease in a hospital ward. PhD thesis, Aberdeen University, 1975.

9 Milton, G. W. Thoughts in mind of a person with cancer. British Medical Journal, 4, 27 Oct 1973, 221–223.

10 Murray, R. Illness as a crisis. [Cancer.] Journal of Practical Nursing, 23 (2), Feb 1973, 20–23.

11 Nursing Forum The psychodynamic process of the oncological experience. [Emotional support of patients and relatives awaiting the outcome of cancer diagnosis.] Nursing Forum, 14 (3), 1975, 264–267.

12 Parkes, C. M. Accuracy of predictions of survival in later stages of cancer. [A study carried out at St. Christopher's Hospice in which nurses were involved.] British Medical Journal, 2, 1 Apr 1972, 29–31.

13 Parsell, S. and Tagliareni, E. M. Cancer patients help each other. [A club for cancer patients.] American Journal of Nursing, 74 (4), Apr 1974, 650–651.

14 Pienschke, D. Guardedness or openness on the cancer unit. [As it affected (1) patients' confidence in doctors and nurses, (2) patient satisfaction with the information given to them and nursing care, and (3) adequacy of the nursing care.] Nursing Research, 22 (6), Nov/Dec 1973, 484–490.

15 Priyadharsini, J. Emotional reaction of adult patients with the diagnosis of cancer. [Abstract of thesis.] Nursing Journal of India, 44 (9), Sep 1973, 312, 323.

16 Smith, G. Home nursing care of the patient with prostatic carcinoma. Nursing Mirror, 139, 12 Dec 1974, 61–62.

17 Stanley, P. M. A Marie Curie educational project. [Home care of the cancer patient.] District Nursing, 15 (7), Oct 1972, 153.

18 Ward, A. W. M. Telling the patient. [A survey in general practice of patients told about their malignant disease.] Journal of the Royal College of General Practitioners, 24, 144, Jul 1974, 465–468.

19 White, J. F. 'Yes, I hear you, Mr. H.' [Case study of a man dying with lung cancer.] American Journal of Nursing, 75 (3), Mar 1975, 410–413.

e SPECIFIC REGIONS

1 Bond, J. V. Wilms' tumour. Nursing Times, 71, 30 Oct 1975, 1731–1733.

2 Campbell, D. Nursing care study. Primary adenocarcinoma of the bladder. [Total cystectomy and ureterocolic diversion.] Nursing Mirror, 138, 10 May 1974, 86–89.

3 Charters, D. Nursing care study. Right lateral nephrectomy [for carcinoma of the kidney]. Nursing Times, 70, 9 May 1974, 703–704.

4 Feit, H. L. The unmentionable rectum. Bedside Nurse, 5 (10), Oct 1972, 26–27.

5 Fergusson, J. D. Carcinoma of the prostate. Nursing Mirror, 139, 12 Dec 1974, 51–54.

6 Freeman, J. F. A series of articles from the Royal Marsden Hospital, London. 1. Wilms' tumour. Nursing Mirror, 134, 12 May 1972, 18–19.

7 Golebiowski, A. Carcinoma of the bronchus. Nursing Times, 69, 9 Aug 1973, 1021–1024.

8 Hanebuth, L. When your patient has multiple myeloma. RN Magazine, 34 (8), Aug 1971, 36, 66, 68, 70.

9 Hart, K. Patient care study. Carcinoma of the bronchus plus secondary deposits. Queen's Nursing Journal, 16 (7), Oct 1973, 146–147.

10 Hendry, W. F. Management of prostatic cancer. Nursing Mirror, 139, 12 Dec 1974, 58–60.

11 Institute of Urology A symposium on prostatic carcinoma. Nursing Mirror, 139, 12 Dec 1974, 51–62.

12 Iredale, P. Nursing care study. Multiple malignant melanoma. [Carcinoma of the skin.] Nursing Times, 70, 17 Oct 1974, 1610–1613.

13 Ive, A. Premalignant conditions and causes of skin cancer. Nursing Mirror, 140, 22/29 May 1975, 56–58.

14 Jackson, K. M. Nursing care study. Multiple sclerosis and carcinoma of the stomach. Nursing Times, 70, 3 Oct 1974, 1532–1534.

15 Jacobs, P. Tumours of bone. Nursing Times, 68, 14 Dec 1972, 1572–1575.

16 Johnson, A. G. Carcinoma of the stomach: early diagnosis and management. Nursing Mirror, 138, 31 May 1974, 54–57.

17 Jones, S. J. Smoking and lung cancer. Nursing Mirror, 141, 18 Sep 1975, 48–49.

18 Kryk, H. and others Grand rounds on brain tumors: specific nursing management of patients who have different types of brain tumors. Canadian Nurse, 71 (9), Sep 1975, 42–46.

19 Lehane, C. P. Nursing care study. Carcinoma of the stomach complicated by metastases. Nursing Mirror, 136, 9 Feb 1973, 38–40.

20 Mass, K. Recent advances in the treatment of lung cancer. Bedside Nurse, 5 (3), Mar 1972, 14–18.

21 Mazzola, R. and Jacobs, G. B. Brain tumors, diagnosis and treatment. RN Magazine, 38 (3), Mar 1975, 42–45.

22 McOuat, F. Acoustic nerve tumors: diagnosis, surgical management and nursing care. Journal of Neurosurgical Nursing, 6 (1), Jul 1974, 20–26.

23 Naylor, H. G. Carcinoma of the colon. Nursing Times, 67, 7 Jan 1971, 12–15; 14 Jan 1971, 50–52.

24 Ophutsky, L. C. and Pohutsky, K. R. Cancer update. Computerized axial tomography of the brain: a new diagnostic tool. American Journal of Nursing, 75 (8), Aug 1975, 1341–1342.

25 Pagliero, K. M. Lung cancer. Nursing Times, 70, 2 May 1974, 667–669.

26 Peckham, M. The non-Hodgkin's lymphomas. Nursing Times, 71, 7 Aug 1975, 1252–1255.

27 Richardson, D. K. Nursing care study. Malignant change in benign tumour [in stomach lining]. Nursing Times, 70, 7 Mar 1974, 339–340.

28 Riches, E. The concerted treatment of cancer of the kidney. Nursing Mirror, 137, 19 Oct 1973, 22–28.

29 Robins, P. Skin cancer: from cause to cure. RN Magazine. 37. Mar 1974. 29–32

30 Shearer, R. J. The investigation of prostatic carcinoma. Nursing Mirror. 139, 12 Dec 1974. 55–57.

31 Southcott, R. D. C. Bladder tumours. Nursing Times, 69, 12 Apr 1973, 466–468.

32 Stanewick, B. Chemosurgery in skin cancer. AORN Journal, 23 (3), Sep 1975, 351–359.

33 Thomson, J. P. S. Carcinoma of the colon. Nursing Times, 71, 15 May 1975, 770–773.

34 Van Lier, M. A. A nursing care study [of inoperable cancer of the abdominal cavity]. New Zealand Nursing Journal, 67 (5), May 1974, 20–23.

f BREAST CANCER (Includes mastectomy, screening)

1 Akehurst, A. C. Post-mastectomy morale. Nursing Mirror, 139, 21 Nov 1974, 66.

2 Barbour, T. I traveled the mastectomy road. [Experiences of a nurse.] Supervisor Nurse, 6 (3), Mar 1975, 40–41, 43.

3 Calvert, A. H. Chemotherapy in the treatment of breast cancer. Nursing Mirror, 141, 16 Oct 1975, 63–65.

4 Carbary, L. J. Breast cancer – curable or deadly? Journal of Practical Nursing, 24 (4), Apr 1974, 20–23.

5 Chew, A. T. Nursing care study. Diabetes mellitus, carcinoma of both breasts. Nursing Mirror, 138, 24 May 1974, 79–81.

6 Davey, J. Breast cancer screening. [Well-Woman Clinic Royal Marsden Hospital.] [Symposium on mastectomy.] Nursing Mirror, 140, Apr 1975, 45–49.

7 Deacon, C. Radioactive yttrium implant to pituitary gland: case study, [as treatment for carcinoma of the breast]. Nursing Mirror, 132, 5 Feb 1971, 31–33.

8 Downie, P. A. Cancerous diseases. 2. Breast surgery. Nursing Times, 70, 22 Aug 1974, 1311–1312.

9 Eardley, A. Triggers to action: a study of what makes women seek advice for breast conditions. [Survey in Manchester started in 1972.] Health Education Journal, 34 (2), 1975, 39–47.

10 Esselstyn, C. B. Selective surgery for breast cancer. AORN Journal, 22 (5), Nov 1975, 731–732.

11 Evans, J. Mastectomy – the patient's point of view. [Symposium on mastectomy.] Nursing Mirror, 140, 3 Apr 1975, 62.

12 Hadfield, G. J. Benign diseases of the breast. Nursing Mirror, 138 (10), 24 May 1974, 68–70.

13 Holt, J. A. G. Thermography in screening [for breast cancer]. Health and Social Service Journal, 83, 10 Feb 1973, 305, 308.

14 Irwig, L. M. Screening for cancer. Breast cancer. [The acceptability and effectiveness of screening.] Lancet, 2, 30 Nov 1974, 1307–1308.

15 Leis, H. P. Risk factors in breast cancer. AORN Journal, 22 (5), Nov 1975, 723–729.

16 Leis, H. P. Surgical procedures for breast cancer. RN Magazine, 37 (1), Jan 1974, OR1–OR2, OR4, OR6.

17 Maguire, P. The psychological and social consequences of breast cancer. [Symposium on mastectomy.] Nursing Mirror, 140, 3 Apr 1975, 54–57.

18 Mamaril, A. P. Preventing complications after radical mastectomy: early intervention to prevent or minimise the physical effects and emotional strains of surgery. American Journal of Nursing, 74 (11), Nov 1974, 2000–2003.

19 Marie Curie Memorial Foundation Advice to patients following mastectomy. The Foundation, 1971. (Education leaflet no. 14.)

20 Mastectomy Association Helpful hints for you and the family. Croydon: The Association, 1971. [And other miscellaneous pamphlets.]

21 Midwife, Health Visitor and Community Nurse Getting it off my chest:a midwife describes her experiences and problems following mastectomy. Midwife, Health Visitor and Community Nurse, 11 (12), Dec 1975, 399–400.

22 Nourse, E. Patient care study. Carcinomatosis [of the breasts]. Queen's Nursing Journal, 18 (5), Aug 1975, 142–143.

23 Nursing Mirror A symposium on mastectomy. Nursing Mirror, 140, 3 Apr 1975, 45–62.

24 Occupational Health Nursing Women's attitudes regarding breast cancer. Occpational Health Nursing. 22 (2). Feb 1974. 20–23.

25 Ritter, B. Breast surgery demands sympathetic nursing. Nursing Care, 7 (8), Aug 1974, 26–29.

26 RN Magazine early detection of breast cancer with mammography. RN Magazine, 37 (12), Dec 1974, 36–38.

27 Roberts, J. M. Mastectomy – a patient's point of view. Nursing Times, 71, 14 Aug 1975, 1290–1291.

28 Torrie, A. Mastectomy – 'the emotional operation'. Nursing Mirror, 132, 28 May 1971, 34–35.

29 Wakeley, C. Tumours occurring in the male breast. Nursing Mirror, 137, 17 Aug 1973, 26–27.

30 Watts, G. T. Non-mutilating mastectomy. Nursing Mirror, 135, 1 Dec 1972, 32–34

g GYNAECOLOGICAL CANCER

1 Allman, S. T. and others The national cervical cytology recall system: report of a pilot study. Health Trends, 6 (2), May 1974, 39–41.

2 Avery, W. and others Vulvectomy. [Removal of the external genitalia as a treatment of vulvar carcinoma.] American Journal of Nursing, 74 (3), Mar 1974, 453–455.

3 Bentall, A. P. Carcinoma of the vulva. Nursing Mirror, 140, 27 Feb 1975, 48–50.

4 Benton, B. D. A. Stilbestrol and vaginal cancer. [Increased risk of cancer of the vagina and cervix in adolescent daughters of women who took diethylstilbestrol during pregnancy.] American Journal of Nursing, 74 (5), May 1974, 900–901.

5 Craddock, F. G. and Husain, O. A. N. A mobile cancer screening service. [Women's National Cancer Control Campaign.] Nursing Mirror, 141, 30 Oct 1975, 48–50.

6 Crichton, C. Nursing care study. Carcinoma of the cervix in pregnancy. Nursing Times, 70, 13 Jun 1974, 906–907.

7 Davidson, C. M. Significance of a positive vaginal smear during pregnancy. Midwife and Health Visitor, 7 (4), Apr 1971, 143–146.

8 Davison, R. L. and Clements, J. E. Why don't they attend for a cytotest? A pilot study among a high risk population. Medical Officer, 125, 25 Jun 1971, 329–330.

9 Elliott, E. M. Calling all women. [Cervical screening campaign at London Transport Acton Works.] Occupational Health, 27 (3), Mar 1975, 98–101.

10 Fitzpatrick, G. Care of the patient with cancer of the cervix. Parts 1 and 2. Bedside Nurse, 4 (1), Jan 1971, 11–18; 4 (2), Feb 1971, 9–16.

11 Gilbert, M. P. Observations at a rural cervical cytology clinic. Maternal and Child Care, 7 (69), Mar/Apr 1971, 30–31.

12 Health and Social Service Journal Screening policy. [Comment on the Government's policy of cervical screening since 1966.] Health and Social Service Journal, 84, 7 Dec 1974, 2813–2814.

13 Hudson, C. N. Cancer of the ovary. Nursing Mirror, 136, 6 Apr 1973, 19–20.

14 Kraft, C. A. and others Where R.Ns run a mobile cancer-detection unit. RN Magazine, 37 (8), Aug 1974, 27–29.

15 Layzell, M. S. Carcinomatosis [arising from bilateral ovarian tumours]. Nursing Times, 69, 19 Apr 1973, 503–504.

16 Milligan, C. and others Cancer update. Screening for cervical cancer. [Colposcopy.] American Journal of Nursing, 75 (8), Aug 1975, 1343–1344.

17 Peck, J. E. Outpatient cervical cryosurgery. Nursing Times, 71, 20 Feb 1975, 314–315.

18 Rodney, M. B. Sexual activity and cervical cancer: the pap test quest. Bedside Nurse, 4 (4), Apr 1971, 14–16.

19 Russo, D. W. Experiments in nursing. Pap testing by RNs? It's effective. [Cervical cancer detection.] RN Magazine, 37 (9), Sep 1974, 69.

20 Sansom, C. D. and others Trends in cytological screening in the Manchester area 1965–1971. Community Medicine, 126 (19), 5 Nov 1971, 253–257.

21 Soika, C. V. Gynecologic cytology. [Screening for cancer.] American Journal of Nursing, 73 (12), Dec 1973, 2092–2094.

22 Taylor, R. W. Cervical cytology. Nursing Mirror, 141, 17 Jul 1975, 58–59.

23 Thomson, J. G. Cervical cytology in England and Wales: some facts. Health Trends, 3 (2), May 1971, 24–25.

24 Vose, P. Nursing care study. Anaplastic neoplasm of the right cervical glands. Nursing Mirror, 139, 23 Aug 1974, 74–75.

25 Wakefield, J. The family doctor and cervical cytology. Health Trends, 3 (3), May 1971, 25–29.

26 Wakefield, J. Seek wisely to prevent: studies of attitudes and action in a cervical cytology programme. HMSO, 1972.

27 Whitfield, A. P. Cancer prevention – recent encouragement in preventive measures. (a) Cervical cancer screening programmes and voluntary support. Royal Society of Health Journal, 92 (6), Dec 1972, 282–287.

h HEAD, FACE AND NECK

1 Barlow, D. Malignant conditions of the oesophagus. Nursing Times, 67, 12 Aug 1971, 979–981.

2 Brown, C. Nursing care study. Total laryngectomy. Nursing Times, 67, 16 Sep 1971, 1144–1147.

3 Chandler, J. R. Cryosurgery of malignant neoplasms of the head and neck. RN Magazine, 36 (5), May 1973, OR 1–2, 4.

4 Cohen, B. Precancerous conditions of the mouth. Nursing Mirror, 134, 4 Feb 1972, 20–25.

5 Daly, K. M. 'Don't wave good-bye'. [Thoughts of a patient treated for cancer of the tongue.] American Journal of Nursing, 74 (9), Sep 1974, 1641.

6 Debul, B. The laryngectomee: a booklet for family and friends. Darville, Illinois: Interstate, 1973.

7 Downie, P. A. Cancerous diseases – 3. Head, neck, oesophageal and thoracic surgery. Nursing Times, 70, 29 Aug 1974, 1354–1355.

8 Gillespie, I. E. Carcinoma of the oesophagus. Nursing Times, 69, 6 Dec 1973, 1644–1647.

9 Goodyear, A. The nurse's role. [Symposium on laryngectomy.] Nursing Mirror, 141, 4 Dec 1975, 51–52.

10 Harvey, T. G. Diagnosis and surgical management. [Symposium on laryngectomy.] Nursing Mirror, 141, 4 Dec 1975, 48–50.

11 Helsper, J. T. Staining techniques: screening tests for oral cancer. RN Magazine, 35 (10), Oct 1972, OR3–4, 8.

12 Keough, G. and Niebel, H. N. Oral cancer detection – a nursing responsibility. American Journal of Nursing, 73 (4), Apr 1973, 684–686.

13 Lauder, E. Toward total rehabilitation [for a laryngectomee]. Nursing Digest, 3 (2), Mar/Apr 1975, 50–51.

14 Moore, A. M. A. Surgical conditions of the head and neck. Nursing Mirror, 132, 19 Feb 1971, 19–23.

15 Nicholson, E. M. Personal notes of a laryngectomee. American Journal of Nursing, 75 (12), Dec 1975, 2157–2158.

16 Nursing Mirror A symposium on laryngectomy – the team approach. Nursing Mirror, 141, 4 Dec 1975, 47–57.

17 O'Dell, A. J. Objectives and standards in the care of the patient with a radical neck dissection. Nursing Clinics of North America, 8 (1), Mar 1973, 159–164.

18 Page, M. L. Nursing care study. Laryngectomy for carcinoma of the larynx. Nursing Mirror, 136, 4 May 1973, 16–20.

19 Pizer, M. E. and Kay, S. Mouth cancer: concepts of treatment. RN Magazine, 35 (10), Oct 1972, OR 12, 15–16.

20 Richards, F. Nursing care study. Terminal care of a patient suffering from carcinomatosis [presenting with an advanced carcinoma of the oesophagus]. Nursing Mirror, 138, 19 Apr 1974, 78–80.

21 Searcey, L. Nursing care of the laryngectomy patient. RN Magazine, 35 (10), Oct 1972, 35–41.

22 Seymour-Jones, A. Carcinoma of the larynx. Nursing Times, 69, 2 Aug 1973, 983–984.

23 Stoker, A. Salivary tumours. Nursing Times, 69, 8 Mar 1973, 302–305.

24 Thomas, B. J. Coping with the devastation of head and neck cancer. RN Magazine, 37, Oct 1974, 25–30.

25 Thomas, K. Carcinoma of the larynx. Nursing Times, 71, 6 Mar 1975, 371–373.

26 Tierney, E. A. Accepting disfigurement when death is the alternative. [Case study of a patient with cancer of the head and neck.] American Journal of Nursing, 75 (12), Dec 1975, 2149–2150.

27 Welty, M. J. and others The patient with maxillofacial cancer. 1. Surgical treatment and nursing care. 2. Psychologic aspects. Nursing Clinics of North America, 8 (1), Mar 1973, 137–158.

28 Williams, R. G. and Penistone, E. Head and neck surgical nursing. Nursing Times, 69, 16 Aug 1973, 1047–1049.

29 Workman, R. Nursing care study. Carcinoma of the post-cricoid region. Nursing Mirror, 137, 6 Jul 1973, 35–37.

30 Zirkle, T. J. and Thompson, R. J. Repairing the face and neck after radical excision. RN Magazine, 37 (10), Oct 1974, OR 9–11.

i LEUKAEMIA AND CHILDHOOD CANCER

1 Benoliel, J. Q. The concept of care for a child with leukemia. Nursing Forum, 11 (2), 1972, 194–204.

2 Blackburn, E. K. Acute leukaemia. Nursing Times, 67, 29 Apr 1971, 509–511.

3 Burton, L. Cancer children. (Parents need help as well as the child when the child is dying. Their reactions, in fact, may make the child feel worse.) New Society, 17, 17 Jun 1971, 1040–1043.

4 Coles, R. M. Acute myeloblastic leukaemia. Nursing Times, 68, 8 Jun 1972, 707–709.

5 Coles, R. M. Nursing care study. Chronic leukaemia. Nursing Times, 68, 15 Jun 1972, 739–740.

6 Crosby, M. H. Control systems and children with lymphoblastic leukemia. Nursing Clinics of North America, 6 (3), Sep 1971, 407–413.

7 Goldstone, A. H. Acute lymphoblastic leukaemia. [Treatment and the nurse's role.] Nursing Times, 71, 13 Mar 1978, 418–420.

8 Graham-Pole, J. Leukaemia in childhood. Nursing Mirror, 133, 23 Jul 1971, 18–20.

9 Greene, P. Acute leukemia in children. American Journal of Nursing, 75 (10), Oct 1975, 1709–1714.

10 Greene, P. The child with leukemia in the classroom. [The part played by the nurse as a mediator.] American Journal of Nursing, 75 (1), Jan 1975, 86–87.

11 Hamlin, D. Nursing care study. A child with acute lymphoblastic leukaemia. [Prize winning essay in nursing care study competition.] Nursing Times, 71, 6 Feb 1975, 210–213.

12 Hugos, R. Living with leukemia. American Journal of Nursing, 72 (12), Dec 1972, 2185–2188.

13 Isler, C. The cancer nurses – Part 2. Care of the pediatric patient with leukemia. RN Magazine, 35 (4), Apr 1972, 30–35.

14 Isler, C. Children are surviving leukemia and lymphoma. [Treatment at Philadelphia's Mercy Catholic Medical Center.] RN Magazine, 38 (11), Nov 1975, 20–25.

15 Journal of Practical Nursing Leukemia – in children and adults. Journal of Practical Nursing, 32 (6), Jun 1972, 22–23, 42.

16 Kikuchi, J. How the leukemic child chooses his confidant. Canadian Nurse, 71 (5), May 1975, 22–23.

17 Lacasse, C. M. A dying adolescent. [Case study of a boy with leukemia.] American Journal of Nursing, 75 (3), Mar 1975, 433–434.

18 Pearson, D. Malignant disease in children. Mother and Child, 45 (5), Sep/Oct 1973, 11–13.

19 Preston, K. O. Nursing children with cancer. Nursing Times, 67, 22 Apr 1971, 467–469.

20 Scott, Sir R. B. Leukaemia. Nursing Mirror, 135, 24 Nov 1972, 24–26.

21 Snell, P. Nursing care study. Acute myeloblastic leukaemia. Nursing Times, 71, 1 May 1975, 693–695.

22 Spiers, A. S. D. Leukaemia and surgery. Nursing Times, 70, 3 Oct 1974, 1535–1537.

23 Stewart, A. Oxford survey of childhood cancers. Nursing Mirror, 133, 22 Oct 1971, 25–26.

24 Taylor, N. R. W. Malignant disease in childhood. Nursing Mirror, 136, 29 Jun 1973, 44–45.

25 Terry, P. B. Nursing care study. [Rhabdomyosarcoma in a girl of 11.] Nursing Mirror, 140, 2 Jan 1975, 45–48.

26 Timmons, A. L. Is it so awful? [Personal experiences of a child with leukaemia.] American Journal of Nursing, 75 (6), Jun 1975, 988.

27 Whitehouse, J. M. A. The leukaemias. 1. Acute leukaemia. 2. Chronic leukaemia. Nursing Times, 68, 8 Jun 1972, 703–706; 15 Jun 1972, 737–738.

83 CARDIOVASCULAR SYSTEM

a GENERAL

1 American Heart Association. Council on Cardiovascular Nursing and American Nurses' Association. Division on medical-surgical nursing practice Standards of cardiovascular nursing practice. Kansas City: American Nurses' Association, 1975.

2 Armington, Sr. C. and Creighton, H. Nursing of people with cardiovascular problems. Boston: Little, Brown, 1971.

3 Ashworth, P. M. and Rose, H. Cardiovascular disorders: patient care. Baillière Tindall, 1973.

4 Daly, J. M. and others Central Venous catherization American Journal of Nursing, 75 (5), May 1975, 820–824.

5 Drake, J. J. Locating the external reference point for central venous pressure determination. [Exploratory study to determine the variable performance of intensive care nurses, using two different methods.] Nursing Research, 23 (6), Nov–Dec 1974, 475–482.

6 Foster, S. B. Self-assessment of current knowledge in cardiopulmonary nursing; 1,337 multiple choice questions and referenced answers. Flushing: Medical Examination Publishing Co. 1975.

7 Grove, L. The microcirculation and shock. Journal of the American Association of Nurse Anesthetists, 60 (3), Jun 1972, 185–192.

8 Krueger, J. M. Monitoring central venous pressure: a programmed sequence. New York: Springer, 1973.

9 Latimer, R. D. and Marcusson, R. W. Central venous catheterization. Nursing Times, 68, 7 Sep 1972, 1124–1126.

10 Lee, P. W. R. Return to nursing. 20. Central venous pressure measurement. Nursing Mirror, 135, 22 Sep 1972, 20–21.

11 Lewis, E. P. Nursing in cardiovascular diseases. New York: American Journal of Nursing Co., 1971. (Contemporary Nursing Series.) Particles selected and reprinted from the American Journal of Nursing, Nursing Research and Nursing Outlook, 1971.

12 Miller, A. Systems of life. Nos 9–12. Cardiovascular system 1–4. Nursing Times, 71, 4 Sep 1975; 2 Oct 1975; 6 Nov 1975; 4 Dec 1975.

13 McKinnon–Mullett, E. L. Circulation research: exploring its potential in clinical nursing research. Nursing Research, 21 (6), Nov/Dec 1972, 494–498.

14 Pallett, F. Circulatory system: physiology and pharmacology. Butterworths, 1971. (Nursing in depth series.)

15 Payne, J. E. and Kaplan, H. M. Alternative techniques for venipuncture. American Journal of Nursing, 72 (4), Apr 1972, 702–703.

16 Redman, B. K. Client education therapy in treatment and prevention of cardiovascular diseases. Cardio-Vascular Nursing, 10 (1), Jan/Feb 1974, 1–6.

17 Rowlands, D. J. Coronary care. 2. Cardiovascular anatomy and physiology. Nursing Times, 70, 10 Jan 1974, 36–39.

b DISEASES

1 Balfour, T. W. Lord dilatation treatment for haemorrhoids. Nursing Mirror, 136, 9 Mar 1973, 29–30.

2 Beshore, J. A. How to prevent – and if necessary, treat – emboli. RN Magazine, 38 (11), Nov 1975, 29–35.

3 Browse, N. L. Ischaemic feet. Nursing Mirror, 138, 31 May 1974, 68–70.

4 Browse, N. L. Prevention of pulmonary embolism. Nursing Times, 69, 20/27 Dec 1973, 1718–1719.

5 Cantor, A. J. Hemorrhoids: patient care essentials. Journal of Practical Nursing, 22 (7), Jul 1972, 20–21, 34.

6 Cawley, M. No cure, just care. [Case study of a patient with severe arteriosclerotic cardiovascular disease.] American Journal of Nursing, 74 (11), Nov 1974, 2010–2013.

7 Chappell, A. G. Pulmonary embolism. Nursing Mirror, 132, 8 Jan 1971, 26–28.

8 Cross, L. Nursing care study. Surgery in arterial occlusion. Nursing Mirror, 141, 30 Oct 1975, 51–53.

9 Daly, C. R. and Kelly, E. A. Prevention of pulmonary embolism: intracaval devices. American Journal of Nursing, 72 (11), Nov 1972, 2004–2006.

10 Derdall, M. J. Basilar aneurysms. Canadian Nurse, 67 (4), Apr 1971, 49–52.

11 Ellis, H. Arteriosclerotic disease of the lower limbs. Nursing Times, 69, 31 May 1973, 698–700.

12 Gallitano, A. L. and others A safe approach to the subclavian vein. RN Magazine, 36 (7), Jul 1973, OR 13–14.

13 Gover, J. and others Doppler examination in peripheral vascular disease. Australian Nurses' Journal, 3 (11), Jun 1974, 30–32, 35.

14 Gernert, C. F. and Schwartz, S. Pulmonary artery catheterization. American Journal of Nursing, 73 (7), Jul 1973, 1182–1185.

15 Hastings, F. Nursing care study. Polyarteritis nodosa. Nursing Mirror, 141, 14 Aug 1975, 53–55.

16 Jackson, B. S. Chronic peripheral arterial disease. American Journal of Nursing, 72 (5), May 1972, 928–934.

17 Jackson, B. S. Nursing decisions. [Experiences in clinical problem solving. Chronic peripheral vascular disease.] RN Magazine, 38 (12), Dec 1975, 33–39.

18 Kirkley, K. Nursing care study. Aortic bifurcation graft. Nursing Times, 71, 31 Jul 1975, 1202–1204.

19 Lawson, L. J. Reconstructive surgery for lower limb ischaemia. Nursing Times, 70, 21 Feb 1974, 261–265.

20 Leutzinger, R. Nursing care study. Polyarteritis nodosa. Improvement was minimal before a chemical sympathectomy. Nursing Times, 70, 3 Jan 1974, 14–16.

21 Lloyd, J. K. Prevention of atherosclerosis in childhood. Nursing Mirror, 139, 26 Sep 1974, 66–67.

22 Lord, P. H. Haemorrhoids – the dilatation procedure and regime. Nursing Times, 71, 19 Jun 1975, 961–963.

23 Low, A. W. Pain in haemorrhoid repair. Nursing Times, 71, 12 Jun 1975, 930–931.

24 Mackenzie, D. M. and others Nursing care study. A patient with an abdominal aneurysm. Nursing Times, 71, 8 May 1975, 720–722.

25 Mayer, G. G. Disseminated intravascular coagulation. American Journal of Nursing, 73 (12), Dec 1973, 2067–2069.

26 Miller, G. A. Pulmonary embolism. Nursing Mirror, 139, 23 Aug 1974, 71–73.

27 Miller, V. M. Femoropopliteal bypass graft with the saphenous vein: nursing care. RN Magazine, 35 (11), Nov 1972, OR1, 4, 7.

28 Partridge, J. P. Treatment of haemorrhoids. Nursing Times, 71, 12 Jun 1975, 928–929.

29 Reynolds, W. Sutureless hemorrhoidectomy. RN Magazine, 36 (5), May 1973, OR 11, 13.

30 Rose, M. A. Home care after peripheral vascular surgery. American Journal of Nursing, 74 (2), Feb 1974, 260–262.

31 Skilton, J. S. Lumbar sympathectomy. [The use in the treatment of vascular disorders.] Nursing Times, 71, 6 Mar 1975, 376–377.

32 Walton, K. W. Atherosclerosis and ischaemic disease. Nursing Mirror, 139, 28 Nov 1974, 48–52.

c DEEP VEIN THROMBOSIS

1 Davies, A. M. Streptokinase therapy for deep vein thrombosis. Nursing Times, 69, 15 Feb 1973, 211–212.

2 Drug and Therapeutics Bulletin Prevention and treatment of deep-vein thrombosis. Drug and Therapeutics Bulletin, 10 (6), March 1972, 21–24.

3 Faris, I. B. and others Temperature chart analysis in the diagnosis of postoperative deep vein thrombosis. Lancet, 2, 14 Oct 1972, 775–776.

4 Hills, N. H. Deep vein thrombosis after surgery. Nursing Mirror, 135, 21 Jul 1972, 29–30.

5 Kline, A. L. and Fegan, W. G. The effect of footwear on venous return. Nursing Times, 67, 30 Dec 1971, 1644–1645.

6 Lau, O. J. Deep vein thrombosis. Clinical features and some modern techniques of diagnosis. Nursing Times, 69, 11 Oct 1973, 1332–1333.

7 Nicholaides, A. M. and others Optimal electrical stimulus for prevention of deep vein thrombosis. [During operations.] British Medical Journal, 3, 23 Sep 1972, 756–758.

8 Powley, J. M. and Doran, F. S. A. Galvanic stimulation to prevent deep-vein thrombosis [during operations]. Lancet, 1, 24 Feb 1973, 406–407.

9 Roberts, V. C. and Cotton, L. T. Prevention of postoperative deep vein thrombosis in patients with malignant disease. British Medical Journal, 1, 2 Mar 1974, 358–360.

10 Thomas, M. L. Pelvic phlebography. Nursing Mirror, 132, 19 Mar 1971, 23–26.

11 Wadsworth, T. G. Postoperative deep vein thrombosis – some points and a suggestion. Nursing Mirror, 134, 28 Jan 1972, 28–29.

12 Wingfield, J. G. Thrombo-embolic phenomena associated with childbirth. Midwives Chronicle, 86, Sep 1972, 280–282.

d HYPERTENSION AND HYPOTENSION (Includes patient teaching, screening)

1 Aagaard, G. N. Treatment of hypertension. American Journal of Nursing, 73 (4), Apr 1973, 620–623.

2 Alexander, M. F. Portal hypertension. Nursing Times, 68, 6 Jan 1972, 9–20.

3 Batterman, B. and others Hypertension. 1. Detection and evaluation. Cardio-Vascular Nursing, 11 (4), Jul/Aug 1975, 35–40.

4 Bernards Case study. Hypertension. New Zealand Nursing Journal, 66 (55), May 1973, 11–15.

5 Carter, A. B. Hypertension – its causes and treatment. Nursing Times, 67, 6 May 1971, 531–533.

6 Cockerill, P. Nursing care study. Independence for Mrs. D. [A patient with hypotension.] Nursing Times, 71, 13 Feb 1975, 260–261.

7 Conte, A. and others Group work with hypertensive patients. [Patient education.] American Journal of Nursing, 74 (5), May 1974, 910–912.

8 Coope, J. A screening clinic for hypertension in general practice. Journal of the Royal College of General Practitioners, 24, Mar 1974, 161–166.

9 Cooper, T. Hypertension the silent killer. 2. Treatment and therapy. Journal of Practical Nursing, 23 (11), Nov 1973, 23–25; (12), Dec 1973, 16–18.

10 Creegan, S. M. A comparison of blood pressure readings taken simultaneously by faculty and students. Nursing Papers, 4 (1), Jul 1972, 36–42.

11 Cumming, A. M. M. Nursing care study. Nursing in clinical research. [Case of a child suffering from hypertension.] Nursing Times, 70, 20 Jun 1974, 962–964.

12 Davidson, W. L. Detecting high blood pressure in an industrial population. Report on a hypertension screening program at Merck & Co. Inc. Occupational Health Nursing, 23 (5), May 1975, 10–13.

13 Del Bueno, D. J. The renal humoral system: a cause of hypertension? RN Magazine, 38 (9), Sep 1975, 109–110, 113.

14 Federspiel, B. Renin and blood pressure. American Journal of Nursing, 75 (9), Sep 1975, 1462–1464.

15 Finnerty, F. A. Aggressive drug therapy in accelerated hypertension. American Journal of Nursing, 74 (12), Dec 1974, 2176–2180.

16 Foley, M. F. Variations in blood pressure in the lateral recumbent position. Nursing Research, 20 (1), Jan/Feb 1971, 64–69.

17 Griffith, E. W. and Madero, B. Primary hypertension: patients' learning needs. American Journal of Nursing, 73 (4), Apr 1973, 624–627.

18 Hamilton, M. Management of hypertension. Nursing Mirror, 132, 15 Jan 1971, 33–37.

19 Hopkins, S. J. New drugs for old 1. Hypertension and cardiac failure. Nursing Times, 68, 6 Jul 1972, 841–843.

20 Lancet Home blood-pressure recording. [Training patients to take their own blood-pressures.] Lancet, 1, 1 Feb 1975, 259–260.

21 Lee, G. M. A rural hypertension control program. [Using nurses and community workers.] American Journal of Nursing, 74 (8), Aug 1974, 1450–1452.

22 McCaugherty, D. Nursing care study. Chronic pyelonephritis with malignant hypertension. Nursing Times, 71, 27 Mar 1975, 492–494.

23 McNally, J. M. Is your number up? Ask the nurse. [A nurse conducts a high blood pressure screening program in a university.] RN Magazine, 38 (12), Dec 1975, 43, 46, 48.

24 Mitchell, P. W. and Van Meter, M. J. Reproducibility of blood pressures recorded on patients' records by nursing personnel. Nursing Research, 20 (4), Jul/Aug 1971, 348–352.

25 Nielson, M. A. Intra-arterial monitoring of blood pressure. American Journal of Nursing, 74 (1), Jan 1974, 48–53.

26 Palmer, E. M. and Griffith, E. W. Effect of activity during bedmaking on heart rate and blood pressure. Nursing Research, 20 (1), Jan/Feb 1971, 17–25.

27 Rahman, J. C. Hypertension. [Effective control of hypertension requires the matching of the patient to his medication.] Occupational Health Nursing, 23 (1), Jan 1975, 17–20.

28 Richardson, J. F. and Robinson, D. Variations in the measurement of blood pressure between doctors and nurses. [At private screening clinics.] Journal of the Royal College of General Practitioners, 21, Dec 1971, 698–704.

29 Robinson, A. M. The RNs. goal: under 90mm Hg. diastolic. RN Magazine, 37 (5), May 1974, 43–49.

30 Rodman, M. J. Drug therapy today. Drugs used in cardiovascular disease. 2. Treating hypertension. RN Magazine, 36 (4), Apr 1973, 41–42, 44, 46, 48, 51, 53–54.

31 Seth, G. S. Original research into normal blood pressures: a study to find the mean arterial pressure in adult females and its variation in different age groups. Occupational Health, 24 (2), Feb 1972, 41–44.

32 Smith S. E. Drugs and hypertension. Nursing Times, 67, 14 Oct 1971, 1287–1288.

33 Smith, S. E. How drugs act. 12. Drugs and hypertension. Nursing Times, 71, 11 Sep 1975, 1474–1475.

34 Ungvarski, P. J. Nursing assessment in hypertension. Occupational Health Nursing, 23 (11), Nov 1975, 9–15.

e VARICOSE VEINS AND ULCERS (See also Nurses' health and welfare)

1 Baluch, R. B. Varicose veins in pregnancy. Midwife and Health Visitor, 9 (3), Mar 1973, 76–77.

2 Brown, G. M. Case study. Varicose ulcer. District Nursing, 15 (3), Jun 1972, 59–60.

3 Cleave, T. L. Varicose veins and venous thrombosis in the legs: their relationship to the colon, hereditary differences in Britain and suggested preventive treatment. Nursing Times, 70, 30 May 1974, 828–829.

4 Cobey, J. C. and Cobey, J. H. Chronic leg ulcers. American Journal of Nursing, 74 (2), Feb 1974, 258–259.

5 Dodd, H. Varicose veins and venous disorders of the lower limb. 1. Introduction to venous disorders. Nursing Mirror, 135, 17 Nov 1972, 42–47.

6 Dodd, H. Varicose veins and venous disorders of the lower limb. 2. Diagnosis and treatment. Nursing Mirror, 135, 24 Nov 1972, 46–51.

7 Fegan, W. G. Bandaging the lower limb. [With particular reference to the treatment of varicose veins by compression sclerotherapy.] Nursing Times, 69, 23 Aug 1973, 1079–1080.

8 Fegan, W. G. Varicose feet. Nursing Mirror, 139, 30 Aug 1974, 55–57.

9 McCarrick, H. Varicose ulcers – a nurse's province? Nursing Times, 69, 18 Jan 1973, 74–75.

10 Stone, L. A. Dressing leg ulcers [using polyether foam]. Nursing Times, 70, 13 Jun 1974, 914–915.

11 Vukovitch, N. A clinic for varicose ulcers. Nursing Times, 68, 31 Aug 1972, 1090–1092.

12 Wakely, Sir C. Ulceration and some uncommon ulcers. Nursing Mirror, 138, 7 Jun 1974, 54–55.

84 CARDIAC AND CORONARY CARE

a CARDIAC DISORDERS

1 Baird, I. M. Management of failing heart. Nursing Mirror, 137, 24 Aug 1973, 30–33.

2 Coats, K. Non-invasive cardiac diagnosis procedures. American Journal of Nursing, 75 (11), Nov 1975, 1980–1985.

3 Conway, N. A pocket atlas of arrythmias for nurses. Wolfe Medical, 1974.

4 Crouchman, M. Idiopathic chylopericardium. Nursing Times, 70, 6 Jun 1974, 874–875.

5 Ismay, G. Congestive cardiac failure. Nursing Times, 68, 29 Jun 1972, 797–800.

6 Mayer, G. G. and Kaelin, P. B. Arrhythmias and cardiac output. American Journal of Nursing, 72 (9), Sep 1972, 1597–1600.

7 Reid, L. Cor pulmonale. Nursing Mirror, 136, 1 Jun 1973, 26–27.

8 Patton, R. D. Arrhythmias that warn of cardiac insult. RN Magazine, 35 (4), Apr 1972, OR 1–4, 6–7, 10, 12.

b CARDIAC NURSING (Includes Cardiogenic shock, Catheterization)

1 Andreoli, K. G. and others Comprehensive cardiac care: a text for nurses, physicians and other health practitioners. 3rd ed. St. Louis: Mosby, 1975.

2 Begley, L. A. External counter-pulsation for cardiogenic shock. American Journal of Nursing, 75 (6), Jun 1975, 967–970.

3 Boyd, J. M. L. Understanding and treating cardiogenic shock. RN Magazine, 38 (4), Apr 1975, 53–54, 56, 58, 60, 62.

4 Breakey, E. J. Intra-aortic balloon pump. Canadian Nurse, 71 (8), Aug 1975, 18–21.

5 Bregman, D. The dual-chambered intra-aortic balloon [used in cardiogenic shock]. RN Magazine, 37 (12), Dec 1974, ICU 1–2.

6 Brown, M. G. American nursing for heart patients. [Author's account of her tour of the USA on a Chest and Heart Association Scholarship.] Health Magazine, 10 (1), Mar 1973, 21–23.

7 Chavigny, K. A comparison of a pilot study to the main research thesis on pulse palpation in acute cardiac patients. International Journal of Nursing Studies, 10 (4), Dec 1973, 229–237.

8 Chow, R. K. Identifying professional nursing practice through research: cardiosurgical patient care. International Journal of Nursing Studies, 9 (3), Aug 1972, 125–134.

9 Clark, H. Nursing care study. Left ventricular failure with acute pulmonary oedema. Nursing Times, 71, 3 Jul 1975, 1040–1042.

10 Cogen, R. Cardiac catheterization: preparing the adult. [Including emotional care.] American Journal of Nursing, 73 (1), Jan 1973, 77–79.

11 Crews, J. Nurse-managed cardiac clinics. Cardio-Vascular Nursing, 8 (4), Jul/Aug 1972, 15–18.

12 Crook, B. R. Cardiac catheterization – what the nurse should know. Nursing Times, 69, 29 Nov 1973, 1608–1609.

13 Dorr, K. S. The intra-aortic balloon pump. [The problems of use for patients and nurses.] American Journal of Nursing, 75 (1), Jan 1975, 52–55.

14 Foster, S. B. Pump failure. [Factors involved and the nurse's responsibility in diagnosis and treatment.] American Journal of Nursing, 74 (10), Oct 1974, 1830–1834.

15 Frost, D. Nursing care study. Paroxysmal ventricular tachycardia complicated by acute retention of urine. Nursing Times, 70, 4 Apr 1974, 499–501.

16 Gillette, E. Heartbeat – the rhythm of life. [Types of coronary heart diseases and nursing care in cardiogenic shock.] Nursing Care, 8 (6), Jun 1975, 24–27.

17 Goldstrom, D. K. Cardiac rest: bed or chair? American Journal of Nursing, 72 (10), Oct 1972, 1812–1816.

18 Gotsman, M. S. and others Principles of cardiac catheterization for the nurse. SA Nursing Journal, 38 (7), Jul 1971, 19, 21, 23–26; (8), Aug 1971, 13–16.

19 Habak, P. A. and others Rotating tourniquets: how effective in left heart failure? RN Magazine, 38 (1), Jan 1975, ICU 1–2, 5.

20 Jones, P. Rotating tourniquets: the nurse's role. RN Magazine, 38 (1), Jan 1975, ICU 6.

21 Lamberton, M. M. Cardiac catheterization: anticipatory nursing care. American Journal of Nursing, 71 (9), Sep 1971, 1718–1721.

22 Lehmann, J. Auscultation of heart sounds. Where to listen, how to listen, and what to listen for in the identification of heart sounds. American Journal of Nursing, 72 (7), Jul 1972, 1242–1246.

23 Leighton-Price, F. R. Nursing care study. Subacute bacterial endocarditis in a patient with a patent ductus arteriosus. Nursing Mirror, 139, 5 Jul 1974, 79–83.

24 McIntyre, H. M., editor Heart disease: new dimensions of nursing care. Garden Grove: Trainex Press, 1974.

25 McIntyre, H. M. How the LP/VN can help prevent heart disease. Journal of Practical Nursing, 21 (9), Sep 1971, 25–29.

26 McIntyre, H. M. and Mason, D. T. The prevention of heart disease: a greater challenge. Cardio-Vascular Nursing, 7 (5), Sep/Oct 1971, 77–81.

27 Martinez-Lopez, J. I. Can you recognize heart sounds in diastole? [Heart sounds influencing the process of patient's diseases.] RN Magazine, 38 (4), Apr 1975, ICU 3, 6, 11.

28 Meyer, M. L. Cardiac catheterization: a challenging parameter in nursing. RN Magazine, 34 (10), Oct 1971, 35–41.

29 Miller, G. A. Cardiac catheterization. Nursing Mirror, 141, 7 Aug 1975, 56–57.

30 Nursing Clinics of North America Symposium on concepts in cardiac nursing. Nursing Clinics of North America, 7 (3), Sep 1972, 411–591.

31 Obuchowski, M. J. The cardiac risk screening program. Occupational Health Nursing, 22 (2), Feb 1974, 10–11.

32 Raby, C. M. Nursing care study. Ineffective endocarditis. Nursing Times, 71, 15 May 1975, 764–766.

33 Robinson, L. A. Patient's information base: a key to care. [A study of eleven cardiac patients.] Canadian Nurse, 70 (12), Dec 1974, 34–36.

34 Scott, E. J. C. Cardiology in Edinburgh. [Including the work of the nurse.] Nursing Times, 68, 5 Oct 1972, 1244–1246.

35 Stude, C. Cardiogenic shock. American Journal of Nursing, 74 (9), Sep 1974, 1636–1640.

36 Woogara, R. Nursing care study. Haemopneumothorax and cardiac tamponade. Nursing Times, 71, 13 Feb 1975, 255–256.

c EDUCATION AND TRAINING

1 Begent, R. H. J. and MacArthur, Y. Training for coronary care with an arrhythmia simulator. Nursing Times, 68, 28 Dec 1972, 1661.

2 Chow, R. K. Developing dynamic scientific sessions for nurses: a three-year retrospective. [With reference to cardiac care.] Cardio-Vascular Nursing, 9 (5), Sep/Oct 1973, 23–26.

3 Gordon, M. S. Learning from a cardiology patient simulator. [Computer programmed animated manikins.] RN Magazine, 38 (8), Aug 1975, ICU 1, 4, 6.

4 Haferkorn, V. Continuing education for the specialty nurse [in the coronary care unit]. Nursing Outlook, 23 (4), Apr 1975, 245–247.

5 McConnell, R. D. Nursing opportunities. [In cardiothoracic nursing including post basic training.] Nursing Mirror, 141 (6), 7 Aug 1975, 51–52.

6 Scheuer, R. Coronary care nurse training program: an evaluation. Nursing Research, 21 (3), May/Jun 1972, 228–232.

7 Schorow, M. and others Training nurses for coronary care practice. Nursing Outlook, 19 (2), Feb 1971, 95–97.

8 Wiener, M. M. and others Nurse training goes modern: a multimedia instructional system for teaching nurses the concepts and techniques of intensive coronary care. Hospitals, 45, 1 Oct 1971, 74, 76, 78, 80.

d CARDIAC MONITORING

1 Armstrong, M. L. Electrocardiograms: a systematic method of reading them. 3rd ed. Bristol: John Wright, 1974.

2 Asbury, A. J. Electronic equipment in nursing. [Includes ECG monitor.] Nursing Times, 69, 5 Jul 1973, 861–863.

3 Butler, H. H. How to read an ECG. Basic interpretations for nurses and other health workers. RN Magazine, 36 (1), Jan 1973, 35, 37–45; 36 (2), Feb 1973, 49–61; 36 (3), Mar 1973, 50–59.

4 Delano, A. and others Monitoring the acutely ill cardiac patient. Cardio-Vascular Nursing, 7 (1), Jan/Feb 1971, 61–64.

5 Hamer, J. An introduction to electrocardiography: a primer for students, graduates practitioners and nurses concerned with coronary care and other forms of intensive care. Pitman, 1975.

6 Hampton, J. R. The ECG made easy. Churchill Livingstone, 1973.

7 Hoffman, I. AYZ is the ABC of ECG: an introduction to QRS-T interpretation for medical students, interns, nurses and ECG technicians. Chicago: Year Book Medical Publishers, 1973.

8 Hubner, P. J. B. Nurses' guide to cardiac monitoring. 2nd ed. Baillière Tindall, 1975.

9 McGuinness, J. B. Displacement cardiography: a new technique for study of cardiac movement. Nursing Times, 70, 18 Jul 1974, 1111–1112.

10 Marks, A. E. Cardiac monitoring technicians. [Use of technicians to look after the machines, giving nurses time to care for their patients.] Nursing Outlook, 20 (6), Jun 1972, 388–389.

11 Meehan, M. EKG primer. Programmed instruction. American Journal of Nursing, 7 (11), Nov 1971, 2195–2202.

12 Nursing Times Comprehensive monitoring. [New system introduced by Kent Cambridge Medical Limited.] Nursing Times, 69, 20/27 Dec 1973, 1747.

13 Owen, S. G. Electrocardiography: a programmed text for self-tuition in the principles of electrocardiography and the interpretation of electrocardiograms. 2nd ed. English University Press, 1973.

14 Pinneo, R. Essentials of cardiac monitoring. Journal of Practical Nursing, 23 (11), Nov 1973, 26–29.

15 Robinson, A. M. Stress testing: key to activity for the heart patient. RN Magazine, 36 (12), Dec 1973, ICU 1, ICU 5.

16 Rowlands, D. J. Coronary care. 4 and 5. Electrocardiography. Nursing Times, 70, 24 Jan 1974, 114–117; 31 Jan 1974, 146–148.

17 Rowlands, D. J. Coronary care. 6. Cardiac electrophysiology. Nursing Times, 70, 7 Feb 1974, 180–183.

18 Schamroth, L. An introduction to electrocardiography. 4th ed. Oxford: Blackwell Scientific, 1971.

19 Schulze, V. E. Electrocardiography and related coronary care: a manual for the nurse. Garden Grove: Trainex Press, 1974.

20 Van Meter, M. and Lavine, P. G. Reading EKGs correctly. Jenkintown: Intermed Communications, 1975. (Nursing 77 skillbook series.)

21 Vos, H. P. The EKG-interpretation of common arrhythmias. Journal of the American Association of Nurse Anesthetists, 41 (5), Oct 1973, 391–406.

e CARDIAC SURGERY (Includes heart transplantation)

1 Batcheldor, S. A. Nursing care following mitral valve replacement. Nursing Mirror, 141, 7 Aug 1975, 59–62.

2 Brener, E. R. Surgery for coronary artery disease. American Journal of Nursing, 72 (3), Mar 1972, 469–473.

3 Busby, J. C. Cardiac surgery, yesterday and today. [Resumé of advances since 1866.] Nursing Times, 71, 11 Dec 1975, 1978–1981.

4 Clarke, N. Case report 2. Open heart surgery on the hemophiliac. RN Magazine, 36 (5), May 1973, 44–47.

5 Cooley, D. A. and Wormuth, C. E. Direct coronary surgery. AORN Journal, 21 (5), Apr 1975, 789–796.

6 Cooper, D. K. C. Transplantation of the heart. Nursing Mirror, 134, 14 Apr 1972, 21–23.

7 Ennis, P. J. A patient with aortic valve incompetence. [Operation for aortic valve replacement with a Starr-Edwards prosthesis.] Nursing Times, 69, 7 Jun 1973, 733–735.

8 Gilbert, R. Heart valve replacement using homografts. Nursing Times, 68, 16 Nov 1972, 1439–1441.

9 Heriza, E. and others Groote Schuur Hospital. The second double heart transplant. SA Nursing Journal, 42 (9), Sep 1975, 29, 12.

10 Hill, D. G. Coronary artery surgery. [For angina pectoris.] Nursing Mirror, 139, 19 Sep 1974, 65–66.

11 Long, M. L. and others Cardiopulmonary bypass. American Journal of Nursing, 74 (5), May 1974, 860–867.

12 Oakley, C. M. Infective endocarditis. Nursing Times, 70, 25 Jul 1974, 1150–1152.

13 Pagliero, K. M. Porcine heterograft heart valves. Nursing Times, 71, 12 Jun 1975, 925–927.

14 Pagliero, K. M. Surgery for coronary artery disease. Nursing Times, 70, 25 Apr 1974, 622–626.

15 Paneth, M. Cardiac valve replacement. Nursing Mirror, 141, 7 Aug 1975, 58–59.

16 Reid, J. M. Pregnancy and cardiac valve prosthesis. Nursing Mirror, 133, 1 Oct 1971, 35–36.

17 Sears, J. A. Groote Schuur Hospital. Heart transplantation: palliative surgery. SA Nursing Journal, 42 (9), Sep 1975, 24–25.

18 Tompsett, E. M. Modern heart surgery. District Nursing, 15 (7), Oct 1972, 139, 144.

19 Tubbs, G. S. The history of cardiothoracic surgery. Nursing Mirror, 141, 7 Aug 1975, 48–50.

20 Ume, G. A. Case study [of the first successful open-heart surgery performed in the University of Nigeria Teaching Hospital, Enugu.] Nigerian Nurse, 6 (3), Jul/Sep 1974, 24–31.

21 Verderber, A. Cardiopulmonary bypass: postoperative complications. American Journal of Nursing, 74 (5), May 1974, 868–869.

22 Wright, J. E. C. The surgical treatment of angina pectoris. Nursing Mirror, 141, 7 Aug 1975, 53–55.

f CARDIAC SURGERY: NURSING

1 Aiken, L. H. and Henrichs, T. F. Systematic relaxation as a nursing intervention technique with open heart surgery patients. Nursing Research, 20 (3), May/Jun 1971, 212–218.

2 Bryant, R. B. The nursing care and management of coronary artery grafts. Australian Nurses' Journal, 3 (5), Nov 1973, 24–26.

3 Chung, T. M. Y. Nursing care study. Mitral valve replacement and aortic valve homograft. Immediate postoperative care. Nursing Times, 70, 5 Sep 1974, 1375–1377.

4 Clareborough, J. K. and Simpson, F. The role of the nurse in modern cardiac surgery. Australian Nurses' Journal, 1 (7), Jan 1972, 24, 27; Nursing Journal of India, 63 (4), Apr 1972, 133–134.

5 Hanton, P. Nursing care study. Aortic valve incompetence. Nursing Times, 69, 13 Dec 1973, 1685–1689.

6 Hodges, L. C. Systems and nursing care of the cardiac surgical patient. Nursing Clinics of North America, 6 (3), Sep 1971, 415–424.

7 King, O. M. Care of the cardiac surgical patient. St. Louis: Mosby, 1975.

8 Merino, D. V. Return to nursing! Cardio-thoracic nursing. 2. Cardiac surgical nursing. Nursing Mirror, 135, 1 Sep 1972, 26–29.

9 National Heart and Chest Hospitals Care of the cardiothoracic patient. A symposium. Nursing Mirror, 141, 7 Aug 1975, 47–65.

10 O'Connor, C. T. Curare in patient care. [Postoperative care of paralysed patient after heart surgery.] American Journal of Nursing, 72 (5), May 1972, 913–915.

11 Stewart, D. M. Nursing care study. Coronary artery bypass graft. Nursing Times, 70, 25 Apr 1974, 627–629.

12 Tompsett, E. M. Nursing care of the patient undergoing cardiac surgery. District Nursing, 15 (10), Jan 1973, 224–225, 235.

13 True, M. Before and after heart surgery: nursing essentials. Journal of Practical Nursing, 23 (11), Nov 1973, 30–31.

14 Welman, E. Intensive nursing care of the cardiac surgery patient. Nursing Mirror, 139, 14 Nov 1974, 75–78.

15 Winward, R. Nursing care study. Closure of ventricular septal defect. Nursing Mirror, 139, 16 Aug 1974, 74–76.

g CARDIAC SURGERY: PATIENT

1 Ellis, R. Unusual sensory and thought disturbances after cardiac surgery. American Journal of Nursing, 72 (11), Nov 1972, 2021–2025.

2 Elsberry, N. L. Psychological responses to open heart surgery: a review. Nursing Research, 21 (3), May/Jun 1972, 220–227.

3 Guthrie, M. Cardiac surgery in the first person. [Patient's experiences.] Canadian Nurse, 69 (9), Sep 1973, 31–33.

4 McFadden, E. H. and Giblin, E. C. Sleep deprivation in patients having open-heart surgery. Nursing Research, 20 (3), May/Jun 1971, 249–254.

5 Meserko, V. Pre-operative classes for cardiac patients. American Journal of Nursing, 73 (4), Apr 1973, 665.

6 **Rushton, G.** My heart operation. Nursing Times, 68, 13 Jan 1972, 37–38.

7 **Swan, J. T.** Coronary bypass. [Experiences of a patient undergoing open heart surgery.] American Journal of Nursing, 75 (12), Dec 1975, 2142–2145.

8 **Trace, D.** Psychiatric side-effects of cardiothoracic surgery. Nursing Mirror, 139, 14 Nov 1974, 71–72.

9 **Walker, B. B.** The postsurgery heart patient: amount of uninterrupted time for sleep and rest during the first, second, and third postoperative days in a teaching hospital. Nursing Research, 21 (2), Mar/Apr 1972, 164–169.

10 **Wise, D. J.** Crisis intervention before cardiac surgery. American Journal of Nursing, 75 (8), Aug 1975, 1316–1318.

11 **Woods, N. F.** Patterns of sleep in postcardiotomy patients. Nursing Research, 21 (4), Jul/Aug 1972, 347–352.

h SURGERY: CHILDREN

1 **Altshuler, A.** Complete transposition of the great arteries. American Journal of Nursing, 71 (1), Jan 1971, 96–98.

2 **Andrews, I.** Nursing care study. Correction of atrial septal defect in a child. Nursing Times, 69, 22 Feb 1973, 238–240.

3 **Beck, M.** Attitudes of parents of pediatric heart patients towards patient care units. Nursing Research, 22 (4), Jul/Aug 1973, 334–338.

4 **Breckenridge, I. M.** Surgical treatment of transposition of the great arteries. Nursing Mirror, 136, 5 Jan 1973, 38–40.

5 **Cortez, A. and others** The utilization of nurses in expanded roles to deliver pediatric cardiology health care. [Children's Heart Program of South Texas.] Pediatric Nursing, 1 (3), May/Jun 1975, 22–29, 32.

6 **Friedberg, D. Z. and Caldart, L.** A center for pediatric cardiovascular patients. [Education of patients, families and professionals involved with the newborn by a nurse educator.] American Journal of Nursing, 75 (9), Sep 1975, 1480–1482.

7 **Garrett, G. E. R.** Nursing care study. Transposition of the great arteries. Nursing Times, 69, 22 Nov 1973, 1564–1566.

8 **Gedge, E. M.** Care of children undergoing cardiac surgery. Nursing Times, 68, 13 Jan 1972, 39–41.

9 **Gedge, E. M.** Transposition of the great vessels. Nursing Mirror, 135, 1 Sep 1972, 34–35.

10 **Hamilton, T.** Major open heart surgery in childhood. Nursing Times, 68, 20 Jan 1972, 70–76.

11 **Heeckeren, D. W. van and Stansel, H. C.** Arterial monitoring of the infant undergoing cardiac surgery. RN Magazine, 35 (6), Jun 1972, OR 25, 27–28.

12 **Hogarth, W.** Cardiopulmonary bypass in infants under two years: the technique used at Harefield Hospital for intracardiac repair of congenital cardiac lesions. Nursing Times, 71, 12 Jun 1975, 921–924.

13 **Hogarth, W.** Division of double aortic arch for respiratory distress. [Nursing care study of open heart surgery on a baby.] Nursing Times, 68, 7 Dec 1972, 1552–1554.

14 **Howarth, E.** Nursing care study. Transposition of the great vessels. Nursing Times, 69, 6 Sep 1973, 1147–1149.

15 **Johnson, A. M.** Congenital heart disease: its effects and treatment. Some anatomical and physiological considerations. Nursing Mirror, 137, 31 Aug 1973, 11–15.

16 **Laycock, D.** Waterston's operation for Fallot's tetralogy. Nursing Times, 68, 25 May 1972, 632–634.

17 **Mantle, F.** Total correction of Fallot's tetralogy and patent foramen ovale. Nursing Times, 68, 27 Jul 1972, 934–936.

18 **Roberts, F. B.** The child with heart disease. American Journal of Nursing, 72 (6), Jun 1972, 1080–1084.

19 **Rydin, L. and Engle, M. A.** The infant with transposition of the great arteries. Cardio-Vascular Nursing, 9 (6), Nov/Dec 1973, 27–30.

20 **Tesler, M. and Hardgrove, C.** Cardiac catheterization: preparing the child. American Journal of Nursing, 73 (1), Jan 1973, 80–82.

21 **West, R.** Familial hypercholesterolaemia in children. [Treatment in an attempt to prevent heart attacks.] Nursing Mirror, 139, 26 Jul 1974, 74–76.

22 **Young, O.** Infant cardiac surgery using profound or deep hypothermia. New Zealand Nursing Journal, 66 (3), Mar 1973, 9–12.

i CORONARY CARE

1 **Bellamy, D.** Mobile coronary care. [Unit started in Belfast 1966.] Health Magazine, 12 (2), Summer 1975, 20–22.

2 **Binnion, P. F.** Coronary artery disease – epidemiology and emergency treatment: the role of the industrial nurse. Occupational Health Nursing, 3 (5), May 1975, 7–9.

3 **Cameron, M. and others** Follow up of emergency ambulance calls in Nottingham: implications for coronary ambulance service. British Medical Journal, 1, 15 Feb 1975, 384–386.

4 **Chamberlain, D. A. and Williams, J. H.** The Brighton experiment. An appraisal of a coronary ambulance system. Health Magazine, 12 (3), Autumn 1975, 11–15.

5 **Clifford, A. H.** Gloucestershire's mobile resuscitation units. Health and Social Service Journal, 84, 2 Mar 1974, 480–481.

6 **Gearty, G. F. and others** Pre-hospital coronary care service. British Medical Journal, 3, 3 Jul 1971, 33–35.

7 **Hall, F. R.** Coronary care in the community. [Coronary Care Ambulance Service, Barnsley.] Royal Society of Health Journal, 93 (2), Apr 1973, 87–88.

8 **Heller, N.** Emergency rescue: CCU nurses at the scene via radio. [Emergency medical system at Doctor's Hospital, Coral Gables, Florida. RN Magazine, 38 (3), Mar 1975, ICU 1, 2, 4, 5.

9 **Holt, P. M.** Assessing British coronary care units. Nursing Mirror, 132, 25 Jun 1971, 14–16.

10 **Joyce, P. M.** Coronary care units stem mortality rates. Australian Nurses' Journal, 2 (11), May 1973, 27–28.

11 **Lennon, M.** Coronary care in Belfast. [Coronary care and mobile units.] Nursing Times, 67, 29 Jul 1971, 921–924.

12 **Morgan, D. M.** The changing coronary care unit – present status and future objectives. Canadian Hospital, 48 (9), Sep 1971, 57–60, 62.

13 **Nursing Mirror** New venture at Aberdeen. [12-bedded coronary care unit.] Nursing Mirror, 133, 3 Sep 1971, 28–29.

14 **Oliver, M. F. and others** Intensive coronary care. Geneva: WHO 1974. (For physicians and nurses.)

15 **Payne, S. and others** Implementation of a problem-oriented system in a CCU. Nursing Clinics of North America, 9 (2), Jun 1974, 255–263.

16 **Roberts, G.** The coronary care unit. [Huddersfield Royal Infirmary.] Nursing Times, 68, 30 Nov 1972, 1507–1508.

17 **Robinson, W.** Mobile coronary care in Barnsley. Nursing Times, 69, 29 Mar 1973, 401.

18 **Rose, G.** The contribution of intensive coronary care. British Journal of Preventive and Social Medicine, 29 (3), Sep 1975, 147–150.

19 **Rowlands, D. J.** Coronary care: a series of 10 articles. Macmillan Journals, 1974.

20 **Rowlands, D. J.** Coronary care. 3. Pathology, clinical features and treatment. Nursing Times, 70, 17 Jan 1974, 78–81.

21 **Rowlands, D. J.** Coronary care. 10. CCU equipment. Nursing Times, 70, 7 Mar 1974, 343–347.

22 **Sandler, G.** Mobile coronary care. [Barnsley.] Royal Society of Health Journal, 93 (2), Apr 1973, 89–91.

23 **Teesside County Borough, Health Department** A study of coronary heart disease. The information is being assembled to provide a data base for planning for a total system of care for coronary cases in the hospital and in the community. Nursing Times, 68, 16 Nov 1972, Occ. papers, 181–182.

24 **Wallace, S. J. M.** Pre-hospital coronary care. [Mobile coronary care units, with particular reference to the scheme at the Royal Victoria Hospital, Belfast.] Nursing Mirror, 139, 14 Nov 1974, 73–75.

25 **White, N. M. and others** Mobile coronary care provided by ambulance personnel. [Scheme in Brighton.] British Medical Journal, 3, 22 Sep 1973, 618–622.

26 **WHO Chronicle** Mobile coronary care units. WHO Chronicle, 25 (2), Feb 1971, 79–82.

j CORONARY CARE NURSING

1 **Argondizzo, N. T. and Reed, P. K.** The legacy of coronary care nursing. [After more than a decade of experience.] Cardio-Vascular Nursing, 11 (3), May/Jun 1975, 35–38.

2 **Charter, D.** CCU – where nurses function on a par with physicians. Canadian Hospital, 48 (3), Mar 1971, 34–38.

3 **Corona, D. F.** After the CCU, what? [Quality of care for the postcoronary patient.] RN Magazine, 36 (6), Jun 1973, 42–43, 68–69, 71–72, 74, 75.

4 **Craig, D. B.** In the CCU, I learned by doing. Nursing Care, 7 (5), May 1971, 29–31.

5 **Deal, J.** Beginner's guide to intensive coronary care. Bowie, Maryland: Charles Press, 1974. [For nurses.]

6 **Deal, J.** It's a big move. From the CCU to the general ward. Bedside Nurse, 4 (7), Jul 1971, 16–20.

7 **Germain, C. P. and Minogue, W. F.** Precoronary care: nursing considerations. Cardiovascular Nursing, 8 (3), May/Jun 1972, 11–14.

8 **Jarvinen, K. A. and Jarvinen, P. H.** Risk of an enema to persons with coronary heart disease. Nursing Mirror, 138, 19 Apr 1974, 81.

9 **Kellberg, E. R.** Coronary care nurse profile. Nursing Research, 21 (1), Jan/Feb, 30–37.

10 **MacDonald, F. G.** Coronary care units and the nurse. Nursing Times, 68, 20 Jul 1972, Occ. papers, 113–116.

11 MacDonald, I. Diet and coronary disease. [Reprinted from Modern Genetics.] Nursing Mirror, 137, 17 Aug 1973, 23–25.

12 Riehl, C. L. Coronary nursing care. New York: Appleton-Century-Crofts, 1971.

13 Rockwell, S. M. Handling those tough questions the nursing books don't answer. [In a cardiovascular care unit.] RN Magazine, 35 (4), Apr 1972, ICU 1–3.

14 Rodman, T. and others The physiologic and pharmacologic basis of coronary care nursing. St. Louis: Mosby, 1971.

15 Rowlands, D. J. Coronary care. 1. The coronary care unit: its organization and the nurse. Nursing Times, 70, 3 Jan 1974, 10–13.

16 Royal College of Nursing. Professional Nursing Department Community coronary care. Report of Conference, London, 4th June 1971. Rcn, 1971.

17 Secor, J. Coronary care: a nursing specialty. New York: Appleton-Century-Crofts, 1971.

18 Taylor, P. M. Coronary care nurse. New Zealand Nursing Journal, 68 (8), Aug 1974, 20–22.

19 Towers, M. Pain in the chest. 2. Clinical presentation of coronary heart disease. Nursing Times, 71, 2 Jan 1975, 19–21.

20 Turner, R. and Ball, K. The nurses' role in preventing coronary artery disease. Nursing Times, 70, 20 Jun 1974, 949–951.

21 Wright, F. H. Nurses at work. Intensive coronary care nursing in a unit without resident medical staff. Australian Nurses' Journal, 2 (4), Oct 1972, 8, 10, 13.

k DRUG THERAPY

1 Allendorf, E. E. and Keegan, M. H. Teaching patients about nitroglycern. [A study of patients with angina to show their existing knowledge and possible benefit of teaching by nurses.] American Journal of Nursing, 75 (7), Jul 1975, 1168–1170.

2 Cooper, P. Drugs for cardiac complaints. Midwife and Health Visitor, 10 (8), Aug 1974, 241; (12), Dec 1974, 383.

3 Deberry, P. and others Teaching cardiac patients to manage medications. American Journal of Nursing, 75 (12), Dec 1975, 2191–2193.

4 DiPalma, J. R. Drug therapy today. Drugs for hyperlipidemia. RN Magazine, 37 (3), Mar 1974, 55–56, 58, 60, 62.

5 Gettes, L. S. The electrophysiologic effect of antiarrhythmic drugs. RN Magazine, 36 (3), Mar 1973, ICU 1–2, 7; (4), Apr 1973, ICU 1–2, 7–8.

6 Gray, I. R. Drugs acting on the heart. Nursing Mirror, 137, 19 Oct 1973, 36–37.

7 Hopkins, S. J. New drugs for old. 1. Hypertension and cardiac failure. Nursing Times, 68, 6 Jul 1972, 841–843.

8 Keegan, L. G. Dispelling the myth of the apical-radial pulse in digitalis therapy. American Journal of Nursing, 72 (8), Aug 1972, 1434–1445.

9 Lancour, J. M. The nurse and cardiovascular drug therapy. Cardiovascular Nursing, 9 (4), Jul/Aug 1973, 19–22.

10 Levitt, B. and others The clinical pharmacology of antiarrhythmic drugs. Cardiovascular Nursing, 10 (5), Sep/Oct 1974, 23–26; (6), Nov/Dec 1974, 27–31.

11 Rasmussen, S. The pharmacology and clinical use of digitalis. Cardiovascular Nursing, 11 (1), Jan/Feb 1975, 23–28.

12 Rodman, M. J. Drug therapy today. Drugs used in cardiovascular disease. 1. Managing cardiac emergencies. RN Magazine, 36 (3), Mar 1973, 71–72, 75–78, 80, 82.

13 Rodman, M. J. Drug therapy today. Drugs used in cardiovascular disease. 3. Treating edema. RN Magazine, 36 (5), May 1973, 55–56, 58, 60, 62, 64–65.

14 Rowlands, D. J. Coronary care. 9. Drug treatment. Nursing Times, 70, 28 Feb 1974, 306–309.

15 Shapiro, R. M. Anticoagulant therapy [in the treatment of thromboembolic disease]. American Journal of Nursing, 74 (3), Mar 1974, 439–443.

16 Sleet, R. A. Drugs used for cardiac disease in domiciliary practice. District Nursing, 14 (8), Nov 1971, 168–169.

17 Smith, S. E. Drugs and the heart. Nursing Times, 68, 16 Mar 1972, 317–318.

18 Smith, S. E. How drugs act. 15. Drugs and the heart. Nursing Times, 71, 2 Oct 1975, 1585–1586.

19 Spencer, R. Problems of drug therapy in congestive heart failure. RN Magazine, 35 (8), Aug 1972, 46–49.

20 Winslow, E. H. Digitalis. American Journal of Nursing, 74 (6), Jun 1974, 1062–1065.

l MYOCARDIAL INFARCTION

1 Bowman, G. S. Myocardial infarction. Results of an experiment – a study in mobilizing patients. Nursing Times, 70, 16 May 1974, 746–747; 23 May 1974, 793–794.

2 Boylan, A. An approach to nursing. 2. Meeting the patient's needs. [An example of the system, considering the theoretical case of a patient with myocardial infarction.] Nursing Times, 70, 21 Nov 1974, 1817–1818.

3 Boyle, D. Early discharge in acute myocardial infarction. Nursing Mirror, 140, 17 Apr 1975, 63–64.

4 Bragg, T. L. Psychological response to myocardial infarction. Nursing Forum, 14 (4), 1975, 383–395.

5 Bunke, B. Respiratory function after acute myocardial infarction: implications for nursing. Cardio-Vascular Nursing, 9 (3), May/Jun 1973, 13–18.

6 Cambier, D. M. Rehabilitation after a myocardial infarction. Queen's Nursing Journal, 16 (11), Feb 1974, 259–261.

7 Clark, J. M. Nursing care study. Myocardial infarction. Nursing Times, 71, 23 Oct 1975, 1699–1701.

8 Cross, S. Nursing care study. Myocardial infarction with cerebral embolus. Nursing Mirror, 141, 23 Oct 1975, 55–57.

9 Davies, I. J. T. Coronary thrombosis and myocardial infarction. District Nursing, 14 (31, Jun 1971, 46–48.

10 Deal, J. CPR and the ABCs. Diagnosis and treatment of the 'sudden death' patient. Bedside Nurse, 4 (3), Mar 1971, 11–17.

11 Felmers, M. C. O. and Dunning, A. I. IM lidocaine injections for myocardial infarction. RN Magazine, 38 (7), Jul 1975, ICU 6–7.

12 Gibson, T. C. A reappraisal of fever in acute MI. RN Magazine, 38 (5), May 1975, ICU 3–4, 6, 11.

13 Haslam, R. H. A. and Jameson, H. D. When cardiac standstill resembles epileptic attacks. RN Magazine, 36, Oct 1973, ICU 8, 12, 16.

14 Heng, F. W. Acute myocardial infarction and its nursing management. Nursing Journal of Singapore, 13 (2), Nov 1973, 83–87.

15 Hochberg, H. M. Effects of electrical current on heart rhythm. American Journal of Nursing, 71 (7), Jul 1971, 1390–1394.

16 Hockenberger, J. M. and Rubin, M. B. Cyclic occurrence of premature ventricular contractions in acute myocardial infarction patients: a pilot study. Nursing Research, 23 (6), Nov/Dec 1974, 489–491.

17 Holt, P. M. Nursing care study. Myocardial infarction. Nursing Times, 70, 13 Jun 1974, 908–910.

18 Keen, L. Current nursing management of myocardial infarction as practiced at Johannesburg Hospital. S. A. Nursing Journal, 52 (12), Dec 1975, 5–6, 8–9.

19 Leach, R. A. Nursing care study. Coronary thrombosis. Nursing Mirror, 136, 26 Jan 1973, 39–40.

20 Morgan, S. Nursing care study. Myocardial infarction followed by cardiac arrest. Nursing Times, 69, 26 Jul 1973, 955–957.

21 Nursing Mirror Computerized medicine in America. [Myocardial Infarction Research Units.] Nursing Mirror, 132, 21 May 1971, 10–12.

22 Nursing Times Measuring myocardial infarction. [Radiological scanning.] Nursing Times, 70, 26 Sep 1974, 1498.

23 Nursing Times Myocardial infarcts [and the optimum time of best rest afterwards]. Nursing Times, 70, 7 Feb 1974, 183.

24 Pentecost, B. L. Acute coronary care in the home. [Myocardial infarction.] Nursing Mirror, 141, 11 Dec 1975, 63–64.

25 Robinson, I. Myocardial infarction. Nursing Times, 68, 16 Nov 1972, 1442–1445.

26 Rowlands, D. J. Coronary care. 7. Complications following myocardial infarction. Nursing Times, 70, 14 Feb 1974, 226–229.

27 Rowlands, D. J. Coronary care. 8. Myocardial infarction (cont.) Cardiac arrest. Nursing Times, 70, 21 Feb 1974, 266–269.

28 Royal College of Nursing Coronary thrombosis. Nursing Times, 67, 17 Jun 1971, 744.

29 Smallbone, D. F. Coronary thrombosis. Occupational Health, 23 (8), Aug 1971, 263–268.

30 Smith, A. M. and others Serum enzymes in myocardial infarction. American Journal of Nursing, 73 (2), Feb 1973, 277–279.

31 Tyzenhouse, P. S. Myocardial infarction and its effect on the family. American Journal of Nursing, 73 (6), Jun 1973, 1012–1013.

32 Wenger, N. K. and Mount, F. An educational algorithm for myocardial infarction. [Patient education.] Cardiovascular Nursing, 10 (3), May/Jun 1974, 11–15.

33 Wild, J. B. Emergency care of ventricular standstill. Nursing Times, 67, 17 Jun 1971, 734–735.

34 Wishart, J. Fat embolism. Nursing Times, 67, 16 Sep 1971, 1140–1141.

m PACEMAKERS

1 Bain, B. Pacemakers and the people who need them. American Journal of Nursing, 71 (8), Aug 1971, 1582–1585.

2 Barstow, R. E. Nursing care of patients with pacemakers. Cardio Vascular Nursing, 8 (2), Mar/Apr 1972, 7–10.

3 Bryant, R. B. and Waddy, J. L. The pacemaker patient and his management. Australian Nurses' Journal, 4 (3), Sep 1974, 29–32, 35.

4 Deal, J. Battery operated. Bedside Nurse, 5 (11), Nov 1972, 12–17.

5 Escher, D. J. W. Medical aspects of artificial pacing of the heart. Cardio Vascular Nursing, 8 (1), Jan/Feb 1972, 1–5.

6 Fan, L. F. The artificial pace maker. Hong Kong Nursing Journal, 11, Nov 1971, 62–65.

7 Geddes, J. S. Pacemakers keep some people ticking. Nursing Times, 68, 6 Jan 1972, 5–8.

8 Germain, C. P. Helping your patient with an implanted pacemaker. RN Magazine, 37 (8), Aug 1974, 30–35.

9 Kos, P. and Culbert, P. Teaching patients about pacemakers. American Journal of Nursing, 71 (3), Mar 1971, 523–527.

10 Nursing Mirror Pacemakers checked by phone. Nursing Mirror, 133, 2 Jul 1971, 10.

11 Roberts, G. Artificial cardiac pacing – the vital stimulus. Nursing Times, 67, 28 Oct 1971, 1336–1338.

12 Shilling, E. Pacemaker evaluation clinic. American Journal of Nursing, 73 (10), Oct 1973, 1710–1714.

13 Siggers, D. C. The implanted cardiac pacemaker. Nursing Times, 68, 23 Mar 1972, 335–337.

14 Sowton, E. and others Ten-year survey of treatment with implanted cardiac pacemaker. British Medical Journal, 3, 20 Jul 1974, 155–159.

15 United States. National Institutes of Health Nursing care of patients with internal or external pacemakers. Washington: US Department of Health, Education and Welfare, 1971.

16 Williams, C. D. The CCU nurse has a pacemaker. [Nurse working in a CCU has pacemaker fitted and teaches patients from own experience.] American Journal of Nursing, 72 (5), May 1972, 900–902.

17 Winslow, E. H. and Marino, L. B. Temporary cardiac pacemakers. American Journal of Nursing, 75 (4), Apr 1975, 586–591.

n PSYCHOLOGICAL ASPECTS

1 Baxter, S. Psychological problems of intensive care. 2. [Patients in coronary care units. Reprinted from British Journal of Hospital Medicine.] Nursing Times, 71, 9 Jan 1975, 63–65.

2 Cassem, N. H. What is behind our masks? [Sources of stress and conflict to nurses working in the CCU.] AORN Journal, 20 (1), Jul 1974, 79, 81–82, 84, 86, 88, 91–92.

3 Cassem, N. H. and Hackett, T. P. Psychiatric consultation in a CCU. RN Magazine, 36 (7), Jul 1973, ICU 1, 4–5.

4 Cassem, N. H. and Hackett, T. P. Sources of tension for the CCU Nurse. American Journal of Nursing, 72 (8), Aug 1972, 1426–1430.

5 Davis, M. Z. Socioemotional component of coronary care. American Journal of Nursing, 72 (4), Apr 1972, 705–709.

6 Gentry, W. D. and Williams, R. B., joint editors Psychological aspects of myocardial infarction and coronary care. St. Louis: Mosby, 1975.

7 Hutchinson, S. Some psychological aspects of CCU nursing. [Psychological care of an anxious patient and his relatives.] RN Magazine, 36 (6), Jun 1973, ICU 1, 4, 9.

8 Lee, R. E. and Ball, P. A. Some thoughts on the psychology of the coronary care unit patient. American Journal of Nursing, 75 (9), Sep 1975, 1498–1501.

9 Royle, J. Coronary patients and their families receive incomplete care. [Nurses should identify and meet their learning needs at all stages of their illness and recovery.] Canadian Nurse, 69 (2), Feb 1973, 21–25.

10 Sczekalla, R. M. Stress reactions of CCU patients to resuscitation procedures on other patients. Nursing Research, 22 (1), Jan/Feb 1973, 65–69.

11 Trimble, M. R. Psychological needs of coronary patients. Nursing Times, 70, 19 Sep 1974, 1464–1465.

12 Twerski, A. J. Psychological considerations on the coronary care unit. Cardio-Vascular Nursing, 7 (2), Mar/Apr 1971, 65–68.

o RESUSCITATION

1 Alter, J. CPR training for everyone? At this hospital, yes! [Inservice program in cardiopulmonary resuscitation.] RN Magazine, 35 (8), Aug 1972, 50–52.

2 American Heart Association Cardiopulmonary resuscitation in basic life support for unwitnessed cardiac arrest. New York: The Association, 1974.

3 American Journal of Nursing Advanced life support. [Special equipment and drugs used in prevention of cardiopulmonary arrest.] American Journal of Nursing, 75 (2), Feb 1975, 242–247.

4 Brown, J. Defibrillation by nursing staff in general medical wards. Nursing Times, 7, 2 Oct 1975, 1572–1573.

5 Deal, J. CPR and the ABCs. Diagnosis and treatment of the 'Sudden Death' patient. Bedside Nurse, (4). Feb 1971, 17–21; (3), Mar 1971, 11–17.

6 Gilston, A. Cardiac arrest. Nursing Times, 67, 13 May 1971, 570–572.

7 Gilston, A. and Resnekov, L. Cardio-respiratory resuscitation. Heinemann Medical, 1971.

8 Palen, C. S. The passage. [A nurse's experience of resuscitation after cardiac arrest which failed.] American Journal of Nursing, 75 (11), Nov 1975, 2004–2005.

9 Pearce, M. Management of cardiac arrest. Nursing Mirror, 133, 6 Aug 1971, 25–28.

10 Poulter, R. R. RP board [for cardiac resuscitation]. Nursing Mirror, 133, 3 Sep 1971, 21.

11 Robinson, J. E. Cardiac arrest and the nurse's duties. Nursing Mirror, 136, 23 Feb 1973, 30–32.

12 Ungvarski, P. J. CPR current practice revised. [Guidelines for cardio pulmonary resuscitation and emergency cardiac care.] American Journal of Nursing, 75 (2), Feb 1975, 236–241.

13 Wilson, P. and Aarvold, J. A. The organization and operational nursing management of cardiac arrest. International Journal of Nursing Studies, 12 (1), Mar 1975, 23–32.

14 Wreford, B. M. Cardiac resuscitation: a new method. Operational Health, 23 (8), Aug 1971, 269–272.

p REHABILITATION

1 Barry, E.M. and others Hospital program for cardiac rehabilitation. American Journal of Nursing, 72 (12), Dec 1972, 2174–2177.

2 Bowar-Ferres, S. Returning to work – another stage of recovery for the MI patient. [Role of the industrial nurse in rehabilitation after myocardial infarction.] Occupational Health Nursing, 23 (11), Nov 1975, 18–25.

3 Borgman, M. F. Coronary rehabilitation – a comprehensive design. International Journal of Nursing Studies, 12 (1), Mar 1975, 13–21.

4 Cay, E. L. and others Psychological influences determining return to work after a coronary thrombosis. Rehabilitation, 81, Apr/Jun 1972, 27–34.

5 Gaskell, D. Physiotherapy [for cardio-thoracic patients.] Nursing Mirror, 141, 7 Aug 1975, 62–65.

6 Germain, C. P. Exercise makes the heart grow stronger. American Journal of Nursing, 72 (12), Dec 1972, 2169–2173.

7 Groden, B. M. Helping a post-coronary patient to manage his future. Health Magazine, 10 (2), Jun 1973, 32–33.

8 Groden, B. M. and Cheyne, A. I. Rehabilitation after cardiac illness. British Medical Journal, 2, 17 Jun 1972, 700–703.

9 Houser, D. Outside the coronary care unit. [Rehabilitation program for cardiac patients.] Nursing Forum, 12 (1), 1973, 96–107.

10 Lawson, B. Easing the sexual fears of the cardiac patient. RN Magazine, 37 (4), Apr 1974, ICU 1–2, 5.

11 Marcus, R. 19 steps to cardiac rehabilitation. RN Magazine, 38 (2), Feb 1975, ICU 1, 2.

12 Murray, A. Cardiac survival and rehabilitation. Physiotherapy, 59 (12), Dec 1973, 383–385.

13 Nixon, P. G. F. Recovery from coronary illness. Rehabilitation, 81, Apr/Jun 1972, 23–25.

14 RN Magazine The cardiac team: smoothing the recovery process. [Work of a cardiac rehabilitation team.] RN Magazine, 38 (7), Jul 1975, ICU 1, 2.

15 Royal College of Physicians and British Cardiac Society Cardiac rehabilitation 1975. Summary of the report of a joint working party. [Editorial comment 394–395.] British Medical Journal, 3, 16 Aug 1975, 417–419.

16 Semple, T. The after care of heart attacks. Rehabilitation, 81, Apr/Jun 1972, 21–23.

17 Smallbone, D. After-care and rehabilitation, following coronary thrombosis. Occupational Health, 23 (10), Oct 1971, 321–324.

18 Stijns, H. J. and others Physical rehabilitation in hospital and at home for patients after an acute myocardial infarction. Rehabilitation, 94, Jul/Sep 1975, 31–36.

85 COMMUNICABLE DISEASES

a GENERAL

1 Anderson, T. Whose responsibility? [Control of infectious diseases.] Public Health, 85 (3), Mar 1971, 99–102.

2 Brown, G. L. Infectious diseases. 'Q' fever. Nursing Mirror, 141, 16 Oct 1975, 46–47.

3 Davies, J. W. and Jessamine, G. Histoplasmosis. Canadian Nurse, 71 (8), Aug 1975, 38–40.

4 Easton, H. G. Infectious-disease units in the future hospital service. Lancet, 1, 16 Jun 1973, 1373–1376.

5 Ferrer, H. P. Epidemiology. Health and Social Service Journal, 83, 17 Mar 1973, 593, 595.

6 Ghosh, S. K. Typhoid fever in present day Britain. Public Health, 88 (2), Jan 1974, 71–78.

7 Goodman, M. The changing pattern of measles. Community Medicine, 126 (24), 10 Dec 1971, 333–336.

8 Haider, S. Infectious diseases. 1. Sore throats. Nursing Mirror, 137, 12 Oct 1973, Supp. 1–8.

9 Haider, S. Infectious diseases. 2. Rashes. Nursing Mirror, 137, 19 Oct 1973, Supp. 1–8.

10 Hime, J. M. Patterns of some diseases transmissible from animals to man – a review. Community Health, 6 (3), Nov/Dec 1974, 161–167.

11 Howard-Jones, N. The end of an epoch. [International efforts to control the spread of infectious diseases.] World Health, Jul 1971, 27–32.

12 Hughes, E. M. A patient with gas gangrene. Nursing Times, 69, 15 Feb 1973, 204.

13 James, D. G. Sarcoidosis. 1. Management of Sarcoidosis. 2. Nursing Times, 68, 13 Jan 1972, 56–59; 20 Jan 1972, 77–79.

14 James, D. G. Sarcoidosis has many faces. Nursing Mirror, 136, 15 Jun 1973, 30–32.

15 Jamieson, W. M. Infectious diseases. Whooping-cough. Nursing Mirror, 141, 13 Nov 1975, 63–65.

16 Laugier, G. V. The control and eradication of animal disease communicable to man. Royal Society of Health Journal, 92 (6), Dec 1972, 299–302.

17 Maudsley, R. H. Gas gangrene and its management. Nursing Times, 69, 15 Feb 1973, 201–203.

18 Millar, E. L. M. Poliomyelitis epidemiology and control. Public Health, 85 (3), Mar 1971, 103–106.

19 Morton, G. The pandemic influenza of 1918. Canadian Nurse, 69, Dec 1973, 25–27.

20 Nursing Times More about gangrenes. Nursing Times, 69, 15 Feb 1973, 205.

21 Nye, F. J. Infectious diseases. Enteric fever, Salmonella and food poisoning. Nursing Mirror, 141, 30 Oct 1975, 58–59.

22 Parry, H. E. Pets and parasites. Nursing Mirror, 134, 21 Jan 1972, 20–24.

23 Parry, W. H. Communicable diseases: an epidemiological approach. 2nd ed. English Universities Press, 1973. (Modern nursing series.)

24 Rosenhouse, L. Can we forget about quarantine? Nursing Care, 6 (12), Dec 1973, 25–28.

25 Rowland, H. A. K. Imported diseases. Nursing Mirror, 134, 16 Jun 1972, 45–47.

26 Smith, H. Nursing of infectious diseases. (NM Conference lecture.) Nursing Mirror, 138, 14 Jun 1974, 65–66.

27 Van Zwanenberg, D. Diphtheria. Nursing Times, 67, 10 Jun 1971, 705–706.

28 Williams, E. Brucellosis in Britain. Nursing Mirror, 134, 18/25 Feb 1972, 39–41.

29 Williams, E. Infectious diseases. Brucellosis. Nursing Mirror, 141, 25 Dec 1975, 45–47.

30 Williams, R. F. Outbreaks of infection and their management. Nursing Times, 67, 27 May 1971, 637.

31 Williamson, F. Man against insect – the fight to control disease. [The work of Ronald Rose and Giovanni Grassi.] Nursing Times, 70, 18 Jul 1974, 1100–1103.

32 Williamson, F. Man against insect. 3. Walter Reed v. yellow fever. Nursing Times, 70, 1 Aug 1974, 1202–1203.

33 Williamson, F. Microbes. I. Antony Leewenhoek – inventor of the microscope. Nursing Times, 69, 15 Nov 1973, 1512–1513.

34 Williamson, F. Microbes. 2. Lazaro Spallanzani: disproving spontaneous life. Nursing Times, 69, 22 Nov 1973, 1576–1577.

35 Wright, A. E. Nursing and the laboratory aspects of immunity. Nursing Times, 69, 20 Sep 1973, 1224–1225.

b IMMUNIZATION AND VACCINATION

1 Baker, B. H. Immunity in action. Nursing Care, 7 (10), Oct 1974, 16–20.

2 British Medical Journal Vaccination against whooping cough. [Leading article.] British Medical Journal, 3, 31 Aug 1974, 539–540.

3 British Medical Journal Whooping cough vaccination. British Medical Journal, 4, 25 Oct 1975, 186–187.

4 Bunting, F. W. Immunity against the infectious diseases. Nursing Times, 67, 27 May 1971, 634–636.

5 Central Health Services Council. Joint Committee on vaccination and immunization and Scottish Health Service Planning Council Whooping-cough vaccine. [Statement showing the hazard of whooping cough is greater than immunization.] British Medical Journal, 3, 20 Sep 1975, 687–688.

6 Community Health Issue on immunization. Community Health, 2 (5), Mar/Apr 1971, 225–249.

7 Cvjetanovic, B. Immunization programmes. WHO Chronicle, 27 (2), Feb 1973, 66–69.

8 Dick, G. Immunization in childhood. Nursing Mirror, 135, 14 Jul 1972, 28–30.

9 Dick, G. Immunization in childhood. Community Medicine, 127 (6), 11 Feb 1972, 73–77.

10 Essex-Cater, A. J. Programmes for protection. [The immunization agents routinely used in the UK and the ages at which they are normally administered to children.] Nursing Times, 69, 6 Dec 1973, 1667–1669.

11 Francis, B. J. Current concepts in immunization. American Journal of Nursing, 73 (4), Apr 1973, 646–649.

12 Frenkiel, A. L. Vaccination and immunization: a task for the primary care team. Queen's Nursing Journal, 16 (4), Jul 1973, 89–92.

13 Griffith, A. H. A fresh look at bacterial vaccines. Public Health, 87 (1/2), Nov 1972/Jan 1973, 17–23.

14 Haider, S. Health protection for travellers. Nursing Mirror, 138, 24 May 1974, 75–76.

15 Hutchinson, A. Diseases subject to the International Health Regulations. Royal Society of Health Journal, 94 (3), Jun 1974, 107–109, 113.

16 Iduna To vaccinate or not to vaccinate? [The problem of neurological complications and the position of the health visitor as regards immunization.] Health Visitor, 47 (11), Nov 1974, 320.

17 Lange, M. Relief work in Kurdistan. [Vaccination of refugees.] Nursing Mirror, 141, 31 Jul 1975, 64–66.

18 Nursing Times A vaccine against mental retardation [to prevent cytomegalovirus infection in utero]. Nursing Times, 70, 7 Feb 1974, 197.

19 Rao, N. M. Health education in immunization of children. Nursing Journal of India, 65 (11), Nov 1974, 291, 293–294.

20 Smith, S. E. How drugs act. 25. Biological drugs and vaccines. Nursing Times, 71, 11 Dec 1975, 1992–1993.

21 Stuart-Harris, Sir C. Human virus diseases. 1. Success and failure. Nursing Mirror, 133, 24 Dec 1971, 9–11.

22 Stuart-Harris, Sir C. Human virus diseases. 3. Chemotherapy. Nursing Mirror, 134, 7 Jan 1972, 27–29.

23 Stuart-Harris, Sir C. Human virus diseases. 4. Immunization. Nursing Mirror, 134, 14 Jan 1972, 33–35.

24 Stuart-Harris, Sir Human virus diseases. 5. Immunization. Nursing Mirror, 134, 21 Jan 1972, 31–33.

25 Taylor, D. Vaccination – the risks and the benefits. Health and Social Service Journal, 84, 9 Nov 1974, 2593–2594.

26 TeWinkle, M. B. Immunization and communicable diseases. Journal of Practical Nursing, 24 (3), Mar 1974, 22–25.

27 WHO Chronicle Immunization against whooping cough. WHO Chronicle, 29 (9), Sep 1975, 365–367.

28 WHO Chronicle Measles vaccination. WHO Chronicle, 27 (3), Mar 1973, 101–102.

c CHOLERA

1 Adeniyi, J. D. Cholera control: problems of beliefs and attitudes. International Journal of Health Education, 5 (4), 1972, 238–245.

2 Davies, J. W. Cholera epidemiology and control. Canadian Nurse, 70 (3), Mar 1974, 25–27.

3 Jegede, S. A. Cholera in Nigeria. Nursing Mirror, 133, 17 Sep 1971, 16–18.

4 Morris, R. J. Cholera: the social disease. New Society, 18, 8 Jul 1971, 52–56.

5 Shuck, W. H. An unwelcome guest. [An account of the cholera epidemic in the town of Sheffield in 1832.] Nursing Mirror, 132, 21 May 1971, 32–35.

d HEPATITIS

1 Allan, M. M. Nursing care study. Liver failure in a child with infective hepatitis. Nursing Times, 69, 13 Dec 1973, 1683–1684.

2 Antoneto, Sr. Infective hepatitis. Nursing Journal of India, 65 (9), Sep 1974, 249–250.

3 Barbara, M. Haemodialysis report: the hepatitis scourge. Australian Nurses' Journal, 2 (5), Nov 1972, 23–24.

4 British Medical Journal Decrease in the incidence of hepatitis in dialysis units associated with prevention programme. Public health laboratory service survey. British Medical Journal, 4, 28 Dec 1974, 751–754.

5 British Medical Journal Hepatitis contracted in the course of employment. British Medical Journal, 4, 4 Dec 1971, 632.

6 British Medical Journal Hepatitis hazard in regular haemodialysis. British Medical Journal, 4, 2 Dec 1972, 501–502.

7 British Medical Journal The several viruses of post-transfusion hepatitis. British Medical Journal, 3, 20 Sep 1975, 663.

8 Cossart, Y. E. Australia antigen and hepatitis. Public Health, 87 (1/2), Nov 1972/Jan 1973, 33–38.

9 Craske, J. and others An outbreak of hepatitis associated with intravenous injection of factor-VIII concentrate. Lancet, 2, 2 Aug 1975, 221–223.

10 Davison, A. M. and others Neuropathy associated with hepatitis in patients maintained on haemodialysis. British Medical Journal, 1, 12 Feb 1972, 409–411.

11 Dempster, G. Infection control. Protection from carriers of hepatitis B. [Safety precautions for staff dealing with hepatitis cases.] Dimensions in Health Service, 52 (12), Dec 1975, 27–29.

12 Department of Health and Social Security and others Advisory Group on Hepatitis and the Treatment of Chronic Renal Failure. Report. The Department, 1973.

13 Drug and Therapeutics Bulletin Hepatitis: preventing the spread of infection. Drug and Therapeutics Bulletin, 11 (5), 2 Mar 1973, 17–20.

14 Frye, C. Viral hepatitis – a risk to nurses. Canadian Nurse, 69 (7), Jul 1973, 33–36.

15 Hawe, B. J. and others Dialysis-associated hepatitis: prevention and control. British Medical Journal, 1, 6 March 1971, 540–543.

16 Heathcote, J. and Sherlock, S. Spread of acute type B hepatitis in London. Lancet, 1, 30 Jun 1973, 1468–1470.

17 Hurst, C. A. Treatment of renal disease. 3. Hepatitis. Nursing Times, 68, 21 Sep 1972, 1181.

18 Kaslow, R. A. and Zelliner, S. R. Infection in patients on maintenance haemodialysis. Lancet, 2, 15 Jul 1972, 117–118.

19 Lancet Australia antigen – the pace quickens. Lancet, 1, 13 Jan 1973, 85–86.

20 Lancet Hepatitis and the treatment of chronic renal failure. [Review of advisory group 1970–1972.] Lancet, 2, 15 Jul 1972, 122.

21 Lucas, C. R. Serum hepatitis. Historical aspects, relationship to Australia Antigen, present status in Victoria, prospects for vaccinal immunity. Australian Nurses' Journal, 2 (8), Feb 1973, 26–27, 43.

22 Lyne, N. M. and Jeffries, D. J. Management of patients with acute hepatitis and carriers of hepatitis B antigen (Australia antigen) in the operating theatre. NATNews, 11 (3), Apr 1974, 12–13.

23 MacConachie, E. Serum hepatitis with polyarteritis nodosa – a personal account. Nursing Times, 68, 24 Aug 1972, 1070–1072.

24 Nursing Times Hepatitis – the elusive viruses. [A short history of research.] Nursing Times, 70, 31 Oct 1974, 1704.

25 Oag, D. A realistic approah to the Rosenheim report. [A survey in seven hospitals to find out to what extent the recommendations of the Rosenheim report on hepatitis have been carried out and how effective they are.] Nursing Times, 70, 31 Oct 1974, 1691–1695.

26 Polakoff, S. A. and others Hepatitis in dialysis units in the United Kingdom. British Medical Journal, 3, 8 Jul 1972, 94–99.

27 Ross, C. A. C. Australia antigen and hepatitis in the West of Scotland (September 1970 – September 1971). Health Bulletin, 30 (2), Apr 1972, 120–122.

28 Rowland, A. J. The epidemiology of infectious hepatitis. Public Health, 87 1/2, Nov 1972/Jan 1973, 25–32.

29 Turner, G. C. A new look at infectious diseases. Hepatitis. British Medical Journal, 1, 24 Feb 1973, 476–479.

30 Warren, W. D. Australian antigen viewed as indicator of hazard of hepatitis transmission. Hospital Topics, 50 (12), Dec 1972, 47–48.

31 Weatherston, L. Outbreak of hepatitis in a renal transplantation unit. Nursing Times, 67, 4 Nov 1971, 1365–1367.

32 Zuckerman, A. J. Hepatitis B vaccine. Safety criteria and non-B infection. Lancet, 1, 26 Jun 1976, 1396–1397.

33 Zuckerman, A. J. Is hepatitis caused by viroids? Lancet, 1, 30 Jun 1973, 1486–1487.

e LEPROSY

1 Bechelli, L. Leprosy today. World Health, Oct 1971, 10–19.

2 Desikan, K. V. Immunology of leprosy. Nursing Journal of India, 65 (10), Oct 1974, 263–264, 281.

3 Fazalbhoy, Z. A. Need of health education programme for control of leprosy. Pakistan Nursing and Health Review, 4, 2, 1973, 17–20.

4 Gabrielle, Sister. Facts about leprosy. 1. Jamaican Nurse, 13 (2), Aug/Sep 1973, 8–10.

5 Gabrielle, Sister. The control and management of leprosy. 2. Jamaican Nurse, 13 (3), Dec 1973/Jan 1974, 35, 40.

6 Hasselblad, O. W. First instalment of a talk [on leprosy with particular reference to Jamaica]. Jamaican Nurse, 14 (3), Dec 1974, 12–14.

7 Hasselblad, O. W. Second instalment of a talk [on the causes and symptoms of leprosy.] Jamaican Nurse, 5 (1), May 1975, 26–27.

8 Johansen, H. Leprosy nursing in the 70's. Nursing Journal of India, 63 (1), Jan 1972, 5, 28.

9 Nursing Journal of India Issue on leprosy in India. Nursing Journal of India, 65 (1), Jan 1974, 11–22.

10 Nursing Mirror A symposium on leprosy. Nursing Mirror, 142, 4 Mar 1976, 47–61.

11 Roberts, K. L. Leprosy, old myths and new methods. Australian Nurses' Journal, 1 (10), Apr 1972, 31–32.

12 Spinelli, R. J. Hansen's disease. Wanted: more than just clinical nursing. [Leprosy.] Journal of Practical Nursing, 22 (12), Dec 1972, 20–21.

13 Thomas, B. J. Leprosy. An ancient scourge – a continuing problem. RN Magazine, 38 (3), Mar 1975, 47–48, 50–51, 53.

14 World Health Organization Isolation unnecessary – 25 facts about leprosy. Nursing Mirror, 138, 29 Mar 1974, 68.

f MALARIA

1 Bright, M. Can malaria be eradicated? World Medicine, 10 (20), 16 Jul 1975, 25, 27–28.

2 Bruce-Chwatt, L. J. and Abela-Hyzler, P. Malaria and its surveillance in the United Kingdom. Health Trends, 7 (1), Feb 1975, 18–23.

3 Bruce-Chwatt, L. J. Transmission of malaria. 75th anniversary of Ronald Ross's discovery. British Medical Journal, 3, 19 Aug 1972, 464–466.

4 Bruce-Chwatt, L. J. and others Malaria in the United Kingdom. British Medical Journal, 2, 29 Jun 1974, 707–711.

5 Glossop, J. M. Nursing care study. Malaria. Nursing Mirror, 135, 15 Dec 1972, 35–37.

6 Maegraith, B. G. and Devlin, M. Crises in malaria. Nursing Mirror, 139, 16 Aug 1974, 52–55.

7 Shute, P. G. and Maryon, M. Malaria in England past, present and future. Royal Society of Health Journal, 94 (1), Feb 1974, 23–29, 49.

8 Stephensen, C. Malaria: coming home with mobile Americans. RN Magazine, 38 (6), Jun 1975, 53–54, 56–60.

g RABIES

1 Joss, G. E. and Brooksby, J. B. International transport of animals: their welfare and the attendant threat to the UK. (a) Air transport. [Disease hazards with particular reference to rabies.] Royal Society of Health Journal, 95 (4), Aug 1975, 219.

2 Macrae, A. D. Rabies. British Medical Journal, 1, 10 Mar 1973, 604–606.

3 Scowen, P. Mad dogs and Englishmen: the background to the new Rabies Act. Nursing Mirror, 139, 26 Jul 1974, 39–40.

4 Stamford, P. Victory over rabies. A battle won in pediatrics. [Case study.] RN Magazine, 37, May 1974, 65 (9 pages).

5 West, G. Rabies in perspective. Nursing Mirror, 141, 17 Jul 1975, 40–42.

6 WHO Chronicle New prospects for rabies control. WHO Chronicle, 28 (1), Jan 1974, 16–24.

7 Wright, W. J. The menace of rabies. Nursing Times, 69, 1 Nov 1973, 1444–1445.

h RESPIRATORY TRACT INFECTIONS

1 Bradbrook, R. A. Mumps. [Clinical features, complications and treatment.] Nursing Times, 70, 12 Dec 1974, 1930–1931.

2 Brocklebank, J. T. Influenza – a virus infection in children. Nursing Mirror, 138, 29 Mar 1974, 74–75.

3 Carbary, L. J. The kissing disease: on the way: a successful vaccine for infectious mononucleosis. Nursing Care, 8 (1), Jan 1975, 22–24.

4 Cross, K. W. and Farmer, R. D. T. Influenza vaccine in the elderly. Community Health, 6, Jan/Feb 1975, 224–228.

5 Giesbrecht, E. Infectious mononucleosis – the kissing disease. Canadian Nurse, 68 (2), Feb 1972, 37–40.

6 Gordon, H. Flu vaccine – money well spent? [Survey among Wandsworth Borough Council staff.] Health and Social Service Journal, 83, 14 Apr 1973, 858–859.

7 Gray, J. A. Infectious diseases. Mumps. Nursing Mirror, 141, 27 Nov 1975, 50–52.

8 Gunn, A. D. G. Glandular fever. Nursing Times, 71, 23 Oct 1975, 1697–1698.

9 Hall, T. S. The fight against 'flu – the work of the common cold unit. [Reprinted from Chemist and Druggist.] Nursing Mirror, 136, 25 May 1973, 48–50.

10 Krushner, J. A. The control of influenza. Queen's Nursing Journal, 18 (6), Sep 1975, 162–163.

11 Miller, D. L. Influenza: current problems and future prospects. Nursing Mirror, 134, 3 Mar 1972, 29–30.

12 Occupational Health Winter's scourge. [Influenza.] Occupational Health, 27 (12), Dec 1975, 534–535.

13 Stuart-Harris, Sir C. Human virus diseases. 2. Colds, influenza, and enteroviral infection. Nursing Mirror, 133, 31 Dec 1971, 25–27.

14 Walker, D. D. Influenza immunization in industry. Occupational Medicine, 21 (3), Jul 1971, 87–92.

15 Williams, W. O. Influenza. [The influenza epidemic: its clinical pattern and management.] Queen's Nursing Journal, 17 (8), Nov 1974, 171–172.

16 Wright, W. J. Ornithosis. [Psittacosis and its effect on humans.] Nursing Mirror, 140, 20 Mar 1975, 81–82.

i RUBELLA

1 Dudgeon, J. A. Recent advances in rubella. Nursing Mirror, 136, 6 Apr 1973, 14–16.

2 Hatcher, J. Rubella during pregnancy. Midwives Chronicle, 85, Aug 1971, 278–279.

3 Hurley, R. Rubella in pregnancy. Midwife and Health Visitor, 10 (8), Aug 1974, 223, 225, 227, 229.

4 Hutchinson, D. N. and others Rubella vaccination of non-immune schoolgirls and young women. Community Medicine, 126 (17), 22 Oct 1971, 225–227.

5 Mais, H. J. Rubella vaccination and termination of pregnancy. Nursing Mirror, 136, 1 Jun 1973, 28–29.

6 Nursing Times Rubella protection – but how? Nursing Times, 67, 14 Jan 1971, 41–42.

7 Platt, A. M. Rubella vaccination in the puerperium. Midwife and Health Visitor, 8 (10), Oct 1972, 343–346.

8 Reid, W. M. Congenital rubella – one approach to prevention. Canadian Nurse, 67 (1), Jan 1971, 38–40.

9 Sutton, R. N. P. Rubella. Nursing Mirror, 141, 25 Sep 1975, 63–65.

10 Wellstead, A. J. The rubella problem. Nursing Mirror, 137, 21 Sep 1973, 34–35.

11 Yates, C. Rubella vaccination. [Association with congenital defects after rubella in pregnancy.] Occupational Health, 28 (3), Mar 1976, 141–146.

j SMALLPOX

1 Dick, G. Vaccination against smallpox. Midwife and Health Visitor, 8 (11), Nov 1972, 380–381.

2 Henderson, D. An end – and a beginning. The success of the Smallpox Eradication Campaign marks the point of departure for new efforts to combat other health problems which beset mankind. Nursing Journal of India, 66 (4), Apr 1975, 76–78.

3 International Nursing Review Goodbye to smallpox. International Nursing Review, 22 (2), Mar/Apr 1975, 54–57.

4 Kavalier, F. Spotting the smallpox. [How a case of smallpox in South London in February 1973 was dealt with.] Nursing Times, 69, 19 Apr 1973, 494.

5 Lancet Smallpox target zero? [WHO's efforts to eradicate smallpox.] Lancet, 4, 23 Feb 1974, 295–296.

6 March, D. C. The personnel problems of opening a smallpox hospital. [Ainsworth Smallpox Hospital, Lancashire.] Hospital and Health Services Review, 70 (11), Nov 1974, 389–392.

7 Nursing Mirror The smallpox contingency. [Procedures at Ainsworth Smallpox Hospital, Bury.] Nursing Mirror, 141, 27 Nov 1975, 41–42.

8 Nursing Mirror Victory over smallpox. [To commemorate World Health Day April 7 – mainly illustrations.] Nursing Mirror, 140, Apr 1975, 39–41.

9 Nursing Times Smallpox: end of an era. [News feature, mainly illustrations, to mark end of WHO campaign.] Nursing Times, 71, 3 Apr 1975, 522–523.

10 Parker, W. S. Smallpox control. Royal Society of Health Journal, 94 (1), Feb 1974, 21–22, 43.

11 Parry, W. H. Control of smallpox. Lancet, 1, 5 May 1973, 989–990.

12 Ramsay, A. M. The epidemiology and clinical features of smallpox. Public Health, 86 (2), 2 Jan 1972, 79–82.

13 Willard, N. India. Eradicating smallpox gently. World Health, Jun 1974, 20–25.

14 WHO Chronicle. Progress in smallpox eradication. WHO Chronicle, 28 (8), Aug 1974, 359–363.

15 World Health Issue devoted to smallpox. World Health, Oct 1972, 3–33.

16 World Health Issue on smallpox. World Health, Feb–Mar 1975, 3–47.

k TETANUS

1 Buganga, J. Nursing care study. Tetanus neonatorum. Nursing Times, 70, 4 Apr 1974, 504–505.

2 Oyediran, A. B. O. O. The control of tetanus in Nigeria. Nigerian Nurse, 4 (3), Jul/Sep 1972, 6–7, 9–10.

3 Watt, S. C. Nursing care study. Tetanus. Nursing Times, 71, 30 Jan 1975, 174–175.

4 Westlund, D. Tetanus: a case study. Canadian Nurse, 70 (7), Jul 1974, 17–21.

l TUBERCULOSIS

1 Alexander, S. and others Caring for the tuberculous patient. Journal of Practical Nursing, 21 (1), Jan 1971, 22–26; (2), Feb 1971, 22–26.

2 Aquinas, M. Tuberculosis today. Hong Kong Nursing Journal, 12, May 1972, 47–49.

3 British Thoracic and Tuberculosis Association Tuberculosis among immigrants related to length of residence in England and Wales. British Medical Journal, 3, 20 Sep 1975, 698–699.

4 Bruce, L. G. Tuberculosis – no place for complacency. Nursing Times, 71, 24 Apr 1975, 651–653.

5 Collins, T. F. B. The modern approach to tuberculosis. S. A. Nursing Journal, 38 (9), Sep 1971, 25–26, 28.

6 Da Silva, A. O. A. The role and function of NA PT in Nigeria. [National Association for the Prevention of Tuberculosis.] Nigerian Nurse, 5 (2), Apr/Jun 1973, 13–15, 16.

7 Ellis, D. A. Nursing care study. Military tuberculosis. Nursing Mirror, 139, 24 Oct 1974, 73–76.

8 Enright, T. The nurse and modern tuberculosis control. Australian Nurses' Journal, 2 (12), Jun 1973, 34.

9 Gardner, P. A. and others Tuberculosis and the immigrant in Blackburn. Public Health, 86 (4), May 1972, 189–197.

10 Gosselin, M. Tuberculosis: why cling to isolation practices? Journal of Practical Nursing, 22 (3), Mar 1972, 22–25.

11 Hanmer, G. A. Tuberculosis then and now. [Nursing care of patients in the late 1920's and early 1930's.] Midwife and Health Visitor, 10 (7), Jul 1974, 191–193; (8), Aug 1974, 233–236.

12 Hitze, K. L. Tuberculosis control: is modern knowledge being applied? WHO Chronicle, 26 (9), Sep 1972, 383–388.

13 Idowu, J. A. Controlling tuberculosis in Western Nigeria. Nigerian Nurse, 5 (2), Apr/Jun 1973, 6–7, 9–12.

14 Kaur, R. Nursing care study. Pulmonary tuberculosis complicated by constrictive pericarditis. Nursing Times, 70, 1 Aug 1974, 1186–1189.

15 Kelly, H. B. Patient population and treatment choices. Nursing Outlook, 19 (8), Aug 1971, 541–542.

16 Kenefick, T. C. Tuberculous ulceration of the mouth. [Case study of oral tuberculosis.] Nursing Times, 70, 26 Sep 1974, 1504–1505.

17 Leggat, P. O. Control of tuberculosis. Nursing Times, 70, 5 Sep 1974, 1385–1387.

18 Lotte, A. Tuberculosis in children: a cooperative study in Europe. WHO Chronicle, 26 (12), Dec 1972, 550–554.

19 Mercenier, P. Evaluation of tuberculosis control programmes. WHO Chronicle, 26 (12), Dec 1972, 547–549.

20 Murphy, P. Satellite clinics for tuberculosis care. Nursing Outlook, 20 (3), Mar 1972, 186–187.

21 Mushlin, I. and Nayer, H. R. Big city approach to tuberculosis control. [New York.] American Journal of Nursing, 71 (12), Dec 1971, 2342–2345.

22 Nursing Journal of India Issue on tuberculosis including nursing care. Nursing Journal of India, 45 (2), Feb 1974, 41–56.

23 Orriss, H. D. Consumer's viewpoint: an experience of hospitalization. [Five months spent in a long-stay hospital with TB.] Social Work Today, 6, 17 Apr 1975, 44–45.

24 Riddle, P. R. Urinary tuberculosis. Nursing Times, 70, 19/26 Dec 1974, 1976–1978.

25 Robinson, A. M. Pulmonary TB: not quite a disease of the past. RN Magazine, 38 (2), Feb 1975, 77–80, 82.

26 Ross, J. D. Use of card system in community control of tuberculosis [in Edinburgh]. Community Health, 6 Jan/Feb 1975, 205–215.

27 Springett, V. H. Tuberculosis. Community Health, 7 (2), Oct 1975, 66–69.

28 Weg, J. G. Tuberculosis and the generation gap. American Journal of Nursing, 71 (3), Mar 1971, 495–500.

29 World Health Organization No beds for TB. Nursing Mirror, 137, 19 Oct 1973, 46–47.

30 WHO Chronicle Tuberculosis control: progress of the new strategy. WHO Chronicle, 29 (4), Apr 1975, 123–133.

31 Wright, M. G. Tuberculosis in the '70s. Canadian Nurse, 68 (6), Jun 1972, 27–29.

m SEXUALLY TRANSMITTED DISEASES

1 Acres, S. E. and Davies, J. W. Venereal disease problem in Canada. Canadian Nurse, 67 (7), Jul 1971, 24–27.

2 Ahern, C. 'I think I have VD'. [Venereal disease among young people.] Nursing Clinics of North America, 8 (1), Mar 1973, 77–90.

3 Allott, F. W. Sexually transmitted diseases. 2. Confidentiality: attitudes of patients. Nursing Times, 69, 17 May 1973, 633–635.

4 Archer, C. A. N. A history of venereal diseases. Community Health, 3 (6), May/Jun 1972, 273–276.

5 Baker, R. VD – the old enemy within.]The role of the nurse.] Nursing Care, 7 (8), Aug 1974, 16–17.

6 Barber, R. M. Education in and prevention of the venereal diseases. Health Visitor, 45 (2), Feb 1972, 37–39.

7 Bernfeld, W. K. Gonorrhoea. Nursing Times, 67, 1 Apr 1971, 382–383.

8 Bernfeld, W. K. Sexually transmitted diseases. Nursing Mirror, 135, 29 Dec 1972, 18–21.

9 Brookes, P. WHO's 1972 balance sheet. VD a world epidemic. Nursing Times, 69, 17 May 1973, 644.

10 Brown, M. A. Adolescents and VD. Nursing Outlook, 21 (2), Feb 1973, 99–103.

11 Brown, M. T. Trichomonal vaginitis. Nursing Mirror, 140, 27 Mar 1975, 60–62.

12 Brown, M. T. Trichomonal vaginitis. A common female complaint. Nursing Times, 169, 17 May 1973, 642–643.

13 Brown, W. J. Acquired syphilis. Drugs and blood tests. American Journal of Nursing, 71 (4), Apr 1971, 713–715.

14 Caldwell, J. G. Congenital syphilis: a nonvenereal disease. American Journal of Nursing, 71 (9), Sep 1971, 1768–1772.

15 Carbary, L. J. VD: US number one epidemic. Journal of Practical Nursing, 24 (6), Jun 1974, 20–23.

16 Csonka, G. W. Reiter's disease. Nursing Mirror, 136, 4 May 1973, 28–30.

17 Dicker, K. The unmentionable diseases. Nursing Times, 67, 21 Jan 1971, 94–95.

18 DiPalma, J. R. Drug therapy today. Keeping up with venereal disease. RN Magazine, 38 (1), Jan 1975, 59–60, 62, 64, 66.

19 Elliott, H. and Ryz, K. Venereal diseases: treatment and nursing. Baillière Tindall, 1972. (Patient care.)

20 Ferrari, H. The nurse and VD control. [Nurse's role in patient education and prevention.] Canadian Nurse, 67 (7), Jul 1971, 28–30.

21 Fluker, J. L. Sexually transmitted infection. Midwife and Health Visitor, 8 (8), Aug 1972, 275–278.

22 Gould, D. Venereal diseases. Education essential. World Health, Jun 1974, 28–31.

23 Harris, J. R. W. Sexually transmitted diseases. 4. Social aspects. Nursing Times, 69, 17 May 1973, 638–639.

24 Harris, M. Special clinic nursing. Queen's Nursing Journal, 17 (4), Jul 1974, 79–80.

25 International Journal of Health Education The sexually transmitted diseases: a challenge to health education. International Journal of Health Education, 18 (3), Jul/Sep 1975, supplement 1–16.

26 Jelinek, G. Gonorrhoea. Nursing Mirror, 137, 20 Jul 1973, 30–32.

27 Jelinek, G. Venereal and sexually transmitted diseases. Queen's Nursing Journal, 16 (8), Nov 1973, 181–182.

28 Lenz, P. E. Women, the unwitting carriers of gonorrhea. American Journal of Nursing, 71 (4), Apr 1971, 716–719.

29 London Borough of Hammersmith The X in sex: don't let the unknown factor result in the hazards of sexual infections. [Publicity campaign for teenagers and their parents.] Nursing Times, 67, 1 Apr 1971, 380–381.

30 McGrath, P. and Laliberte, E. B. Level of basic venereal disease knowledge among junior and senior high school nurses in Massachusetts. A survey. Nursing Research, 23 (1), Jan/Feb 1974, 31–37.

31 Marshall, J. Sexually transmitted diseases. Mother and Child, 44 (6), Nov/Dec 1972, 5–8.

32 Morton, R. S. Sexually transmitted diseases. 1. Clinical aspects. Nursing Times, 69, 17 May 1973, 630–633.

33 Morton, R. S. Venereal diseases. District Nursing, 14 (11), Feb 1972, 231–232.

34 Neeson, J. D. Herpes virus genitalis: a nursing perspective. Nursing Clinics of North America, 10 (3), Sep 1975, 599–607.

35 Oates, J. K. Sexually transmitted diseases. Nursing Times, 68, 6 Jul 1972, 832–834.

36 Parker, J. D. J. Herpes simplex of the genitals. Nursing Times, 71, 11 Dec 1975, 1975–1977.

37 Plumb, B. Sexually transmitted diseases. 5. The seamen's dispensary, Liverpool. The nurse's role. Nursing Times, 69, 17 May 1973, 639–641.

38 Schofield, M. VD and the young. New Society, 26, 18 Oct 1973, 135–137.

39 Shaw, W. E. Sexually transmitted diseases. 3. Nursing and nurse training in venereology. Nursing Times, 69, 17 May 1973, 635–638.

40 Walsh, F. A. VD – The LP/VN's role in prevention. Journal of Practical Nursing, 22 (1), Jan 1972, 18–21, 30.

41 Whyte, S. B. VD – the new danger. Nursing Mirror, 141, 28 Aug 1975, 41.

42 World Health Issue on sexually transmitted diseases. World Health, May 1975, 3–33.

43 World Health Organization Ignorance and indifference: 25 facts about venereal diseases. Nursing Mirror, 138, 19 Apr 1974, 59.

86 DERMATOLOGY

a GENERAL

1 Alsop, J. A. Necrobiosis lipoidica diabeticorum. Nursing Times, 67, 11 Feb 1971, 168–170.

2 Baker, H. Epidermal growth and renewal. Nursing Mirror, 139, 26 Sep 1974, 71–73.

3 Baker, H. Psoriasis. Nursing Mirror, 136, 8 Jun 1973, 16–19.

4 Brown, J. K. Dermatology, past and present. Queen's Nursing Journal, 17 (4), Jul 1974, 83–84.

5 Bunney, E. H. Control of plantar warts. Nursing Mirror, 136, 2 Feb 1973, 30–33.

6 Burton, J. L. Acne is good for you. Nursing Mirror, 136, 27 Apr 1973, 33–34.

7 Burton, J. L. Acne vulgaris. Occupational Health, 23 (7), Jul 1971, 227–232.

8 Carter, M. Nursing care study. How John learned to smile again. [Nursing care study of a 13 year old pemphigus vulgaris patient.] Nursing Times, 69, 11 Oct 1973, 1329–1330.

9 Champion, R. H. Urticaria. [Hives.] Nursing Mirror, 139, 23 Aug 1974, 55–56.

10 Cobb, J. Psychosomatic factors in skin disease. Nursing Mirror, 137, 3 Aug 1973, 26–29.

11 Cooper, P. Drugs for scalp disorders. Midwife, Health Visitor and Community Nurse, 11 (8), Aug 1975, 269.

12 Cooper, P. Progress in therapeutics. Drugs for superficial mycoses. Midwife, Health Visitor and Community Nurse, 11 (11), Nov 1975, 367.

13 Copeman, P. W. M. Ill effects of drug treatment on the skin. Nursing Mirror, 138, 12 Apr 1974, 51–54.

14 Cunliffe, W. J. Itching – mechanism, causes and treatment. Nursing Times, 68, 23 Mar 1972, 356–357.

15 Dave, V. K. Contact dermatitis. Nursing Times, 67, 29 Apr 1971, 504–506.

16 Ellis, A. Nursing care study. Pemphigus neonatorum. [Bullous impetigo.] Nursing Mirror, 136, 6 Apr 1973, 38–40.

17 Fry, P. R. Dermatology. Nursing Times, 70, 24 Jan 1974, 112–113.

18 Hanron, J. S. Directing your care to the lupus patient's needs. RN Magazine, 38 (5), May 1975, 46–49.

19 Harmon, V. M. and Steele, S. M. Nursing care of the skin: a developmental approach. New York: Appleton-Century-Croft, 1975.

20 Holt, S. B. Dermatoglyphics. Nursing Mirror, 137, 20 Jul 1973, 16–19.

21 Huckbody, E. Early foundations of dermatology. Nursing Times, 69, 21 Jun 1973, 803–805.

22 Ingram, J. T. Functional disorders of the skin. Nursing Times, 69, 25 Jan 1973, 116–118.

23 Ingram, J. T. Skin diseases common to animals and to man. Nursing Times, 69, 8 Feb 1973, 181.

24 Ingram, J. T. The magic of dermatology. 1. Acute and chronic infections of the skin. Impetigo, erysipelas, perionychia, tuberculosis, syphilis. Nursing Times, 69, 4 Jan 1973, 5–7.

25 Ingram, J. T. The magic of dermatology. 2. Itching. Nursing Times, 69, 11 Jan 1973, 54–55.

26 Ingram, J. T. The magic of dermatology. 3. Animal parasites. Nursing Times, 69, 18 Jan 1973, 86–87.

27 Ingram, J. T. The magic of dermatology. 5. Malignant diseases of the skin. Nursing Times, 69, 1 Feb 1973, 139–141.

28 Jaffe, G. and Cowley, V. Wearing tights: a clinical trial of pHisoHex in prevention and treatment of skin disorders resulting from occlusive clothing. Nursing Times, 68, 31 Aug 1972, 1098–1099.

29 Jenner, E. A. Nursing care study. Psoriasis: a threat to promotion. Nursing Times, 69, 5 Jul 1973, 856–858.

30 Keane, E. Nursing care study. Atopic eczema. Nursing Times, 71, 18 Dec 1975, 2013–2015.

31 Keenan, A. and Alexander, J. O'd. Dermatology. Heinemann Medical, 1971. (Modern practical nursing series no. 4.)

32 Kinmont, P. D. C. Pruritus. Nursing Mirror, 136, 11 May 1973, 34–37.

33 Knight, A. G. Candidiasis. Nursing Times, 71, 2 Oct 1975, 1579–1581.

34 Leider, M. Some principles of dermatologic nursing. RN Magazine, 35 (5), May 1972, 48–53.

35 Lyell, A. Toxic epidermal necrolysis. Nursing Mirror, 136, 12 Jan 1973, 42–45.

36 Michaelides, C. and Lyons, G. The effects of hair cosmetics [on the hair and scalp]. Queen's Nursing Journal, 17 (12), Mar 1975, 263–264.

37 Mitchell, D. M. Eczema. Nursing Mirror, 136, 2 Mar 1973, 37–40.

38 Munro-Ashman, D. The effect of cosmetics on the skin. Nursing Mirror, 140, 13 Mar 1975, 54–56.

39 Nursing Times Systems of life. 1. The skin. [Mainly diagrams.] Nursing Times, 71, 2 Jan 1975, [4 pages.]

40 Oates, J. K. Ulceration of the genitalia. Nursing Mirror, 136, 23 Mar 1973, 25–27.

41 Rice, A. K. Common skin infections in school children. American Journal of Nursing, 73 (11), Nov 1973, 1905–1909.

42 Roberts, S. L. Skin assessment for color and temperature. American Journal of Nursing, 75 (4), Apr 1975, 610–613.

43 Rodman, M. J. Drug therapy today. Systemic and topical drugs for psoriasis and acne. RN Magazine, 38 (4), Apr 1975, 63–70.

44 Rook, A. Alopecia in young women. Nursing Mirror, 133, 19 Nov 1971, 18–20.

45 Roxburgh, R. C. Infantile eczema. Nursing Times, 71, 24 Jul 1975, 1166–1167.

46 Sarkany, I. Coping with psoriasis. Nursing Mirror, 133, 30 Jul 1971, 28–30.

47 Sarkany, I. Detergents and hand eczema. Nursing Times, 67, 30 Sep 1971, 1211–1212.

48 Szur, L. Radiotherapy in benign skin disease. Nursing Times, 69, 25 Oct 1973, 1413–1415.

49 Thorne, N. Return to nursing. 15. Changes in dermatology. Nursing Mirror, 133, 3 Sep 1971, 30–35.

b INDUSTRIAL DERMATOLOGY

1 Engel, H. O. Industrial dermatitis. Nursing Times, 71, 11 Sep 1975, 1450–1453.

2 Holland, J. Conditions of the hand. Prescribed hand diseases. Occupational Health, 27 (7), Jul 1975, 286–292.

3 Holland, J. Dermatitis of the hand. Occupational Health, 27 (6), Jun 1975, 244–247.

4 Thomson, W. Occupation and the skin. Nursing Times, 68, 6 Jul 1972, 835–837; 13 Jul 1972, 873–875.

87 DIGESTIVE SYSTEM

a GENERAL AND DISORDERS (Includes endoscopy)

1 Altshuler, A. Esophageal varices in children. American Journal of Nursing, 72 (4), Apr 1972, 687–693.

2 Bewick, M. The pancreas. 1. Anatomy, physiology and investigation. Nursing Times, 69, 16 Aug 1973, 1052–1055.

3 Bewick, M. The pancreas. 2. Trauma, fistulae and pancreatitis. Nursing Times, 69, 23 Aug 1973, 1087–1090.

4 Bewick, M. The pancreas. 3. Cysts and tumours and diabetes. Nursing Times, 69, 30 Aug 1973, 1111–1115.

5 Bono, J. A. and others Fiberoptic endoscopy of the UGI [and of the colon]. RN Magazine, 38 (9), Sep 1975, OR 1, 4, 7.

6 Bullock, J. Refresher course. Dysphagia. Nursing Times, 71, 4 Dec 1975, 1928–1930.

7 Cherry, F. M. The Boerema Button. [Emergency procedure for patients with bleeding oesophageal varices.] Nursing Times, 71, 9 Oct 1975, 1615–1617.

8 Clark, M. L. Malabsorption. Nursing Mirror, 140, 26 Jun 1975, 48–50.

9 Corman, M. L. and others Cathartics. American Journal of Nursing, 75 (2), Feb 1975, 273–279.

10 Cotton, P. and others A new look inside the gut: fibre-optic endoscopy. Nursing Mirror, 136, 12 Jan 1973, 22–23.

11 Creamer, B. Adult coeliac disease. Nursing Mirror, 138, 14 Jun 1974, 47–49.

12 Edwards, D. A. W. Diagnosis of oesophageal disorders. Nursing Mirror, 136, 19 Jan 1973, 17–19.

13 Ellis-Brown, R. S. Oesophageal hiatus hernias. Nursing Mirror, 135, 21 Jul 1972, 17–20.

14 Gaffney T. W. and Campbell, R. P. Feeding techniques for dysphagic patients. American Journal of Nursing, 74 (12), Dec 1974, 2194–2195.

15 Griffin, K. M. and others Teaching the dysphagic patient to swallow: two rehabilitation specialists and a nurse explain the steps used. RN Magazine, 37 (9), Sep 1974, 60–63.

16 Harmon, M. L. and Waye, J. D. Fiber optics: photography in the stomach. RN Magazine, 34 (7), Jul 1971, 46–51.

17 Heimlich, H. J. Esophagoplasty with reversed gastric tube. RN Magazine, 35 (6), Jun 1972, OR 1, 4, 7, 9.

18 Joannides, S. C. Anatomical drawings. 2 and 3. Organs of the digestive system 1 and 2. Nursing Mirror, 71, 9 Oct 1975, 1620–1621; 71, 16 Oct 1975, 1659–1660.

19 Johnson, A. G. Gall-stone dyspepsia – a functional illness? Nursing Mirror, 141, 2 Oct 1975, 57–58.

20 Jones, J. and Stewart, J. S. Coeliac disease. Nursing Times, 69, 20 Sep 1973, 1213–1215.

21 Lee, F. I. Gastroscopy. Nursing Times, 69, 22 Nov 1973, 1567–1569.

22 Midgley, J. W. and Osterhage, R. A. Effect of nursing instruction and length of hospitalization on postoperative complications in cholecystectomy patients. Nursing Research, 22 (1), Jan/Feb 1975, 69–72.

23 Miller, J. Endoscopy review. AORN Journal, 16 (11), Nov 1972, 146–156.

24 Notman, E. M. Planning an endoscopy room. Nursing Times, 70, 6 Jun 1974, 886–889.

25 Pagliero, K. M. Oesophageal strictures and their management. Nursing Times, 69, 6 Dec 1973, 1641–1643.

26 Parbhoo, S. P. Ascites. Nursing Times, 71, 16 Oct 1975, 1651–1653.

27 Preinfalk, H. Nursing care of the patient undergoing biliary tract surgery. [Pre- and postoperative care.] Nursing Mirror, 141, 2 Oct 1975, 59–60.

28 Purewal, R. K. Nursing care study. Cholecystectomy. Nursing Times, 70, 19 Sep 1974, 1452–1455.

29 Pyle, B. Nursing care study. A baby with oesophageal atresea. Nursing Times, 69, 12 Jul 1973, 889–891.

30 Ritchie, H. D. Surgical jaundice. Nursing Mirror, 137, 12 Oct 1973, 54–56.

31 Ryall, R. The digestive system. Harmondsworth: Penguin Education, 1973. (Penguin library of nursing.)

32 Salmon, P. R. Fibre-optic endoscopy. Pitman, 1974.

33 Tinckler, L. Nasogastric tube management. Nursing Times, 69, 4 Jan 1973, 12–15.

34 Trace, A. Nursing care study. Pancreatic dermatosis. Nursing Times, 69, 27 Oct 1973, 1400–1402.

35 Trapnell, J. E. Acute pancreatitis. Nursing Mirror, 139, 19 Dec 1974, 52–54.

36 Wakeley, C. Gall-stone disease. Nursing Mirror, 137, 2 Nov 1973, 10–12.

37 Wallace, E. D. and Young, D. G. Oesophageal atresia and tracheo-oesophageal fistula. 1. Immediate repair. 2. Delayed repair. Nursing Mirror, 137, 26 Oct 1973, 22–24; 2 Nov 1973, 34–36.

b GASTROINTESTINAL DISORDERS

1 Askew, A. R. Appendicetomy. Nursing Times, 71, 2 Oct 1975, 1570–1571.

2 Barlow, D. Hiatus hernia. Nursing Mirror, 133, 31 Dec 1971, 9–13.

3 Bates, M. Hiatus hernia. Nursing Mirror, 141, 4, Sep 1975, 50–55.

4 Bouchier, I. A. D. Ulcerative colitis. Nursing Times, 67, 14 Jan 1971, 45–47.

5 British Medical Jouranl Any questions? Screening nursing staff after gastroenteritis. British Medical Journal, 3, 29 Sep 1973, 689.

6 Buchan, D. J. Mind-body relationships in gastrointestinal disease. Canadian Nurse, 67 (3), Mar 1971, 35–37.

7 Cartwright, R. Y. Commensal bacteria of the human gastrointestinal tract. Nursing Times, 70, 9 May 1974, 705–706.

8 Charlesworth, D. Acute abdomen in the elderly. Nursing Times, 69, 12 Apr 1973, 469–471.

9 Cherkofsky, N. and Buckley, D. M. Dx: ulcerative colitis. Nursing Care, 8 (1), Jan 1975, 11–14.

10 Cornell, S. A. and others Comparison of three bowel management programs during rehabilitation of spinal cord injured patients. Nursing Research, 22 (4), Jul/Aug 1973, 321–328.

11 Cotton, P. B. Diagnosis of epigastric problems. Nursing Times, 70, 14 Feb 1974, 232–235.

12 Cox, A. G. Bowel preparation [before surgery]. Nursing Times, 70, 4 Apr 1974, 502–503.

13 De Dombal, F. T. Early surgery for severe ulcerative colitis. Nursing Mirror, 133, 12 Nov 1971, 32–33.

14 De Dombal, F. T. Pregnancy and . . . ulcerative colitis. Nursing Mirror, 136, 11 May 1973, 11–14.

15 Devlin, B. Congenital abnormalities causing intestinal obstruction in adult patients. Nursing Mirror, 138, 10 May 1974, 76–79.

16 Donn, M. Theatre nursing care study. Massive bowel resection for acute ischaemic disease. Nursing Times, 71, 27 Feb 1975, 333–337.

17 Dorgu, R. Bowel function: disorders and management. Butterworths, 1971. (Nursing in depth series.)

18 Douglas, A. P. Diarrhoea. Nursing Times, 71, 18 Dec 1975, 2022–2023.

19 Duthie, H. L. The appendix. Nursing Times, 69, 7 Jun 1973, 723–725.

20 Earlam, R. Epigastric pain. Nursing Mirror, 136, 16 Mar 1973, 30–32.

21 Emmanuel, L. S. Basic surgery. 2. Techniques of hiatal hernia repair. RN Magazine, 37 (9), Sep 1974, OR 1–2, 6.

22 Fielding, J. F. Regional enteritis. (Crohn's disease.) Nursing Mirror, 137, 5 Oct 1973, 42–44.

23 Gilmore, O. J. A. Appendicitis diagnostic problems and errors. [Study of 444 patients in Reading district general hospitals.] Nursing Mirror, 141, 18 Dec 1975, 51–53.

24 Given, B. A. and Simmons, S. J. Nursing care of the patient with gastrointestinal disorders. St. Louis: Mosby, 1971. 2nd ed. 1975.

25 Gunning, A. J. Hiatus hernia in adults. Nursing Times, 67, 14 Oct 1971, 1280–1283.

26 Haider, S. Infectious diseases. 3. Acute infective gastro-enteritis in adults. Nursing Mirror, 137, 26 Oct 1973, 9–11.

27 Hudson, C. Intestinal disorders in pregnancy. Midwife and Health Visitor, 10 (12), Dec 1974, 378–381.

28 Jackson, B. Ulcerative colitis from an etiological perspective. American Journal of Nursing, 73 (2), Feb 1973, 258–261.

29 Keusch, G. Bacterial diarrheas. American Journal of Nursing, 73, (6), Jun 1973, 1028–1032.

30 Knight, R. Diarrhoeal illness among travellers. Nursing Times, 69, 14 Jun 1973, 769–770.

31 Knight, R. Intestinal parasitic infections in Britain. Nursing Mirror, 134, 19 May 1972, 33–34.

32 Lytle, W. J. Femoral hernia diagnosis and operation procedure. Nursing Times, 67, 7 Oct 1971, 1246–1247.

33 McCallum, D. I. Dermatological complications of Crohn's disease. Nursing Times, 68, 9 Mar 1972, 280–282.

34 Milton-Thompson, G. J. Constipation. Nursing Mirror, 132, 2 Apr 1971, 30–33.

35 Naish, J. M. Discomfort after food. Nursing Times, 71, 25 Dec 1975, 2060–2062.

36 Naish, J. M. Stagnation in the small intestine. [Stagnant loop syndrome.] Nursing Times, 70, 4 Jul 1974, 1033–1035.

37 Neely, J. Postoperative ileus. Nursing Mirror, 138, 10 May 1974, 82–84.

38 Priestley, J. W. A nurse's role in a gastro-enterology investigation unit. Nursing Times, 68, 13 Jan 1972, 47–49.

39 Testa, J. Preoperative evaluation of a patient with intestinal obstruction. AANA Journal, 43 (5), Oct 1975, 496–499.

40 Timbury, G. C. and Tate, M. Management of constipation in psychiatric patients. Nursing Times, 69, 16 Aug 1973, 1050–1051.

41 Watkinson, G. Ulcerative colitis. Nursing Mirror, 141, 24 Jul 1975, 50–53.

42 Wharton, B. A. Management of gastroenteritis at home. Health Visitor, 48 (4), Apr 1975, 110–111.

43 Willacke, J. Bowel sounds. American Journal of Nursing, 73 (12), Dec 1973, 2100–2101.

44 Williams, J. Crohn's disease. Nursing Times, 67, 8 Jul 1971, 822–824.

45 Williams, L. F. Jr. The acute abdomen. American Journal of Nursing, 71 (2), Feb 1971, 299–303.

46 Williamson, J. A comparative trial of a new laxative. [In patient survey carried out in a geriatric hospital.] Nursing Times, 71, 23 Oct 1975, 1705–1707.

47 Wright, I. Bowel function in hospital patients. Royal College of Nursing, 1974. (Rcn Study of nursing care project reports, series 1, no. 4.)

48 Wright, P. A. Diarrhoea. A specific treatment programme in Palestinian Refugee Camps. Nursing Times, 67, 29 Jul 1971, 915–918.

c COLON AND RECTUM

1 Aylett, S. Prolapse of the rectum. Nursing Mirror, 140, 19 Jun 1975, 50–52.

2 Belinksy, I. and others Colonofiberoscopy: technique in colon examination. American Journal of Nursing, 73 (2), Feb 1973, 306–308.

3 Bleasdale, A. Abdominoperineal resection of the rectum. Nursing Times, 68, 10 Feb 1972, 186–188.

4 Brooke, B. N. Management of acute colonic obstruction. Nursing Mirror, 137, 3 Aug 1973, 42–45.

5 Curtis, C. Colonoscopy: the nurse's role. American Journal of Nursing, 75 (3), Mar 1975, 430–432.

6 Eastwood, M. and Mitchell, W. D. Diverticular disease. Nursing Times, 71, 9 Jan 1975, 68.

7 Feit, H. L. The unmentionable rectum. Bedside Nurse, 5 (10), Oct 1972, 26–27.

8 Hawkins, C. Diverticular disease of the colon: a disease of civilization. Nursing Mirror, 135, 6 Oct 1972, 35–37.

9 Hunt, T. Colonic irrigation. Nursing Mirror, 139, 5 Jul 1974, 76–77.

10 Le Brun, H. I. Surgery of the rectum and colon. Nursing Times, 69, 14 Jun 1973, 758–762.

11 Painter, N. S. Diseases of the colon and diet. Nursing Mirror, 136, 29 Jun 1973, 26–29.

12 Painter, N. S. Diverticular disease of the colon and constipation and their relationship to our diet. Nursing Times, 68, 4 May 1972, 536–537; 11 May 1972, 564–565; 18 May 1972, 620–621.

13 Rogers, B. H. Colonoscopy: the OR nurse's function. AORN Journal, 19 (3), Mar 1974, 656–670.

14 Smith, S. E. Drug therapy, 1972–8. Drugs and the colon. Nursing Times, 68, 20 Jul 1972, 907–908.

15 Smith, S. E. How drugs act – 22. Drugs and the colon. Nursing Times, 71, 20 Nov 1975, 1860–1861.

16 Wastell, C. Fissure-in-ano. Nursing Times, 71, 13 Feb 1975, 258–259.

17 Wells, C. Rectal prolapse. Nursing Times, 67, 25 Mar 1971, 345–347.

18 Williams, C. B. Colonoscopy. [New diagnostic technique.] Nursing Times, 69, 25 Jan 1973, 108–110.

19 Wilson, A. and others Geriatric faecal incontinence: a drug trial conducted by nurses. [Stobhill General Hospital, Glasgow.] Nursing Mirror, 140, 17 Apr 1975, 50–52.

d LIVER DISEASE (Includes transplantation)

1 Bowman, G. S. Liver biopsy. Nursing Times, 68, 6 Jul 1972, 839–840.

2 Lancet Liver transplantation. Lancet, 2, 6 Jul 1974, 29–30.

3 Murray-Lyon, I. M. Transplantation of the liver. Nursing Times, 67, 1 Jul 1971, 798–799.

4 Watt, E. A. Nursing care study. Liver transplant. Nursing Times, 70, 28 Mar 1974, 466–467.

5 Williams, R. Liver transplantation at King's College Hospital, London. Physiotherapy, 57 (8), Aug 1971, 362–364.

e PEPTIC ULCER

1 Clark, C. G. Surgery for peptic ulcer. Nursing Times, 67, 29 Jul 1971, 928–930.

2 Clark, M. L. Medical treatment of peptic ulcer. Nursing Mirror, 139, 6 Sep 1974, 48–50.

3 Emmanuel, S. Basic surgery. 4. Surgery for peptic ulcer. RN Magazine, 38 (4), Apr 1975, OR 5, 9, 12.

4 Johnston, D. A. Duodenal ulcers. Surgical treatment of duodenal ulceration. Nursing Mirror, 136, 11 May 1973, 24–26.

5 Langman, M. J. S. Duodenal ulcers. Nursing Mirror, 136, 4 May 1973, 38–39.

6 Librach, I. M. Peptic ulcer: facts and figures. Nursing Mirror, 134, 16 Jun 1972, 23–24.

7 Wastell, C. Chronic duodenal ulcer – a continuing challenge. Nursing Mirror, 136, 12 Jan 1973, 37–41.

f CHILDREN'S DISEASES

1 Arneil, G. C. Dehydration in babies. Nursing Times, 68, 10 Aug 1972, 992–995.

2 Dickson, J. A. S. Hernias in children. Nursing Times, 69, 2 Aug 1973, 989–990.

3 Haider, S. Infectious diseases. 4. Infantile gastro-enteritis. Nursing Mirror, 137, 2 Nov 1973, 26–27.

4 Hammond, J. E. Risks that follow childhood vomiting. Nursing Mirror, 139, 19 Dec 1974, 50–51.

5 Kuzemko, J. A. Recurrent diarrhoea in children. Nursing Mirror, 141, 10 Jul 1975, 54–58.

6 Lewis, G. M. Vomiting in infancy. Nursing Times, 68, 13 Apr 1972, 435–439.

7 Martin, E. J. and Young, D. G. Nursing care study. A baby with extrinsic duodenal obstruction. Nursing Times, 69, 23 Aug 1973, 1081–1083.

8 Patterson, A. The management of an infant with Hirschsprung's disease. Nursing Times, 67, 30 Sep 1971, 1203–1206.

9 Pyle, B. Nursing care study. A baby with oesophageal atresea. Nursing Times, 69, 12 Jul 1973, 889–891.

10 Strang, R. Intussusception in infants. Nursing Times, 70, 7 Mar 1974, 348–349.

11 Taylor, M. L. and others Neonatal jaundice and phototherapy. Nursing Mirror, 135, 6 Oct 1972, 38–41.

12 Woodcock, S. C. Neonatal Hirschsprung's disease. Nursing Mirror, 135, 28 Jul 1972, 28–30.

g STOMA CARE: GENERAL

1 Ahnafield, A. Ileostomies and urinary ostomies: preoperative and postoperative care. Journal of Practical Nursing, 22 (3), Mar 1972, 30–34, 40–41.

2 American Journal of Nursing Ostomy care. New York: American Journal of Nursing Company, 1972.

3 Barwin, B. N. and others Ileostomy and pregnancy. British Journal of Clinical Practice, 28 (7), Jul 1974, 256–258.

4 Clarke, T. K. Other developments in ostomy care. [A new dressing – Stomahesive – and a new appliance – Translet Freedom.] Nursing Mirror, 136, 8 Jun 1973, 26–27.

5 Connors, M. Ostomy care: a personal approach. Appliances, skin care and irrigations by a nurse who is a successfully rehabilitated ostomate. American Journal of Nursing, 74 (8), Aug 1974, 1422–1425.

6 Cosper, B. Physiological colostomy. [A diet of a synthetically formulated product Vivonex for three months avoids the need for a colostomy.] American Journal of Nursing, 75 (11), Nov 1975, 2014–2015.

7 Devlin, H. B. Stoma care. A surgeon's viewpoint. Nursing Times, 70, 18 Apr 1974, 576–577.

8 Gibbs, G. E. and White, M. Stomal care. American Journal of Nursing, 72 (2), Feb 1972, 268–271.

9 Jagelman, D. G. and Reeves, K. Postoperative ileostomy management. Nursing Mirror, 136, 1 Jun 1973, 33–34.

10 Jeter, K. Urinary ostomy in childhood. Journal of Practical Nursing, 24 (12), Dec 1974, 30–32, 38.

11 Meyer, A. H. Efficient, economical management of ostomy appliances and supplies [by a central supply department]. Hospital Topics, 52 (5), May 1974, 10, 12–14.

12 Mundy, P. The 'ostomy' patient: stomal care. Australian Nurses' Journal, 4 (6), Dec/Jan 1975, 28, 33, 44.

13 Murray, B. S. The patient has an ileal conduit. Nursing Mirror, American Journal of Nursing, 71 (8), Aug 1971, 1560–1565.

14 Neyegon, M. E. Nursing care study. Transplantation of ureters and total cystectomy. Nursing Mirror, 136, 23 Feb 1973, 39–41.

15 Oates, G. D. and others Stoma care. Queensborough, Kent: Abbott Laboratories, 1973.

16 Philippart, A. I. and Eraklis, A. J. Transverse colostomy in the infant. RN Magazine, 35 (6), Jun 1972, OR 13, 15.

17 Schauder, M. R. and Jaffrey, I. S. Better management of fecal fistulas with stoma bags. RN Magazine, 37 (5), May 1974, 56–57, 59.

18 Schauder, M. R. Ostomy care: come irrigations. American Journal of Nursing, 74 (8), Aug 1974, 1424–1425.

19 Shapbell, N. J. and Sweigart, J. E. A urinary device for patients with problem stomas. Nursing Clinics of North America, 9 (2), Jun 1974, 383–386.

20 Tuffill, S. G. Urinary diversion. Nursing Mirror, 134, 14 Jan 1972, 17–22.

21 Wallace, D. M. Urinary diversion. Nursing Times, 67, 2 Dec 1971, 1502–1505.

22 Watt, R. C. Urinary diversion. American Journal of Nursing, 74 (10), Oct 1974, 1806–1811.

h STOMA CARE: NURSE AND PATIENT

1 Alexander, N. B. Towards independence with an ostomy. Queen's Nursing Journal, 16 (1), Feb 1974, 250–251, 253.

2 Baum, M. E. Everything you always wanted to know about an ostomy but were afraid to ask. Nursing Care, 7 (10), Oct 1974, 14–15.

3 Binder, D. P. Sex, courtship and the single ostomate. Los Angeles: United Ostomy Association, 1973.

4 Cressy, M. K. Pyschiatric nursing intervention with a colostomy patient: a case presentation. Perspectives in Psychiatric Care, 10 (2), Jun 1972, 69–71.

5 Curlee, F. and others Ostomy manual for nursing staff. Minnesota: Rochester Methodist Hospital, 1974.

6 Davis, F. Coping with a colostomy – the importance of the nurse. Nursing Times, 70, 18 Apr 1974, 580–582.

7 Dawson, A. M. A step forward in stoma care. [Stoma clinic at St. Bartholomew's Hospital.] Nursing Times, 67, 22 Apr 1971, 477–478.

8 Devlin, H. B. Colostomy care. From a lecture given at the London Nursing Exhibition Oct 25, 1974. [Includes a history of colostomy.] Nursing Mirror, 139, 7 Nov 1974, 60–65.

9 Devlin, H. B. and others The community and the colostomy patient. District Nursing, 13 (12), Mar 1971, 234–235.

10 Dominguez, B. C. and Perrin, J. C. S. Advocate for the crippled child. [Nurse 'stomatologist'.] American Journal of Nursing, 73 (10), Oct 1973, 1750–1751.

11 Dott, N. M. and Fraser, J. Personal points of view – colostomy after-care and the Stoma Clinic. Health Bulletin, 30 (2), Apr 1972, 162–165.

12 Finn, B. Training the stoma care nurse. Nursing Times, 70, 18 Apr 1974, 579.

13 Gallagher, A. M. Body image changes in the patient with a colostomy. Nursing Clinics of North America, 7 (4), Dec 1972, 669–676.

14 Gambrell, E. Sex and the male ostomate. Los Angeles: United Ostomy Association, 1973.

15 Goligher, J. C. and Pollard, M. The care of your colostomy. 2nd ed. Baillière Tindall, 1973.

16 Goodard, G. M. The patient with a colostomy. Nursing Mirror, 134, 31 Mar 1972, 43–44.

17 Gross, L. Ostomy care: a letter to parents. [Advice on how to help children adjust to ostomy surgery, extracted from the book 'Ileostomy: a Guide.'] American Journal of Nursing, 74 (8), Aug 1974, 1427–1428.

18 Gutowski, F. Ostomy procedure: nursing care before and after. [Includes pre-operative teaching.] American Journal of Nursing, 72 (2), Feb 1972, 262–267.

19 Hughes, E. S. R. and others All about an ileostomy, 4th ed. Sydney: Angus and Robertson, 1972.

20 Jackson, B. S. Colostomates: the mosaic of stress and implied care. [Results of an observation study of six colostomates during hospitalization.] Australian Nurses' Journal, 4 (10), May 1975, 24–27.

21 Lancet Stomal-therapy specialists. [The training of nurses.] Lancet, 1, 9 Feb 1974, 204.

22 Larson, D. Living comfortably with your ileostomy. Minneapolis: Sister Kenny Institute, 1973. (Rehabilitation publication no. 718).

23 Lennon, M. A second chance. [The Colostomy Welfare Group.] Nursing Times, 67, 22 Apr 1971, 482.

24 McEvoy, P. Nursing care study. An elderly patient with intestinal obstruction. [Adaptation to a colostomy.] Nursing Times, 70, 18 Apr 1974, 583–584.

25 Norris, C. and Gambrell, E. Sex, pregnancy and the female ostomate. Los Angeles: United Ostomy Association, 1972.

26 Nursing Times Nursing care study. Mr. Brown and Miss Smith. [Home treatment of a colostomy patient after discharge from hospital.] Nursing Times, 69, 29 Mar 1973, 399–400.

27 Nursing Times A slightly neglected area? [The work of a stoma adviser.] Nursing Times, 69, 25 Jan 1973, 126–127.

28 St. Bartholomew's Hospital. Stoma Therapy Department Care of the ileostomy. The Hospital, 1974.

29 Seales, J. Stoma care. [Project presented for a practical work instructors' course, giving four case studies.] Queen's Nursing Journal, 18 (1), Apr 1975, 19–20.

30 Saunders, H. B. Stoma care. Stoma care nurse – a new role. Nursing Times, 70, 18 Apr 1974, 578–579.

31 Saunders, B. The work of the nurse – stoma therapist. Nursing Times, 67, 22 Apr 1971, 478–481.

32 Spraggon, E. M. Urinary diversion stomas: a guide for patients and nurses. 2nd ed. Edinburgh: Churchill Livingstone, 1975.

33 Thornton, M. E. A chance for applied research. [Experiences of a nurse researching into stoma care.] Nursing Times, 71, 20 Feb 1975, 291–292.

88 EAR, NOSE, THROAT AND MOUTH

a GENERAL

1 Carbary, L. J. Tips on tonsillectomies. Nursing Care, 8 (7), Jul 1975, 12, 14.

2 Chadwick, D. L. Treatment of ENT conditions. Nursing Times, 70, 21 Mar 1974, 424–425.

3 Gates, N. Planning and staffing an ENT unit. Nursing Mirror, 140, 1 May 1975, 52–57.

4 Gibb, A. G. Antral puncture. Nursing Times, 67, 15 Jul 1971, 851–852.

5 Gibb, M. E. Eptistaxis. Nursing Times, 67, 8 Apr 1971, 403–405.

6 Harrison, D. F. N. Tonsillectomy. Care of the child undergoing tonsillectomy from pre-admittance preparation to postoperative care. Nursing Times, 71, 22 May 1975, 808–811.

7 Holden, H. Cryosurgery. [The use of cryosurgery in the treatment of various ENT conditions.] Nursing Mirror, 140, 6 Feb 1975, 50–52.

8 Leacey, D. Facilitating ear, nose and throat examination. Nursing Times, 70, 17 Oct 1974, 1608–1609.

9 Marshall, S. and Oxlade, Z. E. Ear, nose and throat nursing. 5th ed. Baillière Tindall, 1972. (Nurses' aids series.)

10 Mechner, F. and others Patient assessment: examination of the head and neck. [Including lymph glands and thyroid.] American Journal of Nursing, 75 (5), May 1975, P. 1. 1–24.

11 Pilgrim, M. C. and Sands, D. Reconstructive nasal surgery. [Including patient care.] American Journal of Nursing, 73 (3), Mar 1973, 451–456.

12 Robinson, D. 'Becoming a patient': mothers' ideas about tonsillectomy. Medical Officer, 125, 15 Jan 1971, 37–41.

13 Rotter, K. The ear, nose and throat for nurses. 3rd ed. Faber, 1972.

14 Shah, N. ENT emergencies. 1. Epistaxis. Nursing Mirror, 134, 10 Mar 1972, 28–30.

15 Shah, N. ENT emergencies. 2. Foreign bodies in ENT. Nursing Mirror, 134, 17 Mar 1972, 39–41.

16 Shah, N. ENT emergencies. 3. Facial paralysis. Nursing Mirror, 134, 24 Mar 1972, 44–45.

17 Shaheen, O. H. Disorders of the sinuses. Nursing Times, 69, 24 May 1973, 673–674.

18 Shaheen, O. H. Disorders of the sinuses. Nursing Mirror, 139, 19 Jul 1974, 51–52.

19 Skipp, E. J. E.N.T.: current practice. Queen's Nursing Journal, 17 (4), Jul 1974, 74–75, 82.

20 Sprung, E. The child and tonsillectomy: nursing care. Bedside Nurse, 4 (7), Jul 1971, 22–23.

21 Taub, S. A different way of seeing the larynx and nasopharynx. AORN Journal, 16 (12), Dec 1972, 50–53.

22 Watson, R. T. Chronic rhinitis. Nursing Times, 70, 19/26 Dec 1974, 1972–1975.

23 White, N. OR nursing in otomicrosurgery. AORN Journal, 22 (6), Dec 1975, 889–897.

24 Wood, B. S. B. Adenoids and tonsils in childhood. Nursing Mirror, 136, 1 Jun 1973, 10–12.

b CLEFT LIP AND PALATE

1 Black, S. Cleft lip and palate. 5. Speech rehabilitation. Nursing Times, 69, 15 Nov 1973, 1526–1527.

2 Huddart, A. G. The care and management of the newborn cleft palate infant. Nursing Mirror, 140, 16 Jan 1975, 61–65.

3 O'Riordan, B. C. Cleft lip and palate. 4. Dental aspects. Nursing Times, 69, 8 Nov 1973, 1480–1482.

4 Pressland, B. M. Nursing care. 2. Cleft lip and palate. Nursing Times, 69, 25 Oct 1973, 1406–1407.

5 Smith, D. I. Cleft lip and palate. 3. Orthodontic aspects. Nursing Times, 69, 1 Nov 1973, 1441–1443.

6 Stranc, M. F. Cleft lip and palate. 1. Surgical treatment. Nursing Times, 69, 18 Oct 1973, 1366–1368.

c EAR DISEASES

1 Blancher, G. C. My trip through the semicircular canals. [A nurse's experience of severe vertigo and sound distortion associated with Meniere's syndrome.] American Journal of Nursing, 74 (10), Oct 1974, 1842–1843.

2 Booth, J. B. Tympanoplasty. Nursing Mirror, 140, 6 Feb 1975, 48–49.

3 Colman, B. H. Chronic mucous otitis. Nursing Times, 69, 15 Mar 1973, 336–338.

4 Cooke, E. T. M. Chronic suppurative otitis media. Nursing Times, 70, 28 Nov 1974, 1846–1847.

5 Denham, D. Nursing care study. Endolymphatic shunt for the treatment of Meniere's disease. Nursing Times, 68, 12 Oct 1972, 1287–1288.

6 Dix, M. R. Treatment of vertigo. Physiotherapy, 60 (12), Dec 1974, 380–384.

7 Fuller, A. P. Meniere's disease. Nursing Mirror, 138, 3 May 1974, 74–76.

8 Hammond, V. Stapedectomy. Nursing Mirror, 140, 6 Feb 1975, 45–48.

9 Malkin, E. A. The middle ear cleft and its acute infections. Nursing Times, 70, 19 Sep 1974, 1466–1467.

10 Mechner, F. Patient assessment: examination of the ear. Programmed instruction. American Journal of Nursing, 75 (3), Mar 1975, P.I. 1–23.

11 Pendrill, L. Pre- and post-operative nursing care in tympanoplasty. Nursing Mirror, 140, 6 Feb 1975, 53–54.

12 Rasmussen, E. M. Examination with the auriscope and syringing of the ear. Queen's Nursing Journal, 16 (6), Sep 1973, 130, 132.

13 Thornton, R. The artificial ear – research into cochlear implants. Nursing Mirror, 141, 31 Jul 1975, 55–58.

d DEAFNESS: GENERAL

1 Bailie, R. W. Deafness – a problem of communication. Nursing Times, 68, 27 Jul 1972, 923–926.

2 Bartha, M. The invisible handicap. [The work of the Royal Association in Aid of the Deaf and Dumb.] Health and Social Service Journal, 85, 1 Mar 1975, 490–491.

3 Beaver, R. Hearing loss in the elderly – a community health perspective. Public Health, 11 (1), Nov 1973, 19–25.

4 Carty, R. Patients who cannot hear. Nursing Forum, 11 (3), 1972, 290–299.

5 Clark, D. Voluntary visitors to the elderly deaf. British Medical Journal, 4, 30 Dec 1972, 766–768.

6 Colman, B. H. Deafness. Nursing Times, 70, 24 Oct 1974, 1661–1663.

7 Cornforth, A. R. T. and Woods, M. M. Deaf people in psychiatric hospitals. 1. Why loss of hearing? Nursing Times, 68, 27 Jan 1972, 101–103.

8 Cornforth, A. R. T. and Woods, M. M. Deaf people in psychiatric hospitals. 2. Disturbed and deaf. Nursing Times, 68, 3 Feb 1972, 139–141.

9 Cornforth, A. R. T. and Woods, M. M. Deaf people in psychiatric hospitals. 3. Subnormal and deaf. Nursing Times, 68, 10 Feb 1972, 177–180.

10 Cornforth, A. R. T. and Woods, M. M. Progressive or sudden hearing loss. Nursing Times, 68, 17 Feb 1972, 205–207.

11 Cornforth, A. R. T. and others Teaching sign language to the deaf mentally handicapped. [Study in four Surrey hospitals.] Nursing Times, 70, 31 Oct 1974, 1696–1697.

12 Department of Health and Social Security. Advisory Committee on Services for Hearing Impaired People Report. . . [on] the rehabilitation of the adult hearing-impaired. DHSS 1975. Chairman: T. Bird.

13 Felstein, I. Lipreading, hearing aids and the elderly. Midwife, Health Visitor and Community Nurse, 11 (7), Jul 1975, 209–210.

14 Herth, K. Beyond the curtain of silence: being deaf means using other senses and learning other ways to communicate. American Journal of Nursing, 74 (6), Jun 1974, 1060–1061.

15 James, E. Calming the deaf-mute's fears of the ED. RN Magazine, 37 (1), Jan 1974, OR 8.

16 Ludman, H. Modern surgery of deafness. Nursing Mirror, 134, 12 May 1972, 36–40.

17 Madell, J. R. The hard of hearing patient: special considerations for nursing care. Journal of Practical Nursing, 23 (12), Dec 1973, 22–24.

18 Nursing Mirror A symposium on the surgery of deafness. Nursing Mirror, 140, 6 Feb 1975, 45–47.

19 Perron, D. M. Deprived of sound. [Care of the deaf in hospital.] American Journal of Nursing, 74 (6), Jun 1974, 1057–1059.

20 Rawson, A. Deafness: report of a Departmental Enquiry into the promotion of research. HMSO, 1973. (Department of Health and Social Security, reports on health and social subjects no. 4.)

21 Royal National Institute for the Deaf Deaf and hard of hearing people. The Institute, 1973.

22 Wilson, C. A. Specialized psychiatric services for the deaf. Nursing Mirror, 133, 17 Sep 1971, 28–31.

e DEAFNESS: CHILDREN

1 Dodds, J. Are babies more difficult to screen for hearing? [The increased exposure of babies to noise may lead them to inhibit their reactions to it: with a survey of 42 families showing some of the weaknesses of the screening system.] Health Visitor, 48 (3), Mar 1975, 72–74.

2 Dodds, J. Testing hearing ability in the under-fives. Nursing Times, 71, 6 Nov 1975, 1791–1792.

3 Lesser, S. R. and Easser, R. Psychiatric management of the deaf child. Canadian Nurse, 71 (10), Oct 1975, 23–25.

4 Midwife, Health Visitor and Community Nurse The story of Graham, by his mother. [The problems of coping with a deaf child with the help of the Nuffield Hearing and Speech Centre.] Midwife, Health Visitor and Community Nurse, 11 (2), Feb 1975, 51–53.

5 Moody, D. and Chesham, I. Hearing tests for young children. Nursing Mirror, 133, 17 Dec 1971, 34–35.

f DENTISTRY AND DENTAL CARE

1 Baric, J. and others A health education approach to nutrition and dental health education. Health Educat Journal, 33 (3), 1974, 79–90.

2 Bates, J. F. and Harrison, A. A survey of housebound persons in Cardiff with special reference to dental care. Public Health, 89 (2), Jan 1975, 57–63.

3 Beal, J. F. and Dickson, S. The attitudes of West Midland Mothers to water fluoridation. Public Health, 87 (3), Mar 1973, 75–80.

4 Berman, D. S. Family practitioner services and management towards an integrated child health service. (a) Dental health in childhood. Royal Society of Health Journal, 94 (4), Aug 1974, 199–202.

5 Bowen, W. H. Aetiology of dental caries. Nursing Mirror, 137, 19 Oct 1973, 14–15.

6 Clewett, J. A. A consideration of dental health education. Health Education Journal, 34 (4), 1975, 115–118.

7 Clewett, J. A. A dental health education exercise. [In a primary school.] Health Education Journal, 32 (4), 1973, 111–114.

8 Doughty, J. F. Dental auxiliaries. Hospital and Health Services Review, 69 (10), Oct 1973, 364–366.

9 Ettinger, R. L. and Manderson, R. D. Dental care of the elderly. [Study of 442 institutionalized elderly in Edinburgh, and a suggested planned oral health policy.] Nursing Times, 71, 26 Jun 1975, 1003–1006.

10 Franks, A. S. T. Dental care and the handicapped person. (c) Dental care of the elderly handicapped. Royal Society of Health Journal, 95 (4), Aug 1975, 180–182.

11 Jaffe, E. Dental care and the handicapped person. (b) The delivery of dental care to handicapped children. Royal Society of Health Journal, 95 (4), Aug 1975, 177–180.

12 Longworth, T. S. School dental records. [An investigation to evaluate the effect of the school service on dental health and total treatment demand.] Health and Social Service Journal, 85, 12 Jul 1975, 1464–1466.

13 Marsland, E. A. Fluoridation – the alternative. (a) Pollution of the oral environment. Royal Society of Health Journal, 93 (5), Oct 1973, 253–256.

14 Murray, J. J. Water fluoridation: a choice for the community. Community Health, 6 (2), Sep/Oct 1974, 75–82.

15 Plowman, R. D. Dentists, too, need nurses. [Role of the dental nurse.] Nursing Times, 70, 25 Apr 1974, 645.

16 Pool, D. Dental care and the handicapped person. (a) The dental needs of handicapped children. Royal Society of Health Journal, 95 (4), Aug 1975, 175–177.

17 Public Health The future of community dentistry. Public Health, 87 (3), Mar 1973, 81–83.

18 Stafford, G. D. Problems associated with providing a dental service for the elderly. Public Health, 87 (1/2), Nov 1972/Jan 1973, 9–15.

19 Sutton, R. B. O. Acute periodontal conditions. Nursing Mirror, 139, 5 Jul 1974, 67–69.

20 Swallow J. N. The child, the dentist and dentistry. Midwife and Health Visitor, 8 (7), Jul 1972, 244–247.

21 Wood, D. G. and Bellman, G. M. A survey of the dental knowledge of nursing staff. Nursing Mirror, 137, 26 Oct 1973, 12–14.

22 World Health Issue on dentistry throughout the world. World Health, Dec 1973, 4–31.

23 World Health Organization Individual action required. 25 facts about dental diseases and oral health. Nursing Mirror, 139, 5 Jul 1974, 70.

g MOUTH CARE

1 DeWalt, E. M. Effect of timid hygienic measures on oral mucosa in a group of elderly subjects. Nursing Research, 24 (2), Mar/Apr 1975, 104–113.

2 Franks, A. S. T. The mouth in old age. Nursing Times, 69, 4 Oct 1973, 1292–1293.

3 Hardman, F. G. Oral surgery for nurses. 2nd ed. Bristol: Wright, 1971.

4 Henderson, W. Complications of infections of the mouth and pharynx in children. Nursing Times, 68, 11 May 1972, 569–570.

5 Howarth, M. H. A study of the mouth care procedure carried out by nurses for the very ill person. MSc thesis, Faculty of Medicine, Manchester University, 1975. Summary in Nursing Times 73, 10 Mar 1977, 354–355.

6 Jones, J. H. Oral ulceration. Nursing Times, 69, 18 Oct 1973, 1361–1363.

7 Levine, P. and Grayson, B. H. Safeguarding your patients against periodontal disease. RN Magazine, 36 (7), Jul 1973, 38–41.

8 Lovelock, D. J. Oral hygiene for patients in hospital. [Advice.] Nursing Mirror, 137, 12 Oct 1973, 39–42.

9 MacLennan, W. D. Oral hygiene in hospital. [Principles and recommended practice.] Nursing Times, 70, 28 Mar 1974, 471–472.

10 Minton, O. H. Oral disease: prevention and dental care. Mother and Child, 46 (1), Feb 1974, 12–17.

11 Pope, W. and others A study of oral hygiene in the geriatric patient. International Journal of Nursing Studies, 12 (2), Jul 1975, 65–72.

12 Reitz, M. and Pope, W. Mouth care. [Recommended procedures.] American Journal of Nursing, 73 (10), Oct 1973, 1728–1730.

13 Smith, C. Infections of the mouth and pharynx. Nursing Times, 68, 11 May 1972, 566–568.

14 Trowbridge, J. E. and Carl, W. Oral care: of the patient having head and neck irradiation. American Journal of Nursing, 75 (12), Dec 1975, 2146–2149.

15 Tuck, F. Nursing care study. Mandibular osteotomy for malocclusion. Nursing Mirror, 141, 13 Nov 1975, 51–53.

89 ENDOCRINE AND METABOLIC SYSTEMS

a GENERAL AND DISORDERS
(Includes Cushing's syndrome, restricted growth, thyroid disorders)

1 Beardwell, C. G. Thyroid diseases and their medical treatment. Nursing Times, 71, 25 Sep 1975, 1536–1538.

2 Davies, A. G. Growth hormone. Nursing Mirror, 137, 7 Sep 1973, 40–43.

3 Davis, R. W. Care of the patient with thyroid disease. Nursing Care, 8 (10), Oct 1975, 10–14.

4 Driscoll, A. E. A teaching aid for endocrine disorders. Paintings can be guides in recognizing signs of endocrine dysfunction. American Journal of Nursing, 73 (11), Nov 1973, 1944–1945.

5 Elliott, D. D. Adrenocortical insufficiency. A self instruction unit. American Journal of Nursing, 74 (6), Jun 1974, 1115–1130.

6 Emmanuel, S. Basic surgery 3. Surgery of the thyroid and parathyroid glands. RN Magazine, 37 (11), Nov 1974, OR-1–2, 4.

7 Ference, R. H. The little people – no small problem. [Achondroplastic dwarfism.] RN Magazine, 37 (9), Sep 1974, 70–71, 74, 80, 82, 86.

8 Hall, R. Hypothyroidism. Nursing Mirror, 135, 6 Oct 1972, 23–24.

9 Havard, C. W. H. Endocrine exophthalmos. Nursing Mirror, 135, 7 Jul 1972, 21–23.

10 Heidt, C. S. The OR nurse's role in transseptal transsphenoidal hypophysectomy. [Removal of pituitary gland.] RN Magazine, 36 (7), Jul 1973, OR 1, 3, 6.

11 Lewis, J. G. The endocrine system. Harmondsworth: Penguin Education, 1973, (Penguin library of nursing).

12 Lindley, M. The small people of Britain. [Association for Research into Restricted Growth.] Nursing Times, 68, 25 May 1972, 635–636.

13 Lozyo, F. Nursing care study – thyroidectomy. The Zambia Nurse Journal, 5 (4), Apr/May 1973, 10–12.

14 McGann, M. Cushing's syndrome: its complexities and care. RN Magazine, 38 (8), Aug 1975, 40–43.

15 McGann, M. Treatment and care of the patient with hyperparathyroidism. RN Magazine, 37 (11), Nov 1974, 48–51.

16 McKelvie, P. Hypophysectomy. [Operative procedure and postoperative care.] [Removal of pituitary gland.] Nursing Times, 71, 10 Apr 1975, 570–573.

17 Manns, L. and Boechler, N. E. Two disorders of the thyroid gland: a description of hypothyroidism and hyperthyroidism, and an up-to-date account of tests used to diagnose disorders of the thyroid gland. Canadian Nurse, 68 (9), Sep 1972, 42–45.

18 May, C. B. Adenomatous goitre. Nursing Times, 67, 4 Feb 1971, 138–140.

19 Munro, D. S. and Duthie, H. L. The management of Cushing's syndrome. Nursing Mirror, 137, 21 Sep 1973, 12–15.

20 Nelson, M. A. The medical challenge. [Of restricted growth.] Nursing Times, 68, 25 May 1972, 636–638.

21 Nelson, M. A. Restricted growth. Nursing Mirror, 141, 14 Aug 1975, 45–47.

22 Newton, G. M. Nursing care study. Clitoroplasty for andrenogenital syndrome. Nursing Times, 72, 27 May 1976, 816–819.

23 Price, W. H. Delayed puberty. Nursing Mirror, 136, 20 Apr 1973, 16–20.

24 Pryor, J. P. Hyperparathyroidism. Nursing Times, 69, 22 Nov 1973, 1558–1559.

25 Russell, P. M. G. Obstetric endocrinology. Nursing Mirror, 133, 26 Nov 1971, 33–34.

26 Small, J. C. and Clarke-Williams, M. J. Endocrinology. Heinemann Medical, 1972. (Modern practical nursing series no. 12).

27 Smith, S. E. Drug therapy 1972.6. Drugs and the thyroid gland. Nursing Times, 68, 6 Apr 1972, 406–407.

28 Smith, S. E. How drugs act.18. Drugs and the thyroid gland. Nursing Times, 71, 23 Oct 1975, 1708–1709.

29 Spencer, R. T. Patient care in endocrine problems. Philadelphia: Saunders, 1973, (Monographs in clinical nursing no. 4).

30 Sprung, E. When Johnny doesn't grow. [Hypopituitary dwarfism.] Nursing Care, 6 (7), Jul 1973, 27–29.

31 Thomson, J. A. Acromegaly. Nursing Mirror, 135, 6 Oct 1972, 26–29.

32 Tweedily, K. H. Phaeochromocytoma – diagnosis and management: a case study. Nursing Mirror, 132, 12 Mar 1971, 42–45.

33 Wood, G. Don't look down on us. Nursing Mirror, 141, 14 Aug 1975, 49–52.

34 Wright, G. M. Phaeochromocytoma: a nursing case study. Nursing Times, 67, 29 Apr 1971, 512–514.

b DIABETES: GENERAL

1 Allan, F. N. Diabetes before and after insulin. Medical History, 16 (3), Jul 1972, 266–273.

2 Burston, G. R. Hyper-osmolar non-ketoacidotic diabetes mellitus. Nursing Mirror, 137, 7 Sep, 19–20.

3 Coleman, V. The history of diabetes. Nursing Mirror, 140, 3 Apr 1975, 70.

4 Fleming, C. A survey of diabetes mellitus in East Fife. District Nursing, 15 (8), Nov 1972, 164–165, 168.

5 Fulton, M. and others Helping diabetics adapt to failing vision. American Journal of Nursing, 74 (1), Jan 1974, 54–57.

6 Garland, C. Diabetic ketosis. Nursing Times, 70, 9 May 1974, 710–711.

7 Grant, D. M. Banting and Best – the men who tamed diabetes. Canadian Nurse, 67 (10), Oct 1971, 27–30.

8 Jarrett, R. J. Treatment of diabetes and its problems. District Nursing, 14 (1), Apr 1971, 9–10.

9 Kula, J. J. Diabetic dietetics. Journal of Practical Nursing, 23 (1), Jan 1973, 16–17.

10 Laufer, I. J. The current status of diabetes mellitus research. Journal of Practical Nursing, 23 (1), Jan 1973, 18–21, 32.

11 Lister, J. Oral drugs in the treatment of diabetes mellitus. Nursing Mirror, 137, 31 Aug 1973, 22–23.

12 McKendry, J. B. R. Idiopathic edema [and its connection with diabetes.] Canadian Nurse, 69 (6', May 1973, 41–43.

13 Marks, V. Hypoglycaemia. Nursing Mirror, 136, 5 Jan 1973, 25–27.

14 Marks, V. Hypoglycaemia and its treatment. Nursing Times, 68, 10 Aug 1972, 989–991.

15 Page, N. McB. Disappearing diabetes. [Case study of a nurse who probably fabricated a diabetic condition.] British Medical Journal, 2, 17 May 1975, 365–366.

16 Queen's Nursing Journal Travel and the diabetic. Queen's Nursing Journal, 18 (4), Jul 1975, 124.

17 Smith, S. E. How drugs act. 19. Antidiabetic drugs. Nursing Times, 71, 30 Oct 1975, 1744–1745.

18 Stowe, S. M. Hypophysectomy for diabetic retinopathy. [Removal of the pituitary gland in the treatment of diabetes.] American Journal of Nursing, 73 (4), Apr 1973, 632–637.

19 Sutcliffe, B. A. Diabetic retinopathy: it's management and social aspects. Nursing Mirror, 138, 17 May 1974, 56–59.

20 Talf, B. Hypoglycemia. A symptom, not a disease. Journal of Practical Nursing, 24 (3), Mar 1974, 16–18.

21 Whelton, M. J. Hyperosmolar non-ketotic diabetic coma. Nursing Mirror, 133, 17 Dec 1971, 17–18.

22 Whittington, T. H. Eyes and eyesight in diabetes. Nursing Times, 67, 23 Sep 1971, 1171–1173.

23 Wolfe, B. M. and Powers, R. Hypoglycemia. Canadian Nurse, 69 (10), Oct 1973, 38–40.

24 World Health Issue devoted to diabetes. World Health, Feb/Mar 1971, 3–45.

25 Wright, A. D. Love and marriage [in diabetics]. [Reprinted from Balance, the newspaper of the British Diabetic Association.] Nursing Mirror, 141, 23 Oct 1975, 57.

c DIABETES: NURSING AND COMMUNITY CARE (Includes nurse practitioner and treatment in general practice)

1 Allison, S. E. A framework for nursing action in a nurse-conducted diabetic management clinic. Journal of Nursing Administration, 3 (4), Jul/Aug 1973, 53–60.

2 Burke, E. L. Insulin injection. The site and the technique. American Journal of Nursing, 72 (12), Dec 1972, 2194–2196.

3 Butterfield, W. J. H. Return to nursing. 12. A modern approach to diabetes. Nursing Mirror, 133, 13 Aug 1971, 11–13.

4 Grancio, S. D. Nursing care of the adult diabetic patient. Nursing Clinics of North America, 8 (4), Dec 1973, 605–615.

5 John Mary, Sister. The nursing care of the diabetic. World of Irish Nursing, 2 (12), Dec 1973, 225–228.

6 Jordan, J. D. The nurse practitioner in a group practice. [Specialising in diabetes.] American Journal of Nursing, 74 (8), Aug 1974, 1447–1449.

7 Jordan, J. D. and Shipp, J. C. The primary health care professional was a nurse. [Diabetic patients.] American Journal of Nursing, 71 (5), May 1971, 922–925.

8 McEvoy, P. Nursing care study. Diabetes mellitus. Nursing Times, 70, 11 Jul 1974, 1074–1075.

9 Malhotra, A. K. Diabetes – some important hints and the role of a nurse in its prevention and management. Nursing Journal of India, 66 (6), Jun 1975, 129–130.

10 Malins, J. M. and Stuart, J. M. Diabetic clinic in a general practice. British Medical Journal, 4, 16 Oct 1971, 161.

11 Malins, J. M. and Stuart, J. M. A diabetic clinic in group practice. Health Magazine, 9 (2), Jun 1972, 9–11.

12 Russell, R. G. The team approach to diabetes. [Including the work of the practice nurse.] Practice Team, no. 41, Oct 1974, 2, 4–6.

13 Stein, G. H. The use of a nurse practitioner in the management of patients with diabetes mellitus. Medical Care, 12 (1), Oct 1974, 885–890.

14 Williams, S. M. Diabetic urine testing by hospital nursing personnel. Nursing Research, 20 (5), Sep/Oct 1971, 444–447.

15 Wilson, P. Nursing care study. The management of diabetic keto-acidosis provoked by sepsis. Nursing Mirror, 140, 13 Mar 1975, 74–77.

d DIABETES: PATIENT AND PATIENT TEACHING

1 British Diabetic Association The diabetic's handbook. The Association, 1972.

2 Burke, B. L. Training program in diabetes care. Nursing Outlook, 19 (8), Aug 1971, 548–549.

3 Burton, J. Management of a new diabetic patient in the home [with a chart to simplify patient teaching]. Queen's Nursing Journal, 18 (3), Jun 1975, 70–71.

4 Canadian Nurse Idea exchange. Teaching insulin administration – no oranges, please. [Using sponge rubber for practice.] Canadian Nurse, 68 (4), Apr 1972, 45.

5 Candau, M. G. Diabetes and living. Occupational Health, 23 (4), Apr 1971, 110–112.

6 Davenport, R. R. and others Dietiticians, nurses teach diabetic patients. Interdisciplinary team provides group and individual instruction for patients and their families. Hospitals, 48, 1 Dec 1974, 81–82.

7 Farquhar, J. W. Notes for the guidance of parents of diabetic children. 2nd ed. Edinburgh: Churchill Livingstone, 1975.

8 Gates, K. A candid evaluation of diabetic teaching. Dimensions in Health Service, 52 (11), Nov 1975, 13–14.

9 Goeller, J. Diabetic teaching in a 200 bed hospital. Dimensions in Health Service, 52 (6), Jun 1975, 44–45.

10 Hollands, M. A. Role of the dietitian in diabetes education. Hospital Administration in Canada, 14 (4), Apr 1972, 42, 44.

11 Hollands, M. A. and Armstrong, J. TRIDEC – a pioneer in shared medical services in Canada. [Tri-Hospital Diabetes Education Centre.] Hospital Administration in Canada, 17 (4), Apr 1975, 28–30, 32.

12 Laugharne, E. Insulin goes metric: a time for review. [The importance of patient education by nurses.] Canadian Nurse, 71 (2), Feb 1975, 22–24.

13 Laugharne, E. The tri-hospital/diabetes education centre. [Patient education scheme in Toronto.] Dimensions in Health Service, 52 (3), Mar 1975, 43–44.

14 Nickerson, D. Teaching the hospitalized diabetic. American Journal of Nursing, 72 (5), May 1972, 935–939.

15 Perks, J. Please nurse, what is diabetes? Nursing Times, 69, 22 Nov 1973, 1585.

16 Salzer, J. E. Classes to improve diabetic self-care. [Conducted by a nurse.] American Journal of Nursing, 75 (8), Aug 1975, 1324–1326.

17 Skelton, J. M. A diabetic teaching tool. [Teaching aid for patients.] Canadian Nurse, 69 (12), Dec 1973, 35–38.

18 Stuart, S. Day-to-day living with diabetes. American Journal of Nursing, 71 (8), Aug 1971, 1548–1550.

19 Thomas, L. R. Patients with diabetes mellitus – the teaching function of the nurse. Nursing Journal of India, 44 (1), Jan 1973, 14, 16.

20 Trayser, L. M. A teaching program for diabetics. American Journal of Nursing, 73 (1), Jan 1973, 92–93.

21 University College Hospital. Diabetic Clinic Notes for diabetics: diets and instructions given to patients attending the Diabetic Clinic, University College Hospital. 8th ed. H. K. Lewis, 1971.

e DIABETES: PREGNANCY

1 Atkins, J. Detecting a diabetic tendancy in pregnancy. Nursing Times, 68, 16 Mar 1972, 322–323.

2 Brearley, B. F. The management of pregnancy in diabetes mellitus. Practitioner, 215, Nov 1975, 644–652.

3 Cranley, M. C. and Frazier, S. A. Preventive intensive care of the diabetic mother and her fetus. Nursing Clinics of North America, 8 (3), Sep 1973, 489–499.

4 Dixon, G. Management of diabetes in pregnancy. Midwife and Health Visitor, 10 (1), Oct 1974, 304–307, 310–312.

5 Guthrie, D. W. and Guthrie, R. A. The infant of the diabetic mother. [Treatment and nursing care.] American Journal of Nursing, 74 (11), Dec 1974, 2008–2009.

6 Laugharne, E. and Duncan, F. Gestational diabetes – when teaching is important. Canadian Nurse, 69 (3), Mar 1973, 34–36.

7 Todd, R. McL. The baby of the diabetic mother. Nursing Times, 69, 11 Oct 1973, 1322–1325.

f DIABETES: CHILDREN AND ADOLESCENTS

1 Barson, C. and MacNamara, G. P. Nursing care study. Neonatal diabetes. Nursing Mirror, 138, 29 Mar 1974, 81–82.

2 Bedford, I. M. Case study of a young diabetic. Occupational Health, 23 (12), Dec 1971, 392–394.

3 Blair, P. Palingswick House – hostel for diabetic children. Health and Social Service Journal, 85, 29 Mar 1975, 710–711.

4 Court, J. M. Your child has diabetes: a guide to parents and to their children who have diabetes. Heinemann Medical, 1972.

5 Craig, J. O. Caring for the diabetic child. Nursing Mirror, 140, 20 Mar 1975, 74–76.

6 Guthrie, D. W. and Guthrie, R. A. Diabetes in adolescence. American Journal of Nursing, 75 (10), Oct 1975, 1740–1744.

7 Guthrie, D. W. and Guthrie, R. A. Juvenile diabetes mellitus. Nursing Clinics of North America, 8 (4), Dec 1973, 587–603.

8 Hearnshaw, J. R. 'Learning to live.' Summer camps for diabetic children. Queen's Nursing Journal, 18 (4), Jul 1975, 102–103, 106.

9 Leahey, M. D. and others Pediatric diabetes: a new teaching approach. Canadian Nurse, 71 (10), Oct 1975, 18–20.

10 Lorich, M. L. and Kaiser, S. A. A diabetic child is still a child – with diabetes. RN Magazine, 38 (10), Oct 1975, 39–43.

11 McFarlane, J. Children with diabetes: special needs during growing years. American Journal of Nursing, 73 (8), Aug 1973, 1360–1363.

12 McFarlane, J. and Hames, C. C. Children with diabetes: learning self-care in camp. American Journal of Nursing, 73 (8), Aug 1973, 1362–1365.

13 O'Reily, E. Diet and the diabetic child. Mother and Child, 43 (5), Sep/Oct 1971, 15–16, 20.

14 Pridham, K. F. Instruction of a school age child with chronic illness for increased responsibility in self-care using diabetes mellitus as an example. International Journal of Nursing Studies, 8 (4), Dec 1971, 237–245.

15 Robinson, W. Home treatment is best for diabetic children. [British Diabetic Association meeting.] Nursing Mirror, 141, 2 Oct 1975, 36.

16 Sprung, E. Diabetes mellitus in children. Nursing Care, 8 (3), Mar 1975, 8–11.

17 Stephens, J. W. Childhood diabetes. Journal of Practical Nursing, 23 (9), Sep 1973, 22–23, 30–31.

18 Wadsworth, M. E. J. and Jarrett, R. J. Incidence of diabetes in the first 26 years of life. [Results of a National Survey of Health and Development study of 5632 children born in 1946.] Lancet, 2, 16 Nov 1974, 1172–1176.

19 Watson, A. A study of family attitudes to children with diabetes. Community Medicine, 128 (5), 19 May 1972, 122–125.

g METABOLIC SYSTEM AND ALLERGY

1 Baker, B. H. Allergy, 1972. Bedside Nurse, 5 (12), Dec 1972, 22–25.

2 Legerman, D. G. What to tell the allergic patient. Nursing Care, 7 (11), Nov 1974, 15–17.

3 Mahon, D. F. Scriver testing for inherited metabolic diseases. Nursing Mirror, 137, 13 Jul 1973, 10–15.

4 Norman, A. P. Allergy in childhood. [Asthma, Eczema, Hay Fever and Food allergy.] Nursing Mirror, 137, 7 Sep 1973, 9–11.

h OBESITY

1 Crow, R. A. and Wright, P. Experimental studies of obesity: relevance to problems of nursing care. Nursing Times, 70, 24 Jan 1974, 103–105.

2 Flatter, P. Nursing care of the jejunoileal bypass patient. [A treatment for severe obesity.] RN Magazine, 37 (3), Mar 1974, 34–39.

3 Fox, Dr. A bit too fat? then play it cool. Nursing Times, 70, 25 Jul 1974, 1144–1145.

4 Gazet, J. C. Surgery for obesity. [Results of 62 jejunal bypass operations at St. George's Hospital.] Nursing Times, 71, 9 Oct 1975, 1618–1619.

5 Hartie, A. Obesity: environmental control of eating. Nursing Mirror, 141, 11 Dec 1975, 47–49.

6 Heydman, A. H. Intestinal bypass for obesity. American Journal of Nursing, 74 (6), Jun 1974, 1102–1104.

7 Honywood, H. The team approach to obesity. Practice Team, no. 34, Mar 1974, 2, 4–5; no. 35, Apr 1974, 6, 8.

8 Kalisch, B. J. The stigma of obesity. American Journal of Nursing, 72 (6), Jun 1972, 1124–1127.

9 Laurent, L. P. E. The management of obesity. Midwife and Health Visitor, 8 (11), Nov 1972, 382–384.

10 Laurent, L. P. E. Obesity. Nursing Mirror, 132, 23 Apr 1971, 21–23.

11 Lindner, D. The nurse's role in a bariatric clinic. RN Magazine, 37 (2), Feb 1974, 28–33.

12 Loxson, R. Changing obesity patterns. [Inservice program on weight control among community health nurses.] Nursing Outlook, 23 (11), Nov 1975, 711–713.

13 Meyerowitz, B. R. and others From massive weight loss to abdominal panniculectomy. RN Magazine, 37 (2), Mar 1974, OR1, OR4.

14 Pescatore, E. A. Personal reaction to weight loss. American Journal of Nursing, 74 (12), Dec 1974, 2227–2229.

15 Richardson, S. An answer to the overweight problem. [Local authority obesity clinic.] Midwife and Health Visitor, 7 (11), Nov 1971, 425, 427.

16 Robinson, W. Obesity. A health farm. [Champneys health resort, Tring.] Nursing Mirror, 141, 11 Dec 1975, 52–53.

17 Ryan, G. C. and Willacker, J. The group way to weight loss. MsS [A disruptive patient and follow up.] American Journal of Nursing, 73 (2), Feb 1973, 273–276.

18 Shumway, S. and Powers, M. The group way to weight loss. American Journal of Nursing, 73 (2), Feb 1973, 269–272.

19 Starkloff, G. B. Surgical treatment of the morbidly obese. [Small-bowel bypass.] RN Magazine, 37 (3), Mar 1974, OR1-OR2, OR5-OR6.

20 Vaughan, M. S. Surgery for the morbidly obese. AORN Journal, 21 (2), Feb 1975, 230–238.

21 Walker, P. Obesity. Dietary control. Nursing Mirror, 141, 11 Dec 1975, 50–51.

22 Whitney, J. A. Surgical weight loss. [Intestinal by-pass procedure.] Nursing Care, 6 (6), Jun 1973, 16–18.

23 Yaffe, M. Inside every fat man. [Social aspects of obesity.] New Society, 24, 21 Jun 1973, 674–676.

i OBESITY: CHILDREN

1 Brook, C. G. D. Obesity in children. Nursing Mirror, 137, 20 Jul 1973, 40–42.

2 Creery, R. D. G. The overweight child. [With particular reference to the role of the health team.] Midwife and Health Visitor, 10 (5), May 1974, 117–120.

3 Hardcastle, D. and others Helping obese schoolgirls to lose weight: Stansted Summer School. Community Medicine, 128, 7, 2 Jun 1972, 167–169.

4 Howarth, E. Nursing care study. Obesity in a child of eleven. Nursing Times, 69, 26 Apr 1973, 534–536.

5 Lloyd, J. K. Obesity in children. Mother and child, 44 (5), Sep/Oct 1972, 7–9, 20.

6 Lloyd, J. K. Obesity in childhood. Nursing Times, 69, 26 Apr 1973, 532–533.

7 Lorber, J. Obesity in children. Nursing Mirror, 138, 22 Mar 1974, 68–72.

8 McLaughlan, G. P. Obesity in childhood. Community Medicine, 127 (5), 4 Feb 1972, 59–64.

9 Robinson, H. L. Learning to count the calories. [Slimming group for Oxford schoolchildren run by a health visitor.] Nursing Times, 71, 3 Jul 1975, 1062–1064.

10 Wheeler, E. F. The problem of obesity in children. Nursing Times, 68, 8 Jun 1972, 710–712.

90 HAEMATOLOGY

a GENERAL AND DISORDERS (Includes blood transfusion)

1 Affara, F. A. Blood gases, Nursing Times, 69, 11 Jan 1973, 43–45; 18 Jan 1973, 80–82.

2 Allen, J. G. Vitae custodes – the volunteer blood doners. Nursing Outlook, 20 (9), Sep 1972, 588–591.

3 Bird, D. W. G. The haemoglobin molecule: disorders of its synthesis and structure. Nursing Mirror, 135, 1 Sep 1972, 36–37.

4 Butcher, G. Some donors are getting their own back. Nursing Times, 67, 5 Aug 1971, 955–958.

5 Child, J. and others Blood transfusions: complications. American Journal of Nursing, 72 (9), Sep 1972, 1602–1605.

6 Child, J. A. Haematology reporting. [Use of electronic counting machines in determining red cell, white cell and platelet counts.] Nursing Times, 71, 3 Jul 1975, 1045–1048.

7 Clack, W. Collecting a blood sample. S A Nursing Journal, 40 (12), Dec 1973, 34–35,

8 Clarke, C. A. Prevention of Rh haemolytic disease. [Inaugural lecture at the 59th London Nursing Exhibition, October 23rd–25th, 1974.] Nursing Mirror, 139, 24 Oct 1974, 57–59.

9 Delamore, I. W. Christmas disease. District Nursing, 14 (9), Dec 1971, 182, 184.

10 Friedman, P. and others The IV laboratory nurse: nurses, rather than lab technologists collect blood specimens. Hospitals, 46 (18), 16 Sep 1972, 102, 104, 106–107.

11 Hall, D. Portable transfusion box. Occupational Health, 24 (2), Feb 1972, 37–38.

12 Harding Rains, A. J. Blood substitutes in the treatment of haemorrhage. Nursing Mirror, 135, 4 Aug 1972, 18–19.

13 Hatcher, J. Blood platelets. Nursing Mirror, 133, 2 Jul 1971, 37.

14 Hatcher, J. Collection of blood cultures. Nursing Mirror, 135, 29 Sep 1972, 34–35.

15 Hatcher, J. The differential leucocyte count. Nursing Mirror, 140, 24 Apr 1975, 65–66.

16 Hatcher, J. The ward ESR. [Blood test.] Nursing Mirror, 134, 4 Feb 1972, 36–37.

17 Horoshak, I. Auto transfusion: promising alternative to donor blood. RN Magazine, 38 (5), May 1975, 33–40.

18 Humphreys, D. Careers extraordinary. The blood brigade. [Nurse in the Blood Transfusion Service.] Nursing Times, 68, 1 Jun 1972, 674–676.

19 Isler, C. Blood: the age of components. [Administration of components, instead of whole blood, to meet increasing demand.] RN Magazine, 36 (6), Jun 1973, 31–41.

20 Jenkins, G. and others A review of transfusion complications. AANA Journal, 43 (4), Aug 1975, 369–374.

21 Krishen, S. Blood donation and the nurse. Nursing Journal of India, 65 (5), May 1974, 145–146.

22 Lippmann, M. and Myhre, B. A. Hazards of massive transfusion. AANA Journal, 43 (3), Jun 1975, 269–277.

23 Marzluf, M. J. A positive approach to being negative. [RH disease in the newborn.] Nursing Care, 7 (1), Jan 1974, 12–15.

24 Marzluf, M. J. Transfusion recipients: new battleground in a 5000 year old cold war. [Serum hepatitis.] Nursing Care, 6 (4), Apr 1973, 12–15.

25 Miller, A. Systems of life. Nos 7 and 8. Blood 1 and 2. Nursing Times, 71, 3 Jul 1975 [4 pages]; 71, 7 Aug 1975 [4 pages].

26 Nursing Clinics of North America Symposium on patients with blood disorders. Nursing Clinics of North America, 7 (4), Dec 1972, 709–826.

27 Osborne, D. J. and others Society at work. Why give blood? [Survey by questionnaire in the Swansea area.] New Society, 34, 23 Oct 1975, 210–211.

28 Pannall, P. Collecting a blood sample for biochemical tests. S A Nursing Journal, 41 (3), Mar 1974, 29–31.

29 Ravenscroft, M. M. Nurse in the haematology unit. Nursing Times, 71, 13 Mar 1975, 420–421.

30 Rock, G. Component therapy. [The use of blood components rather than whole blood, in the treatment of disease.] Canadian Nurse, 70 (9), Sep 1974, 24–27.

31 Shelley, U. Blood disorders in childhood. Nursing Mirror, 133, 31 Dec 1971, 16–21; 134, 7 Jan 1972, 20–22.

32 Smith, S. E. Drugs and the blood. Nursing Times, 68, 30 Mar 1972, 383–385.

33 Smith, S. E. How drugs act – 17. Drugs and the blood. Nursing Times, 71, 16 Oct 1975, 1665–1666.

34 Swift, M. H. Nursing care study. Timothy. [Case of severe anaphylactoid purpura – Henoch-Schoenlein syndrome.] Nursing Times, 70, 2 May 1974, 674–676.

35 **United States Department of Health Education and Welfare** National Institutes of Health. Clinical Center. Nursing Department. Nurse's role in blood component transfusion procurement. Washington: DHEW, 1975.

36 **White, E. H.** Blood transfusion therapy. Nursing Care, 8 (6), Jun 1975, 18, 30–31.

b ANAEMIA AND SICKLE CELL DISEASE

1 **Baird, I. M.** Iron deficiency anaemia. Nursing Times, 69, 19 Apr 1973, 495–497.

2 **Boyd, R. V.** Drugs related to the anaemias. District Nursing, 14 (8), Nov 1971, 162–164.

3 **Carter, Y. A.** Nursing management in sickle cell disease. RN Magazine, 38 (10), Oct 1975, 47–50.

4 **Davis, R. W.** The patient with sickle cell anemia. Bedside Nurse, 5 (9), Sep 1972, 22–24.

5 **England, J. M.** Pernicious anaemia. Nursing Mirror, 139, 30 Aug 1974, 52–54.

6 **Foster, S.** Sickle cell anaemia: closing the gap between theory and therapy. American Journal of Nursing, 71 (10), Oct 1971, 1952–1956.

7 **Hedge, U. M.** Sickle cell anaemia. Nursing Mirror, 140, 26 Jun 1975, 45–47.

8 **Johnson, F. P. and Hatcher, W.** The patient with sickle cell disease. Nursing Forum, 13 (3), 1974, 259–288.

9 **Journal of Practical Nursing** A look at a sickle cell clinic. [In Jamaica.] Journal of Practical Nursing, 23 (2), Feb 1973, 18–19.

10 **Markson, J. L.** The anaemias. 1. Introduction. Nursing Times, 67, 9 Dec 1971, 1523–1524.

11 **Markson, J. L.** The anaemias. 2. Pernicious anaemia. Nursing Times, 67, 16 Dec 1971, 1562–1564.

12 **Markson, J. L.** The anaemias. 3. Haemolytic anaemia. Nursing Times, 67, 23 Dec 1971, 1611–1613.

13 **Markson, J. L.** The anaemias. 4. Aplastic anaemia. Nursing Times, 67, 30 Dec 1971, 1624–1625.

14 **Nursing Mirror** Fight against sickle cell anaemia. Nursing Mirror, 137, 14 Sep 1973, 44.

15 **Ogston, D.** Pernicious anaemia. Nursing Times, 71, 27 Feb 1975, 338–339.

16 **Pochedly, C.** Sickle cell anemia: recognition and management. American Journal of Nursing, 71 (10), Oct 1971, 1948–1951.

17 **Simpson, E.** Understanding sickle cell anemia. Journal of Practical Nursing, 23 (2), Feb 1973, 16–17.

18 **Sloman, M. J.** Guide to thalassaemia. [The nature of an hereditary anaemia.] Nursing Times, 70, 19/26 Dec 1974, 1968–1970.

19 **Sloman, M. J.** Homozygous beta thalassaemia. [Nursing care study of a child with anaemia.] Nursing Times, 70, 19/26 Dec 1974, 1970–1971.

20 **Stern, P.** APA: insidious foe of an aging Swede. [Addison's pernicious anemia.] American Journal of Nursing, 73 (1), Jan 1973, 111–113.

21 **Strelling, M. K.** Anaemia in infants of low birth-weight. Nursing Mirror, 135, 1 Dec 1972, 24–28.

22 **Waters, W. E.** Anaemia in women. Nursing Mirror, 134, 28 Apr 1972, 20–21.

c HAEMOPHILIA

1 **Anscombe, A. R.** Surgery in haemophilia. Nursing Mirror, 132, 23 Apr 1971, 17–18.

2 **Bentley, G.** Haemophilia. 1. Incidence, inheritance and management. Nursing Times, 71, 4 Dec 1975, 1926–1927.

3 **Bentley, G.** Haemophilia. 2. Chronic haemophilic arthropathy. Nursing Times, 71, 11 Dec 1975, 1984–1986.

4 **Clarke, N.** Case report. 2. Open heart surgery on the hemophiliac. RN Magazine, 36 (5), May 1973, 44–47.

5 **Davies, C.** A nurse in a haemophilia centre. Nursing Times, 68, 17 Aug 1972, 1030–1033.

6 **Davio, E.** Nursing management of the youngster with a coagulation disorder. Journal of Practical Nursing, 21 (3), Mar 1971, 32–35, 48–49.

7 **Eyster, M. E.** Emergency care of the hemophiliac. RN Magazine, 38 (10), Oct 1975, OR 3–5, 6.

8 **Jones, P.** Answering the needs of haemophiliac children and their families. Community Medicine, 128 (15), 28 Jul 1972, 351–354.

9 **Jones, P.** Nursing the haemophiliac. Nursing Mirror, 136, 23 Feb 1973, 33–36.

10 **Le Quesne, B. and others** Home treatment for patients with haemophilia. Lancet, 2, 31 Aug 1974, 507–510.

11 **Massie, R. and Massie, S.** Journey. [Parents experience of child's haemophilia.] Gollancz, 1975.

12 **Sergis, E. and Hilgartner, M. W.** Hemophilia. [Home care programs in which patients transfuse themselves during bleeding episodes.] American Journal of Nursing, 72 (11), Nov 1972, 2011–2020.

13 **Shafran, R.** Case report. 1. Increasing freedom for the hemophiliac. [Pre- and post-operative care in open heart surgery.] RN Magazine, 36 (5), May 1973, 39–43.

91 MUSCULOSKELETAL SYSTEM

a GENERAL AND DISEASES

1 **Aladjem, H.** The sun is my enemy: one woman's victory over a mysterious and dreaded disease. [Lupus erythematosus.] New Jersey: Prentice-Hall, 1972.

2 **Brower, P. and Hicks, D.** Maintaining muscle function in patients on bed rest. American Journal of Nursing, 72 (7), Jul 1972, 1250–1253.

3 **Cantrell, T.** Describing hand function. Nursing Times, 71, 2 Oct 1975, 1577–1578.

4 **Davidson, J. K. and Griffiths, P. D.** Caisson disease of bone. Nursing Times, 67, 26 Aug 1971, 1049–1052.

5 **Delaney, T. J.** Connective tissue diseases. [Lupus erythematosus, systemic sclerosis, dermatomyositis and rheumatoid arthritis.] Nursing Mirror, 139, 28 Nov 1974, 60–63.

6 **DiPalma, J. R.** Drug therapy today. Recent developments in bone-disease treatment. RN Magazine, 36 (1), Jan 1973, 63–72, [7 pages.]

7 **Ehtisham, M.** Osteoporosis. Nursing Times, 70, 3 Oct 1974, 1544–1546.

8 **Evanson, J. M.** Paget's disease of the bone. Nursing Times, 71, 5 Jun 1975, 878–880.

9 **Fox, J. A.** A case of corrosion. [Case study of a chronic leg ulcer from osteomyelitis caused by corrosion of a metal plate.] Nursing Times, 70, 25 Jul 1974, 1156–1157.

10 **Golding, D. N.** Polyarteritis. Nursing Times, 69, 12 Apr 1973, 464–465.

11 **Griffin, A. J. and Mowat, A. G.** Shoulder-hand syndrome. Nursing Times, 71, 10 Apr 1975, 580–582.

12 **Gumpel, J. M.** Systematic lupus erythematosus. Nursing Times, 71, 17 Apr 1975, 609–611.

13 **Hartley, B.** I've got a wolf by the ears. [A patient with systemic lupus erythematosus.] Canadian Nurse, 70 (1), Jan 1974, 28–31.

14 **Haslock, I. and Wright, V.** The diffuse connective tissue diseases. [Systemic lupus erythematosus, systemic sclerosis polymyositis and polyarteritis nodosa.] Nursing Mirror, 141, 14 Aug 1975, 56–60.

15 **Heap, L.** The preservators. Two hand splints designed by a patient with a 30 year history of syringomyelia. Nursing Times, 69, 24 May 1973, 666–667.

16 **Helal, B.** Replacement of fingers. Nursing Times, 70, 29 Aug 1974, 1348–1352.

17 **Holland, T.** Conditions of the hand. Prescribed hand diseases. [Through occupation.] Occupational Health 27 (7), Jul 1975, 286–292.

18 **Miller, A.** Systems of life, 2 and 3. Bones Nursing Times, 71, 6 Feb 1975; [4 pages] 6 Mar 1975, [4 pages].

19 **Miller, A.** Systems of life. Joints. Nursing Times, 71, 3 Apr 1975, [4 pages].

20 **Muckle, D. S.** Soft tissue injuries. Nursing Mirror, 136, 9 Feb 1973, 24–26.

21 **Pendleton, T. and Grossman, B. J.** Rehabilitating children with inflammatory joint disease. American Journal of Nursing, 74 (12), Dec 1974, 2223–2226.

22 **Proctor, H.** The painful shoulder. [Soft tissue injuries.] Nursing Mirror, 138, 14 Jun 1974, 60–64.

23 **Soika, C. V.** Combatting osteoporosis. [Diet and exercise to counteract.] American Journal of Nursing, 73 (7), Jul 1973, 1193–1197.

24 **Wright, V. and others** Structure and function of joints. Nursing Mirror, 138, 26 Apr 1974, 70–73.

b BACK DISORDERS (Includes surgery; see also Nurses' back problems, Lifting patients)

1 **Amundsen, M. A.** A look at the back: a clinical review. Occupational Health Nursing, 21 (10), Oct 1973, 21–24.

2 **Barnes, J.** Backache in women. Nursing Mirror, 134, 31 Mar 1972, 28–29.

3 **Bell, E. J.** Laminectomy. Nursing Mirror, 133, 3 Sep 1971, 13–16.

4 **Brannon, M.** The problem back service. [Special unit for patients with prolonged chronic back disabilities.] American Journal of Nursing, 75 (8), Aug 1975, 1295–1297.

5 **Carbary, L. J.** Low back pain. Nursing Care, 7 (8), Aug 1974, 12–15.

6 **Cooper, S. B.** Low back pain caused by rupturing of the nucleus pulposus. ONA Journal, 2 (9), Sep 1975, 224–230.

7 **Evans, C.** Chemonucleolysis. [Injecting chymopapain into the nucleus pulposus of a ruptured intervertebral disc.] Nursing Times, 71, 25 Sep 1975, 1539–1541.

8 **Golding, D. N.** Acute backache. Nursing Times, 70, 7 Feb 1974, 184–185.

9 **Harrold, A. J.** Laminectomy for disc disorders. Nursing Times, 67, 8 Apr 1971, 406–408.

10 **Higgins, C.** Oh, my aching back. Occupational Health Nursing, 21 (1), Jan 1973, 9–11.

11 Hodgson, S. Anatomy of back pain. Occupational Health, 25 (1), Jan 1973, 9–12.

12 Huncke, B. H. and Wallen, J. A. Chemonucleolysis – promising treatment for disc disease. RN Magazine, 36 (12), Dec 1973, OR3 – OR4, OR6.

13 Lettin, A. W. F. Back injury. Surgical treatment of low back pain. Nursing Times, 70, 7 Nov 1974, 1732–1735.

14 Maddison, R. Nursing care study. Prolapsed intervertebral disc. Nursing Times, 70, 18 Apr 1974, 585–587.

15 Mulhall, C. Nursing care study. Back pain – and a laminectomy operation. Australian Nurses' Journal, 2 (5), Nov 1972, 27–29.

16 ONA Journal The psychological evaluation and treatment of the chronic back pain patient: a new approach. ONA Journal 2 (7), Jul 1975, 163–165.

17 Stuart, E. Persistent dislocation of cervical vertebrae 5 and 6. Nursing Times, 68, 2 Nov 1972, 1376–1378.

18 Twomey, M. R. Recent advances in the treatment of spinal deformities. Nursing Times, 69, 20 Sep 1973, 1216–1219.

19 Warr, A. C. Acute low back pain. Nursing Mirror, 137, 14 Sep 1973, 47–49.

20 Whincup, M. Back injuries and legal remedies. Occupational Health, 23 (4), Apr 1971, 120–123.

21 Wiener, C. L. Pain assessment on an orthopedic ward. [Assessment of the degree of low back pain.] Nursing Outlook, 23 (8), Aug 1975, 508–516.

c NEUROMUSCULAR DISORDERS (Includes myasthenia gravis and muscular dystrophy)

1 Blount, M. and Kinney, A. B. Myasthenia gravis: nursing essentials. Journal of Practical Nursing, 22 (6), Jun 1972, 26–32.

2 Gardner-Medwin, D. Children with neuromuscular disease. Muscular Dystrophy Group of Great Britain, 1974.

3 Lange, M. J. Myasthenia gravis. Nursing Times, 70, 29 Aug 1974, 1345–1347.

4 Liverani, L. and Osserman, R. S. Myasthenia gravis: a nursing care plan. Nursing Clinics of North America, 7 (1), Mar 1972, 185–195.

5 Matthews, W. B. Myasthenia gravis. Nursing Times, 71, 13 Nov 1975, 1807–1809.

6 Muscular Dystrophy Group of Great Britain The muscular dystrophy handbook. The Group, 1975.

7 Myasthenia Gravis Foundation Myasthenia gravis: a manual for the nurse. New York: The Foundation, 1975.

8 Nursing Times Myasthenia gravis – a personal account. Nursing Times, 71, 13 Nov 1975, 1809–1812.

9 Skirm, L. Myasthenia gravis. A time of quiet desperation. Journal of Practical Nursing, 25 (12), Dec 1975, 21–23, 35.

10 Stackhouse, J. Myasthenia gravis. Canadian Nurse, 69 (12), Dec 1973, 28–31.

11 Turner, P. A. Case study. Muscular dystrophy. [The role of the district nurse.] District Nursing, 15 (7), Oct 1972, 147–149.

d RHEUMATIC DISEASES

1 Ansell, B. M. Rheumatoid arthritis – medical management. Nursing Mirror, 133, 10 Sep 1971; 20–23.

2 Ansell, B. M. Still's disease. Nursing Mirror, 134, 3 Mar 1972, 36–41.

3 Ansell, B. M. Still's disease. Nursing Times, 69, 10 May 1973, 596–600.

4 Arden, G. P. Surgical treatment of Still's disease. Nursing Mirror, 138, 31 May 1974, 62–67.

5 Arthritis Foundation. Allied Health Professions Section Arthritis manual for allied health professionals. New York: The Foundation, 1973.

6 Barnes, C. G. Treatment of gout. Nursing Mirror, 136, 6 Apr 1973, 21–24.

7 Block, S. R. Juvenile rheumatoid arthritis. Journal of Practical Nursing, 24 (12), Dec 1974, 20–23.

8 Boyle, M. T. and Kaufman, A. Strep screening to prevent rhematic fever. [Health education program using student nurses needing clinical community experience.] American Journal of Nursing, 75 (9), Sep 1975, 1487–1488.

9 Brewerton, D. HL-A 27 and arthritis, [Hereditary factors in rheumatic diseases.] Nursing Mirror, 141, 17 Jul 1975, 54–55.

10 Broadley, H. M. Management of the foot in the rheumatoid arthritis. British Journal of Occupational Therapy, 37 (1), Jan 1974, 4–9.

11 Brooks, P. M. and Stephens, M. E. B. How safe are anti-rheumatic drugs? A study of possible iatrogenic deaths in patients with rheumatoid arthritis. Health Bulletin, 33 (3), May 1975, 108–111.

12 Chobin, N. and others Strep screening to prevent rheumatic fever. From project to ongoing program. [Three year project using school nurses.] Amerian Journal of Nursing, 75 (9), Sep 1975, 1489–1490.

13 Coleman, V. The top drugs. Indocid – combating arthritic pains. Nursing Times, 69, 17 May 1973, 648.

14 Cooper, P. Progress in therapeutics. Treatment of rheumatic disease. Midwife, Health Visitor and Community Nurse, 11 (5), May 1975, 155.

15 Doyle, E. F. Rheumatic fever – a continuing problem. Cardiovascular Nursing, 10 (4), Jul/Aug 1974, 17–21.

16 Feeney, R. Preventing rheumatic fever in school children. American Journal of Nursing, 73 (2), Feb 1973, 265.

17 Grahame, R. Rheumatoid disease. 1. Clinical aspects. Nursing Times, 67, 3 Jun 1971, 664–667.

18 Grahame, R. Rheumatoid disease. 2. Caring for patients. Nursing Times, 67, 10 Jun 1971, 701–704.

19 Grossman, B. J. Rheumatic fever: declining but still dreaded. Journal of Practical Nursing, 24 (2), Feb 1974, 23–26, 30.

20 Hamilton, A. The rehabilitation of the arthritic patient. Queen's Nursing Journal, 17 (7), Oct 1974, 142–146.

21 Hart, F. D. Management of patients with rheumatoid arthritis. Nursing Mirror, 132, 5 Feb 1971, 25–27.

22 Hart, F. D. Menopausal arthritis. Nursing Mirror, 132, 30 Apr 1971, 26–28.

23 Hart, F. D. Pain in osteoarthrosis. Practitioner, 212, Feb 1974, 244–250.

24 Haslock, I. and Champney, B. Osteoarthrosis. Nursing Mirror, 139, 21 Nov 1974, 57–62.

25 Haslock, I. and others Drug therapy in rheumatic disease. Nursing Mirror, 149, 24 Apr 1975, 52–57.

26 Haslock, I. and others Gout. Nursing Mirror, 140, 23 Jan 1975, 49–53.

27 Haslock, I. and others Infective arthritis. Nursing Mirror, 140, 10 Apr 1975, 54–57.

28 Haslock, I. and others Rheumatic fever. Nursing Mirror, 140, 13 Mar 1975, 50–53.

29 Helal, B. Replacement of fingers. Nursing Times, 70, 29 Aug 1974, 1348–1352.

30 Hoffman, A. L. Psychological factors associated with rheumatoid arthritis: review of the literature. Nursing Research, 23 (3), May/Jun 1974, 218–234.

31 Huskisson, E. C. and Hart, F. D. Pain threshold and arthritis. British Medical Journal, 4, 28 Oct 1972, 193–195.

32 Jessop, J. D. Rheumatoid arthritis. Nursing Mirror, 137, 13 Jul 1973, 42–46.

33 Langstaff, S. R. Nursing care study. Rheumatoid arthritis treated with penicillamine. Nursing Times, 71, 12 Jun 1975, 918–919.

34 Lewis, R. C. Home care of arthritis. Philadelphia: Lippincott, 1971.

35 Loxley, A. K. The emotional toll of crippling deformity. [Arthritis.] American Journal of Nursing, 72 (10), Oct 1972, 1839–1841.

36 McCarrick, H. Aids for the disabled. Learning to live with it. [Rheumatoid arthritis.] Nursing Times, 70, 11 Jul 1974, 1078–1081.

37 McNamee, A. Rheumatoid hand reconstruction with Swanson prosthesis. [Role of OR nurse.] Hospital Administration in Canada, 15 (2), Feb 1973, 33–34.

38 MacRae, I. Arthritis – its nature and management. Nursing Clinics of North America, 8 (4), Dec 1973, 643–652.

39 Mowat, A. G. and Davies, L. J. F. Rheumatoid arthritis 1. Some aspects of current medical treatment. Nursing Times, 71, 4 Sep 1975, 1400–1401.

40 Mowat, A. G. and Davies, L. J. F. Rheumatoid arthritis. 2. Some aspects of current surgical treatment. Nursing Times, 71, 4 Sep 1975, 1402–1405.

41 Nicolle, F. V. and Calnan, J. S. Artificial finger joints for rheumatoid arthritis. NATNews, 8 (2), Summer 1971, 8–9.

42 O'Dell, A. J. Hot packs for morning joint stiffness, for patients with arthritis. [A study which illustrates the value of applying research methods to aspects of patient care.] American Journal of Nursing, 75 (6), Jun 1975, 986–987.

43 Pendleton, T. and Grossman, B. J. Rehabilitating children with inflammatory joint disease. American Journal of Nursing 74 (12) Dec 1974, 2223–2226.

44 Pigett, D. C. Still's disease. [A case study by a student nurse.] New Zealand Nursing Journal, 67 (12), Dec 1974, 19–20.

45 Ruffell, J. and Honywood, H. The team approach to arthritic diseases. Practice Team, 32, Jan 1974, 6, 8; 33, Feb 1974, 2, 4, 6.

46 Schissel, C. The needs of the occupational health nurse in relation to arthritis. Occupational Health Nursing, 22 (2), Feb 1974, 17–19.

47 Scott, J. T. The fight against the rheumatic diseases. Nursing Mirror, 138, 26 Apr 1974, 66–68.

48 Scott, M. M. Diagnosis of rheumatoid arthritis. Bedside Nurse, 4 (5) May 1971, 10–13.

49 Spinks, E. The patient's viewpoint. [A nurse who is an arthritic.] Rehabilitation, 95, Oct/Dec 1975, 33–34.

50 Thomas, B. J. Recognizing and treating arthritis in the young. RN Magazine, 37 (9), Sep 1974, 64–68.

51 Weaver, A. L. Management of rheumatoid arthritis. Bedside Nurse, 4 (5), May 1971, 14–18.

52 Wright, V. Oiling human joints. Nursing Mirror, 133, 23 Jul 1971, 30–33.

53 Wright, V. and others Rheumatic diseases in the community. Nursing Mirror, 139, 17 Oct 1974, 56–60.

54 Wright, V. and others The surgery of arthritis. Nursing Mirror, 141, 17 Jul 1975, 50–53.

e SPINAL DISEASES

1 Cyriax, J. Cervical spondylosis. Butterworths, 1971.

2 Gumpel, J. M. Ankylosing spondylitis. Nursing Times, 70, 22 Aug 1974, 1308–1310.

3 Hart, F. D. Ankylosing spondylitis. Nursing Mirror, 133, 2 Jul 1971, 23–26.

4 Moll, J. M. H. Ankylosing spondylitis. Nursing Times, 69, 2 Aug 1973, 985–988.

5 Raynolds, N. Teaching parents home care after surgery for scoliosis. American Journal of Nursing, 74, Jun 1974, 1090–1092.

6 Reid, U. V. Screening for adolescent idiopathic scoliosis. Canadian Nurse, 71 (11), Nov 1975, 13–15.

7 Sells, C. J. and May, E. A. Scoliosis screening in public schools. American Journal of Nursing, 74 (1), ᵀan 1974, 60–62.

8 Simmons, E. H. and Brown, M. E. Surgery and kyphosis in ankylosing spondylitis. Canadian Nurse, 68 (5), May 1972, 24–29.

9 Wilkinson, M., editor Cervical spondylosis. Nursing Mirror, 133, 29 Oct 1971, 30–32.

10 Williams, E. Syringomyelia and its surgical treatment. Nursing Times, 69, 24 May 1973, 662–665.

11 Wright, V. Ankylosing spondylitis. Nursing Mirror, 141, 16 Oct 1975, 66–68.

f CHIROPODY

1 Bender, M. P. and Johnston Elderly problem clients in chiropody. Chiropodist, 30 (11), Nov 1975, 307–311.

2 Brodie, B. S. Aspects of pain. [Implications for chiropody.] Chiropodist, 30 (12), Dec 1975, 334–337.

3 Carbary, L. J. Foot problems. Nursing Care, 8, (6) Jun 1975, 10–14, 16.

4 Cawley, M. I. D. and Smidt, L. A. The physical care of the rheumatoid foot. Chiropodist, 29 (11), Nov 1974, 345–354.

5 Denvir, V. J. A school foot health service after ten years. Community Medicine, 126 (14), 1 Oct 1971, 185–188; Chiropodist, 27 (8), Aug 1972, 291–301.

6 French, G. J. Chiropody and the rheumatic patient. Chiropodist, 29 (10), Oct 1974, 315–323.

7 French, G. J. The professions supplementary to medicine. Chiropody. Nursing Mirror, 141, 30 Oct 1975, 54–56.

8 Ivers, J. H. B. and Gardiner, R. Feet of school children. Health and Social Service Journal, 83, 21 Jul 1973, 1641–1643.

9 Nott, M. G. Painful feet. Nursing Times, 69, 13 Sep 1973, 1190–1191.

10 Robb, S. Bunion surgery: appropriate client teaching can shorten the convalescent and rehabilitation period. American Journal of Nursing, 74 (12), Dec 1974, 2181–2184.

11 Robb, S. Bunion surgery. Canadian Nurse, 71 (8), Aug 1975, 40–44.

12 Samman, P. D. Fungal feet. Nursing Mirror, 138, 29 Mar 1974, 42–44.

13 Swallow, A. W. Feet in winter. [Chilblains.] Queen's Nursing Journal, 17 (8), Nov 1974, 173–174.

14 Wildbore, H. Children's feet. Mother and Child, 44 (5), Sep/Oct 1972, 13–17.

15 Witting, M. R. The place of chiropody in the National Health Service. Community Health, 4 (6), May/Jun 1973, 290–293.

92 ORTHOPAEDICS

a GENERAL AND NURSING

1 Bosanko, L. A. Immediate postoperative prosthesis. American Journal of Nursing, 71 (2), Feb 1971, 280–283.

2 Brown, S. Orthopedic nursing. 1. Easing the burden of traction and casts. RN Magazine, 38 (2), Feb 1975, 36–41.

3 Cresswell, P. M. Nursing care study. Total shoulder replacement. Nursing Times, 70, 18 Apr 1974, 593–594.

4 Griffin, W. and others Group exercise for patients with limited motion. [In an orthopaedic unit.] American Journal of Nursing, 71 (9), Sep 1971, 1742–1743.

5 Guy, F. M. Implants used in orthopaedic surgery. Nursing Times, 68, 20 Apr 1972, 463–466; 27 Apr 1972, 500–503.

6 Helal, B. Joint replacement. Nursing Mirror, 135, 1 Sep 1972, 18–21.

7 Hogberg, A. Orthopedic nursing. 2. Preventing orthopedic complications. RN Magazine, 38 (3), Mar 1975, 34–37.

8 Jones, S. L. Orthopedic injuries: illness and deviance. American Journal of Nursing, 75 (11), Nov 1975, 2030–2033.

9 Lanham, R. H. Surgery of the foot: essentials of nursing care. Journal of Practical Nursing, 22 (11), Nov 1972, 22–24, 34.

10 Little, J. M. An immediate prosthesis. Nursing Mirror, 133, 1 Oct 1971, 17–19.

11 Moerane, H. P. I. Report of a course in orthopaedic nursing undertaken at the Robert and Agnes Hunt Orthopaedic Hospital, Shropshire, England. [Joint Board of Clinical Nursing Studies post registration course.] SA Nursing Journal, 42 (11), Nov 1975, 17.

12 Morris, R. Planning the care of the orthopedic patient. Nursing Care, 8 (1), Jan 1975, 19–21.

13 Murray, R. I. Superb orthopaedic centre for Musgrave. Nursing Mirror, 132, 26 Mar 1971, 34–37.

14 Organ, P. M. Nursing care study: correction of pectus excavatum. Nursing Mirror, 134, 30 Jun 1972, 29–31.

15 Parks, V. J. M. Arthroscopy. NATNews, 12 (9), Dec 1975, 8.

16 Pope, D. P. Orthopaedic nursing. Nursing Times, 68, 9 Mar 1972, Occ. papers, 37–39.

17 Powell, M. Orthopaedic nursing 11. Nursing Mirror, 133, 6 Aug 1971, 15–21.

18 RN Magazine Orthopedic nurses, 1200 strong, plan first national congress. RN Magazine, 36 (10), Oct 1973, OR 21.

19 Roaf, R. and Hodkinson, L. J. Textbook of orthopaedic nursing. 2nd ed. Oxford: Blackwell, 1975.

20 Sankaran, B. Modern nursing care in orthopedics – some facets. Nursing Journal of India, 44 (8), Aug 1973, 269–270, 278.

21 Schubert, W. and Gunn, N. Adapting nursing histories for orthopedics. ONA Journal, 1 (4), Nov 1974, 96–97.

22 Smith, C. Closed injuries of the ankle. Nursing Times, 69, 28 Jun 1973, 820–825.

23 Trantham, S. Behavioural objectives for orthopedic nursing personnel. ONA Journal, 2 (3), Mar 1975, 66–69; (4), Apr 1975, 87–90.

24 Vorhees, J. Orthopedic nursing. 3. The lingering danger of head injuries. RN Magazine, 38 (4), Apr 1975, 43–45.

25 Webb, K. J. Early assessment of orthopedic injuries [to prevent permanent disabilities]. American Journal of Nursing, 74 (6), Jun 1974, 1048–1052.

26 Wells, L. B. Seven steps to take in orthopedic emergencies. RN Magazine, 37 (10), Oct 1974, OR 14, OR 18, OR 20, OR 22.

b CHILDREN

1 Dunn, B. H. Common orthopedic problems of children. Pediatric Nursing, 1 (6), Nov/Dec 1975, 7–10.

2 Fixsen, J. A. Common postural deformities in children. Nursing Times, 68, 31 Aug 1972, 1086–1088.

3 Fixsen, J. A. Orthopaedic examination of the newborn. Nursing Times, 139, 31 Oct 1974, 57–60.

4 Hawkins, D. Orthopaedic adventure in Ghana. [Voluntary service overseas at an orthopaedic training centre for handicapped children.] Nursing Mirror, 139, 2 Aug 1974, 66–68.

5 Johnson, J. E. and others Altering children's distress behaviour during orthopedic cast removal. [Testing the hypothesis that discrepancy between expected and experienced physical sensations causes distress.] Nursing Research, 24 (6), Nov/Dec 1975, 404–410.

6 Nursing Mirror A symposium on diseases of the hip in childhood. Nursing Mirror, 140, 6 Mar 1975, 45–63.

7 Rankin, E. A. Aspects of orthopaedic management of the hospitalized child. Journal of Practical Nursing, 24 (12), Dec 1974, 24–25.

8 Roberts, G. C. L. Developments in orthopaedic surgery in childhood. Nursing Mirror, 135, 11 Aug 1972, 33–35.

9 Savage, J. H. The red arrow. [Trolley developed in the Paediatric Unit, Book Hospital, as a means of self propulsion for children following hip treatment.] Nursing Times, 71, 20 Nov 1975, 1869.

10 Walker, G. Minor orthopaedic problems of childhood. Chiropodist, 29 (7), Jul 1974, 197–209.

c CONGENITAL MALFORMATIONS

1 Boshoff, C. Congenital dislocation of the hip. SA Nursing Journal, 41 (5), May 1974, 16–17, 19–20.

2 Brown, A. Congenital dislocation of the hip. Nursing Times, 70, 25 Apr 1974, 618–621.

3 Cartner, M. J. Congenital club foot. Nursing Mirror, 141, 20 Nov 1975, 58–62.

4 Catterall, A. The management of congenital dislocation of the hip. Nursing Mirror, 140, 6 Mar 1975, 45–49.

5 Cote, D. M. Independence for phocometic children. [Thalidomide children in Canada.] Canadian Nurse, 69 (12), Dec 1973, 19–24.

6 Dunn, P. M. Congenital postural deformities: perinatal associations. Nursing Mirror, 136, 27 Apr 1973, 26–29.

7 Edwards, D. H. Problems of children with dysmelia. [Congenital deficiencies of the limbs.] Nursing Mirror, 138, 3 May 1974, 64–66.

8 Gifford, M. E. A do-it-yourself CDH pram. Nursing Times, 67, 1 Jul 1971, 806.

9 Gray, D. Williams' rods: insertion for osteogenesis imperfecta. Nursing Times, 69, 22 Nov 1973, 1560–1561.

10 Justis, E. J. Congenital anomalies of the hand. Journal of Practical Nursing, 22 (11), Nov 1972, 18–21.

11 Kemp, H. B. S. Perthes' disease. Nursing Mirror, 140, 6 Mar 1975, 58–63.

12 Paterson, C. R. Osteogenesis imperfecta. Midwives Chronicle, 87, Nov 1974, 380–382.

13 Richards, H. J. Deformities of the feet. [Congenital abnormalities.] Queen's Nursing Journal, 17 (2), Feb 1975, 239–241.

14 Smith, C. Talipes. 1. Anatomy of the foot. [Congenital abnormality of the locomotor system.] Nursing Times, 71, 23 Jan 1975, 138–139.

15 Smith, C. Talipes. 2. Clinical features of talipes equinovarus. Nursing Times, 71, 30 Jan 1975, 176–177.

16 Smith, C. Talipes. 3. Nursing care of a child wearing a splint. Nursing Times, 71, 6 Feb 1975, 222–223.

17 Smith, C. Talipes. 4. Further types of talipes deformity. Nursing Times, 71, 13 Feb 1975, 270.

18 Smithells, R. W. Defects and disabilities in thalidomide children. British Medical Journal, 1, 3 Feb 1973, 269–272.

19 Stewart, J. M. The story of an incredible journey. [Education of a limbless child.] SA Nursing Journal, 41 (2), Feb 1974, 24–26.

20 Sundaram, S. Club foot. Management and nursing responsibilities [at the Government General Hospital, Madras.] Nursing Journal of India, 65 (9), Sep 1974, 237, 250–251.

21 Swinson, N. Congenital subluxation of the hip – nursed at home. Nursing Times, 68 (1), 6 Jan 1972, 26–27.

22 Young, M. Nursing treatment of congenital dislocation of the hip. Nursing Mirror, 140, 6 Mar 1975, 50–51.

d AMPUTATION

1 Anders, R. L. and Purol, R. M. Amputee discussion program. [Psychiatric treatment of army amputee patients.] Journal of Psychiatric Nursing, 10 (4), Jul/Aug 1972, 12–15.

2 Browse, N. L. Amputation of the lower limb. Nursing Mirror, 138, 7 Jun 1974, 63–65.

3 Chilvers, A. S. and Browse, N. L. The social fate of the amputee. Lancet, 2, 27 Nov 1971, 1192–1193.

4 Clarke-Williams, M. J. Lower limb amputation in the elderly. Nursing Times, 70, 12 Dec 1974, 1939–1941.

5 Davis, B. C. Rehabilitation of the lower-limb amputee. Nursing Mirror, 138, 7 Jun 1974, 70–73.

6 Hamilton, A. The management of the geriatric amputee. Rehabilitation, no. 89, Apr/Jun 1974, 5–9.

7 Hamilton, A. The rehabilitation of the geriatric amputee. Rehabilitation, no. 87, Oct/Dec 1973, 5–8.

8 Hamilton, E. A. and Nichols, P. J. R. Rehabilitation of the elderly lower-limb amputee. British Medical Journal, 2, 8 Apr 1972, 95–99.

9 Harding, J. M. Amputation of the lower limb. Nursing Times, 70, 4 Jul 1974, 1025–1027.

10 Humm, W. Care of the lower limb amputee. [Nursing care and rehabilitation.] Nursing Times, 70, 12 Dec 1974, 1935–1938.

11 Jeglijewski, J. M. Target: outside world. Physical and psychological wounds must heal if the amputee, civilian or soldier, is to have a successful transition from hospital to everyday living. American Journal of Nursing, 73 (6), Jun 1973, 1024–1027.

12 Jones, C. Nursing care study. Above knee amputation. Nursing Mirror, 138, 7 Jun 1974, 77–80.

13 McVittie, C. K. Nursing care study. Traumatic amputation of the right arm. Nursing Mirror, 141, 28 Aug 1975, 47–48.

14 Parkes, C. M. Reaction to the loss of a limb. [Report of a DHSS research project.] Nursing Mirror, 140, 2 Jan 1975, 36–40.

15 Saylor, Rev. D. E. The disorientated patient. Reorienting reactions: phantom limb. Journal of Practical Nursing, 23 (1), Jan 1973, 24–25.

16 Scott, R. N. Myo-electric control – one more aid for the amputee. Canadian Nurse, 67 (4), Apr 1971, 44–48.

17 Stuart, E. Nursing care study. Amputation for osteogenic sarcoma. Nursing Times, 68, 16 Nov 1972, 1453–1454.

18 Weiss, M. Physiologic amputation. Rehabilitation, no. 82, Jul/Sep 1972, 17–26.

19 Welch, D. C. and Helsby, R. Lower limb amputations in the elderly: an analysis of physical and social conditions. Nursing Times, 68, 15 Jun 1972, 743–744.

20 Wild, G. B. Amputation hastens return to work. Occupational Health, 24 (3), Mar 1972, 97.

21 Wood, M. A. Nursing care of the elderly lower-limb amputee. Nursing Mirror, 138, 7 Jun 1974, 66–67.

22 Zalewski, N. and others Hemipelvectomy. The triump of Ms. A. American Journal of Nursing, 73 (12), Dec 1973, 2073–2077.

e FRACTURES

1 Adamson, P. D. An accident at home. [Fractured femur.] Nursing Times, 69, 9 Aug 1973, 1025–1026.

2 Bradley, D. Common fractures near to the elbow joint. Nursing Times, 70, 5 Sep 1974, 1381–1384.

3 Bradley, D. Fractures of the ankle joint. Nursing Times, 68, 7 Sep 1972, 1115–1119.

4 Bradley, D. Fractures of the patella. Nursing Times, 67, 9 Dec 1971, 1531–1534.

5 Bradley, D. Fractures of the pelvis. Nursing Times, 68, 30 Mar 1972, 376–379.

6 Brown, A. Supracondylar fractures of the humerus. Nursing Times, 71, 18 Dec 1975, 2016–2018.

7 Campbell, W. Fractures of the bones of the face. Nursing Times, 70, 21 Nov 1974, 1813–1816.

8 Devas, B. Stress fractures in athletes. Nursing Times, 67, 25 Feb 1971, 227–232.

9 Dwyer, N. St. J. P. Engineers solve long-bone fracture problem. [East Birmingham Hospital's use of external compression clamps.] Nursing Times, 69, 29 Nov 1973, 1601–1602.

10 Esah, M. Fractures and the tibia and fibula. Nursing Times, 68, 2 Mar 1972, 258–261.

11 Jones, G. J. Nursing care study. Intensive care following multiple fractures. Nursing Mirror, 137, 10 Aug 1973, 35–38.

12 Leonard, J. Nursing care study. Dislocated axis [in a two-year old girl]. Nursing Times, 70, 10 Oct 1974, 1576–1577.

13 Lindsay, T. Nursing care study. A new lease of life for Mrs. H. [Geriatric patient with a fractured lumber vertebrae.] Nursing Mirror, 141, 24 Jul 1975, 72–74.

14 May, A. Internal fixation of fractures: improvements in engineering and aseptic techniques. Nursing Times, 70, 14 Nov 1974, 1777–1779.

15 Nursing Mirror Pseudarthrosis of the tibia. Nursing Mirror, 134, 2 Jun 1972, 13.

16 Percy, A. J. Slipping of the upper femoral epiphysis. Nursing Mirror, 140, 6 Mar 1975, 52–56.

17 Rowe, J. W. Fracture of the olecranon. Nursing Times, 70, 28 Nov 1974, 1854–1855.

18 Rowe, N. L. and Beetham, M. D. Fractures of the mandible. Nursing Times, 67, 2 Sep 1971, 1083–1086.

19 Ryan, J. Compression in bone healing: rigid fixation of bone fragments promotes healing. American Journal of Nursing, 74 (11), Nov 1974, 1998–1999.

20 Simpson, H. A. S. Fractured femur and patella complicated by cerebral fat embolism. Nursing Times, 68, 13 Apr 1972, 431–434.

21 Smith, C. Nursing care study. Colles' fracture. Nursing Mirror, 139, 26 Sep 1974, 76–79.

22 Smith, C. Supracondylar fractures of the humerus. Nursing Times, 69, 27 Sep 1973, 1244–1247.

23 Stone, K. H. Fractures of the shaft of the humerus. Nursing Mirror, 134, 30 Jun 1972, 26–27.

24 Sweetman, R. J. Avulsion fracture of the lesser trochanter. Nursing Times, 68, 27 Jan 1972, 122–123.

25 Thomas, T. G. and Stevens, R. S. Social effects of fractures of the neck of the femur. British Medical Journal, 3, 17 Aug 1974, 456–458.

26 Twist, P. Reduction of fractures – the valium and pethidine technique. Nursing Times, 69, 15 Mar 1973, 344–345.

27 Young, M. Nursing care of slipped femoral epiphysis. Nursing Mirror, 140, 6 Mar 1975, 57.

f PLASTER CASTS, SPLINTS AND APPLIANCES

1 Bradley, D. Checking a plaster – how and why. [Checking a plaster cast the day after its application.] Nursing Times, 70, 1 Aug 1974, 1190–1192.

2 Carpenter, E. M. Equipment for children in plaster. Occupational Therapy, 35 (10), Oct 1972, 749–756.

3 Frankland, J. C. and others Polyurethane foam splintage. A new technique. Practitioner, 209, Dec 1972, 831–834.

4 Johnson, H. W. Thomas's splint with a difference. Nursing Mirror, 132, 12 Mar 1971, 32.

5 Lancet Acrylic cement and the cardiovascular system. [Report of working party on acrylic cement in orthopaedic surgery.] Lancet, 2, 26 Oct 1974, 1002–1004.

6 Metcalfe, J. W. and Johnson, R. The Liverpool jacket. [Turnbuckle collars incorporated into a plaster of Paris body case in the postoperative management of spinal surgery.] British Journal of Clinical Practice, 25 (11), Nov 1971, 496–498.

7 Roberts, E. Polyurethane foam leg troughs. Nursing Times, 67, 15 Apr 1971, 447–448.

8 Scrutton, D. Orthopaedic splints and appliances. Nursing Mirror, 139, 31 Oct 1974, 73–75.

9 Shorland, M. A. Southlands temporary walking aid. Nursing Mirror, 133, 13 Aug 1971, 18–20.

10 Williams, M. An aid to patient care. [Oswestry abduction working splint used after Charnley low friction arthroplasty.] Nursing Times, 69, 15 Feb 1973, 214–215.

g TRACTION

1 Courtial, D. C. How to care for the patient with pelvic traction. Hospital Management, 112 (3), Aug 1971, 16.

2 Dimoh, J. H. and Donahoo, C. Nursing care of the patient in traction. Journal of Practical Nursing, 22 (9), Sep 1972, 18–19, 30, 32.

3 Hilt, N. T. Use of the Bradford frame in pediatric orthopedic nursing care. ONO Journal, 1 (1), Aug 1974, 10–15.

4 Law, John Nursing care study. Use of Dunlop traction. Nursing Times, 71, 3 Apr 1975, 537–539.

5 McArdle, D. Recent advances in skin traction. Australian Nurses' Journal, 1 (11), May 1972, 31–32.

6 Owen, R. Indications and contra-indications for limb traction. Physiotherapy, 58 (2), Feb 1972, 44–45.

7 Perkins, G. The George-Perkins traction. World Medicine, 9 (9), 30 Jan 1974, 17–19, 21.

8 Powell, M. Application of limb traction and nursing management. Physiotherapy, 58 (2), Feb 1972, 46–51.

9 Powell, M. Limb traction: some aspects of nursing management. Nursing Mirror, 137, 27 Jul 1973, 26–32.

10 Savage, J. H. A traction frame for a child's cot. Nursing Times, 70, 6 Jun 1974, 880–881.

h HIP AND KNEE JOINT REPLACEMENT SURGERY

1 Bennage, B. A. and Cummings, M. E. Nursing the patient undergoing total hip arthroplasty. Nursing Clinics of North America, 8 (1), Mar 1973, 107–116.

2 Bridgwater, S. E. Nursing care study. Charnley hip replacement. Nursing Times, 71, 26 Jun 1975, 1000–1002.

3 Cunningham, L. Bilateral Charnley's total hip replacement. Australian Nurses' Journal, 1 (12), Jun 1972, 42–44.

4 Davis, R. W. Surgery for osteoarthritis of the hip. Bedside Nurse, 5 (5), May 1972, 24–26.

5 Donn, M. C. Nursing care study. Right total hip replacement. Nursing Times, 70, 24 Oct 1974, 1654–1657.

6 Eyre, M. K. Total hip replacement. American Journal of Nursing, 71 (7), Jul 1971, 1384–1387.

7 Graves, S. and Vincent, S. Total hip replacement is a family affair. RN Magazine, 34 (6), Jun 1971, 35–41.

8 Gwilliam, S. Total knee arthroplasty. Canadian Nurse, 70 (9), Sep 1974, 33–36.

9 Harrold, A. J. Internal derangements of the knee. Nursing Times, 67, 16 Dec 1971, 1575–1577.

10 Harwood, J. Nursing care study. The surgical correction of genu valgum. [Knock knee.] Nursing Times, 69, 18 Oct 1973, 1372–1373.

11 ___ · C. M. E. Nursing care study. Complications after hip replacement. Nursing Times, 71, 11 Dec 1975, 1973–1974.

12 Johnson, C. F. and Convery, F. R. Preventing emboli after total hip replacement. American Journal of Nursing, 75 (5), May 1975, 804–806.

13 Krystowski, K. and Nelson, C. L. Total hip-replacement arthroplasty: postoperative care of patient. Hospital Topics, 49 (11), Nov 1971, 69–72.

14 Marmor, L. Surgical insertion of the modular knee. [Including the roles of OR nurses.] RN Magazine, 36 (9), Sep 1973, OR 1 – OR 6.

15 Molinari, M. G. and others Total hip replacement: special guidelines for a special procedure. Journal of Practical Nursing, 21 (8), Aug 1971, 20–21, 30.

16 Monty, C. P. Arthroplasty. [Includes history of hip joint replacement.] Nursing Mirror, 137, 31 Aug 1973, 24–26.

17 Monty, C. P. The history of arthroplasty. NAT-News, 9 (5). Oct 1972, 30, 32, 34.

18 Park, V. J. M. Arthroscopy. [Endoscopic examination of the knee joint.] Nursing Times, 71, 25 Dec 1975, 2058–2059.

19 Ramsden, V. J. Pre and post-operative assessment of hip function. Occupational Therapy, 36 (2), Feb 1973, 147–149.

20 Ring, P. A. Total replacement of the hip. Nursing Mirror, 132, 11 Jun 1971, 20–23.

21 Shiers, L. G. P. Total replacement of knee joint. Nursing Times, 69, 8 Nov 1973, 1477–1479.

22 Shoemaker, R. R. Total knee replacement. Procedure and results. Nursing Clinics of North America, 8 (1), Mar 1973, 117–125.

23 Short, M. A. Nursing care study. Charnley arthroplasty. Nursing Mirror, 136, 1 Jun 1973, 22–25.

24 Thomas, B. J. Total knee: new surgical miracle. [Includes two histories.] RN Magazine, 36 (9), Sep 1973, 35–39.

25 Townley, C. and Hill, L. Total knee replacement. American Journal of Nursing, 74 (9), Sep 1974, 1612–1617.

26 Twomey, M. R. Triple tenodesis of the knee. Nursing Times, 71, 27 Nov 1975, 1889–1891.

27 Wilmot, A. Total knee joint replacement. Nursing Times, 69, 17 May 1973, 626–628.

93 NERVOUS SYSTEM. 1.

a NEUROLOGY AND NURSING

1 Bell, M. and others Nursing involvement with monitoring of ICP. [Intracranial pressure.] Journal of Neurosurgical Nursing, 7 (1), Jul 1975, 28–31.

2 Bickerstaff, E. R. Neurology for nurses. 2nd ed. English Universities Press, 1971. (Modern nursing series.)

3 Blackwell, C. A. PEG and angiography: a patient's sensations. [Reactions to carotid arteriogram and pneumoencephalogram.] American Journal of Nursing, 75 (2), Feb 1975, 264–266.

4 Carini, E. and Owens, G. Neurological and neurosurgical nursing. 6th ed. St. Louis: Mosby, 1974.

5 Gibson, J. A guide to the nervous system. 3rd ed. Faber and Faber, 1974.

6 Hewitt, W. Basic organization of a nervous system. Nursing Times, 67, 1 Jul 1971, 790–793.

7 Hewitt, W. The fate of sensory impulses. 1. Receptor organs and the reflex arc. Nursing Times, 67, 22 Jul 1971, 892–895.

8 Hewitt, W. The fate of sensory impulses. 3. The central sensory pathways. Nursing Times, 67, 29 Jul 1971, 925–927.

9 Hewitt, W. The fate of sensory impulses. 4. The special senses. The auditory and vestibular pathways. Nursing Times, 67, 5 Aug 1971, 959–962.

10 Hewitt, W. The fate of sensory impulses. 5. The visual pathways. Nursing Times, 67, 12 Aug 1971, 982–984.

11 Hewitt, W. Functional neuroanatomy. Nursing Times, 1972. [Reprint of articles in Nursing Times, Jun/Aug 1971].

12 Hewitt, W. The peripheral nervous system. 1. The cerebrospinal nervous system. Nursing Times, 67, 15 Jul 1971, 853–857.

13 Hugh, A. E. Nervous system and endocrine glands. Butterworths, 1972. (Nursing in depth series.)

14 Jeavons, P. M. Electroencephalography. Nursing Times, 67, 28 Jan 1971, 106–109.

15 Jimm, L. R. Nursing assessment of patients for increased intracranial pressure. Journal of Neurosurgical Nursing, 6 (1), Jul 1974, 27–38.

16 Jolly, V. Lumbar puncture and related tests. Butterworths, 1972. (Nursing in depth series.)

17 Langelaan, D. G. Neurological assessment. [Guidance for the nurse.] Nursing Times, 70, 17 Jan 1974, 70–72.

18 Mechner, F. and others Patient assessment: neurological examination. Programmed instruction. American Journal of Nursing, 75 (9), Sep 1975, PI 1–24; (11) Nov 1975, PI 1–24.

19 Nikas, D. L. and Konkoly, R. Nursing responsibilities in arterial and intracranial pressure monitoring. Journal of Neurosurgical Nursing, 7 (2), Dec 1975, 116–122.

20 Nursing Clinics of North America Symposium on neurologic and neurosurgical nursing. Nursing Clinics of North America, 9 (4), Dec 1974, 591–772.

21 Osoff, A. Caring for the child with familial dysautonomia. American Journal of Nursing, 75 (7), Jul 1975, 1158–1162.

22 Russo, B. A. Neurology and neurosurgical nursing continuing education review. Flushing, New York: Medical Examination Publishing Co., 1974.

23 Sandanasamy, G. and Ramamurthi, B. Utilization of patients' relatives in neurological nursing. Nursing Journal of India, 65 (5), May 1974, 137, 149.

24 Shaw, K. Some chronic neurological disorders in 1974. Queen's Nursing Journal, 17 (5), Aug 1974, 98–99, 109.

25 Shearer, D. and others Preparing a patient for EEG American Journal of Nursing, 75 (1), Jan 1975, 63–64.

26 Smelt, M. Higher nervous activity. 1. Conditioned and unconditioned reflexes. Nursing Times, 71, 14 Aug 1975, 1308–1309.

27 Smelt, M. Higher nervous activity. 2. Human behaviour. Nursing Times, 71, 21 Aug 1975, 1347–1348.

28 Smith, S. E. Drugs and the parasympathetic nervous system. Nursing Times, 68, 2 Mar 1972, 256–257.

29 Smith, S. E. How drugs act. 13. Drugs and the parasympathetic nervous system. Nursing Times, 71, 18 Sep 1975, 1505–1506.

30 Snyder, M. and Baum, R. Assessing station and gait. [A tool to evaluate neurological patients' station and gait.] American Journal of Nursing, 74 (7), Jul 1974, 1256–1257.

31 World Federation of Neurological Nurses. New Zealand Nursing Journal, 68 (7), Jul 1974, 11.

b NEUROSURGERY AND NURSING

1 Aorn Journal Issue on micro neurosurgery. AORN Journal, 20 (3), Sep 1974, 385–472.

2 Bader, D. C. H. Microtechnical nursing in neurosurgery. Journal of Neurosurgical Nursing, 7 (1), Jun 1975, 22–24.

3 Bucy, P. C. Neurosurgical nursing. Journal of Neurosurgical Nursing, 6 (1), Jul 1974, 42–46.

4 Chester, J. E. Neurosurgical instrumentation – a review and current trends. Journal of Neurosurgical Nursing, 6 (2), Dec 1974, 62–71.

5 Ehni, G. The surgical nurse and neurological surgery. Journal of Neurosurgical Nursing, 6 (1), Jul 1974, 7–13.

6 Fink, R. A. Add another: NICUs make their debut. [Neurological intensive care at Herrick Memorial Hospital, Berkeley.] RN Magazine, 38 (1), Jan 1975, ICU 8.

7 Gibson, R. M. Some recent advances in neurosurgery. Physiotherapy, 58 (11), 10 Nov 1972, 377–381.

8 Grima, M. R. Nursing care study. Bilateral cervical sympathectomy for acrocyanosis. Nursing Times, 71, 20 Nov 1975, 1850–1852.

9 Koenen, A. J. The scope of a neurosurgical unit in Australia in reference to a neurosurgical training program. Journal of Neurosurgical Nursing, 6 (2), Dec 1974, 89–91.

10 MacIntyre, M. M. J. Nursing care study. Neurosurgical emergency in early pregnancy. Nursing Times, 70, 10 Oct 1974, 1572–1575.

11 Madeja, C. Neurosurgical clinician provides continuity of care. [A patient's care from his first visit, through hospital confinement and clinic follow-up.] AORN Journal, 20 (3), Sep 1974, 426–427, 429, 432.

12 Madeja, C. and others The neurosurgical nurse as a departmental assistant. [Work at Cleveland Clinic, Ohio.] Journal of Neurosurgical Nursing, 7 (2), Dec 1975, 99–101.

13 Marshall, A. M. What are we doing? Where are we going? [Presidential address at the World Federation of Neurosurgical Nurses Congress, 1973.] Journal of Neurosurgical Nursing, 6 (1), Jul 1974, 39–41.

14 Morrison, F. Dorsal column stimulator: nursing aspects. Journal of Neurosurgical Nursing, 7 (1), Jul 1975, 18–21.

15 Odachowski, S. Cerebrospinal fluid acid base balance: importance in neurosurgical nursing. Journal of Neurosurgical Nursing, 6 (2), Dec 1974, 117–121.

16 Runnells, J. B. Adapting OR techniques to microneurosurgery. RN Magazine, 38 (8), Aug 1975, OR 1, 2, 4.

17 Stephens, O. J. and Parsons, M. C. A delicate balance: managing chronic airway obstruction in a neurosurgical patient. American Journal of Nursing, 75 (9), Sep 1975, 1492–1497.

18 White, E. H. The concept of neurosurgical care in a general hospital. Journal of Neurosurgical Nursing, 7 (2), Dec 1975, 82–86.

19 White, E. H. Observe your neurosurgical patient. Journal of Practical Nursing, 24 (8), Aug 1974, 28–29.

c NERVOUS SYSTEM DISORDERS

1 Bierbauer, E. Tips for parents of a neurologically handicapped child. American Journal of Nursing, 72 (10), Oct 1972, 1872–1874.

2 Carter, A. B. Bell's palsy. Nursing Mirror, 136, 25 May 1973, 22–24.

3 Davis, M. The Landry-Guillian Barré Syndrome. SA Nursing Journal, 52 (12), Dec 1975, 22–23.

4 Flewett, T. H. Acute polyneuritis. Nursing Times, 68, 2 Mar 1972, 266–267.

5 Heathfield, K. Peripheral neuritis. Nursing Times, 71, 24 Apr 1975, 648–650.

6 Morgan-Hughes, J. A. The Landry-Guillain Barré syndrome. Nursing Mirror, 140, 10 Apr 1975, 51–52.

7 Naiman, H. Screening for Tay-Sachs disease. [Program in Brookline to test the carrier state in married couples of child bearing age. .] American Journal of Nursing 75 (3), Mar 1975, 436–439.

8 Needham, N. E. Nursing care study. Jakob-Creutzfeld disease. Nursing Mirror, 140, 9 Jan 1975, 71–73.

9 Smith, A. J. Nursing care study. Motor neurone disease. Nursing Mirror, 140, 19 Jun 1975, 75–76.

10 Tavener, D. Bell's palsy. [Cause of illness and method of treatment.] Nursing Times, 71, 5 Jun 1975, 892–893.

11 Thompson, N. Techniques and triumphs of muscle transplantation [in treatment of Bell's palsy.] Nursing Mirror, 136, 25 May 1973, 25–27.

12 Yeoman, P. M. Traction injuries of the brachial plexus. Nursing Mirror, 132, 22 Jan 1971, 26–29.

d BRAIN DAMAGE AND DISORDERS

1 Adams, J. H. Brain damage caused by cerebral hypoxia. Nursing Times, 71, 24 Apr 1975, 654–656.

2 Bates, R. M. E. Nursing care study. Monika: a patient with viral meningitis. Nursing Mirror, 138, 5 Apr 1974, 76–78.

3 Beasley, N. Hope for brain damaged children? Nursing Mirror, 134, 30 Jun 1972, 17–19.

4 Bellam, G. The nursing challenge of the child with neurological problems: how to use toys and play to assess the neurological progress of the brain-damaged child. Nursing Forum, 11 (4), 1972, 396–418.

5 Bokhoree, L. Nursing care study. Chronic otogenic cerebral abscess. Nursing Times, 69, 22 Feb 1973, 236–237.

6 Cassidy, F. M. Adult hydrocephalus. American Journal of Nursing, 72 (3), Mar 1972, 494–499.

7 Christie, A. B. The treatment of pyogenic bacterial meningitis. Nursing Mirror, 141, 20 Nov 1975, 64–65.

8 Chubb, E. Nursing care study. Meningitis in a child. Nursing Times, 70, 25 Jul 1974, 1146–1148.

9 Cragg, C. E. Nursing care of the child with purulent meningitis. Canadian Nurse, 68 (7), Jul 1972, 27–30.

10 Cruickshank, W. M. The brain-injured child in home, school and community. British ed. Pitman, 1971.

11 Eglin, D. Nursing care study. Meningitis – a paediatric emergency. Nursing Times, 70, 11 Apr 1974, 541–544.

12 Fowler, R. S. and Fordyce, W. E. Adapting care for the brain-damaged patient. American Journal of Nursing, 72 (10), Oct 1972, 1832–1835; (11), Nov 1972, 2056–2059.

13 Fredette, S. The art of applying theory to practice. [Goldstein's holistic personality theory applied to a brain-damaged patient.] American Journal of Nursing, 74 (5), May 1974, 856–859.

14 Fretwell, J. E. Nursing care study. A child dies. [A case of glioma of the thalamus.] Nursing Times, 69, 5 Jul 1973, 867–871.

15 Furr, S. C. Subacute schlerosing panencephalitis: care of the child. American Journal of Nursing, 72 (1), Jan 1972, 93–96.

16 Gardner, H. The shattered mind: the person after brain damage. New York: Vintage Books, 1974.

17 Hayter, J. Patients who have Alzheimer's disease. American Journal of Nursing, 74 (8), Aug 1974, 1460–1463.

18 Holmes, A. E. Cerebral aneurysm. Nursing Times, 68, 22 Jun 1972, 777–780.

19 Jennett, B. and Plum, F. Persistent vegetative state after brain damage. RN Magazine, 35 (10), Oct 1972, ICU 1-2, 4.

20 Jones, A. G. Nursing implications in the administration of urea (for lowering intracranial pressure]. Journal of Neurosurgical Nursing, 7 (1), Jul 1975, 37–41.

21 Jones, C. Nursing care study. Chronic meningococcal meningitis. Nursing Mirror, 139, 2 Aug 1974, 73–76.

22 Keech, P. A. Nursing care study. Communicating hydrocephalus. Nursing Mirror, 136, 27 Apr 1973, 23–25.

23 Lamerton, R. Vegetables? [The care of brain-damaged patients.] Nursing Times, 70, 1 Aug 1974, 1184–1185.

24 Loetterle, N. and others Cerebellar stimulation: pacing the brain. [Implantation of brain pacemakers can relieve symptoms of stroke, cerebral palsy and epilepsy.] American Journal of Nursing, 75 (6), Jun 1975, 958–960.

25 Maddox, M. Subarachnoid hemorrhage. American Journal of Nursing, 74 (12), Dec 1974, 2199–2201.

26 Malembeka, G. Nursing care study. Meningitis. Nursing Times, 69, 22 Feb 1973, 241–242.

27 Meadows, S. P. Subarachnoid haemorrhage. Nursing Mirror, 132, 4 Jun 1971, 19–23.

28 Metcalfe, J. Nursing care study. Subarachnoid haemorrhage. Nursing Times, 70, 15 Aug 1974, 1264–1266.

29 Nursing Mirror Recovery following craniotomy. [Case study.] Nursing Mirror, 138, 3 May 1974, 62–63.

30 Pinel, C. Alzheimer's disease. Nursing Times, 71, 16 Jan 1975, 105–106.

31 Reeves, K. R. Beware of Reye's syndrome. [Encephalopathy with fatty degeneration of the viscera.] American Journal of Nursing, 74 (9), Sep 1974, 1621–1622.

32 Schick, C. Occult hydrocephalus in adults. Canadian Nurse, 67 (3), Mar 1971, 47–50.

33 Taylor, F. New trends in neurosurgical nursing: a discussion of continuous recording and control of ventricular fluid pressure and its significance in nursing severely brain injured patients. Hospital Administration in Canada, 16 (5), May 1974, 45–47.

34 Tolley, M. Janie remembered. [Case study of a patient with brain damage after a car accident.] American Journal of Nursing, 75 (6), Jun 1975, 984–985.

35 Williamson, S. Hydrocephalus. Nursing Times, 71, 4 Dec 1975, 1934–1936.

e UNCONSCIOUS PATIENT

1 Bracher, L. M. Nursing care study. A day lost for ever. [The care of an unconscious patient.] Nursing Mirror, 139, 9 Aug 1974, 80–82.

2 Canning, M. Care of the unconscious patient. Nursing Mirror, 139, 9 Aug 1974, 61–62.

3 Cautier-Smith, P. C. Management of prolonged coma. Nursing Times, 70, 1 Aug 1974, 1196–1198.

4 Edmondson, E. Care of the unconscious. Butterworth, 1971. (Nursing in depth series.)

5 Ellwanger, K. and Johnson, E. Caring for the comatose patient. Journal of Practical Nursing, 22 (5), May 1972, 23, 27, 30.

6 Gifford, R. M. R. and Plaut, M. R. Abnormal respiratory patterns in the comatose patient caused by intracranial dysfunction. Journal of Neurosurgical Nursing, 7 (1), Jul 1975, 57–61.

7 Teasdale, G. Acute impairment of brain function. 1. Assessing 'conscious level.' [Using the Glasgow coma scale.] Nursing Times, 71, 12 Jun 1975, 914–917.

8 Teasdale, G. and others Acute impairment of brain function. 2. Observation record chart. Nursing Times, 71, 19 Jun 1975, 972–973.

9 Teasdale, G. and Jennett, B. Assessment of coma and impaired consciousness. A practical scale. Lancet, 2, 13 Jul 1974, 81–84.

f CEREBRAL PALSY

1 Avery, M. Primary care for handicapped children. [Follow-up clinic for children with cerebral palsy.] American Journal of Nursing, 73 (4), Apr 1973, 658–661.

2 Bobath, K. Nursing the child with cerebral palsy. Nursing Mirror, 135, 29 Sep 1972, 20–23.

3 Brockley, J. and Miller, G. Feeding techniques with cerebral-palsied children. Physiotherapy, 51 (7), 10 Jul 1971, 300–308.

4 Lumsden, H. Caring for the cerebral palsy child. Morden, Surrey: Trade and Technical Press, 1971.

5 Pilling, D. The child with cerebral palsy: social, emotional and educational adjustment: an annotated bibliography. Slough, NFER Publishing, 1973, (A National Children's Bureau report.)

6 Thomas, L. Caring for the hospitalized cerebral palsy patient. Journal of Practical Nursing, 25 (12), Dec 1975, 24–25.

g EPILEPSY

1 Bagley, C. The social psychology of the child with epilepsy. Routledge, 1971.

2 Bartha, M. Chalfont Centre for epilepsy. [History and current role]. Nursing Times, 69, 15 Mar 1973, 332–335.

3 Branson, H. K. The epileptic – how you can help. RN Magazine, 35 (6), Jun 1972, 48–51, 55–56, 58.

4 Branson, H. K. The epileptic mother. Nursing Care, 6 (6), Jun 1973, 19–21.

5 Brennan, K. S. W. Epilepsy. Nursing Times, 67, 15 Apr 1971, 435–438.

6 British Medical Journal Epilepsy in the elderly. British Medical Journal, 2, 7 Jun 1975, 524.

7 Cooper, P. Progress in therapeutics. Complications in treatment of epilepsy. Midwife, Health Visitor and Community Nurse, 11 (9), Sep 1975, 307.

8 Dawson, W. The British Epilepsy Association and what it is doing for epileptics and their families. Nursing Times, 67, 15 Apr 1971, 440.

9 Epilepsy Foundation of America. The role of the nurse in the understanding and treatment of epilepsy. Washington: The Foundation, 1974.

10 Garcia, W. A. When your patient suffers a seizure. [Procedures for observing and reporting.] RN Magazine, 38 (2), Feb 1975, 45–47.

11 Harkness, L. Bringing epilepsy out of the closet. [Stigma of epilepsy and organization of group of epileptics to fight discrimination.] American Journal of Nursing, 74 (5), May 1974, 875–876.

12 Holt, J. A. Caring for epileptics. [A nurse examines the needs and problems of epileptics by a questionnaire to teenage girls.] Nursing Times, 71, 24 Jul 1975, 1172–1174.

13 Jeavons, P. M. Television epilepsy. Nursing Mirror, 135, 18 Aug 1972, 24–25.

14 Koshy, K. T. A comprehensive look at epilepsy. Nursing Times, 71, 26 Jun 1975, 1013–1015.

15 Laidlaw, J. Epilepsy and environment. [Roles of Chalfont Centre for Epilepsy and National Hospital-Chalfont Special Centre.] Nursing Times, 71, 16 Jan 1975, 119–120.

16 Laidlaw, J. Living with epilepsy – a case history. [Young woman in Chalfont Centre for Epilepsy.] Nursing Times, 70, 19 Sep 1974, 1456–1458.

17 Manuel, J. Epilepsy in industry. Occupational Health, 23 (3), Mar 1971, 93–95.

18 Occupational Health Tutorial. Employment of epileptics. Occupational Health, 26 (12), Dec 1974, 488–489.

19 Office of Health Economics Epilepsy in society. The Office, 1971.

20 Ounsted, C. A special centre for children with seizures. [Children's Epilepsy Centre, Park Hospital, Oxford.] Health Trends, 6 (4), Nov 1974, 69–71.

21 Scott, D. F. Epilepsy – how it affects mother and baby. Midwife and Health Visitor, 8 (8), Aug 1972, 271–274.

22 Shope, J. T. The clinical specialist in epilepsy. Patients, problems and nursing intervention. Nursing Clinics of North America, 9 (4), Dec 1974, 761–772.

23 Simpson, J. A. Epilepsy. Nursing Mirror, 137, 6 Jul 1973, 27–29.

24 Taylor, D. C. Nursing the epileptic child. Nursing Times, 71, 6 Mar 1975, 396–397.

25 Udall, R. 'Be grateful you're epileptic'. [Personal account by a nurse of her life and restrictions on her activities.] Nursing Times, 67, 15 Apr 1971, 438–439.

26 Williams, D. The nurse and epilepsy. British Epilepsy Association, 1971.

h HUNTINGTON'S CHOREA

1 Catchpole, D. Our life with Huntington's chorea. Nursing Times, 70, 17 Oct 1974, 1616–1618.

2 Hart, M. Huntington's chorea. [Lack of provision for sufferers from this disease with a typical case quoted as an example.] New Society, 30, 24 Oct 1974, 213–214.

3 Palmer, I. O. Huntington's chorea. [Case study.] Nursing Times, 69, 9 Aug 1973, 1015–1020.

i MIGRAINE AND HEADACHE

1 Barrie, M. A. Migraine – a disabling disorder. Nursing Times, 68, 25 May 1972, 640–642.

2 Freese, A. S. The new headache clinics [in United States]. Nursing Care, 8 (4), Apr 1975, 10–13.

3 Furness, J. A. Methods of treating acute migraine in the City Migraine Clinic. Nursing Times, 67, 8 Apr 1971, 414–415.

4 Gladstone, R. M. Headache – diagnosis and management. Canadian Nurse, 67 (12), Dec 1971, 36–38.

5 Hill, J. More than just a headache. [A nurse's experiences of migraine.] Nursing Mirror, 139, 5 Dec 1974, 64–65.

6 Hoskins, L. M. Vascular and tension headaches. American Journal of Nursing, 74 (5), May 1974, 846–851.

7 Livesley, B. The Alice in Wonderland Syndrome. [Effect of his work on Lewis Carroll's experience of migraine.] Nursing Times, 69, 7 Jun 1973, 730–732.

8 Matts, S. G. F. Headache. Nursing Times, 68, 14 Dec 1972, 1584.

9 Migraine Trust Focus on migraine. The Trust, 1971.

10 Migraine Trust Migraine. [Research work.] Queen's Nursing Journal, 16 (4), Jul 1973, 83.

11 Migraine Trust Migraine, mystery and misery. The Trust, 1975.

12 Office of Health Economics Migraine. The Office, 1972 (Studies on current health problems no. 41.)

13 Oxbury, J. M. Migraine. Nursing Mirror, 136, 9 Feb 1973, 33–34.

14 Patten, J. The problems of migraine. Nursing Mirror, 137, 12 Oct 1973, 34–36.

15 Thomas, B. J. Modern treatment for an old complaint. Headache. RN Magazine, 38 (10), Oct 1975, 20–23.

16 Wall, M. C. Dixarit – a treatment for migraine. Nursing Times, 69, 15 Nov 1973, 1520.

17 Wall, M. C. Ergotamine tartrate in migraine and the dangers of overdose. Nursing Times, 68, 14 Dec 1972, 1585.

94 NERVOUS SYSTEM. 2.

a MULTIPLE SCLEROSIS

1 Ashworth, B. Multiple sclerosis. District Nursing, 13 (11), Feb 1971, 216, 219.

2 Braddell-Smith, S. Patient care study multiple sclerosis. Queen's Nursing Journal, 18 (2), May 1975, 44, 48.

3 Colver, D. Multiple sclerosis. [Case study.] Nursing Times, 69, 3 May 1973, 565–567.

4 Dillon, A. M. Nursing care of the patient with multiple sclerosis. Nursing Clinics of North America, 8 (4), Dec 1973, 653–664.

5 Evans, B. Multiple sclerosis and melancholia. [Case study.] District Nursing, 13 (11), Feb 1971, 217.

6 Ford, J. V. Case history: a multiple sclerosis patient. New Zealand Nursing Journal, 69 (6), Jun 1975, 15–16.

7 Jackson, K. M. Nursing care study. Multiple sclerosis and carcinoma of the stomach. Nursing Times, 70, 3 Oct 1974, 1532–1534.

8 Jontz, D. L. Prescription for living with MS. American Journal of Nursing, 73, May 1973, 817–818.

9 Lyon, J. B. A case of multiple sclerosis. Nursing Times, 67, 23 Dec 1971, 1601–1602.

10 Matthews, W. B. Multiple sclerosis: the mysterious disease. Nursing Times, 69, 12 Jul 1973, 887–888.

11 Multiple Sclerosis Society Still at home with multiple sclerosis. The Society, 1972.

12 Office of Health Economics Multiple sclerosis. The Office, 1975. (Studies on current health problems no. 52.)

13 Pauls, P. D. Memories and analysis. [Personal story of a nurse with multiple sclerosis.] Australian Nurses' Journal, 3 (6), Dec/Jan 1973/1974, 29–30.

14 Pinel, C. Multiple sclerosis. Nursing Times, 71, 31 Jul 1975, 1214–1216.

15 Pulton, T. W. Multiple sclerosis: experiences of personal alienation. Canadian Nurse, 71 (7), Jul 1975, 16–18.

16 Robinson, W. Mary's Mead holiday home (for multiple sclerosis patients]. Nursing Times, 69, 27 Sep 1973, 1260–1261.

17 Russell, W. R. Multiple sclerosis. Nursing Mirror, 135, 29 Dec 1972, 24–25.

18 Smith, S. M. Interdependence or independence? The contrasting ways in which two women have adapted their lives to deal with multiple sclerosis. Nursing Times, 71, 31 Jul 1975, 1217–1219.

19 Waine, A. Holiday schemes for MS patients. Nursing Mirror, 139, 21 Nov 1974, 71–72.

20 Wilson, H. J. Nursing care study. Advanced disseminated sclerosis in a young woman. Nursing Mirror, 140, 20 Mar 1975, 83–84.

b PARKINSON'S DISEASE

1 Calne, D. B. L-dopa and Parkinsonism. Nursing Mirror, 133, 8 Oct 1971, 26–27.

2 Carroll, B. Fingers to toes. [Exercise for patients with Parkinson's disease.] American Journal of Nursing, 71 (3), Mar 1971, 550–551.

3 Cooper, P. Advances in the treatment of Parkinsonism. Midwife and Health Visitor, 8 (6), Jun 1972, 220.

4 Cox, A. M. Shy-Drager syndrome. [A nursing care study of a woman with a rare form of Parkinson's disease.] Nursing Times, 71, 13 Mar 1975, 415–417.

5 Dinning, T. A. R. The surgical treatment of Parkinson's disease. Australian Nurses' Journal, 1 (6), Dec 1971, 28–30.

6 Erb, E. Improving speech in Parkinson's disease. American Journal of Nursing, 73 (11), Nov 1973, 1910–1911.

7 Godwin-Austen, R. B. Parkinson's disease: a booklet for patients and their families. Parkinson's Disease Society, 1972.

8 Kay, E. and Boone, E. Stereotactic surgery for Parkinson's disease. American Journal of Nursing, 72 (12), Dec 1972, 2200–2205.

9 Laight, S. Nursing care study. The case of Mr. P. versus Parkinsonism. Nursing Times, 70, 12 Sep 1974, 1414–1416.

10 Marks, J. The treatment of Parkinsonism with L-dopa. Lancaster: Medical and Technical Publishing, 1974.

11 Office of Health Economics Parkinson's disease. OHE, 1974. (Studies of current health problems no. 51.)

12 Parkes, J. D. Parkinson's disease. District Nursing, 13 (11), Feb 1971, 214–215.

13 Pinel, C. Parkinsonism: the causes of this syndrome and its treatment. Nursing Times, 70, 25 Apr 1974, 630–631.

14 Redden, M. Paralysis agitans and L-dopa drug therapy. [Treatment of Parkinsonism.] Nursing Times, 68, 2 Mar 1972, 262–265.

15 Robinson, M. B. Levodopa and Parkinsonism. American Journal of Nursing, 74, Apr 1974, 656–661.

16 Seevers, G. The transformation of Elizabeth. [Case study of a patient with Parkinson's disease.] Journal of Practical Nursing, 23 (4), Apr 1973, 26–27.

17 Smith, S. E. How drugs act. 21. Drugs and Parkinsonism. Nursing Times, 71, 13 Nov 1975, 1828–1829.

18 Strouthidis, T. M. Parkinsonism and its treatment. Nursing Mirror, 139, 19 Sep 1974, 44–48.

19 Tyler, E. Management of Parkinson's disease with L-dopa therapy. Canadian Nurse, 67 (4), Apr 1971, 41–42.

20 Watford, A. E. Nursing care study. Parkinson's disease complicated by fracture. Nursing Times, 71, 17 Apr 1975, 607–608.

21 Williams, A. Parkinson's disease: discussion and implications for nursing care. International Journal of Nursing Studies, 8 (1), Feb 1971, 5–13.

c SPINAL INJURIES (Includes bladder and bowel training)

1 Armstrong, K. Nursing care study. Spinal injury. Nursing Times, 71, 10 Jul 1975, 1092–1094.

2 Beauchamp, E. F. Patient care study: spastic paraplegia. Queen's Nursing Journal, 16 (5), Aug 1973, 109–110.

3 Bedbrook, G. M. Basic principles of management of spinal paralysis. 1. Anatomy, physiology and medical and nursing care. Australian Nurses' Journal, 2 (1), Jul 1972, 23–24, 36.

4 Bedbrook, G. M. Basic principles of management of spinal paralysis. 2. Nursing of neurogenic bladder. Australian Nurses' Journal, 2 (2), Aug 1972, 27–28.

5 Bromley, I. Physiotherapy in spinal cord injuries. [Symposium at Stoke Mandeville Hospital.] Nursing Mirror, 141, 6 Nov 1975, 58–60.

6 Burridge, R. A paraplegic reflects. . . American Journal of Nursing, 75 (4), Apr 1975, 643–644.

7 Cleminson, K. Spinal injuries. Australian Nurses' Journal, 3 (6), Dec/Jan 1973, 25–27, 40; (7), Feb 1974, 12–14.

8 Cornell, S. A. Development of an instrument for measuring the quality of nursing care: a two-dimension Q instrument to measure the quality of nursing care given to spinal cord injured patients. Nursing Research, 23 (2), Mar/Apr 1974, 108–117.

9 Cornell, S. A. and others Comparison of three bowel management programs during rehabilitation of spinal cord injured patients. Nursing Research, 22 (4), Jul/Aug 1973, 321–328.

10 Cox, L. A. The spinal paralysed female: a look at urinary control devices. Australian Nurses' Journal, 4 (5), Nov 1974, 31–33.

11 Deokali, M. Bladder training in spinal paraplegia. SA Nursing Journal, 38 (6), Jun 1971, 21–23.

12 Deokali, M. Bowel training in spinal paraplegia and tetraplegia. SA Nursing Journal, 38 (10), Oct 1971, 20–21.

13 Deokali, M. Prevention of pressure sores in spinal paraplegia and tetraplegia. SA Nursing Journal, 38 (4), Apr 1971, 14–18.

14 Dyson, R. Spinal disc lesions. Nursing Mirror, 133, 3 Dec 1971, 26–30.

15 Fallon, B. So you're paralysed. Spinal Injuries Association, 1975.

16 Foldes, M. S. and Woods, M. E. Crisis intervention: the patient with interruption of spinal cord integrity. [A case study illustrating nursing care of a paralysed patient and his family.] Journal of Neurosurgical Nursing, 7)2), Dec 1975, 72–81.

17 Footitt, B. Nursing care study. Nursing a tetraplegic patient at home. Nursing Times, 70, 22 Aug 1974, 1300–1302.

18 Ford, J. R. Rehabilitation of a quadriplegic. Canadian Nurse, 67 (8), Aug 1971, 37–38.

19 Frankel, H. L. Traumatic paraplegia. [Paper in symposium on spinal injuries.] Nursing Mirror, 141, 6 Nov 1975, 48–52.

20 Grabois, M. Nursing guidelines for the rehabilitation of the quadriplegic and paraplegic patient. Journal of Practical Nursing, 21 (4), Apr 1971, 22–24.

21 Guttmann, L. Sport and the spinal cord sufferer. [Paper in symposium on spinal injuries.] Nursing Mirror, 141, 6 Nov 1975, 64–65.

22 Hopkins, R. B. In a spinal injuries unit. [Christchurch Hospital.] New Zealand Nursing Journal, 69 (10), Oct 1975, 20–21.

23 Humphreys, M. Nursing care in paraplegia and tetraplegia. [Paper in symposium on spinal injuries.] Nursing Mirror, 141, 6 Nov 1975, 52–55.

24 Jones, C. F. Nursing care study. Paraplegia due to spinal lesion. Nursing Mirror, 140, 5 Jun 1975, 79–80.

25 Keane, F. X. Mechanical aids to nursing paraplegics. Nursing Times, 67, 23 Dec 1971, 1603–1607.

26 Kersenbrock, M. Nursing care of the patient with spinal cord injury. RN Magazine, 36 (12), Dec 1973, 25–31.

27 McArdle, D. The nursing management of spinal injuries. Australian Nurses' Journal, 1 (8), Feb 1972, 28–30.

28 Mahoney, M. F. Treating the spinal cord injured patient. Nursing Care, 7 (3), Mar 1974, 17–19; 7 (4), Apr 1974, 12–15.

29 Marshall, A. M. The nurse and acute spinal injury. Journal of Neurosurgical Nursing, 7 (1), Jul 1975, 1–9.

30 Marshall, T. Learning to live with paraplegia. [Written by a patient.] International Journal of Nursing Studies, 10, 1973, 253–257.

31 Nashold, B. S. Electromicturition in paraplegia. [Implementation of a neuroprosthesis.] Nursing Times, 70, 3 Jan 1974, 22–23.

32 Nursing Mirror A symposium on spinal injuries from the National Spinal Injuries Centre, Stoke Mandeville Hospital. Nursing Mirror, 141, 6 Nov 1975, 47–65.

33 Pratt, R. The nursing care of acute spinal paraplegia. 5. Bowel management. Nursing Times, 67, 27 May 1971, 638–639.

34 Pratt, R. Nursing care of paraplegic patients. Macmillan Journals, 1971. Reprint of Nursing Times articles, 29 Apr–10 Jun 1971.

35 Pratt, R. The nursing management of acute spinal paraplegia. 4. Management of the bladder. Nursing Times, 67, 20 May 1971, 604–607.

36 Richards, B. Rehabilitation into the community. [Paper in symposium on spinal injuries.] Nursing Mirror, 141, 6 Nov 1975, 60–63.

37 Sadlick, M. and Penta, F. B. Changing student nurse attitudes towards quadriplegics by use of television. [University of Illinois School of Nursing.] Medical and Biological Illustration, 25 (3), Aug 1975, 129–132.

38 Stansfield, P. From Moscow to Stoke Mandeville. Nursing Times, 67, 17 Jun 1971, 725–726.

39 Stewart, P. Through the webwork: side by side. [The work of a clinical nurse specialist in a Spinal Injury Clinic.] Journal of Neurosurgical Nursing, 6 (1), Jul 1974, 14–19.

40 Thomas, D. I learned to live with quadriplegia. Queen's Nursing Journal, 16 (10), Jan 1974, 226, 228.

41 Vanderlinden, R. G. and others Electrophrenic respiration in quadriplegia: how team members worked together to help a young quadriplegic regain some measure of independence. Canadian Nurse, 70 (1), Jan 1974, 23–26.

42 Vincent, P. J. and others Treatment of patients with spinal cord injuries. [Special care unit, Toronto.] Canadian Nurse, 71 (8), Aug 1975, 26–30.

43 Wray, G. Injuries of the spinal cord – primary nursing management. Nursing Times, 70, 2 May 1974, 663–666.

d STROKE: GENERAL AND NURSING

1 Adams, G. F. Principles of the treatment of stroke. Nursing Mirror, 135, 7 Jul 1972, 12–13.

2 Alcock, M. E. Recovery from 'stroke.' District Nursing, 3 (4), May 1972, 30–31.

3 Ballantyne, G. L. Problems of the stroke patient. New Zealand Nursing Journal, 68 (8), Aug 1974, 14–15.

4 Bearden, F. C. The CVA patient as an indication of general patient need. Journal of Psychiatric Nursing and Mental Health Services, 11 (4), Jul/Aug 1973, 25–26.

5 Benedetto, M. D. Optimal care for the severely involved stroke patient. Rehabilitation, no. 91, Oct/Dec 1974, 27–35.

6 Burt, B. and others Mildred Jones walks again. [Case study of a patient suffering from a cerebrovascular accident.] Canadian Nurse, 70 (12), Dec 1974, 37.

7 Coe, M. The damage is more than physical. [Cerebral vascular accidents.] Nursing Care, 7 (5), May 1974, 16–18.

8 Health Visitor A stroke of misfortune. [Inadequacy of immediate treatment available for stroke patients.] Health Visitor, 48 (7), Jul 1975, 249.

9 Jacobansky, A. M. Stroke. American Journal of Nursing, 72 (7), Jul 1972, 1260–1263.

10 Larsen, G. L. After stroke. Optokinetic nystagmus. American Journal of Nursing, 73 (11), Nov 1973, 1897–1898.

11 Macauley, C. and Anderson, A. D. The nurse as primary therapist in the management of the patient with stroke. Cardio-Vascular Nursing, 10 (2), Mar/Apr 1974, 7–10.

12 McNeil, F. Stroke: nursing insights from a stroke-nurse victim. RN Magazine, 38 (9), Sep 1975, 75–81.

13 Marshall, J. Radiology in the investigation of strokes. Nursing Times, 71, 27 Mar 1975, 511–513.

14 Miller, C. and others Measurement of stroke care nursing proficiency. [Research.] International Journal of Nursing Studies, 2 (4), Dec 1974, 211–222.

15 Palmer, M. E. Patient care conferences: an opportunity for meeting staff needs. [A verbatim report of a conference to discuss the care of a patient who has had a cerebral vascular accident.] Journal of Nursing Administration, 3 (2), Mar/Apr 1973, 47–53.

16 Patrick, G. Forgotten patients on the medical wards. [Study of the nursing care given to six hemiplegic patients who had experienced cerebrovascular accidents.] Canadian Nurse, 68 (3), Mar 1972, 27–31.

17 Pye, I. F. Lesions in cerebrovascular disease. Nursing Mirror, 135, 11 Aug 1972, 15–16.

18 Rainer, W. G. and others Strokes and cerebrovascular insufficiency in young employees. Occupational Health Nursing, 21 (7), Jul 1973, 20–24.

19 RN Magazine Guidelines to stroke-patient care. RN Magazine, 38 (9), Sep 1975, 83–84, 89–91.

20 Suggs, K. M. Coping and adaptive behavior in the stroke syndrome. [Case histories.] Nursing Forum, 10 (1), Jan 1971, 101–111.

21 Whitehouse, F. A. Stroke: the present challenge. Nursing Forum, 10 (1), 1971, 90–99.

22 Wilkinson, M. Treatment of hemiplegia in the acute stage. Nursing Mirror, 139, 9 Aug 1974, 59–61.

e STROKE: REHABILITATION

1 Berni, R. Stroke patient rehabilitation: a new approach. Journal of Practical Nursing, 22 (6), Jun 1972, 18–20.

2 Bowers, J. Counter-stroke. [Patient's experiences of rehabilitation after a stroke.] Occupational Therapy, 35 (5), May 1972, 315–317.

3 Bullock, E. A. Return to fitness. (a) Post stroke rehabilitation. Royal Society of Health Journal, 95 (6), Dec 1975, 284–286.

4 Bullock, E. A. and Lupton, D. Later stages of rehabilitation in hemiplegia. Physiotherapy, 60 (12), Dec 1974, 370–374.

5 D'Alton, A. Physiotherapy in the early rehabilitation of the hemiplegic patient. Nursing Mirror, 139, 9 Aug 1974, 62–64.

6 Draper, J. Long-term care of the hemiplegic patient in the home. Nursing Mirror, 139, 9 Aug 1974, 76–78.

7 Ellis, R. After stroke. Sitting problems. American Journal of Nursing, 73 (11), Nov 1973, 1898–1899.

8 Falknor, H. M. and Harris, B. J. Resocializing the stroke patient through a stroke club. Nursing Outlook, 21 (12), Dec 1973, 778–780.

9 Feldman, J. L. and Schultz, M. E. Rehabilitation after stroke. Cardiovascular Nursing, 11 (2), Mar/Apr 1975, 29–34.

10 Griffith, V. E. A creative approach to the management of a 'stroke' patient's life. Health Magazine, 9 (4), Dec 1972, 32–34.

11 Griffith, V. E. Volunteer scheme for dysphasia and allied problems in stroke patients. [Project sponsored by the Chest and Heart Foundation exploring the use of volunteers for visiting patients at home.] British Medical Journal, 3, 13 Sep 1975, 633–635.

12 Hackler, E. N. and Howell, A. T. Resocializing the stroke patient by trained volunteers. Nursing Outlook, 21 (12), Dec 1973, 776–779.

13 Jones, I. Nursing care study. Rehabilitation of a hemiplegic. Nursing Times, 70, 28 Feb 1974, 310–311.

14 Keane, W. Occupational therapy for the hemiplegic patient. Nursing Mirror, 139, 9 Aug 1974, 69–73.

15 Kisly, C. A. Striking back at stroke: a series of group meetings helps patients and their families find constructive ways of dealing with the psychosocial components of stroke. Hospitals, 47 (22), 16 Nov 1973, 64, 66, 68, 70, 72.

16 Kratz, C. R. Doctors, nurses and patients with stroke. [A study to examine what doctors expect of district nurses dealing with stroke patients.] Health Magazine, 12 (1), Spring 1975, 16–18.

17 Kratz, C. R. Problems of care of the long term sick in the community with particular reference to patients with stroke. PhD thesis, Manchester University, 1974.

18 Langridge, J. C. Rehabilitation – a team approach. [Rehabilitation of the stroke patient.] Nursing Mirror, 139, 9 Aug 1974, 65–66.

19 Millard, J. B. Medical aspects of rehabilitation. [In early treatment of the hemiplegic.] Physiotherapy, 60 (12), Dec 1974, 368–369.

20 Nursing Mirror A symposium on the rehabilitation of the stroke patient. Nursing Mirror, 139, 9 Aug 1974, 57–78.

21 Oradei, D. M. and Waite, N. S. Group psychotherapy with stroke patients during the immediate recovery phase. Nursing Digest, 3 (3), May/Jun 1975, 26–29.

22 Pfaudler, M. After stroke. Motor skill rehabilitation for hemiplegic patients. American Journal of Nursing, 73 (11), Nov 1973, 1892–1896.

23 Schultz, L. C. M. Nursing care of the stroke patient. Rehabilitative aspects. Nursing Clinics of North America, 8 (4), Dec 1973, 633–642.

24 Small, R. G. The rehabilitation of 'stroke' patients: the roles of the local authorities and the voluntary organizations. Health, 8 (2), Summer 1971, 48–50.

25 Summerville, J. G. Rebuilding the stroke patient's life. Nursing Mirror, 139, 9 Aug 1974, 57–58.

26 Todd, J. M. Physiotherapy in the early stages of hemiplegia. Physiotherapy, 60 (11), Nov 1974, 336–342.

27 Underwood, C. S. Occupational therapy in the early stages of hemiplegia. Physiotherapy, 60 (11), Nov 1974, 343–345.

28 Westropp, C. Rehabilitation of the stroke patient. [Role of the occupational therapist.] Health Magazine, 12 (2), Summer 1975, 16–19.

29 Whittet, M. M. Psychological aspects of 'stroke' illness. Health, 8 (2), Summer 1971, 46–47.

30 Whycherley, J. Group therapy in the treatment of the hemiplegic patient. Nursing Mirror, 139, 9 Aug 1974, 73–76.

31 Wilson, K. S. Rehabilitation of a stroke patient. [At Mount Royal Special Hospital for the Aged.] UNA Nursing Journal, 70, May/Jun 1972, 11–16.

f STROKE: SPEECH THERAPY

1 American Journal of Nursing Re-thinking stroke. Aphasic patients talk back. [Three articles on rehabilitating the stroke patient.] American Journal of Nursing, 75 (7), Jul 1975, 1140–1147.

2 Brocklehurst, J. C. Guidelines for rehabilitating stroke patients. 1. Dysphasia – and the nurse. Nursing Mirror, 133, 22 Oct 1971, 17–19.

3 Dalton, P. Learning to speak again. [After 'stroke' illness.] Health Magazine, 10 (2), Jun 1973, 37–39.

4 Ellams, J. Speech therapy for the hemiplegic patient. Nursing Mirror, 139, 9 Aug 1974, 66–69.

5 Hopkins, A. The need for speech therapy for dysphasis following stroke. Health Trends, 7 (3), Aug 1975, 58–60.

6 Ison, P. M. Dysphasia. [Problems for the speech therapist and the patient's family.] Rehabilitation, no. 94, Jul/Sep 1975, 45–47.

7 Leche, P. M. The speech therapist and hemiplegia. Physiotherapy, 60 (11), Nov 1974, 346–349.

8 Mitchell, J. Guidelines for rehabilitating stroke patients. 2. Early management of the aphasic patient. Nursing Mirror, 133, 22 Oct 1971, 19–21.

95 OPHTHALMOLOGY

a GENERAL AND DISORDERS

1 Abrams, J. D. The nature of glaucoma. Nursing Times, 68, 22 Jun 1972, 767–770.

2 Arnott, E. J. Ultrasonic technique for removing the cataractous lens. Nursing Mirror, 136, 2 Feb 1973, 27–28.

3 Arnott, E. J. and Calcutt, C. L. Strabismus. Nursing Mirror, 138, 17 May 1974, 52–55.

4 Bankes, J. L. K. Modern ophthalmic precision surgery. NATNews, 11 (6), Aug 1974, 10–11.

5 Bedford, M. A. Retinoblastoma. Nursing Times, 68, 23 Mar 1972, 340–343.

6 Brennan, M. E. and Knox, E. G. The incidence of cataract and its clinical presentation. Community Health, 7 (1), Jul/Aug 1975, 13–20.

7 Cairns, J. E. Glaucoma. Nursing Mirror, 140, 22/29 May 1975, 53–55.

8 Campbell, A. A series of articles from the Royal Marsden Hospital, London. 2. Tumours of the eye and orbit in childhood. [Intra-ocular and orbital.] Nursing Mirror, 134, 19 May 1972, 26–29.

9 Carbary, L. J. The miracle of corneal transplant surgery. Nursing Care, 7 (12), Dec 1974, 11–13, 15.

10 Catford, G. V. Recent advances in cataract treatment. Nursing Times, 69, 16 Aug 1973, 1060–1061.

11 Elkington, A. R. Disorders of the lacrimal system. Nursing Mirror, 140, 20 Feb 1975, 53–55.

12 Emery, J. M. Cataract treatment and rehabilitation. AORN Journal, 20 (6), Dec 1974, 992–995.

13 Fernsebner, W. Early diagnosis of acute angle-closure glaucoma. American Journal of Nursing, 75 (7), Jul 1975, 1154–1155.

14 Fernsebner, W. Etiology, treatment of glaucoma. AORN Journal, 20 (6), Dec 1974, 996–1001.

15 Graham, M. Cataract extraction. Nursing Times, 70, 23 May 1974, 789–790.

16 Jones-Ashton, I. Microscopes in ophthalmology. Nursing Times, 68, 10 Feb 1972, 173–175.

17 Kwitko, M. L. New lenses for old: a promising method of treating cataracts. [Intraocular lens implantation.] Canadian Nurse, 71 (11), Nov 1975, 34–38.

18 Ledney, D. Understanding the cataract patient. Bedside Nurse, 5 (12), Dec 1972, 11–12.

19 McWilliam, R. J. Infection of the eye. [Conjunctivitis, corneal abrasions and corneal ulcer.] Nursing Times, 69, 1 Feb 1973, 145–146.

20 Naunton, W. J. Treating non-malignant corneal conditions by radiotherapy. Nursing Times, 70, 25 Jul 1974, 1149.

21 O'Riordan, M. D. Modern ocular prosthetics. Queen's Nursing Journal, 16 (5), Aug 1973, 107–108.

22 Pereira, P. Screening for glaucoma. Nursing Times, 68, 22 Jun 1972, 771–774.

23 Pilgrim, M. and Sigler, B. Phaco-embulsification of cataracts. American Journal of Nursing, 75 (6), Jun 1975, 976–977.

24 Rosen, D. A. Argon laser photocoagulation for retinal vascular disease. Canadian Nurse, 69 (5), May 1973, 36–38.

25 Ruben, M. Keratoprosthetics. District Nursing, 14 (4), Jul 1971, 80–81.

26 Samuel, B. A. Corneal grafting. Nursing Times, 69, 1 Mar 1973, 268–271.

27 Sellors, P. J. H. Glaucoma. NM Conference lecture. Nursing Mirror, 131, 4 Sep 1970, 20–23.

28 Sutcliffe, B. A. Fluorescein angiography in perspective. Nursing Mirror, 138, 24 May 1974, 45–49.

29 Weinstein, G. W. Signs and symptoms of ocular disease. Occupational Health Nursing, 19 (5), May 1971, 7–12.

30 Zorab, E. C. The ageing eye. District Nursing, 14 (4), Jul 1971, 70–71.

b NURSING

1 Been, L. M. Some practical aspects in the nursing care of the ophthalmic patient. SA Nursing Journal, 38 (6), Jun 1971, 11, 14.

2 Duncan, M. Nursing care study. Central retinal artery occlusion. Nursing Times, 71, 10 Jul 1975, 1095–1096.

3 Harris, J. A. and others Making a film loop. An exercise in education. [Subject of the loop is irrigating an eye.] Nursing Times, 68, 25 May 1972, 649–651.

4 Havener, W. H. Insight into ophthalmic nursing. Retinal detachment. Journal of Practical Nursing, 23 (3), Mar 1973, 26–29.

5 Havener, W. H. Insights into ophthalmic nursing. Journal of Practical Nursing, 23 (4), Apr 1973, 16–19.

6 Heinrich, U. Space and serenity-sought and achieved in Portsmouth new eye unit. Nursing Mirror, 134, 10 Mar 1972, 44–46.

7 Kavalier, F. A hospital isolated from its community. [Ophthalmic Hospital in Jerusalem of the Order of St. John.] Nursing Times, 69, 5 Jul 1973, 864–866.

8 Mechner, F. and others Patient assessment: examination of the eye. American Journal of Nursing, 74 (11), Nov 1974, 1–24; 75 (1), Jan 1975, 1–24.

9 Ohno, M. I. The eye-patched patient. American Journal of Nursing, 71 (2), Feb 1971, 271–274.

10 Rooke, F. C. E. Ophthalmic nursing. Queen's Nursing Journal, 17 (4), Jul 1974, 81–82.

11 Sherman, S. E. Eye care is a nurse's responsibility too. Nursing Care, 6 (7), Jul 1973, 13–14.

12 Smith, J. S. Care of patients with glaucoma. District Nursing, 14 (4), Jul 1971, 72, 75.

13 Tyler, I. C. A glaucoma screening and study by nurses. Occupational Health Nursing, 19 (9), Sep 1971, 11–12.

14 Wall, M. Nursing care study. Enucleation of the eye. Nursing Mirror, 138, 17 May 1974, 79–80.

15 Weinstock, F. J. Tonometry screening. American Journal of Nursing, 73 (4), Apr 1973, 656–657.

16 Whatley, M. Nursing care study. Cataract extraction. Nursing Times, 70, 23 May 1974, 791–792.

17 White, A. M. W. Ophthalmic community nurse. [A hospital based scheme in Liverpool to provide expert ophthalmic nursing care to patients in their own homes.] Nursing Times, 70, 28 Feb 1974, 324–327.

c BLINDNESS AND PARTIAL SIGHT

1 Ammon, L. L. Surviving enucleation. [The psychological effect of the loss of an eye.] American Journal of Nursing, 72 (10), Oct 1972, 1817–1821.

2 Branson, H. K. The blind mother. [Problems of labour and early infant care.] American Journal of Nursing, 75 (3), Mar 1975, 414–416.

3 Cookson, P. The blind leading the blind. [Experimentation in the rehabilitation of the blind in a psychiatric hospital – Whittingham Hospital, near Preston.] Nursing Mirror, 139, 28 Nov 1974, 64–65.

4 Davies, E. T. Making life easier for the blind. Queen's Nursing Journal, 18 (3), Jun 1975, 83–84.

5 Fawkes, M. A world of shadows. [Case study of the surgical treatment of a road accident victim, resulting in partial sight.] Nursing Times, 70, 26 Sep 1974, 1496–1498.

6 Froehlich, W. That the sightless may see. World Health, Aug/Sep 1972, 12–17.

7 Havener, W. H. What can you do to help prevent blindness. Nursing Care, 7 (3), Mar 1974, 29–31.

8 Horseman, K. Prevention of blindness in Rhodesia. Rhodesian Nurse, 6 (1), Mar 1973, 2–3, 5, 7.

9 Neu, C. Coping with newly diagnosed blindness. American Journal of Nursing, 75 (12), Dec 1975, 2161–2163.

10 Perks, J. Nursing a blind patient. [Advice for nurses by a blind person.] Nursing Times, 71, 30 Oct 1975, 1728–1729.

11 Shafar, J. Episodic blindness. Nursing Times, 71, 30 Jan 1975, 168–170.

12 Sharpe, A. Helping parents in the developmental rearing of a blind child. Maternal-Child Nursing Journal, 2 (1), Spring, 1973, 23–28.

13 Simmons, J. The personal touch. [Experiences of a blind person in hospital.] Nursing Times, 71, 30 Oct 1975, 1729–1730.

14 Sorsby, A. Prevention of blindness: present prospects. Health Trends, 5 (1), Feb 1973, 7–9.

15 Trevor-Davis, R. Industrial rehabilitation. 4. The newly blind. Health Trends, 4 (2), May 1972, 40.

16 WHO Chronicle Prevention of blindness. WHO Chronicle, 27, Jan 1973, 21–27.

17 Woods, H. Preventing blindness: a lot more than meets the eye. [Causes of blindness.] Journal of Practical Nursing, 24 (11), Nov 1974, 28–29, 34.

18 World Health Facts about river blindness. World Health, Oct 1973, 10–11.

19 Zucnick, M. Care of an artificial eye. American Journal of Nursing, 75 (5), May 1975, 835.

d VISION DISORDERS

1 Belsey, R. L. So you think you need glasses? Or sight testing explained. Nursing Times, 67, 21 Oct 1971, 1303–1306.

2 Chaloner, L. Contact lenses. Nursing Times, 70, 10 Jan 1974, 61.

3 Clements, D. B. Management of squint in childhood. Nursing Times, 70, 8 Aug 1974, 1229–1231.

4 Dayneswood, G. The five senses. Sight. Life seen dimly but lived fully. District Nursing, 14 (5), Aug 1971, 90–92.

5 Gardiner, P. A. Squint diagnostic clinic. [Left hand column.] Community Medicine, 127 (9), 3 Mar 1972, 117.

6 Hiles, D. A. Strabismus. American Journal of Nursing, 74 (6), Jun 1974, 1082–1089.

7 Kane, A. H. A study of colour vision tests in young school children. Health Visitor, 47 (2), Feb 1974, 34–35.

8 Lindeman-Meester, H. H. M. Fluids for soft contact lenses, tested by the Kelsey-Sykes and Maurer methods. Nursing Times, 70 (35), 29 Aug 1974, Suppl. 5–6.

9 Magauran, I. M. Errors of refraction and the use of glasses. District Nursing, 14 (4), Jul 1971, 76, 81.

10 Perry, J. The professions supplementary to medicine. Orthoptics. Nursing Mirror, 141, 13 Nov 1975, 54–56.

11 Ruben, M. Contact lenses. Nursing Mirror, 138, 17 May 1974, 49–51.

12 Ruben, M. Contact lenses, shells and prosthetics. Nursing Times, 68, 3 Feb 1972, 133–136.

13 Voke, J. Colour vision and the pill. Nursing Times, 70, 31 Jan 1974, 139.

14 Voke, J. Defective colour vision. Nursing Times, 70, 31 Jan 1974, 136–138.

e EYE INJURIES AND OCCUPATIONAL HEALTH

1 Adams, P. and others Foreign bodies in the eyes. [A study assessing the use of Albucid, Chloromycetin and inactive base ointment in patients aged 15–64.] Nursing Times, 71, 11 Sep 1975, 1444–1446.

2 Carr, C. F. Eye injuries? How many can be prevented? Occupational Health, 23 (3), Mar 1971, 75–79.

3 Carr, C. F. and others Eyes at work: a symposium. Occupational Health, 23 (3), Mar 1971, 75–89.

4 Cutajar, S. and others Foreign bodies in the eyes – an experiment. [Conducted by the British Steel Corporation Medical Department, to compare Albucid and Chloromycetin.] Nursing Times, 71, 9 Jan 1975, 55–56.

5 Drysdale, R. S. Safety – care of the eyes. Occupational Health, 23 (1), Jan 1971, 23–24.

6 Elkington, A. R. Eye injuries. 1. Non-perforating wounds. 2. Perforating wounds. 3. Intra-ocular foreign bodies. Nursing Times, 69, 22 Nov 1973, 1562–1563; 69, 29 Nov 1973, 1597–1598; 6 Dec 1973, 1638–1639.

7 Elkington, A. R. and Kanski, J. J. The hammer and the eye: beware. British Medical Journal, 1, 20 Jan 1973, 156–157.

8 Morgan, A. Minor eye injuries. Nursing Mirror, 140, 13 Feb 1975, 68–70.

9 Nursing Times The hen's secret weapon. [Conjunctivitis in broiler factory workers.] Nursing Times, 70, 14 Feb 1974, 222.

10 Occupational Health Care of eyes in 1975. [Effects of the 'Protection of Eyes Regulations 1974.'] Occupational Health, 27 (6), Jun 1975, 253–255.

11 Perkin, M. and Swan, I. L. Moorfields Eye Hospital course. [For occupational health nurses.] Occupational Health, 23 (1), Jan 1971, 13–15.

12 Phaneuf, M. C. Vision conservation for occupational health nurses: a context. Occupational Health Nursing, 23 (12), Dec 1975, 9–36.

13 Phillips, J. H. Eye emergencies: self-operating irrigation equipment. Occupational Health, 23 (3), Mar 1971, 90–91.

14 Ure, A. W. Vested interest in visual welfare. Occupational Health, 23 (3), Mar 1971, 85–89.

15 Weinstock, F. J. Emergency treatment of eye injuries. American Journal of Nursing, 71 (10), Oct 1971, 1928–1931.

16 Whitehead, K. P. Chemical burns of the eye. Nursing Times, 67, 24 Jun 1971, 759–762.

96 RENAL DISEASE

a GENERAL

1 Baillod, R. A. Treatment of renal failure – Hobson's choice. Nursing Times, 69, 28 Jun 1973, 830–832.

2 Berlyne, G. M. A course in renal disease. 4th ed. Blackwell Scientific, 1974.

3 Bingham, S. Dietary treatment of renal failure. Nursing Mirror, 139, 12 Sep 1974, 65–69.

4 Booth, E. M. Dietary treatment in renal disease. Nutrition, 27 (6), Dec 1973, 375–380.

5 Bowman, G. S. Renal biopsy. Nursing Times, 68, 31 Aug 1972, 1083–1085.

6 Champion, P. R. H. Treatment of renal disease. 2. Dietary management in renal dialysis. 1972. Nursing Times, 68, 14 Sep 1972, 1151–1153.

7 Cole, I. Congenital absence of the left kidney. Nursing Mirror, 130, 17 Apr 1973, 33–35.

8 DiPalma, J. R. Drug therapy today. Preventing drug toxicity in renal failure. RN Magazine, 38 (6), Jun 1975, 65–69.

9 Frye, C. Toxic nephropathy. Canadian Nurse, 68 (6), Jun 1972, 45–47.

10 Goggin, M. J. Drug therapy in renal failure. District Nursing, 14 (8), Nov 1971, 170–172.

11 Hyne, B. E. B. Medical aspects of nutrition in renal failure. Nursing Mirror, 139, 12 Sep 1974, 63–65

12 Jennings, J. End-stage renal failure. Nursing Times, 67, 28 Oct 1971, 1334–1335.

13 McCaugherty, D. Dietetics in renal failure – the patients' viewpoint. Nursing Mirror, 139, 12 Sep 1974, 72–74.

14 Nursing Mirror The RAF's renal unit, [at Princess Mary's RAF Hospital, Halton.] Nursing Mirror, 139, 26 Jul 1974, 53–54.

15 Nursing Times Treatment of Renal Disease Macmillan Journals, 1972; Nursing Times, 68 7 Sep 1972, 1120–1123.

16 Sato, F. F. Trials with cyclophosphamide in SLE. [To combat renal damage caused by systemic lupus erythematosus.] American Journal of Nursing, 72 (6), Jun 1972, 1077–1079.

17 Sherlock, J. E. Kidney dialysis and transplantation. AORN Journal, 20 (5), Nov 1974, 823–824, 826, 828.

18 Taber, S. M. Addenbrookes hospital finds the answer! An effort to improve communications between a dialysis unit and a transplant unit. Nursing Times, 70, 9 May 1974, 724–725.

19 Waters, W. E. Analgesics and the kidney. Nursing Times, 69, 27 Sep 1973, 1241–1243.

20 Watson, S. Nephrogenic diabetes insipidus. Nursing Times, 68, 17 Aug 1972, 1027–1029.

21 Williams, D. G. Glomerulonephritis. Nursing Mirror, 138, 14 Jun 1974, 50–52.

22 Yuill, G. M. The treatment of renal failure. Manchester University Press, 1975.

b NURSING

1 Beckett, J. Role of the nurse in managing the patient's diet [in renal failure.] Nursing Mirror, 139, 12 Sep 1974, 69–71.

2 Cullinan, J. The making and meaning of EDTNA. [European Dialysis and Transplant Association.] Nursing Times, 69, 28 Jun 1973, 819.

3 European Dialysis and Transplant Nurses' Association EDTNA meeting – Tel Aviv. Finding an identity. [Third annual meeting.] Nursing Times, 70, 14 Nov 1974, 1762–1763.

4 European Dialysis and Transplant Nurses' Association Research at work. [Research papers presented at the European renal nurses conference.] Nursing Times, 71, 4 Sept 1975, 1396–1397.

5 European Dialysis and Transplant Nurses' Association Proceedings: Volume 1. The Association, 1973.

6 Fennell, S. E. Percutaneous renal biopsy: evaluation before, and close observation after. American Journal of Nursing, 75 (8), Aug 1975, 1291–1294.

7 Finn, B. Post-basic training in renal nursing. Nursing Times, 69, 28 Jun 1973, 833.

8 Hansen, G. L. Caring for patients with chronic renal disease: a reference guide for nurses. New York: Rochester Regional Medical Program and University of Rochester Medical Centre, 1972.

9 Harrington, J. D. and Brener, E. R. Patient care in renal failure. Philadelphia: Saunders, 1973.

10 Morgan, D. M. Intensive care nursing for renal patients. Canadian Hospital, 48 (10), Oct 1971, 18–20, 22, 26–27.

11 Nursing Clinics of North America Symposium on care of the patient with renal disease. Nursing Clinics of North America, 10 (3), Sep 1975, 411–516.

12 Schlotter, L., editor Nursing and the nephrology patient: a symposium on current trends and issues. Flusing: Medical Examination Publishing Co., 1973.

13 Uldall, R. Renal nursing. Blackwell Scientific, 1972.

c RENAL DIALYSIS

1 Ascott, J. R. Haemodialysis and renal transplantation. Health Trends, 5 (3), Aug 1975, 56–58.

2 Baldwin, J. Viewpoint. Dialysis or transplant? Nursing Times, 69, 29 Nov 1973, 1594–1596.

3 Bradford, K. S. General management: nursing care. (Peritoneal dialysis.) Nursing Mirror, 133, 9 Jul 1971, 26–29.

4 Burrows, K. Treatment of renal disease. 8. Peritoneal dialysis. Nursing Times, 68, 2 Nov 1972, 1381–1382.

5 Casey, J. D. and Koerner, S. OR care of hemodialysis patients. AORN Journal, 20 (5), Nov 1974, 817–821.

6 Foster, M. A. and Stocks, P. A comparison of washback techniques in haemodialysis. Nursing Times, 69, 2 Dec 1971, 1496–1498.

7 Fung, J. H. Y. Haemodialysis. Hong Kong Nursing Journal, (12), May 1972, 31–45.

8 Gillette, E. A patient during a dialysis treatment. Nursing Care, 6 (1), Jan 1973, 17–18.

9 Goodwin, F. and others An exercise in teamwork [Hanbury Dialysis Unit.] Nursing Times, 68, 23 Jun 1972, 1481–1485.

10 Gutch, C. F. and Stoner, M. H. Review of haemodialysis for nurses and dialysis personnel. St. Louis, Mosby, 1971, 2nd ed, 1975.

11 Hurst, C. A. Treatment of renal disease, 4. Shunt and fistula care. Nursing Times, 68, 28 Sep 1972, 1214–1216.

12 Large, B. Treatment of renal disease. 5. Haemodialysis. Nursing Times, 68, 12 Oct 1972, 1282–1286.

13 Large, B. Treatment of renal disease. 6. Complications during dialysis. Nursing Times, 68, 19 Oct 1972, 1330–1331.

14 Lazarus, J. M. and Morgan, A. P. Vascular access in hemodialysis. AORN Journal, 20 (5), Nov 1974, 810–815.

15 Lennon, P. Nursing care study. A foreign patient suffering from acute renal failure. Nursing Times, 70, 31 Oct 1974, 1688–1690.

16 Manohar, E. Peritoneal dialysis. Nursing Journal of India, 44 (1), Jan 1973, 17–18.

17 Marson, S. N. A programmed approach to staff and patient training in a haemodialysis unit. International Journal of Nursing Studies, 10 (4), Dec 1973, 259–267.

18 Moxon, V. Nursing care study. Peritoneal dialysis in a neonate. Nursing Times, 70, 20 Jun 1974, 952–954.

19 Peachey, J. Peritoneal dialysis by machine. Nursing Mirror, 133, 9 July 1971, 23–27.

20 Perry, E. Ethical problems hard to solve. (Rcn Haemodialysis and Transplant Group Conference.] Nursing Mirror, 140, 1 May 1975, 35.

21 Read, M. and Mallison, M. External arteriovenous shunts. American Journal of Nursing, 72 (1), 1972, 81–85.

22 Royal College of Nursing Haemodialysis and Transplant Nursing Group. [Summary of working party report on haemodialysis.] Rcn, 1975.

23 Scurrell, A. M. Peritoneal dialysis – a five year evaluation. Nursing Times, 69, 19 Jul 1973, 929–931.

24 Soffer, R. A. The nurse and hemodialysis. Nursing Care, 6 (10), Oct 1973, 14–18.

25 Whelpton, D., editor Renal dialysis. Sector Publishing, 1974.

26 Wing, A. J. Regular dialysis treatment: the nurse's role. Nursing Mirror, 134, 14 Apr 1972, 29–32.

27 Wing, A. J. and Magowan, M. The renal unit. Macmillan, 1975.

d CHILDREN

1 Arneil, G. C. Nephritis and nephrosis in children. Nursing Mirror, 132, 22 Jan 1971, 17–22.

2 Arneil, G. C. Renal failure in children. Nursing Mirror, 132, 29 Jan 1971, 34–39.

3 Arneil, G. C. and Gow, L. Infection and abnormalities of the renal tract in children. Nursing Mirror, 132, 5 Feb 1971, 34–37.

4 Chantler, C. The nephrotic syndrome in childhood. District Nursing, 14 (2), May 1971, 36–37.

5 Hoover, P. M. and others Adjustment of children with parents on haemodialysis. [Research by interview carried out in Seattle.] Nursing Times, 71, 28 Aug 1975, 1374–1376.

6 Horoshak, I. A special kind of kidney patient. [Children with end-stage renal disease.] RN Magazine, 38 (10), Oct 1975, 55–59.

7 Neff, J. A. Autonomy concerns of a child on dialysis. Maternal-Child Nursing Journal, 4 (2), Summer 1975, 101–108.

8 Neff, J. A. Psychological adaptation to renal transplantation. [In a fifteen year old child.] Maternal-Child Nursing Journal, 2 (2), Summer 1973, 111–119.

9 Parsons, C. M. Nursing care study. Elizabeth. [Nephrotic syndrome with impending renal failure in a young child.] Nursing Times, 70, 30 May 1974, 822–824.

10 Royal College of Nursing Renal dialysis in context. Parents speak at Rcn specialist group conference. Nursing Times, 71, 1 May 1975, 674.

e PATIENT AND FAMILY, AND HOME DIALYSIS

1 Barker, D. Transplant or dialysis? A patient's view. Nursing Times, 70, 11 Apr 1974, 549.

2 Bazzato, G. and Onesti, G. Hemodialysis in the home: techniques and clinical results. Springfield: Thomas, 1975.

3 Campling, J. Life on a kidney machine. New Society, 32, 26 Jun 1975, 770–772.

4 Cocks, J. Home dialysis – domiciliary training. Queen's Nursing Journal, 16 (6), Sep 1973, 131–132.

5 D'Afflitti, J. G. and Swanson, D. Group sessions for the wives of home-hemodialysis patients: a mutual support system evolved during these group sessions.] American Journal of Nursing, 75 (4), Apr 1975, 633–635.

6 Fitzmaurice, E. M. and Fowles, D. M. Tubes – lines – and bubble traps on the district. [Dialysis.] Nursing Times, 67, 23 Sep 1971, 1196–1197.

7 Gower, P. E. and Stubbs, R. K. T. Some administrative problems in adaptation of houses for home dialysis. British Medical Journal, 2, 12 Jun 1971, 637–641.

8 Hall, G. H. Home dialysis for chronic renal failure. Royal Society of Health Journal, 92 (3), Jun 1972, 135–138.

9 Hassall, C. Treatment of renal disease. 1. Psychological problems in long-term care. Nursing Times, 68, 7 Sep 1972, 1120–1122.

10 Hassett, M. Teaching hemodialysis to the family unit. Nursing Clinics of North America, 7 (2), Jun 349–362.

11 Holmes, A. Treatment of renal disease. 7. Home dialysis. Nursing Times, 68, 26 Oct 1972, 1354–1355.

12 Jackle, M. J. Life satisfaction and kidney dialysis. [A study of 30 dialysis patients to test their reactions to the quality of life on dialysis.] Nursing Forum, 13 (4), 1974, 360–370.

13 Levy, N. B., editor Living or dying: adaptation to hemodialysis. Springfield: Thomas, 1974.

14 Levy, N. B. and Wynbrandt, G. D. The quality of life on maintenance haemodialysis. [Interview with 18 patients at State University Hospital, Brooklyn, New York.] Lancet, 1, 14 Jun 1975, 1328–1330.

15 Oberley, E. T. and Oberley, T. D. Understanding your new life with dialysis: a patient guide for physical and psychological adjustment to maintenance dialysis. Springfield: Thomas 1975.

16 Rapaport, F. T., editor A second look at life: transplantation and dialysis patients, their own stories. New York: Grune & Stratton, 1973.

17 Santopietro, M. C. S. Meeting the emotional needs of hemodialysis patients and their spouses. [An analysis of six areas in which nurses can help.] American Journal of Nursing, 75 (4), Apr 1975, 629–630.

18 Schaffer, E. Do-it-yourself dialysis. [Patient teaching in a self-care dialysis centre.] Canadian Nurse, 69 (7), Jul 1973, 29–32.

19 Scottish Hospital Centre Home dialysis. Edinburgh: The Centre, 1972.

20 Sweatman, A. J. and others Comparison of home dialysis and other treatments for chronic renal failure. Practitioner, 212, Jan 1974, 56–66.

21 Walser, D. Behavioral effects of dialysis. [Implications of home dialysis for the patient, his family and the nurse.] Canadian Nurse, 70 (5), May 1974, 23–25.

22 White, P. Renal dialysis at home. District Nursing, 14 (11), Feb 1972, 241.

f TRANSPLANTATION

1 Barr, E. Your help today may save a life tomorrow. [Story of the Kidney Research Unit for Wales Foundation.] Nursing Mirror, 133, 10 Dec 1971, 42–44.

2 Bickerstaff, H. F. Renal transplantation: case study. Nursing Mirror, 132, 30 Apr 1971, 30–32.

3 Bingham, D. M. Kidney transplant: a personal view. AORN Journal, 20 (4), Oct 1974, 703–704, 706, 708, 710, 712.

4 Cholerton, C. A. Nursing care study. Left nephroureterectomy. Nursing Mirror, 141, 20 Nov 1975, 51–52.

5 Collins, B. E. Intensive care assignment: renal transplant. New Zealand Nursing Journal, 67 (5), May 1974, 4–7.

6 George, M. Renal transplants in India. Nursing Journal of India, 62 (12), Dec 1971, 393–394, 409.

7 Jennings, J. Nursing care of the renal transplant patient. Nursing Mirror, 132, 25 Jun 1971, 26–27, 31.

8 Jones, K. Study documents effect of primary nursing on renal transplant patients. [The effect of assigning one nurse to each patient compared with team nursing.] Hospitals, 49 (24), 16 Dec 1975, 85–86, 88–89.

9 Leonard, M. Nephrology nursing: interplay of skills. [Nursing care of the kidney transplant patient.] AORN Journal, 20 (4), Oct 1974, 597–601.

10 McCabe, R. E. and White, P. Recovery, preservation of cadaver kidneys. AORN Journal, 20 (4), Oct 1974, 603–611.

11 McLean, J. P. Nursing care study. Bilateral nephrectomy. Nursing Mirror, 136, 9 Mar 1973, 31–34.

12 Maguire, K. Treatment of renal disease. 9. Kidney transplantation. [Includes list of manufacturers of renal dialysis equipment.] Nursing Times, 68, 9 Nov 1972, 1430–1433.

13 Merchant, F. Pyelolithotomy. Nursing Mirror, 134, 24 Mar 1972, 36–39.

14 Nursing Times Nurses could be asked to authorise kidney removal. Circular HSC (1s) 156 on the working of the Human Tissue Act 1961.] Nursing Times, 71, 3 Jul 1975, 1030.

15 O'Gilvie, J. Nursing care study of renal transplantation. Jamaican Nurse, 12 (3), Dec 1972, 16–17, 38–40.

16 Olsson, C. A. and Krane, R. J. Extracorporeal surgery: new route to greater kidney salvage. RN Magazine 37 (6), Jun 1974, OR 1–2.

17 Royal College of Nursing Transplant risk still high. [Report of the Rcn Dialysis and Transplant Nursing Group meeting.] Nursing Times, 70, 12 Dec 1974, 1916.

18 Schumann, D. The renal donor. [Problems of a living kidney donor.] American Journal of Nursing, 74 (1), Jan 1974, 105–110.

19 Shaw, R. E. Initial surgical management of renal failure. Nursing Mirror, 139, 26 Jul 1974, 48–50.

20 Smith, L. and Ellcome, J. Three transplants from one donor. [Liver and kidney transplants from cadaver donor.] Nursing Times, 67, 1 Jul 1971, 800–802.

21 Taylor, V. W. The physiotherapist in the renal transplant unit. Physiotherapy, 59 (5), May 1973, 151.

22 Willey, M. Care of the patient with a kidney transplant. Nursing Clinics of North America, 8 (1), Mar 1973, 127–135.

97 REPRODUCTIVE SYSTEM

a GYNAECOLOGY

1 Amias, A. G. Aspects of sexual medicine. Sexual life after gynaecological operations. 1. [Includes hysterectomy.] British Medical Journal, 2, 14 Jun 1975, 608–609.

2 Baird, D. T. Ovulation. Nursing Mirror, 141, 23 Oct 1975, 62–65.

3 Barnes, J. Cryosurgery in gynaecology. Nursing Times, 70, 20 Jun 1974, 947–948.

4 Beardall, P. J. Laparoscopy. Canadian Nurse, 69 (4), Apr 1973, 34–36.

5 Brookes, P. The menopause: a neglected part of nursing. Nursing Times, 71, 21 Aug 1975, 1341.

6 Cairney, J. and Cairney, J. Gynaecology for student of nursing. 5th ed. edited and revised by Trevor C. Svensen. Christchurch, New Zealand: Peryer, 1972.

7 Carbary, L. J. The menopause: facts and fallacies. Nursing Care, 7 (7), Jul 1974, 24–25, 27.

8 Carbary, L. J. Menstruation . . . and its problems. Nursing Care, 7 (5), May 1974, 26–28.

9 Daus, A. D. and Hafez, E. S. E. Candida albicans in women. [A study of 92 pregnant and non-pregnant patients to isolate factors affecting the incidence and severity of vaginal candidiasis.] Nursing Research, 24 (6), Nov/Dec 1975, 430–433.

10 Fiedler, D. E. Emotional aspects of gynecological disturbances as related to industry. Occupational Health Nursing, 19 (5), May 1971, 19, 43.

11 Galloway, K. The middle years. The change of life. American Journal of Nursing, 75 (6), Jun 1975, 1006–1011.

12 Graber, E. A. and Barber, H. R. K. The case for and against estrogen therapy. American Journal of Nursing, 75 (10), Oct 1975, 1766–1771.

13 Hall, A. A self-help clinic for women. Canadian Nurse, 70 (5), May 1974, 33–36.

14 Hector, W. and Bourne, G. Modern gynaecology with obstetrics for nurses. 5th ed. Heinemann, 1974.

15 Holmes, M. M. Nursing care study. Uterus didelphys. Nursing Times, 70, 7 Feb 1974, 178–179.

16 Joannides, S. C. Anatomical drawing. 7. Female reproductive organs, and the kidney. Nursing Times, 71, 13 Nov 1975, 1821–1822.

17 Martin, I. C. A. Blood, sweat and tears: some psychiatric aspects of menstrual disorder. Nursing Times, 71, 13 Nov 1975, 1830–1832.

18 Matthews, A. E. B. Endometriosis. Nursing Mirror, 139, 5 Jul 1974, 65–66.

19 Michie, E. A. Urinary oestrogen assays in obstetrics. Nursing Mirror, 136, 5 Jan 1973, 30–32.

20 Newton, J. and Williams, C. V. Menstrual disorders. Nursing Mirror, 140, 30 Jan 1975, 49–53.

21 Price, W. H. Delayed puberty. Nursing Mirror, 136, 20 Apr 1973, 16–20.

22 Roberts, L. A. M. Premenstrual tension syndrome. Nursing Times, 71, 13 Feb 1975, 272–273.

23 Rosseinsky, D. Once a blessing? Premenstrual tension and menstrual synchrony are discussed in the light of some new evolutionary ideas. Nursing Times, 71, 6 Mar 1975, 393–395.

24 Smith, D. F. Endometriosis. Nursing Times, 71, 31 Jul 1975, 1207–1211.

25 Spano, L. and Lamont, J. A. Dyspareunia: a symptom of female sexual dysfunction. Canadian Nurse, 71 (8), Aug 1975, 22–25.

26 Wooket, B. E. P. Well-woman clinic in a group practice. [Screening.] Nursing Mirror, 134, 4 Feb 1972, 33–35.

b HYSTERECTOMY

1 Coope, J. The post-hysterectomy syndrome. Nursing Times, 71, 14 Aug 1975, 1285–1286.

2 Dewhurst, J. E. Nursing care study. Modified Wertheim's hysterectomy. Nursing Mirror, 139, 28 Nov 1974, 71–73.

3 Holm, L. A. Nursing care of patients having a hysterectomy. Canadian Nurse, 67 (7), Jul 1971, 36–37.

4 Levine, R. U. Hysteroscopy – no passing fad. RN Magazine, 38 (11), Nov 1975, OR 1, 2.

5 Mauro, J. D. The threat of hysterectomy. Journal of Practical Nursing, 23 (4), Apr 1973, 28–29.

6 Nursing Times A gynaecological experience. [Hysterectomy on a severely disabled spastic. By the patient concerned.] Nursing Times, 69, 19 Jul 1973, 927–928.

7 Richards, D. H. Depression after hysterectomy. Lancet, 2, 25 Aug 1973, 430–432.

8 Richards, D. H. A post-hysterectomy syndrome. Lancet, 2, 26 Oct 1974, 983–985.

9 Steele, S. J. and Goodwin, M. F. A pamphlet to answer the patient's questions before hysterectomy. [Prepared by the Academic Department of Obstetrics and Gynaecology, Middlesex Hospital.] Lancet, 2, 13 Sep 1975, 492–493.

10 Thomas, B. J. The great debate: elective hysterectomy for sterilization. RN Magazine, 36 (4), Apr 1973, OR 3–4.

11 Williams, M. A. Cultural patterning of the feminine role. A factor in the response to hysterectomy. Nursing Forum, 12 (4), 1973, 378–387.

c INFERTILITY

1 Bishop, P. M. F. Problems of subfertility. Nursing Mirror, 136, 30 Mar 1973, 30–32.

2 Kistner, R. W. The infertile woman. American Journal of Nursing, 73 (11), Nov 1973, 1937–1943.

3 Kuku, S. B. and others Infertility and its consequences in the Nigerian society. Nigerian Nurse, 6 (4), Oct/Dec 1974, 11–13.

4 London, D. R. Male infertility. Nursing Mirror, 137, 31 Aug 1973, 28–29.

5 Newill, R. Infertile marriage. Harmondsworth: Penguin, 1974.

6 Phillip, E. Childlessness: its causes and what to do about them. Arrow, 1975.

7 Ricquier, R. Artificial reproduction [for infertile marriages]. Nursing Times, 70, 4 Apr 1974, 496–498.

8 Robinson, A. M. Infertility and what can be done about it. RN Magazine, 36 (4), Apr 1973, 24–29.

9 Scott, L. S. Childless marriage: investigation and management of the husband. Nursing Times, 69, 13 Sep 1973, 1182–1184.

10 Steele, S. J. Infertility and sub-fertility. Mother and Child, 44 (3), May/Jun 1972, 16–18, 20.

11 Taylor, R. W. Infertility – the role of the fallopian tubes. Nursing Mirror, 133, 3 Sep 1971, 22–23.

d MALE GENITAL SYSTEM

1 Andreou, A. Nursing care study. Prostate gland enlargement. Nursing Times, 71, 7 Aug 1975, 1243–1244.

2 Blandy, J. P. Benign prostatic enlargement. Nursing Mirror, 134, 11 Feb 1972, 12–15.

3 Carbary, L. J. Problems of the prostate. Nursing Care, 8 (8), Aug 1975, 13–15.

4 Cooper, Impotence – causes and management of the male 'curse'. Nursing Mirror, 136, 18 May 1973, 16–18.

5 Crisp, K. L. Nursing care study. Suprapubic prostatectomy. Nursing Mirror, 139, 12 Dec 1974, 63–66.

6 Drexler, C. A four-year old boy experiences surgery for a genital defect. Maternal-Child Nursing Journal, 4 (3), Fall 1975, 197–205.

7 Pryor, J. P. Patient care after prostatectomy. Nursing Times, 69, 11 Oct 1973, 1326–1328.

8 Reece, A. J. Nursing care study. An unusual penile injury. [Rupture of the anterior urethra.] Nursing Times, 70, 4 Jul 1974, 1038.

9 Scott, L. S. Maldescent of the testicle. Nursing Times, 67, 22 Jul 1971, 883–885.

e SEX

1 Benjamin, H. and Ihlenfeld, C. L. Transsexualism. American Journal of Nursing, 73, (3), Mar 1973, 457–461.

2 Brown, P. T. Developments in the treatment of sexual dysfunction. Midwife, Health Visitor and Community Nurse, 11 (3), Mar 1975, 74–76.

3 Comarr, A. E. and Gunderson, B. B. Sexual function in traumatic paraplegia and quadriplegia. American Journal of Nursing, 75 (2), Feb 1975, 250–255.

4 **Costello, M. K.** Sex, intimacy and aging. American Journal of Nursing, 75 (8), Aug 1975, 1330–1332.

5 **Dressen, S. E.** The middle years. The sexually active middle adult. [Counselling by nurses.] American Journal of Nursing, 75 (6), Jun 1975, 1001–1005.

6 **Fortune, S. E.** Sex and community health. Community Health, 5 (4), Jan/Feb 1974, 189–192.

7 **Golub, S.** When your patient's problem involves sex. [A sex counsellor's view on how nurses can deal with patients.] RN Magazine, 38 (3), Mar 1975, 27–31.

8 **Jacobson, L.** Illness and human sexuality. [Nursing of the whole patient must consider the sexual problems, created by disorders and their treatment.] Nursing Outlook, 22 (1), Jan 1974, 50–53.

9 **Krizinofski, M. T.** Human sexuality and nursing practice. Nursing Clinics of North America, 8 (4), Dec 1973, 673–681.

10 **Lawrence, J. C.** Homosexuals, hospitalization and the nurse. Nursing Forum, 14 (3), 1975, 305–317.

11 **Leese, S. M.** Sexual urges in adolescents. Nursing Times, 70, 19 Sep 1974, 1475.

12 **Lindley, P.** Nurse-therapists at work: six case studies. 6. Sexual deviation in a young man. [Symposium at Maudsley Hospital.] Nursing Mirror, 140, 8 May 1975, 63–64.

13 **MacCulloch, M. J.** Review of sexual difficulties in clinical practice. Nursing Mirror, 136, 29 Jun 1973, 12–16.

14 **Nursing Clinics of North America** Symposium on human sexuality. Nursing Clinics of North America, 10 (3), Sep 1975, 517–597.

15 **Russell, L. K.** Sexual counselling: an approach to the integration of sexual counselling into the antepartal management of teenagers. [Project in two New York hospitals.] Journal of Nurse-Midwifery, 20 (1), Spring 1975, 24–29.

16 **Strait, J.** The transsexual patient after surgery. American Journal of Nursing, 73 (3), Mar 1973, 462–463.

17 **Tunnadine, P.** Psycho-sexual problems. Mother and Child, 45 (1), Jan/Feb 1973, 17–20.

18 **Van Bree, N. S.** Sexuality, nursing practice and the person with cardiac disease. Nursing Forum, 14 (4), 1975, 396–411.

19 **Williams, G.** An approach to transsexual surgery. Nursing Times, 69, 21 Jun 1973, 787.

98 RESPIRATORY SYSTEM

a GENERAL AND DISEASES

1 **Asbury, J.** Lungs and automatic ventilation. 1. Anatomy and physiology. Nursing Times, 70, 3 Jan 1974, 19–21.

2 **Ayres, S. M. and Lagerson, J.** Pulmonary physiology at the bedside: oxygen and carbon dioxide abnormalities. Cardiovascular Nursing, 9 (1), Jan/Feb 1973, 1–6.

3 **Branton, P. and Hornsby, M.** Two nursing care studies specially for midwives. 1. Spontaneous pneumothorax in pregnancy. Nursing Mirror, 135, 17 Nov 1972, 26–28.

4 **Cartwright, R. Y.** Commensal bacteria of the human respiratory tract. Nursing Times, 70, 21 Mar 1974, 418–419.

5 **Chrisman, M.** Dyspnea. American Journal of Nursing, 74 (4), Apr 1974, 643–646.

6 **Clarke, S. W.** Fibreoptic bronchoscopy. Nursing Mirror, 141, 27 Nov 1975, 47–49.

7 **Davies, P. D. B.** Spontaneous pneumothorax. Nursing Mirror, 133, 10 Dec 1971, 19–21.

8 **Flenley, D. C.** Acute pulmonary oedema. Nursing Times, 67, 11 Nov 1971, 1408–1410.

9 **Foley, M. F.** Pulmonary function testing. American Journal of Nursing, 71 (6), Jun 1971, 1134–1139.

10 **Heycock, J. B.** Acute infections of the lower respiratory tract in infancy. Nursing Times, 69, 26 Jul 1973, 962–963.

11 **Hinden, E.** Respiratory disease in children. Nursing Mirror, 133, 26 Nov 1971, 19–20.

12 **James, D. G.** Sarcoidosis. Nursing Times, 68, 13 Jan 1972, 56–59; 20 Jan 1972, 77–79.

13 **Litten, H.** Refresher Course. Haemoptysis. [First in a series of information on practical nursing subjects for revision purposes.] Nursing Times, 71, 6 Nov 1975, 1764–1765.

14 **Marici, F. N.** The flexibile fiberoptic bronchoscope. American Journal of Nursing, 73 (10), Oct 1973, 1776–1778.

15 **Oswald, N.** Honeycomb lungs. [Cysts in the lung.] Nursing Mirror, 139, 10 Oct 1974, 51.

16 **Robertson, G.** Nursing care study. Lobar pneumonia. Nursing Mirror, 139, 6 Sep 1974, 75–78.

17 **Sedlock, S. A.** Detection of chronic pulmonary disease. American Journal of Nursing, 72 (8), Aug 1972, 1407–1411.

18 **Seyfried, M. T.** Recognizing respiratory acidocis and alkalosis. RN Magazine, 37 (7), Jul 1974, 48–49.

19 **Stark, J. E.** Patterns of abnormality of lung function. Nursing Times, 71, 18 Sep 1975, 1500–1501.

20 **Stark, J. E.** Testing the function of the lungs. Nursing Times, 71, 11 Sep 1975, 1447–1449.

21 **Stone, E. W. and Zuckerman, S.** The esophageal obturator airway. American Journal of Nursing, 75 (7), Jul 1975, 1148–1149.

22 **Stott, N. C. H.** Respiratory diseases in general practice. Queen's Nursing Journal, 17 (8), Nov 1974, 166–168.

23 **Thompson, R.** An acute case of bilateral lobar pneumonia: nursing care study. Nursing Times, 67, 23 Sep 1971, 1191–1193.

24 **Tordoff, J.** Right pneumothorax treated by intubation: case study. Nursing Mirror, 132, 11 Jun 1971, 32–33.

25 **Towers, M.** Pain in the chest. 1. Causes of pain and determination of a diagnosis. Nursing Times, 70, 19/26 Dec 1974, 1965–1967.

26 **Traver, G. A.** Assessment of thorax and lungs. American Journal of Nursing, 73 (3), Mar 1973, 466–471.

27 **Traver, G. A.** Living with chronic respiratory disease. American Journal of Nursing, 75 (10), Oct 1975, 1777–1781.

28 **Woogara, R.** Nursing care study. Haemopneumothorax and cardiac tamponade. Nursing Times, 71, 13 Feb 1975, 255–256.

b NURSING

2 **Delpizzo, A.** A new look at respiratory stimulants. Journal of the American Association of Nurse Anesthetists, 41 (5), Oct 1973, 411–420.

2 **Foss, G.** Postural drainage. American Journal of Nursing, 73 (4), Apr 1973, 666–669.

3 **Kennedy, P.** Postural drainage. Queen's Nursing Journal, 16 (6), Sep 1973, 126–128.

4 **Lagerson, J.** Teaching your patient to cough. RN Magazine, 37 (7), Jul 1974, ICU 1 [4 pages].

5 **Marshall, M.** Take a deep life-saving breath. [A deep-breathing regime to prevent respiratory failure in patients with chronic chest disease.] Nursing Times, 70, 11 Apr 1974, 545–546.

6 **Mullins, E. and Irvine, J.** Helping the respiratory care patient to help himself. RN Magazine, 37 (10), Oct 1974, ICU 1–2, 4–5.

7 **Nursing Clinics of North America** Symposium on care in respiratory disease. Nursing Clinics of North America, 9 (1), Mar 1974, 97–207.

8 **Slessor, G.** Auscultation of the chest – a clinical nursing skill. Canadian Nurse, 69 (4), Apr 1973, 40–43.

9 **Smith, S. E.** How drugs act. 14. Drugs and the bronchi. Nursing Times, 71, 25 Sep 1975, 1546–1547.

10 **Stevens, C.** Nursing care study. Respiratory failure. Nursing Times, 70, 16 May 1974, 751–752.

11 **Stromborg, M. F.** Preparation for respiratory disease nursing. Nursing Outlook, 19 (11), Nov 1971, 741–743.

c ALLERGIC DISEASES

1 **Buisseret, P. D.** Hay fever. Nursing Times, 70, 6 Jun 1974, 856–858.

2 **Chapman, M.** Nursing care of patients with acute asthma. Nursing Mirror, 139, 12 Jul 1974, 80.

3 **Clark, T. J. H.** Management of acute asthma. Nursing Mirror, 139, 12 Jul 1974, 75–76.

4 **Cooper, P.** Progress in therapeutics. Advances in allergic respiratory tract disease. Midwife and Health Visitor, 9 (3), Mar 1973, 88.

5 **Davies, R. J.** Occupation and asthma. Health Magazine, 11 (2), Summer/Autumn 1974, 11–16.

6 **Dewey, J.** How you can help the asthmatic patient. Nursing Care, 7 (2), Feb 1974, 10–13.

7 **Flavel Matts, S. G.** Asthma. Nursing Mirror, 134, 26 May 1972, 19–21.

8 **Frankland, A. W.** Chronic asthma. Nursing Mirror, 139, 12 Jul 1974, 73–74.

9 **Innocenti, D. M.** Physiotherapy in the management of acute asthma. Nursing Mirror, 139, 12 Jul 1974, 77–79.

10 **Lee, H. Y.** Extrinsic allergic alveolitis. Nursing Mirror, 137, 26 Oct 1973, 31–32.

11 **McAllen, M. K.** Hay fever. Nursing Mirror, 138, 24 May 1974, 63–65.

12 **Maher-Loughnan, G. P.** Psychological aspects of asthma. Nursing Mirror, 136, 16 Feb 1973, 21–22.

13 **Manners, B. T. and others** Allergic respiratory tract disease. Diagnosis in general practice. Nursing Times, 69, 13 Sep 1973, 1185–1186.

14 **Milne, M.** Pressurized bronchodilator aerosols [for the treatment of asthma]. Nursing Mirror, 139, 12 Jul 1974, 83–86.

15 **Moody, L.** Asthma. Physiology and patient care. American Journal of Nursing, 73 (7), Jul 1973, 1212–1217.

16 **Pepys, J.** Hyposensitization. [Preparation and use of allergens in treatment of hay fever, asthma and perennial rhinitis.] Nursing Mirror, 141, 18 Dec 1975, 57–58.

17 Pepys, J. and Simmonds, S. P. Allergic reactions – to alcoholic beverages. Nursing Mirror, 139, 12 Jul 1974, 81–82.

18 Reynolds, G. J. Summer allergy. Queen's Nursing Journal, 18 (4), Jul 1975, 104–106.

19 Senior, R. M. and others How to loosen the grip of status asthmaticus. RN Magazine, 38 (12), Dec 1975, OR 4, 6.

20 Sprung, E. Asthma in children. Bedside Nurse, 5 (2), Feb 1972, 16–17.

21 Symons, C. Causes and treatment of asthma. Nursing Mirror, 136, 27 Apr 1973, 18–20.

22 Ward, M. A day at Pilgrims'. [Pilgrims' School for severely asthmatic boys in Sussex.] Nursing Mirror, 135, 5 Jan 1973, 42–43.

d OBSTRUCTIVE LUNG DISEASES

1 Beatty, C. J. Guess who's dying at dinner. [Emergency procedure for acute airway obstruction.] RN Magazine, 35 (11), Nov 1972, 52–53.

2 Blancher, G. C. Caring for the patient with advanced emphysema. RN Magazine, 37 (8), Aug 1974, 41 (9 pages).

3 Bradley, J. Nursing care study. Acute airways obstruction. Nursing Mirror, 137, 24 Aug 1973, 24–27.

4 Dirschel, K. M. Respiration in emphysema patients. Nursing Clinics of North America, 8 (4), Dec 1973, 617–622.

5 Dromgoole, D. M. Nursing care study. Chronic bronchitis, emphysema and cor pulmonale. Nursing Times, 71, 9 Oct 1975, 1608–1610.

6 Fagerhaugh, S. Y. Getting around with emphysema. American Journal of Nursing, 73 (1), Jan 1973, 94–99.

7 Freedman, S. Air pollution and chest diseases. District Nursing, 15 (9), Dec 1972, 195–199.

8 Gloor, E. M. Chronic obstructive pulmonary disease and the role of the public health nurse in instituting a programme of home care services. [Research study in the United States.] International Journal of Nursing Studies, 10 (2), May 1973, 111–112.

9 Hugh-Jones, P. Emphysema. Nursing Mirror, 139, 12 Jul 1974, 61–65.

10 Lindau, M. Nursing care requirements for chronic emphysema patients. Hospital Progress, 53 (10), Oct 1972, 74–77.

11 McCallum, H. P. Emphysema: what is known and what remains obscure. Canadian Nurse, 68 (2), Feb 1972, 27–33.

12 McCallum, H. How I live with emphysema. Canadian Nurse, 68 (2), Feb 1972, 34–36.

13 Nariman, S. Chronic bronchitis. Nursing Times, 70, 22 Aug 1974, 1303–1304.

14 Nield, M. A. The effect of health teaching on the anxiety level of patients with chronic obstructive lung disease. Nursing Research, 20 (6), Nov/Dec 1971, 537–541.

15 Pasch, S. and Jamieson, T. Going home with cold: is your patient ready? [Teaching a patient with chronic obstructive lung disease.] Canadian Nurse, 71 (7), Jul 1975, 24–25.

16 Pracy, R. The diagnosis of respiratory obstruction in infants and small children. Nursing Times, 68, 27 Jul 1972, 930–933.

17 Stuart-Harris, C. Chronic bronchitis. Nursing Mirror, 137, 10 Aug 1973, 26–29.

18 Thomas, H. E. Acute and chronic bronchitis. Prevention and cure. Nursing Times, 68, 30 Nov 1972, 1519–1520.

19 Woodford, P. The foreign body. Nursing Times, 67, 7 Jan 1971, 24.

e SURGERY (Includes pleural drainage; tracheostomy)

1 Andreou, A. Underwater seal drainage [in chest surgery]. Nursing Times, 70, 27 Jun 1974, 1000–1001.

2 Andrews, I. Nursing care study. Chest surgery and chronic disability. Nursing Times, 68, 19 Oct 1972, 1332–1333.

3 Bevan, D. R. Tracheostomy. [Surgical technique and its problems.] Nursing Times, 71, 28 Aug 1975, 1371–1373.

4 Conner, G. H. and others Tracheostomy. [Series of articles on when it is needed; how it is done; postoperative care; care with a cuffed tube.] American Journal of Nursing, 72 (1), Jan 1972, 68–77.

5 Davies, I. J. T. Mini-tracheostomy. Nursing Times, 67, 3 Jun 1971, 674.

6 Deal, J. When breathing becomes work. 2. [Case study of nursing care after a lung operation.] Nursing Care, 6 (12), Dec 1973, 12–16.

7 Gurevich, I. Some new concepts in tracheostomy suctioning. RN Magazine, 35 (9), Sep 1972, 52–55.

8 Humm, W. Emergency chest therapy for the conscious patient. Nursing Times, 71, 8 May 1975, 728–729.

9 Jacquette, G. To reduce hazards of tracheal suctioning. American Journal of Nursing, 71 (12), Dec 1971, 2362–2364.

10 Kaler, J. and Kaler, H. Michael had a tracheostomy. [Study of a child living at home, written by his parents.] American Journal of Nursing, 74 (5), May 1974, 852–855.

11 Lawless, C. A. Helping patients with endotracheal and tracheostomy tubes communicate. American Journal of Nursing, 75 (12), Dec 1975, 2151–2153.

12 Manchester, G. H. and others A simple method for emergency orotracheal intubation. RN Magazine, 36 (4), Apr 1973, OR 8, 11.

13 Merino, D. V. Return to nursing. 18. Cardio-thoracic nursing. 1. General thoracic surgery. Nursing Mirror, 135, 25 Aug 1972, 29–32.

14 Moghissi, K. Pleural drainage. 1. The pleural cavity and its drainage. Nursing Times, 70, 12 Sep 1974, 1420–1421.

15 Moghissi, K. Pleural drainage. 2. Underwater sealed drainage system. Nursing Times, 70, 19 Sep 1974, 1459–1460.

16 Moghissi, K. Pleural drainage. 3. General care of pleural drains. Nursing Times, 70, 26 Sep 1974, 1508–1509.

17 Moghissi, K. Pleural drainage. 4. Special cases. Nursing Times, 70, 3 Oct 1974, 1538–1539.

18 Moghissi, K. Pleural drainage. 5. After pneumonectomy. Nursing Times, 70, 10 Oct 1974, 1583–1584.

19 Morgan, C. V. and Orcutt, T. W. The care and feeding of chest tubes. [In thoracic surgical nursing.] American Journal of Nursing, 72 (2), Feb 1972, 305–308.

20 Morrell, S. G. Tracheostomy suction system. Nursing Mirror, 135, 6 Oct 1972, 44–45.

21 Shah, N. ENT Emergencies. 4. Respiratory obstruction and tracheostomy. Nursing Mirror, 134, 31 Mar 1972, 35–38.

22 Walker, W. C. Pleural effusion. Nursing Times, 69, 8 Mar 1973, 312–314.

23 Weber, B. Eating with a trach. [Effect of head position on swallowing.] American Journal of Nursing, 74 (8), Aug 1974, 1439.

f INTENSIVE CARE AND VENTILATION

1 Asbury, J. Lungs and automatic ventilation. 2. Types of ventilation. Nursing Times, 70, 10 Jan 1974, 42–43.

2 Asbury, J. Lungs and automatic ventilation. 3. The patient on the ventilator. Nursing Times, 70, 17 Jan 1974, 85–86.

3 Association of Respiratory Therapy Annual meeting. Report on two programs organized to provide intensive respiratory therapy to patients in the hospital and at home. Hospitals, 48, 16 Jan 1974, 59, 62, 64.

4 Bothamley, V. A. Communication and the ventilated patient. [Problems of care necessitate a close relationship between nurse and patient.] Nursing Times, 71, 17 Apr 1975, 628–630.

5 Davis, S. E. Ventilator therapy. SA Nursing Journal, 41 (1), Jan 1974, 34–35.

6 Drain, C. B. A vigilant you can reverse respiratory distress. [Role of observation in respiratory intensive care.] RN Magazine, 38 (12), Dec 1975, ICU 7–8, 12.

7 Koon, G. T. Respirator and the nursing management of a patient on a respirator. Nursing Journal of Singapore, 13 (1), May 1973, 59–64.

8 McAlister, E. A respiratory and intensive care unit. [Royal Victoria Hospital, Belfast.] Nursing Times, 68, 17 Feb 1972, 203–204.

9 Mullins, E. and Irvine, J. Helping the respiratory care patient to help himself. RN Magazine, 37 (10), Oct 1974, ICU 1–2, 4, 5.

10 Pope, B. Principles of mechanical ventilation. New Zealand Nursing Journal, 66 (1), Jan 1973, 25–26.

11 Priyadharsini, J. Mechanical ventilation and the nurse. Nursing Journal of India, 44 (1), Jan 1973, 19–20.

12 Robinson, A. M. Respiratory ICU; learning a new nursing specialty. RN Magazine, 37 (11), Nov 1974, ICU 1–2, 5.

13 Robinson, A. M. When the ARIT is an RN. [Registered inhalation therapist.] RN Magazine, 36 (12), Dec 1973, 40–41.

14 Tinker, J. H. and Wehner, R. The nurse and the ventilator. American Journal of Nursing, 74 (7), Jul 1974, 1276–1278.

99 URINARY SYSTEM

a GENERAL (Includes urinary tract infection)

1 Backhouse, N. Trial and error in the development of urology. Nursing Mirror, 139, 26 Sep 1974, 63–65.

2 Brant, H. A. Pregnancy and urinary tract infections. Nursing Times, 69, 19 Jul 1973, 919–921.

3 British Medical Journal Urinary tract diseases. Articles published in the British Medical Journal. BMJ, 1971.

4 Brocklehurst, J. C. Bladder outlet obstruction in elderly women. Nursing Mirror, 135, 11 Aug 1972, 36–39.

5 Carbary, L. J. Cyctitis: a painful nuisance. Nursing Care, 8 (11), Nov 1975, 24–27.

6 Cattell, W. R. The management of urinary tract infection in adult women. Nursing Mirror, 138, 28 Jun 1974, 65–68.

7 Charlton, C. A. C. The urological system. Harmondsworth: Penguin Education (Penguin library of nursing), 1973.

8 Cleave, T. L. E. coli infections of the urinary tract. Nursing Times, 71, 9 Jan 1975, 66–67.

9 Cooper, P. Drugs for urinary tract infections. Midwife and Health Visitor, 8, May 1972, 180.

10 Davis, C. A new technique for treating growths in the bladder. Helmstein's balloon therapy. Nursing Times, 69, 23 Aug 1973, 1084–1086.

11 Downs, A. W. and Cleland, V. S. Bacteriuria and urinary tract infection in infancy and childhood – a review. Nursing Research, 20 (2), Mar/Apr 1971, 131–139.

12 Droller, H. Urinary infections in the elderly. Nursing Times, 68, 1 Jun 1972, 667–671.

13 Ellis, H. History of the bladder stone. Nursing Mirror, 132, 5 Mar 1971, 30–33.

14 Gray, W. M. Surgical disorders of the genitourinary tract. Physiotherapy, 59 (5), May 1973, 138–141.

15 Hendry, W. F. Urinary tract injuries in gynaecology. Nursing Mirror, 136, 2 Mar 1973, 15–18.

16 Hole, R. Urinary problems. Nursing Mirror, 137, 26 Oct 1973, 33–34.

17 Khan, A. J. and Pfyles, C. V. Urinary tract infection in children. American Journal of Nursing, 73 (8), Aug 1973, 1340–1343.

18 Kilmartin, A. Understanding cystitis. Heinemann Health Books, 1973.

19 Kunin, C. M. Detection, prevention and management of urinary tract infections: a manual for the physician, nurse and allied health worker. Philadelphia: Lea and Febiger, 1972. 2nd ed. 1974.

20 Lowthian, P. Portable urinals for women. Nursing Times, 71, 30 Oct 1975, 1739–1741.

21 Manners, B. T. B. Diagnosis in general practice of urinary infection among women. Nursing Times, 69, 28 Jun 1973, 828–829.

22 Merchant, F. Pyelolithotomy. Nursing Mirror, 134, 24 Mar 1972, 36–39.

23 Newsham, J. E. and Petrie, J. J. B. Urology and renal medicine. 2nd ed. Edinburgh:, Churchill Livingstone, 1975.

24 Reece, A. J. Spontaneous rupture of the male urethra. Nursing Times, 70, 10 Oct 1974, 1578–1579.

25 Reece, A. J. Traumatic rupture of the male urethra. Nursing Times, 70, 30 May 1974, 836–837.

26 Riddle, P. R. Urinary tuberculosis. Nursing Times, 70, 19/26 Dec 1974, 1976–1978.

27 Rodman, M. J. Drug therapy today. Fighting the second most frequent infections. [Urinary tract infections.] RN Magazine, 38 (10), Oct 1975, 75–77; (11), Nov 1975, 91, 92, 95.

28 Stirling, M. W. A. and Scott, R. Urology. Heineman Medical, 1971. (Modern practical nursing series no. 5.)

29 Wilson, G. M. Modern diuretic therapy. Nursing Mirror, 138, 24 May 1974, 61–62.

b NURSING

1 Ansell, D. and Dixon, E. Training in urological patient care. [For nurses and technicians.] Nursing Mirror, 140, 5 Jun 1975, 55–56.

2 Burke, C. W. Timed urinary tests – the nurse's role. [Different types of tests carried out by the laboratory staff.] Nursing Times, 71, 13 Nov 1975, 1813–1815.

3 Campbell, D. Nursing care study. Primary adenocarcinoma of the bladder. [Total cystectomy and ureterocolic diversion.] Nursing Mirror, 138, 10 May 1974, 86–89.

4 Crabtree, M. K. How to assess a patient's urologic complaint. RN Magazine, 38 (11), Nov 1975, 79, 81, 83, 85, 86.

5 Fielding, P. and Wells, T. J. Urinary collecting device: a clinical trial among female geriatric patients. Nursing Times, 71, 23 Jan 1975, 136–137.

6 Hatcher, W. J. The dip-slide method of urine specimen collection. Midwives Chronicle, 84, Apr 1971, 124–125.

7 Jackaman, F. R. and others The dip-slide in urology. British Medical Journal, 1, 27 Jan 1973, 207–208.

8 Quinn, S. J. Nursing care study. Bilateral ruptured ureters due to blunt trauma. Nursing Times, 71, 27 Nov 1975, 1892–1894.

9 Robinson, J. O. Modern urology for nurses. 2nd ed. Heinemann, 1972.

10 Soo, B. and others Bedpan anxiety. [Reactions of 306 patients.] Nursing Journal of Singapore, 15 (1), May 1975, 22–23.

11 Stanton, G. V. Nursing care study. A patient with pelviureteric junction obstruction. Nursing Times, 70, 19/26 Dec 1974, 1982–1983.

12 Stirling, M. W. A. and Scott, R. Urology. Heinemann Medical, 1971. (Modern practical nursing series no. 5), 1971.

13 Ullathorne, M. M. Collecting urine from small children. Nursing Times, 67, 21 Jan 1971, 72–74.

14 Winter, C. C. and Barker, M. R. Nursing care of patients with urologic diseases. 3rd ed. St. Louis: Mosby, 1972.

c INCONTINENCE

1 Bromley, I. Urinary incontinence associated with organic nervous disorders. Physiotherapy, 59 (11), Nov 1973, 360–363.

2 Caldwell, K. P. S. Urinary incontinence. Sector Publishing, 1975.

3 Dobson, P. Management of incontinence in the home: a survey. Disabled Living Foundation, 1974. Follow up conference reported in Nursing Times, 70, 14 Nov 1974, 1759.

4 Dobson, P. Urinary incontinence: social aspects. Physiotherapy, 59 (11), Nov 1973, 358–359.

5 Doyle, P. T. Urinary incontinence – diagnosis and treatment. Nursing Times, 69, 15 Nov 1973, 1521–1523.

6 Edmondson, E. Nursing the incontinent. Butterworth, 1971, (Nursing in depth series.)

7 Edwards, L. E. Incontinence. Practitioner, 214, Jan 1975, 46–55.

8 Elphick, L. On incontinence. Mental Health, Spring 1971, 44–48.

9 Gusfa, A. and others Patient teaching: one approach. [Account of a 'Patient teaching programs manual' with instruction on indwelling urinary catheter, given as an example.] Supervisor Nurse, 6 (12), Dec 1975, 17, 19, 22.

10 Harrison, S. Physiotherapy in the treatment of stress incontinence. Nursing Mirror, 141, 10 Jul 1975, 52–53.

11 Harrison, S. M. Urinary incontinence of non-neurogenic origin. Physiotherapy, 59 (11), Nov 1973, 363–365.

12 Jorow, M. How to teach patients to catheterize themselves. RN Magazine, 38 (12), Dec 1975, 19–21.

13 McQuire, W. A. Electrotherapy and exercises for stress incontinence and urinary frequency. Physiotherapy, 61 (10), Oct 1975, 305–307.

14 Mandelstam, D. Society at work. A common complaint. [Incontinence.] New Society, 32, 29 May 1975, 537–538.

15 Pennefather, M. E. and Tanner, E. R. Spending a 'new penny'. [Stress incontinence.] Nursing Times, 67, 27 May 1971, 640–641.

16 Reid, E. A. Incontinence and nursing practice: an investigation of the nursing management of soiling in non bedfast patients. M Phil thesis, Edinburgh University, 1974.

17 Stone, H. Adult bed wetters and their problems: a road to homelessness? Canterbury: Cyrenians, 1973.

18 Tanner, E. R. Muscle function in the incontinent patient. Queen's Nursing Journal, 16 (7), Oct 1973, 158, 161.

19 Warrell, D. W. Incontinence of urine in women. Nursing Times, 71, 11 Sep 1975, 1470–1473.

20 Warrell, D. W. Stress incontinence. Nursing Mirror, 141, 10 Jul 1975, 51–52.

21 Willington, F. L. Incontinence. Macmillan Journals, 1975. [Reprint of articles from Nursing Times, 1975.]

22 Willington, F. L. Incontinence. 1. Significance of incompetence of personal sanitary habits. Nursing Times, 71, 27 Feb 1975, 340–341.

23 Willington, F. L. Incontinence. 2. Problems in the aetiology of urinary incontinence. Nursing Times, 71, 6 Mar 1975, 378–381.

24 Willington, F. L. Incontinence. 3. Psychological and psychogenic aspects. Nursing Times, 71, 13 Mar 1975, 422–423.

25 Willington, F. L. Incontinence. 4. The nursing component in diagnosis and treatment. Nursing Times, 71, 20 Mar 1975, 464–467.

26 Willington, F. L. Incontinence. 5. Training and retraining for continence. Nursing Times, 71, 27 Mar 1975, 500–503.

27 Willington, F. L. Incontinence. 6. The prevention of soiling. Nursing Times, 71, 3 Apr 1975, 545–548.

28 Young, G. C. and Turner, R. K. Nocturnal enuresis in childhood. Health and Social Service Journal, 83, 7 Apr 1973, 793–795.

d INCONTINENCE: CATHETERIZATION

1 American Journal of Nursing Indwelling catheters: preventing infection. New York: American Journal of Nursing Company, 1972 (Reprint).

2 Birum. L. H. and Zimmerman, D. S. Catheter plugs as a source of infection. American Journal of Nursing, 71 (11), Nov 1971, 2150–2152.

3 **Blandy, J. P.** Catheterization. Nursing Mirror, 134, 2 Jun 1972, 26–29.

4 **Castle, M. and Osterhout, S.** Urinary tract catheterization and associated infection. Nursing Research, 23 (2), Mar/Apr 1974, 170–174.

5 **Chapman, J.** Management of indwelling catheters. Nursing Times, 71, 6 Nov 1975, 1776–1777.

6 **Chavigny, K. H.** The use of polymixin B as a urethral lubricant to reduce the post instrumental incidence of bacteriuria in females: an exploratory study. International Journal of Nursing Studies, 12 (1), Mar 1975, 33–42.

7 **Clark, C. L.** Catheter care in the home. [Teaching relatives care of indwelling catheter including irrigation.] American Journal of Nursing, 72 (5), May 1972, 922–924.

8 **Cleland, V. and others** Prevention of bacteriuria in female patients with indwelling catheters. Nursing Research, 20 (4), Jul/Aug 1971, 309–318.

9 **Degroot, J. and Kunin, C. M.** Indwelling catheters. [An investigation revealing specific problems with practical solutions.] American Journal of Nursing, 75 (3), Mar 1975, 448–449.

10 **Eppink, H.** Catheterizing the maternity patient. American Journal of Nursing, 75 (5), May 1975, 829.

11 **Langford, T. L.** Nursing problem: bacteriuria and the indwelling catheter. American Journal of Nursing, 72 (1), Jan 1972, 113–115.

12 **Morgan, D. M.** Urinary tract infection in hospitalized patients. [Due to indwelling catheters.] Canadian Hospital, 50 (12), Dec 1973, 27, 29, 32.

13 **Poole, P. M.** Continuous bladder drainage. Nursing Mirror, 135, 24 Nov 1972, 42–43.

14 **Schneckloth, N. W.** Indwelling catheter nursing care. AORN Journal, 21 (4), Apr 1975, 695–696, 698–699.

15 **Smith, L.** Long-term catheterization. [Tests of the Bard Silicone Elastome coated balloon catheter showed a saving of nurses' time and more comfort for the patients.] Nursing Times, 71, 14 Aug 1975, 1283–1284.

16 **Wastling, G.** A genito-urinary liaison scheme. [A scheme for transferring the work of changing indwelling catheters of long-term patients from the hospital out-patients department to district nurses.] Nursing Times, 68, 7 Sep 1972, 1128–1130.

17 **Wastling, G.** Long-term catheterization. [Assessment of a hospital liaison scheme in Reading nurses look after patients with indwelling catheters in their homes.] Nursing Times, 70, 3 Jan 1974, 17–18.

e INCONTINENCE: OTHER METHODS

1 **British Medical Journal** Treating incontinence electrically. British Medical Journal, 2, 17 Jun 1972, 670–671.

2 **Broad, J. W.** Urinary incontinence – a new method of control. [Research project at Stretton Hall Hospital in cooperation with the Synthetic Fibres Laboratory at Courtaulds to advise suitable garments to aid the control of incontinence.] Nursing Times, 68, 28 Sep 1972, 1212–1213.

3 **Caldwell, K. P. S.** Sphincter stimulators to prevent incontinence. [Electronic device.] Nursing Times, 69, 15 Nov 1973, 1524–1525.

4 **d'Entrecasteaux, J. S.** Electronic control of urinary incontinence. Nursing Mirror, 132, 15 Jan 1971, 43.

5 **Eckstein, H. B.** Treatment of incontinence by electrical stimulation. Nursing Times, 71, 4 Sep 1975, 1423–1424.

6 **Forsythe, W. I. and others** A controlled clinical trial of trimipramine and placebo in the treatment of enuresis. British Journal of Clinical Practice, 26 (3), Mar 1972, 119–121.

7 **Forsythe, W. I. and others** Enuresis and psychoactive drugs. British Journal of Clinical Practice, 26 (3), Mar 1972, 116–118.

8 **Glen, E. S. and Rowan, D.** Enuretic alarm trainer for night and day. [Bedside alarm device using disposable pads worn within pants such as Kanga marsupial incontinence pants.] Lancet, 2, 26 Oct 1974, 987–988.

9 **Hartie, A. and Black, D.** A dry bed is the objective. [Positive reinforcement programme based on operant conditioning applied to five frequently incontinent long-stay psychiatric patients.] Nursing Times, 71, 20 Nov 1975, 1874–1876.

10 **Henderson, D. J. and Rogers, W. F.** Hospital trials of incontinence underpads. Nursing Times, 67, 4 Feb 1971, 141–143.

11 **Morgan, T. T. and Young, G. C.** The treatment of enuresis: merits of conditioning methods. Community Medicine, 128, 19 May 1972, 119–121.

12 **Nashold, B. S.** Electromicturition in paraplegia. [Implementation of a neuroprosthesis.] Nursing Times, 70, 3 Jan 1974, 22–23.

13 **Nursing Mirror** SertaN – incontinence control. [Female control device.] Nursing Mirror, 132, 11 Jun 1971, 14–15.

14 **Patterson, D. and Schuster, P. A.** Artificial urinary sphincter. [A new approach to the treatment of incontinence involving a patient education program at Foothills Hospital, Calgary.] Canadian Nurse, 71 (11), Nov 1975, 27–31.

15 **Smith, P. H.** Incontinence pads containing carboxymethylcellulose. Practitioner, 207, Nov 1971, 644–648.

16 **Tierney, A. J.** Toilet training: a report of an evaluation of the implementation of an experimental behaviour modification programme in toilet training with a group of severely subnormal patients. Nursing Times, 69, 20–27 Dec 1973, 1740–1745.

17 **Tong, D. P. and others** Comparative evaluation of the cost and comfort of bed pads. [Disposable incontinence bed pads.] Health and Social Service Journal 83, 26 May 1973, 1202–1203.

18 **Willington, F. L. and others** Marsupial pants for urinary incontinence. Nursing Mirror, 135, 18 Aug 1972, 40–41.

19 **Willington, F. L.** Marsupial principle in maintenance of personal hygiene in urinary incontinence. British Medical Journal, 3, 22 Sep 1973, 626–628.

20 **Wilson, M. F.** Bladder training for the chronically ill. [Teaching patients to function without indwelling catheters.] RN Magazine, 38 (6), Jun 1975, 36–37.

f INCONTINENCE: ELDERLY
(See also Spinal injuries)

1 **Bridgewater, J. and Christie, H.** Glyme – 'A silk purse . . .' [A joint study on the control of urinary incontinence in elderly patients at Glyme Ward, Littlemore Hospital, Oxford.] Nursing Mirror, 139, 26 Jul 1974, 58–61.

2 **Brocklehurst, J. C.** Incontinence in the elderly. Nursing Mirror, 136, 1 Jun 1973, 30–32.

3 **Kings Fund Centre** Incontinence in the elderly. Nursing Mirror, 132, 1 Jan 1971, 12–13.

4 **Meers, J. M.** Successful management of incontinence in domiciliary care of the elderly. Midwife and Health Visitor, 7 (4), Apr 1971, 151–154.

5 **Pinel, C.** Disorders of micturition in the elderly. Nursing Times, 71, 18 Dec 1975, 2019–2021.

6 **Wells, T.** Promoting urinary continence in the elderly in hospital. Nursing Times, 71, 27 Nov 1975, 1908–1909.

g INCONTINENCE: CHILDREN

1 **Brennan, K. S. W.** Child psychiatry: a nursing aid. [Device attached to the bed used for the incontinent in a ward for the severely mentally handicapped at St. Joseph's Hospital, Sheffield.] British Medical Journal, 3, 22 Sep 1973, 628–629.

2 **British Medical Journal** Enuresis again. [Comparison of imipramine, electric buzzer and a placebo in the treatment of children.] British Medical Journal, 2, 14 Apr 1973, 69.

3 **Dische, S.** Bedwetting and its treatment. Nursing Mirror, 134, 18–25 Feb 1972, 46–47.

4 **Doyle, P. T.** Enuresis – causes and treatment. Nursing Times, 71, 13 Mar 1975, 424–425.

5 **Hodes, C.** Enuresis – a study in general practice. Journal of the Royal College of General Practitioners, 23, Jul 1973, 520–524.

6 **Kolvin, I.** Enuresis in childhood. Practitioner, 214, Jan 1975, 33–45.

7 **Lowthian, P. T.** Enuresis in the home – protecting the bed. Nursing Times, 69, 29 Mar 1973, 408–410.

8 **McDonagh, M. J.** Is operant conditioning effective in reducing enuresis and encopresis in children? Perspectives in Psychiatric Care, 9 (1), Jan/Feb 1971, 17–23.

9 **Mann, R. W. and others** The treatment of nocturnal enuresis by bell and pad in general practice. Health Visitor, 48 (2), Feb 1975, 40–43, 45–46.

10 **Reece, A. J.** Nursing care study. Ileocystoplasty for enuresis. Nursing Mirror, 135, 29 Dec 1972, 29–31.

11 **Rosenhouse, L.** Bed-wetting. Nursing Care, 8 (6), Jun 1975, 20–21.

12 **Rowan, R. L.** Bed-wetting: a guide for parents. Saint James Press, 1974.

13 **Tyrrell, S.** Some problems of incontinent children attending ordinary school. Public Health, 89 (1), Jan 1975, 77–80.

14 **Young, G. C. and Morgan, R. T. T.** Childhood enuresis: termination of treatment by patients. Community Medicine, 129, 29 Dec 1972, 247–250.

15 **Young, G. C. and Morgan, R. T. T.** Non-attending enuretic children. Community Medicine, 127, 24 Mar 1972, 158–159.

AUTHOR INDEX

Authors are listed alphabetically with their subject reference(s).
Titles are listed where there are no known authors.

AUTHOR INDEX

Grima, M. R. 93b8
Grime, J. 5a16
Grime, P. 29g7
Grimes, O. F. 67g7
Groden, B. M. 84p7, 84p8
Gross, I. N. 20i7
Gross, L. 87h17
Gross, P. F. 28i17
Grossenbacher, G. 39d7
Grossman, B. J. 91a21, 91d19, 91d43
Grossman, H. T. 24b10, 27e3
Grosvenor, P. 46a19
Group, T. M. 5b8, 5i11
Grove, G. J. 39g11
Grove, L. 83a7
Grove Park 81e15
Grover, E. 78e4
Grover, V. M. 50a10
Groves, L. 76b11
Groves, W. H. 17c10
Groves, W. J. B. 35c3
Gruendemann, B. 23c5
Gruendemann, B. J. 18b2, 65d16
Gruer, R. 52c9
Grundy, P. F. 32a12
Guan, H. K. 10d7
Gubert, S. 28e78
Gudermuth, S. 45c18
Gudmundsen, A. 20c8
Guest, D. 70i3
Guichard, M. T. 28f13
Guilleminault, C. 79j6
Guiver, P. 34g7
Gullo, S. V. 19a6
Gumpel, J. M. 91a12, 91e2
Gunderson, B. B. 56d1, 97e3
Gunn, A. D. G. 52b6, 52b7, 73f4, 73g10, 73g11, 85h8
Gunn, I. P. 63e8, 63e9
Gunn, N. 92a21
Gunning, A. J. 87b25
Gunter, L. M. 53b3
Gunther, M. 45f19
Gunther, M. H. D. 45f20
Gunton, G. F. 33d3
Gunzburg, H. C. 81a15, 81a16, 81c18, 81c19
Gurel, M. 38d10
Gurevich, I. 98e7
Gurhy, E. 39g12
Gusfa, A. 99c9
Gutch, C. F. 96c10
Guthneck, M. 33b1
Guthrie, D. W. 89e5, 89f6, 89f7
Guthrie, M. 84g3
Guthrie, R. A. 89e5, 89f6, 89f7
Gutowski, F. 87h18
Guttmann, L. 56e9, 94c21
Guy, F. M. 92a5
Gwaltney, B. H. 26c16
Gwilliam, S. 92h8
Gwynne, G. V. 49d7
Gyulay, J. E. 48f6, 48f7

Haas, L. 45e11
Habak, P. A. 84b19
Habeeb, M. C. 75h13
Hack, K. A. 22a12
Hackett, T. P. 84n3, 84n4
Hackitt, B. S. 37a11
Hackler, E. N. 94e12
Hackshaw, S. M. 21b6
Hadfield, G. J. 82f12
Hadley, B. 65a8
Hadley, R. D. 9l3, 75i9

Haferkorn, V. 84e4
Hafez, E. S. E. 97a9
Haffner, C. 76a8
Hagan, J. M. 45f21
Hagerdorn, R. 62c2
Haggerty, V. C. 15b2
Hagopian, G. 12g9, 21d12
Haider, S. 85a8, 85a9, 85b14, 87b26, 87f3
Haigh, E. 33a13
Haiman-Elkind, H. 10h6
Haines, A. J. 32d2
Haldane, J. D. 44d18–20
Hale, C. B. 2 29
Hales-Tooke, A. 48c12, 48e11, 48e13
Halim, N. F. 28h32
Hall, A. 97a13
Hall, B. A. 75j11
Hall, C. 3c13, 30a19
Hall, C. M. 5g7
Hall, D. 90a11
Hall, D. J. 22a6
Hall, F. R. 84i7
Hall, G. H. 96e8
Hall, J. 20c9
Hall, J. N. 25a6, 25b3, 75d9, 76a9
Hall, K. D. 63d9
Hall, M. E. 80b7
Hall, M. H. 67f3
Hall, M. S. 32c4
Hall, R. 89a8
Hall, S. M. 48b6
Hall, T. 32a13
Hall, T. S. 85h9
Hallam, R. S. 76a10, 79f2, 79f3
Hallas, C. H. 3a6, 81a17
Hallas, J. 29b2, 29f11, 29g8
Haller, L. L. 76d3
Hallett, C. P. 73g12
Halliburton, P. M. 52e14, 52e15
Halliday, N. P. 40h4
Hallman, H. W. 18b3
Hall-Patch, E. 73i1
Hallum, J. L. 39b7
Halman, H. B. 45e12
Halsbury, Earl of 8e5
Halter, H. H. L. E. 11g13
Hambling, E. 7d11, 15b1
Hamby, R. G. 38h6
Hamer, J. 84d5
Hames, C. C. 89f12
Hamil, E. 43a2
Hamilton, Lady 56a14
Hamilton, A. 91d20, 92d6, 92d7
Hamilton, D. 10i14, 11c3
Hamilton, E. A. 92d8
Hamilton, J. 31o9, 71a7
Hamilton, J. M. 68e5
Hamilton, M. 70f1, 70g6, 70j2, 72 11, 73b3, 73d1, 73f5, 73h13, 83d18
Hamilton, P. 66c15
Hamilton, P. M. 47a9
Hamilton, T. 84h10
Hamilton, V. 56a14
Hamilton, W. J. 40g7
Hamlett, J. D. 41d6
Hamlin, D. 82i11
Hammersmith Health Department 42c10
Hammond, G. 8c6, 71a8, 71a9, 72 12
Hammond, H. 53a14
Hammond, J. E. 87f4
Hammond, V. 88c8
Hampe, S. O. 19b10
Hampton, J. R. 84d6
Hampton, P. J. 9c13, 9i2, 15a17, 22b12, 31g11

Hampton, R. A. 31g11
Hamson, L. 57f14
Hancock, C. 6a16
Hancock, W. 11g44
Handby, J. G. 29c6
Handley, K. A. 20h1
Handley, N. 42c11
Hanebuth, L. 82e8
Hanid, T. K. 5c19, 45a12
Hankoff, L. D. 67c5
Hanley, T. 55b13
Hanmer, G. A. 85l11
Hannam, L. 50b5
Hannan, J. F. 82d4
Hannigan, L. 38c21
Hannington-Kiff, J. G. 59b4
Hanrahan, K. A. 8f7, 11c4, 21d13
Hanron, J. S. 86a18
Hansard 3a7, 9f12
Hansen, G. L. 96b8
Hansen, J. 52e16
Hansen, R. E. 38a8
Hanson, E. T. 75f5
Hanson, G. C. 17c5, 17c6
Hanson, J. 44e5
Hanson, R. L. 27f6 27f7
Hanson, S. 15a19, 31n8
Hanton, P. 84f5
Hague, G. 77a5
Har, K. K. 39e12
Harbert, W. B. 81c20
Harboard, W. E. 29c7
Hardcastle, D. 89i3
Hardgrove, C. 45f22, 84h20
Hardgrove, C. B. 48c13, 48c14
Hardial, M. 79e8
Hardie, M. C. 29a9, 29g9
Hardie, M. W. 53b4
Hardiman, M. A. 15b3
Hardin, D. 37c12
Harding, B. 20a11
Harding, E. H. 24c6
Harding, J. M. 92d9
Harding, L. 30d6, 61e9
Harding, V. 48e12
Harding Rains, A J. 90a12
Hardley, P. 50a11
Hardman, F. G. 88g3
Hardwick, R. O. F. 49d2
Hardy, G. 26a2
Hardy, J. 13b8, 15d7
Hardy, M. E. 6c14, 6c15
Hare, E. J. 79i8
Hare, F. 16d12
Hare, R. 57g8
Haren, M. 12j8
Hargreaves, A. G. 52b8
Hargreaves, I. 12b5
Haring, P. W. 75d17
Harkin, J. P. 78a14
Harkiss, K. J. 63f11
Harkness, L. 93g11
Harling, M. 57f15
Harlow, F. W. 63a3
Harmon, M. L. 87a16
Harman, V. 16d18
Harmon, V. M. 86a19
Harnor, J. 54g8
Harper, H. E. 39g13
Harper, M. W. 43d13
Harries, A. J. 70h3
Harries, C. J. 75b7, 75d10, 78h12
Harrington, J. A. 78h13
Harrington, J. D. 96b9

228